THE IOC MANUAL OF SPORTS INJURIES

THE IOC MANUAL OF SPORTS INJURIES

An Illustrated Guide to the Management of Injuries in Physical Activity

EDITED BY

ROALD BAHR, MD PHD
Department of Sports Medicine
Oslo Sports Trauma Research Center
Norwegian School of Sport Sciences
Oslo
Norway

ASSOCIATE EDITORS

Paul McCrory, MBBS PhD
Robert F. LaPrade, MD PhD
Willem Meeuwisse, MD PhD
Lars Engebretsen, MD PhD

MEDICAL ILLUSTRATOR

Tommy Bolic

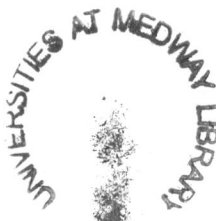

WILEY-BLACKWELL

A John Wiley & Sons, Ltd., Publication

This edition first published 2012 © 2012 by the International Olympic Committee

Wiley-Blackwell is an imprint of John Wiley & Sons, formed by the merger of Wiley's global Scientific, Technical and Medical business with Blackwell Publishing.

Registered office: John Wiley & Sons, Ltd, The Atrium, Southern Gate, Chichester, West Sussex, PO19 8SQ, UK

Editorial offices: 9600 Garsington Road, Oxford, OX4 2DQ, UK
111 River Street, Hoboken, NJ 07030-5774, USA

For details of our global editorial offices, for customer services and for information about how to apply for permission to reuse the copyright material in this book please see our website at www.wiley.com/wiley-blackwell

Designations used by companies to distinguish their products are often claimed as trademarks. All brand names and product names used in this book are trade names, service marks, trademarks or registered trademarks of their respective owners. The publisher is not associated with any product or vendor mentioned in this book. This publication is designed to provide accurate and authoritative information in regard to the subject matter covered. It is sold on the understanding that the publisher is not engaged in rendering professional services. If professional advice or other expert assistance is required, the services of a competent professional should be sought.

The contents of this work are intended to further general scientific research, understanding, and discussion only and are not intended and should not be relied upon as recommending or promoting a specific method, diagnosis, or treatment by physicians for any particular patient. The publisher and the author make no representations or warranties with respect to the accuracy or completeness of the contents of this work and specifically disclaim all warranties, including without limitation any implied warranties of fitness for a particular purpose. In view of ongoing research, equipment modifications, changes in governmental regulations, and the constant flow of information relating to the use of medicines, equipment, and devices, the reader is urged to review and evaluate the information provided in the package insert or instructions for each medicine, equipment, or device for, among other things, any changes in the instructions or indication of usage and for added warnings and precautions. Readers should consult with a specialist where appropriate. The fact that an organization or Website is referred to in this work as a citation and/or a potential source of further information does not mean that the author or the publisher endorses the information the organization or Website may provide or recommendations it may make. Further, readers should be aware that Internet Websites listed in this work may have changed or disappeared between when this work was written and when it is read. No warranty may be created or extended by any promotional statements for this work. Neither the publisher nor the author shall be liable for any damages arising herefrom.

Library of Congress Cataloging-in-Publication Data
The IOC manual of sports injuries / edited by Roald Bahr.
p. ; cm
Includes bibliographical references and index.
ISBN 978-0-470-67416-1 (hardback : alk. paper)
I. Bahr, Roald, 1957- II. International Olympic Committee.
[DNLM: 1. Athletic Injuries –diagnosis. 2. Athletic Injuries–therapy.QT 261]
617.1'027–dc23 2012009756

A catalogue record for this book is available from the British Library.

Wiley also publishes its books in a variety of electronic formats. Some content that appears in print may not be available in electronic books.

Cover image: © Medical Illustrator Tommy Bolic, Sweden.
Cover design by Opta Design

Set in 9.5/12pt ConcordeBQ by Aptara® Inc., New Delhi, India
Printed and bound in Malaysia by Vivar Printing Sdn Bhd

1 2012

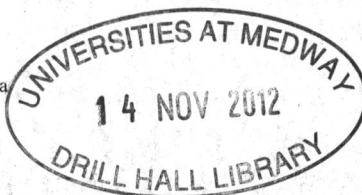

Contents

Contributors List

Håkan Alfredson, MD PhD
Sports Medicine Unit
University of Umeå
Sports Medicine Umeå Inc.
Umeå
Sweden

Juan-Manuel Alonso Martín, MD PhD
Real Federación Española de Atletismo
International Association of Athletics Federations (IAAF)
Madrid
Spain

Ned Amendola, MD
Department of Orthopaedics and Rehabilitation
UI Sports Medicine
University of Iowa
Iowa City, IA
USA

James R. Andrews, MD
Women's and Children's Center and
Andrews Sports Medicine and Orthopaedic Center
Birmingham, AL
USA

Elizabeth Arendt, MD
Department of Orthopedic Surgery
Univeristy of Minnesota
Minneapolis, MN
USA

Arne Kristian Aune, MD PhD
Department of Orthopedics and Sports Medicine
Drammen Private Sykehus
Drammen
Norway

Roald Bahr, MD PhD
Department of Sports Medicine
Oslo Sports Trauma Research Center
Norwegian School of Sport Sciences
Oslo
Norway

Vaughan Bowen, MD
Faculty of Medicine, University of Calgary
Foothills Medical Centre
Calgary, AB
Canada

Karen K. Briggs, MPH
Steadman Philippon Research Institute
Vail, CO
USA

Jens Ivar Brox, MD PhD
Orthopaedic Department
Oslo University Hospital, Rikshospitalet
Sognsveien
Oslo
Norway

Tom Clanton, MD
The Steadman Clinic
Vail, CO
USA

Jill Cook, PT PhD
School of Primary Health Care
Faculty of Medicine, Nursing and Health Sciences
Monash University
Frankston, VIC
Australia

Ann Cools, PT PhD
Department of Physical Therapy and Motor
  Rehabilitation
Ghent University
Gent
Belgium

C. Niek van Dijk, MD PhD
Department of Orthopedic Surgery
Orthopedic Research Center Amsterdam
Academic Medical Center
Amsterdam
The Netherlands

Lars Engebretsen, MD PhD
Department of Sports Medicine
Oslo Sports Trauma Research Center
Norwegian School of Sport Sciences
Oslo
Norway

Éanna Falvey, MB BCh MRCPI MMedSci
Director of Sports and Exercise Medicine
Sports Surgery Clinic
Dublin
Ireland

Bjørn Fossan, PT MT
Olympiatoppen
Oslo
Norway

Andrew Franklyn-Miller, MBBS MRCGP
Aspetar, Qatar Orthopaedic and Sports Medicine
  Hospital
Doha
Qatar

Hilde Fredriksen, PT MT MSc
Olympiatoppen
Oslo
Norway

Toru Fukubayashi, MD PhD
Faculty of Sports Sciences
University of Waseda
Tokorozawa
Saitama
Japan

William E. Garrett, Jr. MD PhD
Department of Orthopaedics
Duke University Medical Center
Durham, NC
USA

Robert Gassner, MD DMD PhD
Department of Oral and Maxillofacial Surgery
Medical University of Innsbruck
Maximilianstrasse
Innsbruck
Austria

Umile Giuseppe Longo, MD MSc
Department of Orthopaedic and Trauma Surgery
University Campus Bio-Medico
Rome
Italy

Jan-Ragnar Haugstvedt, MD PhD
Department of Orthopedics
Østfold Hospital Trust
Moss
Norway

Mark R. Hutchinson, MD
University of Illinois at Chicago
Chicago, IL
USA

Markku Järvinen, MD PhD
Department of Orthopaedics
University of Tampere
Tampere
Finland

Tero Järvinen, MD PhD
Department of Orthopaedics and Traumatology
University of Tampere
Tampere
Finland

Karen M. Johnston, MD PhD
Division of Neurosurgery
University of Toronto
Concussion Management Program AESM
Toronto, ON
Canada

Jon Karlson, MD PhD
Department of Orthopaedics
Sahlgrenska University Hospital/Mölndal
Mölndal
Sweden

Gino M.M.J. Kerkhoffs, MD PhD
Department of Orthopedic Surgery
Orthopedic Research Center Amsterdam
Academic Medical Center
Amsterdam
The Netherlands

Karim Khan, MD PhD
UBC Department of Family Practice and School of
  Kinesiology
Centre for Hip Health and Mobility
Vancouver, BC
Canada

W. Ben Kibler, MD
Lexington Clinic Orthopedics, Sports Medicine Center
Lexington, KY
USA

Ingunn R. Kirkeby, MD PhD
Department of Neurosurgery
Oslo University Hospital, Rikshospitalet
Sognsveien
Oslo
Norway

Michael Kjær, MD PhD
Institute of Sports Medicine Copenhagen
Bispebjerg Hospital
and
Faculty of Health Sciences
University of Copenhagen
Copenhagen
Denmark

Oddvar Knutsen, Manualtherapist
Lia Terapi Trysil
Trysil
Norway

Henning Langberg, PT PhD DSc MSc SSPT
Institute of Sports Medicine Copenhagen
Bispebjerg Hospital
and
Faculty of Health Sciences
University of Copenhagen
Copenhagen
Denmark

Robert F. LaPrade, MD PhD
Sports Medicine and Complex Knee Surgery
The Steadman Clinic
and
Steadman Philippon Research Institute
Vail, CO
and
Department of Orthopaedic Surgery
University of Minnesota
Minneapolis, MN
USA

Peter D. le Roux, MD
Penn Neurosurgery at Pennsylvania Hospital
University of Pennsylvania
Philadelphia, PA
USA

Domhnall MacAuley, MD PhD
Ulster Sports Academy
Faculty of Life and Health Science
University of Ulster
Jordanstown
UK

Leonard Macrina, PT SCS
Champion Sports Medicine
Birmingham, AL
USA

Sverre Mæhlum, MD PhD
Hjelp24 NIMI
Oslo
Norway

Glenn Maron, DDS
Emory University School of Medicine
Atlanta, GA
USA

Gordon Matheson, MD PhD
Sports Medicine Center
Department of Orthopaedic Surgery
Stanford University
Stanford, CA
USA

Frank McCormick, MD
Harvard Combined Orthopedic Residency Program
Massachusetts General Hospital
Boston, MA
USA

Paul McCrory, MBBS PhD
Centre for Health, Exercise and Sports Medicine and
the Florey Neurosciences Institutes
University of Melbourne
Melbourne, VIC
and
The Australian Centre for Research into Sports Injury
  and its Prevention
Monash Injury Research Institute
Monash University
Frankston, VIC
Australia

David McDonagh, MD
Accident Department
St. Olavs Hospital
Trondheim
Norway

Willem Meeuwisse, MD PhD
Sport Medicine Centre
University of Calgary
Calgary, AB
Canada

Nicholas Mohtadi, MD MSc
Department of Kinesiology
University of Calgary Sport Medicine Centre
Calgary, AB
Canada

David Mulder, MD
Montreal General Hospital
Montreal, QC
Canada

Grethe Myklebust, PT PhD
Oslo Sports Trauma Research Center
Norwegian School of Sport Sciences
Oslo
Norway

Loris Pegoli, MD
Hand Unit Sport Service
Plastic Surgery Department
University of Milan
Milano
Italy

Mark J. Philippon, MD
Steadman Philippon Research Institute
The Steadman Clinic
Vail, CO
USA
and
Department of Surgery
McMaster University
Hamilton, ON
Canada
and
Department of Orthopedic Surgery
University of Pittsburgh Medical Center
Pittsburgh, PA
USA

Casey M. Pierce, MD
Department of Clinical Research
Steadman Philippon Research Institute
Vail, CO
USA

Babette M. Pluim, MD PhD
Royal Netherlands Lawn Tennis Association
Amersfoort
The Netherlands

Matthew T. Provencher, MD MC USN
Department of Orthopaedic Surgery
Naval Medical Center San Diego
San Diego, CA
USA

Per Renström, MD PhD
Department of Molecular Medicine and Surgery
Center for Sports Trauma Research and Education
Karolinska Institutet
Stockholm
Sweden

May Arna Risberg, PT PhD
Norwegian Research Center for Active Rehabilitation
Department of Sport Medicine
Norwegian School of Sport Sciences
Oslo
Norway

Gil Rodas, MD
Medical Services
Futbol Club Barcelona
Barcelona
Spain

Marc R. Safran, MD
Department of Orthopaedic Surgery
Stanford University
Redwood City, CA
USA

Per Skjelbred, MD DDS PhD Dr.h.c.
Department of Maxillofacial Surgery and Hospital
   Dentistry
Oslo University Hospital
Oslo
Norway

Roger Sørensen, MD
Orthopaedic Department
Oslo University Hospital, Rikshospitalet
Sognsveien
Oslo
Norway

Kathrin Steffen, PhD
Department of Sports Medicine
Oslo Sports Trauma Research Center
Norwegian School of Sport Sciences
Oslo
Norway

Roland Thomée, PT PhD
Department of Orthopaedics
Lundberg Laboratory for Orthopaedic Research
Sahlgrenska University Hospital
Göteborg
Sweden

Michael Turner, MBBS
British Horseracing Authority
London
UK

Stein Tyrdal, MD PhD
Department of Orthopaedics
Hand and Upper Extremity Unit
Oslo University Hospital
Oslo
Norway

Evert Verhagen, PhD
Department of Public and Occupational Health
EMGO+ Institute for Health and Care Research
VU University Medical Center
Amsterdam
The Netherlands

Geoffrey M. Verrall, MD
Sportsmed SA
Sports Medicine Centre
Adelaide, SA
Australia

Robert G. Watkins III, MD
Marina Spine Center
Marina del Rey, CA
USA

Robert G. Watkins IV, MD
Marina Spine Center
Marina del Rey, CA
USA

Kevin E. Wilk, PT DPT
Champion Sports Medicine
Birmingham, AL
USA

Mike Wilkinson, MB BCh MBA Dip Sports Med
Allan McGavin Sports Medicine Center
Vancouver, BC
Canada

Foreword

The extensive involvement of athletes both in training sessions and competitive events exposes them to numerous possibilities for injury. The potential for injuries that could place limitations on training and could hamper competitive performance constitutes a major concern for each and every athlete. It is, therefore, vitally important that those involved with the health and welfare of athletes are highly knowledgeable with respect to the diverse injuries that can be sustained by the athletes when they are involved in the various sports on the Olympic programme.

This Manual presents comprehensive information related to the assessment and treatment of injuries in chapters organised according to body regions. Each chapter contains sections arranged according to the "presenting symptoms" for both acute and overuse injuries, and includes information regarding rehabilitation and procedures for returning to training and competition.

Dr Roald Bahr has assembled a highly knowledgeable and experienced group of associate editors and contributing authors to produce this comprehensive coverage of a highly important topic. We welcome this splendid contribution to the international literature on sports medicine.

Dr Jacques Rogge
IOC President

Preface

One of the most important medical advances is the understanding that regular physical activity substantially reduces the risk of premature mortality as well as coronary heart disease, hypertension, colon cancer, diabetes, and obesity. In fact, recent studies have shown inactivity and low cardiorespiratory fitness are more important mortality and morbidity predictors than the better known risk factors such as obesity, smoking, elevated cholesterol levels, or elevated blood pressure.

Regular physical activity is the critical factor for optimal health from cradle to grave; it is necessary for normal development during childhood and adolescence and essential for the maintenance of functional ability and independence in later years.

And there is more good news. As people are becoming aware that their daily energy demands are decreasing due to reduced opportunity and increased mechanization at home, at work and during leisure time, they are taking to physical activity and sports in increasing numbers. However, sports participation also entails a risk for injuries. So if we are to succeed in encouraging our patients to become more physically active, it demands us to take this side effect seriously.

This book is meant as a tool to aid not just specialist sports physicians and physical therapists, but also primary care physicians, ER physicians, general physical therapists, athletic trainers, nurse practitioners, physician's assistants, and all those involved in assessing and treating the active individual with injuries sustained in sports and physical activity.

One important point is that the contents of this book are not meant for the elite athlete alone. Modern sports medicine has developed assessment and treatment algorithms—particularly through its focus on early, active rehabilitation—which will benefit all patients, whether the injury was sustained in professional sports, on the school playground, or by just being outdoors enjoying an active lifestyle.

The IOC Manual of Sports Injuries is based on the highly acclaimed *Idrettsskader* (Gazette Bok/Fagbokforlaget: Oslo, Norway), which was written by a group of Norwegian specialists in 2000 and has been published in several languages (Norwegian, English, Spanish, Swedish, Greek, and simplified and traditional Chinese). The English-language version was heralded as "Book of the year!" by the British Journal of Sports Medicine in 2006.

Since 2000, there have been a number of significant developments in our understanding of sports injuries—what they are, how they should be assessed, and how they should be treated. To ensure that *The IOC Manual of Sports Injuries* accurately reflects these advances, we have recruited an international cast of world-leading experts as co-editors and authors.

We have deliberately used a problem-oriented approach to guide the practitioner through a standardized and structured approach to the assessment and management of injuries in physical activity. We cover the various body regions, hoping to distinguish the common from the less common, to link history taking and physical examination to the diagnosis, and to provide detailed guidance on management of the most common injuries and disorders. An added value lies in the exceptional artwork by our medical illustrator, Tommy Bolic; the many illustrations can be used as a tool to improve communication with patients about what their injury represents.

I would like to thank everyone involved for their many contributions to this book—none mentioned, none forgotten. It is our hope that *The IOC Manual of Sports Injuries* will become a valuable clinical guide for practitioners and a helpful teaching tool for students and patients world-wide in years to come.

Roald Bahr
Editor

2012

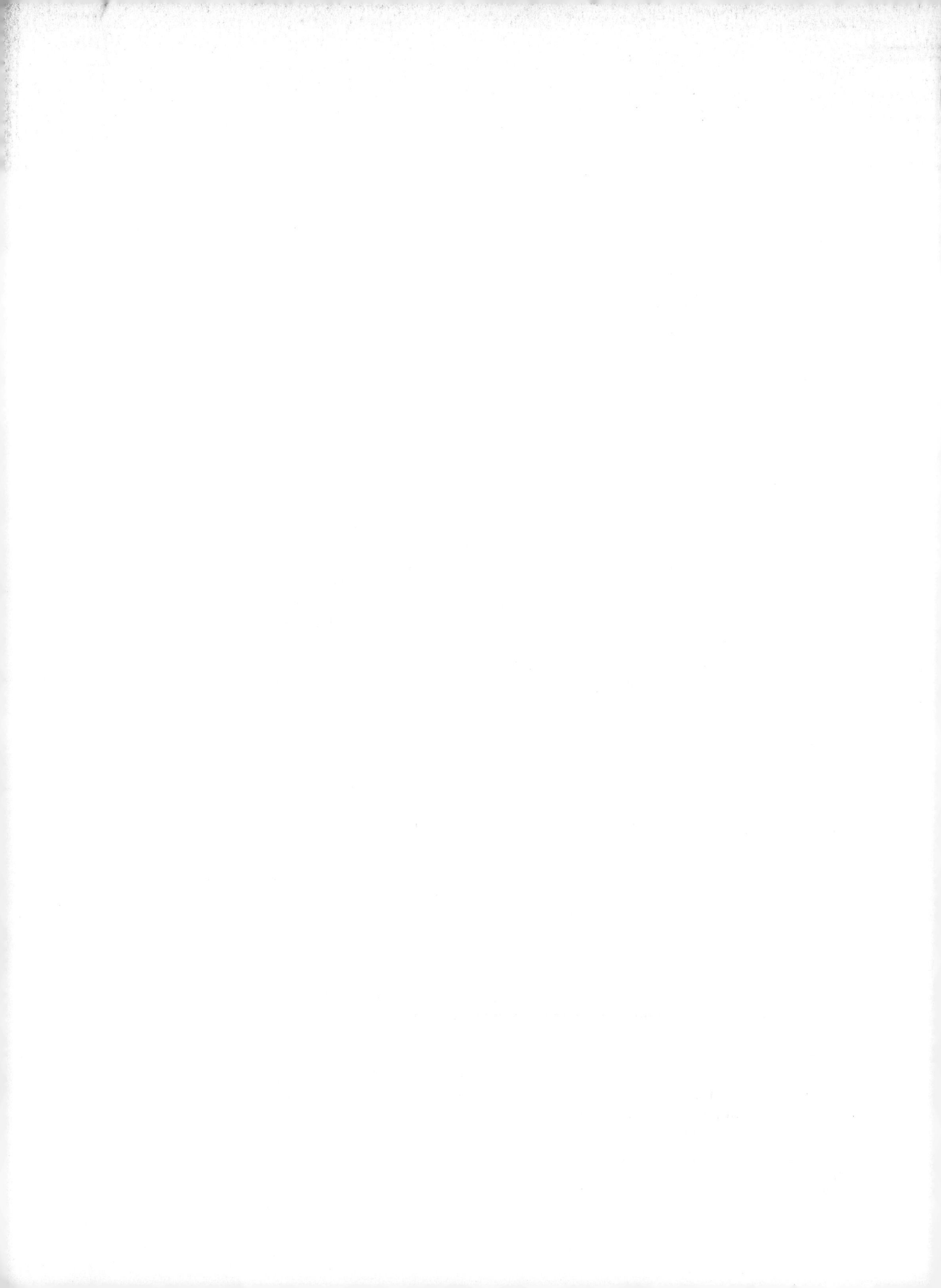

1 Types and Causes of Injuries

Roald Bahr[1], Håkan Alfredson[2], Markku Järvinen[3], Tero Järvinen[3], Karim Khan[4],
Michael Kjær[5], Gordon Matheson[6], and Sverre Mæhlum[7]

[1]Norwegian School of Sport Sciences, Oslo, Norway
[2]University of Umeå, Sports Medicine Umeå Inc., Umeå, Sweden
[3]University of Tampere, Tampere, Finland
[4]Centre for Hip Health and Mobility, Vancouver, BC, Canada
[5]Bispebjerg Hospital, Copenhagen, Denmark
[6]Stanford University, Stanford, CA, USA
[7]Hjelp24 NIMI, Oslo, Norway

Exercise and physical activity are the most important determinants of health in developing and transitioning countries, and sedentary living is the fourth independent risk factor for morbidity and mortality from noncommunicable disease. Regular physical activity reduces the risk of early death in general, and of cardiovascular disease, high blood pressure, type 2 diabetes, and even some types of cancer. Indeed, physical *in*activity can present as great a risk to health as smoking, being overweight, high cholesterol, or high blood pressure. Furthermore, intense exercise is not necessarily more effective than other forms of exercise for prevention and treatment of chronic disease. Significant health benefits can be achieved through moderate physical activity; as a matter of fact, standing as opposed to sitting will also incur health benefits. This holds true even at an advanced age. The least fit people are the ones who can derive the greatest health benefit from regular physical activity.

Unfortunately, exercise and physical activity also have some unfortunate side effects. Injuries are a particular risk. Nevertheless, the net health effect is positive–the benefits of physical activity far exceed the problems caused by injuries.

Acute Injuries and Overuse Injuries

A sports injury may be defined as damage to the tissues of the body that occurs as a result of sport or exercise. In this book, the term applies to any damage that results from any form of physical activity. Physical activity can be defined as moving or using the body, and it includes numerous forms of activity such as working, fitness exercise, outdoor activity, playing, training, getting in shape, working out, and physical education.

Sport injuries can be divided into acute injuries and overuse injuries, depending on the injury mechanism and onset of symptoms. In most cases, it is easy to classify an injury as acute or overuse, but in some cases it may be difficult. Acute injuries occur suddenly and have a clearly defined cause or onset. Overuse injuries occur gradually. However, an important concept with overuse injuries is that they exist along a spectrum whcrc the inciting events are below the threshold for clinical symptomatology, but if not rectified, they eventually produce sufficient tissue damage to result in clinical symptoms. This is important for physicians, therapists, and patients to understand, because it is not uncommon to "react" to "new" clinical symptoms the same way one reacts to acute injuries. Such a response may ignore the underlying clinical symptomatology and thus may interfere with effective treatment. For example, an athlete with a stress fracture (a fatigue fracture) in the foot will often state that the symptoms originated during a specific run, perhaps even from a specific step. The injury may accordingly be misclassified as an acute injury. However, the actual cause of the stress fracture is that the specific run was a precipitating event on top of the underlying spectrum of tissue damage on the skeleton from overuse over time. Therefore, these types of injuries should be classified as overuse injuries.

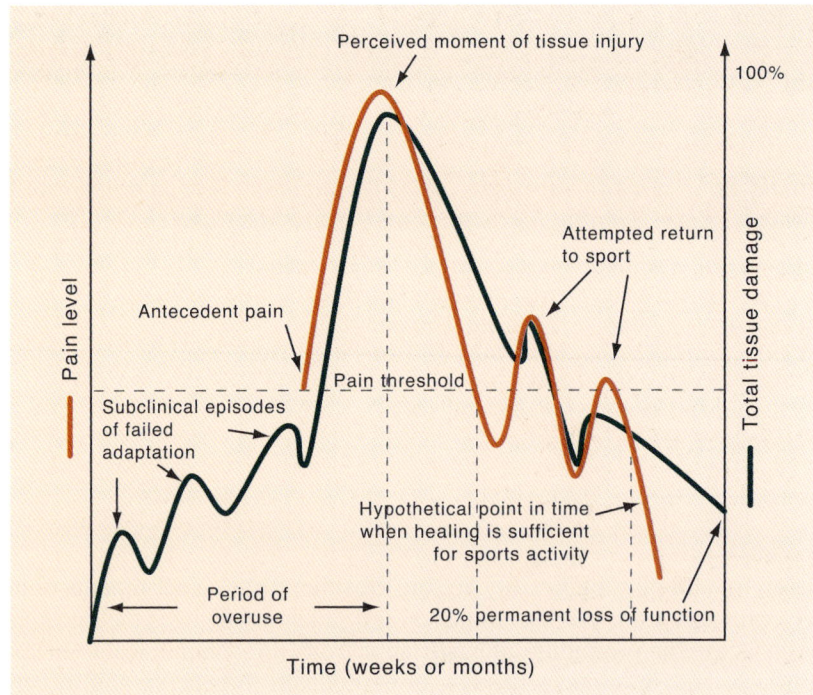

Figure 1.1 Hypothetical overview of pain and tissue injury in a typical overuse injury. (Reproduced with permission from the Norwegian Sports Medicine Association.)

As shown in Figure 1.1, the pathological process is often under way for a period of time before the athlete notices the symptoms. Repetitive low-grade forces that lead to microtrauma in the tissues cause overuse injuries. In most cases, the tissue will repair without demonstrable clinical symptoms. However, if this process continues, the ability of the tissue to repair can be exceeded, resulting in a clinical overuse injury with symptoms. It is vitally important that athletes as well as therapists and physicians understand this concept so that correct treatment can be initiated.

The difference between acute injuries and overuse injuries can also be described in biomechanical terms. Dynamic or static muscle action creates internal resistance in the loaded structures (stress) that counteracts deformation (strain) of the tissue. All tissue has a characteristic ability to tolerate deformation and stress, and injuries occur when the tolerance level is exceeded. An acute injury occurs when loading is sufficient to cause irreversible deformation of the tissue, whereas an overuse injury occurs as a result of repeated overloading either in the loading itself or through inadequate recovery time between loadings. Each incidence, alone, is not enough to cause irreversible deformation, but the repeated actions can result in an injury over time.

Acute injuries are most common in sports in which the speed is high and the risk of falling is great (e.g., downhill skiing) and in team sports where there is much contact between players (e.g., ice hockey and soccer). Overuse injuries make up the large portion of injuries in aerobic sports that require long training sessions with a monotonous routine (e.g., long-distance running, bicycling, or cross-country skiing). But a large number of overuse injuries also occur in technical sports, in which the same movement is repeated numerous times (e.g., tennis, javelin throwing, weightlifting, and high jumping).

Why Do Injuries Occur?

The basic principle for training is that the body reacts to a specific physical training load with specific predictable adaptation. Loading that exceeds what an athlete is used to will cause the tissue that is being trained to attempt to adapt to the new loading. For example, training provides a stimulus that causes the muscles to increase the production of contractile proteins, the muscle fibers become larger (and more numerous), and the muscle fibers specifically adapt to whether the training requires primarily endurance or maximum strength. This principle applies to all types of tissue. The skeleton, tendons, ligaments, and cartilage adapt accordingly. The tissue becomes stronger and tolerates more (Figure 1.2).

However, if the training load exceeds the tissue's ability to adapt, injuries will occur. The risk of overuse injuries increases when training load increases. This could result from an increase in the duration of individual training sessions or an increase in training intensity or the frequency of training sessions. Often the duration, intensity, and frequency of training increase at the same time, such as at a training camp or at the beginning of the season. Therefore, it is common to say that overuse injuries are due to "too much, too often, too quickly, and with too little rest," which means that training load increases more quickly than the tissue is able to adapt.

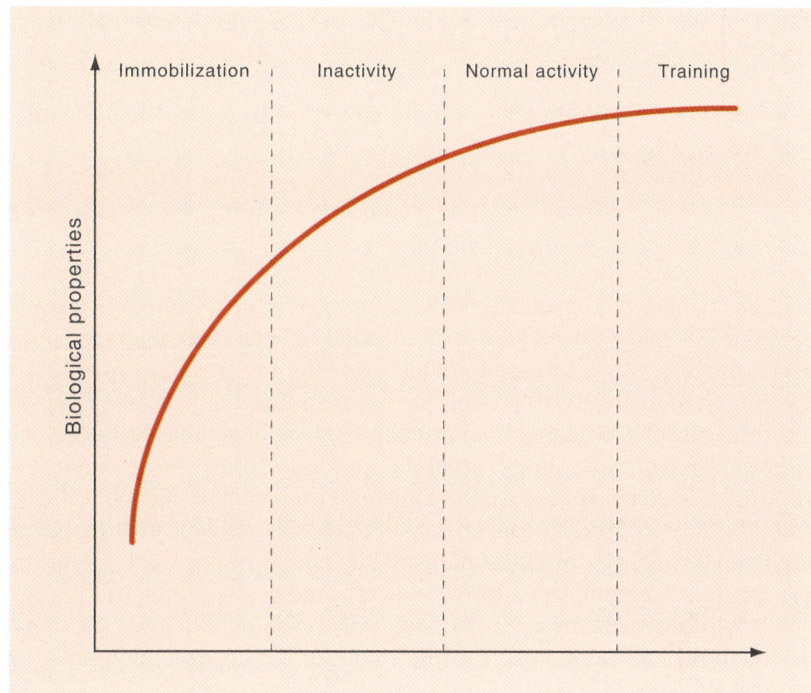

Figure 1.2 Adaption to training. Immobilization significantly weakens the biological properties of the tissue, whereas exercise improves function. (Reproduced with permission from the Norwegian Sports Medicine Association.)

Various Types of Injuries

Sport injuries can be divided into *soft-tissue injuries* (cartilage injuries, muscle injuries, tendon injuries, and ligament injuries) and *skeletal injuries* (fractures). The various types of tissue have distinctly different biomechanical properties and their ability to adapt to training also varies. This chapter examines the characteristics of the various types of tissue and the ways in which the skeleton, cartilage, muscles, tendons, and ligaments can be injured.

Ligaments

Structure and Function

Ligaments consist of collagen tissue that connects one bone to another. Their primary function is passive stabilization of the joints. In addition, the ligaments serve an important proprioceptive function.

Ligaments consist primarily of cells, collagen fibers, and proteoglycans. Fibroblasts are the most important cell type, and their main function is to produce collagen (primarily type I but several other types as well). The amount of proteoglycan is much lower than the amount found in cartilage. While the collagen fibers in tendons are organized in a parallel manner (in the longitudinal direction of the muscles), the orientation of the fibers in ligaments can be parallel, oblique, or even spiral (e.g., the anterior cruciate ligament). The organization of fiber direction is specific to the function of each ligament. In addition, ligaments contain slightly more elastic fibers than tendons.

Ligaments may insert directly or indirectly into the bone: directly with a transition zone consisting of fibrocartilage first and mineralized fibrocartilage last (including specialized collagen fibers that go down into the bone vertically), or indirectly by growing into the surrounding periosteum.

Ligaments may be intra-articular (localized within a joint inside the joint capsule), capsular (where the ligament projects as a thickening of the joint capsule), or extra-capsular (localized outside the joint capsule). The cruciate ligaments are intra-artic-ular ligaments. The anterior talofibular ligament is a capsular ligament, where it may be difficult to distinguish between the ligament and the rest of the capsule, whereas the calcaneofibular ligament is an extracapsular ligament. The type of ligament is important for the healing potential after a total rupture. Following total rupture of an intra-articular ligament, such as the anterior cruciate ligament, healing will not take place, whereas the capsular ligaments have excellent healing potential. Blood supply to ligaments also differs. Capsular ligaments have a good blood supply, just as the surrounding joint capsule does, whereas the blood supply to intra-articular liga-ments enters proximally or distally, typically resulting in a midzone of marginal vas-cularization. The blood supply is important for the healing potential after an injury.

Ligaments contain a number of different nerve endings that supply the nervous sys-tem with information about body position, movement, and pain. This information is key in controlling the muscles that surround a joint such as the knee. Even if the main function of ligaments is passive stabilization of the joint, much evidence indicates that the proprioceptive function of ligaments is more impor-tant than previously thought. Liga-ment injuries may reduce the ability to register the position and move-ments of the joint, even when the injury does not result in significant mechanical instability. This may in-crease the risk of recurrent injuries.

Figure 1.3 shows how ligaments re-act to stretching. At first, the wavy pattern of the microscopic colla-gen fibers straightens out and mini-mal force is required to cause a significant change in length. As force increases further, the collagen fibers will be stretched, and the relation-ship between load and deformation is linear. This means that the liga-ment serves as an ideal spring in the elastic zone, as long as the change in length does not exceed about 4%. If a force causes a change in length in ex-

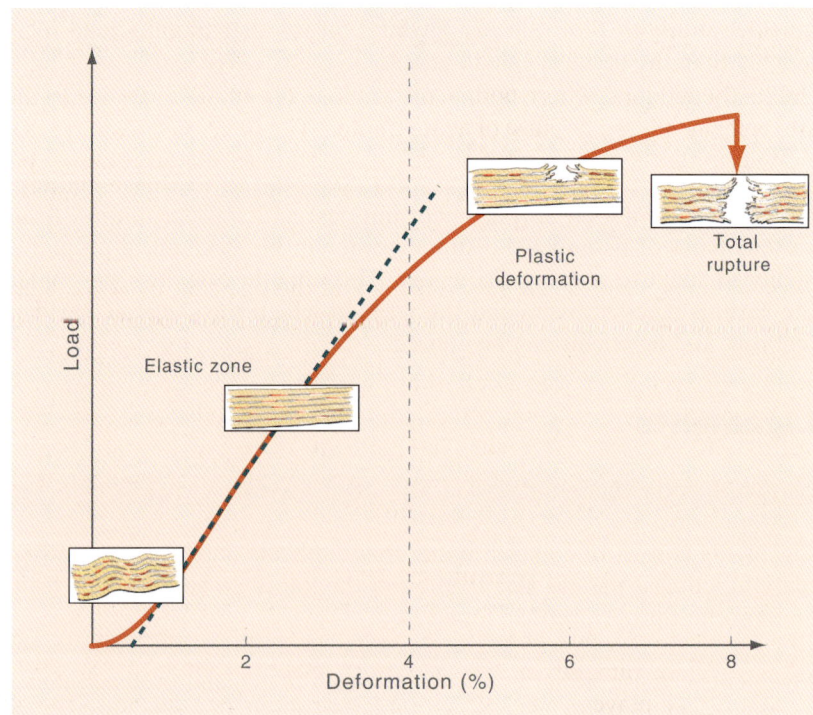

Figure 1.3 Acute stress–deformation curve for ligaments. (© Medical Illustrator Tommy Bolic, Sweden.)

cess of this, the collagen fibers will rupture—first single fibers and then all of the fibers will fail (a total rupture). The strength and stiffness of a ligament depends on the longi-tudinal and cross-sectional area. The greater the cross-sectional area, the stronger and stiffer the ligament. A longer ligament is less stiff, but the maximum tensile strength does not change if the cross-sectioned area is the same.

Adaption to Training

Connective tissue adapts slowly to increased loading but weakens rapidly as a result of immobilization (Figure 1.4). The ligaments adapt to training by increasing the cross-sectional area, as well as by changing the material properties so that they become stronger per unit area. Normal everyday activity (without specific training) is apparently sufficient to maintain 80–90% of the ligament's mechanical properties. Systematic training increases ligament strength by 10–20%. In contrast, the negative effect of immobilization sets in quickly. After a few weeks, strength is reduced to about half. Systematic training causes strength in the ligament substance to return after several weeks, but the tensile strength in the ligament–bone junction will remain at a reduced level for several months despite systematic retraining.

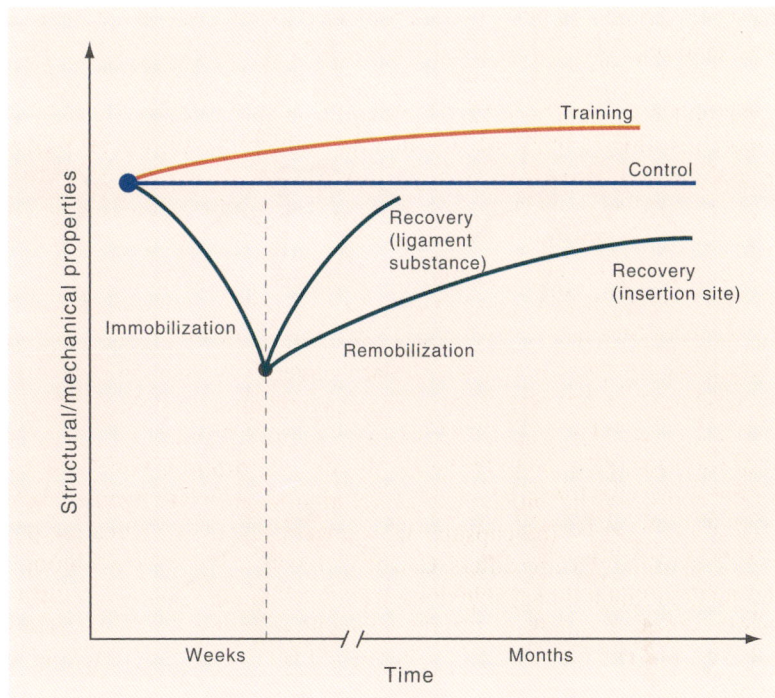

Figure 1.4 Schematic representation of the relationship between training, immobilization, and remobilization on the structural and mechanical properties of the ligaments. (Reproduced with permission from the Norwegian Sports Medicine Association.)

Ligament Injuries

Unlike the tendons, where both acute and overuse injuries can occur, the ligaments are typically injured because of acute trauma. The injury mechanism is sudden overloading, where the ligament is stretched with the joint in an extreme position. For example, inversion trauma in the ankle may cause the lateral ligaments—primarily the anterior talofibular ligament—to rupture.

Ruptures may occur in the midsubstance of the ligament or at the ligament–bone junction (Figure 1.5). Sometimes avulsion fractures also occur, which means that the ligament pulls a piece of the bone with it, usually with an eggshell shape. Several factors determine the location of the rupture, including the age of the patient. Children often sustain avulsion fractures, while midsubstance ruptures commonly occur in adolescents and adults. The ligament–bone junction can be the weak point in middle-aged patients, and avulsion fractures are most common in the elderly, particularly if the skeleton is osteoporotic.

Overuse injuries in the ligaments are rare, and symptomatic inflammatory conditions hardly ever occur. Nevertheless, overuse injuries may occur as the ligament is gradually stretched out, probably because of repetitive microtrauma. One example is the shoulder joint, where throwers (e.g., javelin throwers and baseball, handball, and volleyball players) may stretch out their anterior ligaments. This may reduce stability in the joint and predispose the athlete to pain because of entrapment of the subacromial structures. However, one must be aware that the primary ligament injury (stretching) is usually asymptomatic. The symptoms only appear if the instability causes muscular dysfunction and/or results in injury to other structures (e.g., the rotator cuff in the shoulder).

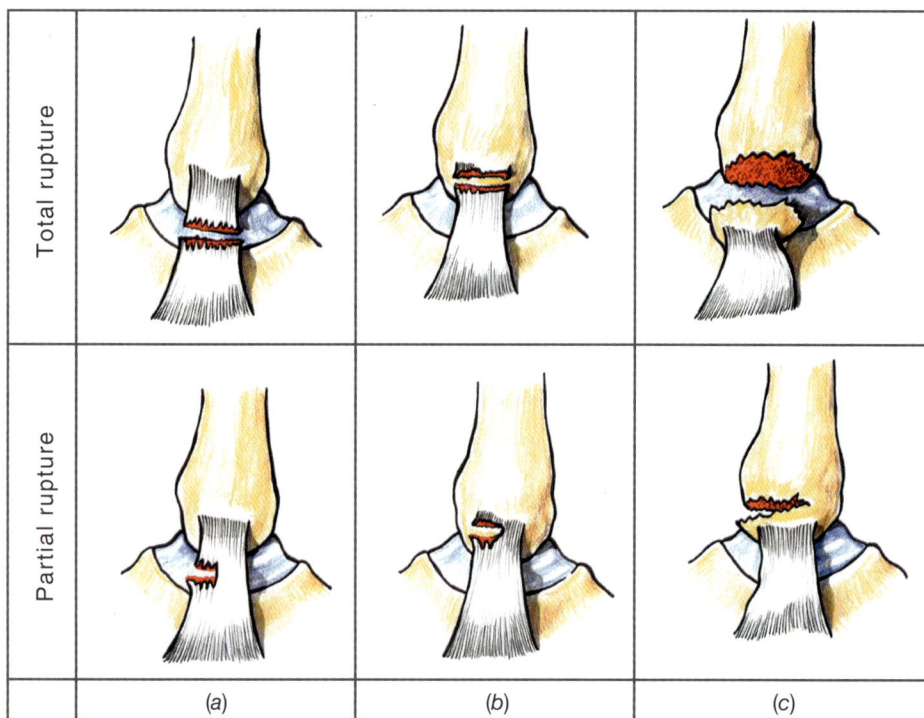

Figure 1.5 Various types of ligament injuries. Total and partial ruptures (a) in the midsubstance, (b) in the ligament–bone junction, and (c) avulsion fractures. (© Medical Illustrator Tommy Bolic, Sweden.)

Internationally, ligament injuries are usually classified as mild (grade 1), moderate (grade 2), or severe (grade 3). Mild injuries only cause structural damage on the microscopic level, with slight local tenderness and no instability. Moderate injuries cause a partial rupture with visible swelling and notable tenderness, but usually with little to no change in stability. Severe injuries cause a complete rupture with significant swelling and instability. Nevertheless, because the relationship between the degree of structural damage, tenderness, and instability is highly variable, this general classification of ligament injuries is very limited for clinical purposes. The use of classification systems developed for the individual ligaments and joints, for which specific tests have been developed, is recommended to grade the degree of the injury. These types of tests and classification systems are described in the discussion of the various regions of the body in Chapters 4–15.

An acute ligament rupture sets off a series of events–the inflammation process–which can be divided into three stages: the inflammatory phase (phase 1), the proliferative phase (phase 2), and the maturation phase (phase 3).

The Inflammation Process

Inflammation ("inflammare" [Lat.]; to set on fire, inflame) is a local tissue response in any vascularized tissue subjected to loading, which results in cell damage. Inflammation consists of a characteristic chain of vascular, chemical, and cellular events that may result in repair, regeneration, or formation of scar tissue. The five cardinal signs of inflammation are *rubor* (redness), *tumor* (swelling), *calor* (heat, increased temperature), *dolor* (pain), and *functio laesa* (loss of function). Among the cardinal signs, pain is generally the most prominent in sport injuries, both as a symptom that the patient experiences subjectively and as a finding, tenderness to palpation. However, it should be noted that painful conditions are not always related to inflammation, as will be described later in the section on tendon injuries. Under normal conditions, erythrocytes, leukocytes, and plasma components are isolated intravascularly. An injury to the vascular endothelium results in leakage of plasma components, erythrocytes, and leukocytes. The inflammation process is activated by a series of different mediators that primarily result in increased vascular permeability, activation of leukocytes, blood platelets, and the coagulation system (Figure 1.6). Vasoactive mediators bind to specific receptors on endothelial cells and smooth muscle cells. This results in vasoconstriction or dilatation. Neutrophils, granulocytes, monocytes, and lymphocytes are attracted to the injury site by chemotactic factors that are released from the activated platelets and the injured cells. These cells release a series of inflammation mediators. Key among these are growth factors, cytokines, chemokines, prostaglandins, and leukotrienes.

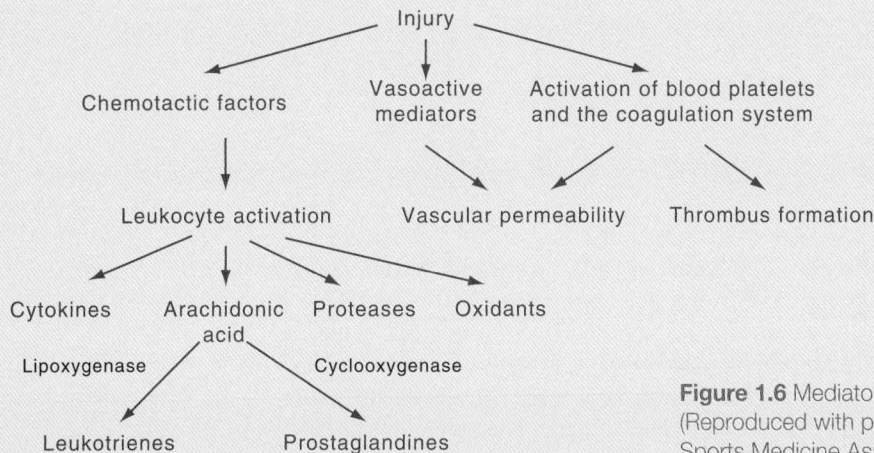

Figure 1.6 Mediators of inflammation. (Reproduced with permission from the Norwegian Sports Medicine Association.)

The Inflammatory Phase (Phase 1)

The inflammatory phase begins with bleeding and the exudation of plasma. Activation of the coagulation cascade causes clotting with a network of fibrin, fibronectin, and collagen blood cells. This network provides some initial strength to the clot. Blood platelets are activated and release a large number of growth factors from their granules. These growth factors function as chemotactic factors recruiting inflammatory cells to the site of the injury. Neutrophil granulocytes release a series of proteolytic enzymes that dissolve the damaged extracellular matrix. Blood platelets and monocytes are recruited into the injured area, invade the tissue and differentiate into macrophages that are actively engaged in the phagocytosis of cell debris and release growth factors that attract pericytes, endothelial cells, and fibroblasts and stimulate cells to the injured area. The inflammatory phase lasts a few days.

The Proliferative Phase (Phase 2)

The proliferative phase is characterized by the accumulation of large numbers of endothelial cells, macrophages, myofibroblasts, and fibroblasts to the site of the injury. Ingrowth of new capillaries (i.e., angiogenesis) begins at the edge of the injury site, and within a few days a rich capillary network supplying oxygen and nutrients is established. The myofibroblasts and fibroblasts organize themselves perpendicular to the direction of capillary ingrowth and an immature granulation tissue is formed. These cells produce an extracellular network that initially consists of fibronectin, type III collagen, and proteoglycans. After a week, the production of type I collagen increases greatly. Some of the fibroblasts transdifferentiate into the contraction-capable cells called myofibroblasts, which are responsible for the scar formation. At the same time, there is continuous breakdown of the initial clot and the injured extracellular early loose connective tissue, and the formation of mechanically stronger newly formed matrix. The macrophages accomplish this by "eating" the superfluous cell components. In addition to that, most of the macrophages transform from inflammatory to anti-inflammatory cells and direct the repair process by secreting growth factors needed for the repair. The continuous deposition and removal of extracellular matrix (with the balance toward deposition) results in remodeling of the injury and increased tensile strength. The proliferation stage lasts a few weeks.

The Maturation Phase (Phase 3)

The final tissue structure is established during the maturation and remodeling stage through continuous remodeling of the scar tissue. The numbers of macrophages and fibroblasts are significantly reduced and the few remaining fibroblasts transform to myofibroblasts, and blood supply is finally established by removal of the capillaries with lowered blood flow and most of the capillaries disappear. The granulation tissue is converted (contracted) by myofibroblasts into a small scar. Thicker collagen fibers are formed in the direction of tension in the tissue from external load, and a network of lateral, cross-bridges providing mechanical strength is established between them. Therefore, the form and function of the scar tissue depend on the degree to which the tissue is subjected to loading during this stage. This stage may last several months, which has important implications for return to sport.

Tendons

Structure and Function

Tendons consist of connective tissue that attaches muscle to bone. Their most important function is to transfer force from the muscles into the skeletal system, thereby contributing to stabilizing the joints. Further, the elasticity of tendon allows for short loading energy stored in the tendon to be released in, for example, jumping activity. Apart from water, the main element in tendons is type I collagen, which makes up 80–90% of the tendinous matrix content. To a large extent, the structure of tendons resembles the structure of ligaments. The collagen is arranged in parallel fibers and the tendons are constructed of increasingly large structures, the tropocollagen, microfibrils, subfibrils, fibrils, and fascicles (Figure 1.7). The strict organization into parallel bundles of various sizes is the main difference between tendons and ligaments. The organization of the ligaments is more variable and dependent on function.

Fascicles are surrounded by a loose connective tissue, endotenon, which makes it easy for them to move in relation to each other. Endotenon also contains veins,

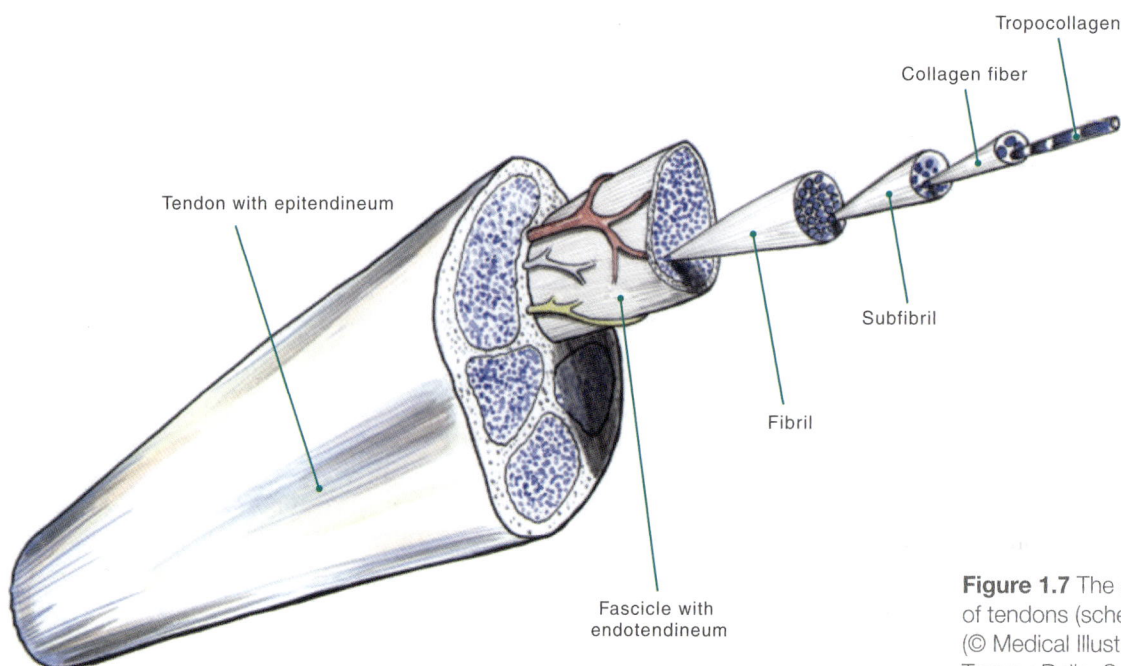

Tropocollagen

Collagen fiber

Tendon with epitendineum

Subfibril

Fibril

Fascicle with endotendineum

Figure 1.7 The structure of tendons (schematic). (© Medical Illustrator Tommy Bolic, Sweden.)

nerve fibers, and lymph vessels. The surface of the tendon is surrounded by a white synovial-like membrane, the epitenon, a loose connective tissue that also supports blood vessels, lymphatics, and nerves. Some tendons are covered by a loose areolar connective tissue, the paratenon, enveloping the tendon. The envelope of tendon is dominated by type IV collagen and acts as an epithelium hindering the tendon to adhere to surrounding tissues.

The muscle cell ends in a number of microscopic membranous infoldings that stick out like small fingers into the myotendinous junction. The collagen fibers creep into the folds that form between the fingers and attach to the basal membrane of the muscle. At the other end, the tendons attach to bone via fibrocartilage and mineralized fibrocartilage. Collagen fibers penetrate the mineralized fibrocartilage into the subchondral bone, contributing to better attachment.

The relationship between stress and deformation of tendons is the same as for the ligaments (Figure 1.3). Initially, the collagen fibers are easily stretched from their normal wavy appearance, in the elastic zone the tendon behaves like an ideal spring, whereas ruptures occur in the deformation zones: first single fibers, then total ruptures.

Adaptation to Training

The tendons adjust to training in the same manner as the ligaments–by increasing the tendon strength through collagen synthesis, cross-link formation and training improved material properties of the tendinous tissue, and if trained sufficiently some increase in tendon cross-sectional area can be seen. Acute exercise results in an increase in collagen synthesis within and around the tendon tissue. Collagen synthesis remains increased for 2–3 days, indicating that training every second or third day is most likely a sufficient stimulus for tendon protein generation. In addition, the relative load intensity required is less than in muscle, which means that also moderate exercise, either concentric or eccentric, will result in elevated formation of new collagen in tendon. Changes in physical activity levels, either increased training or detraining/immobilization, quickly (within 1–3 weeks) alter mechanical properties, most likely through increased or decreased cross-link formation, respectively. In contrast, changes in collagen-rich fibril structures require several months to years to occur.

Tendon Injuries

Tendons can be injured in several different ways, both as acute injuries and as overuse injuries. Because tendons are usually superficial, they can be severed by a penetrating stab or a cut, such as one caused by the edge of a skate. Acute tendon ruptures occur if force is generated in excess of the tendon's ability to tolerate it. These types of tendon ruptures usually occur in connection with eccentric force generation, such as in the Achilles tendon when pushing off at the start of a sprint run. Tendon ruptures may be partial or total, and they usually occur in the midtendon substance but may also occur in the bone–tendon junction or as avulsion fractures. Acute tendon injuries are most common in athletes and recreational exercisers between 30 and 50 years of age in explosive sports, often without previous symptoms or warning. Some studies reveal that structural and degenerative changes can be seen in the tendon prior to exercise.

Tendons are the type of tissue that is most often affected by overuse injuries. Several different terms are habitually used to describe these overuse injuries: tendinitis (tendon inflammation), tenosynovitis (tendon sheath inflammation), tenoperiostitis (inflammation of tendon insertions and origins), periostitis (periosteal inflammation), and bursitis/hemobursitis (bursal inflammation, possibly with bleeding). All these terms describe the parts of the tendon or the surrounding tissue that is affected, and all have the ending "itis," indicating the pathophysiological condition of inflammation.

Even though the concept of inflammation has been used traditionally, the pathogenesis for overuse injuries in tendons is uncertain. Although tendon loading does not normally cause more than a 4% change in length (i.e., within the physiological elastic zone), some sports require repetitive loading in excess of this (4–8% change in length), which may cause collagen fibrils to rupture. Therefore, a potential explanation of what is called tendinitis is that repetitive microtrauma causes injuries that are greater than the fibroblasts are able to repair, resulting in inflammation. It is also possible that cumulative microtrauma can affect collagen cross-bridges, other matrix proteins, or microvascular elements in the tendon. Also, loading that extends the tendon less than 4% can lead to overuse symptoms, and it is likely caused by inadequate time to adapt to each training load.

One problem with explaining tendon overuse as inflammation is that the histological findings do not match those seen with inflammation–surgical specimens are devoid of inflammatory cells. However, degenerative changes, changed fibril organization, reduced cell count, vascular ingrowth, and, occasionally, local necrosis with or without calcification are seen. The concept of tendinosis was introduced to describe these types of focal degenerative changes. Because the relationship between degenerative changes and symptoms is unclear, the terms "tendinosis" or "tendinopathy" are now commonly used to describe chronic tendon pain. Table 1.1 provides an overview of old and new terminology for tendon disorders and injuries. The new terminology emphasizes the need for the terminology to correspond to the histological findings.

New	Old	Definition	Histologic findings
Paratenonitis	Tenosynovitis Tenovaginitis Peritendinitis	An inflammation of only the paratenon, either lined by synovium or not	Inflammatory cells in paratenon or peritendinous areolar tissue
Paratenonitis with tendinosis	Tendinitis	Paratenon inflammation associated with intratendinous degeneration	Same as above, with loss of tendon collagen, fiber disorientation, scattered vascular ingrowth, but no prominent intratendinous inflammation
Tendinosis	Tendinitis	Intratendinous degeneration due to atrophy (aging, microtrauma, vascular compromise, etc.)	Noninflammatory intratendinous collagen degeneration with fiber disorientation, hypocellularity, scattered vascular ingrowth, occasional local necrosis, and/or calcification
Tendinitis	Tendon strain or tear (a) acute (less than 2 weeks) (b) subacute (4–6 weeks) (c) chronic (over 6 weeks)	Symptomatic degeneration of the tendon with vascular disruption and inflammatory repair response	Three recognized subgroups. Each displays variable histology from pure inflammation with hemorrhage and tear, to inflammation superimposed upon preexisting degeneration, to calcification and tendinosis changes in chronic conditions. In chronic stage there may be: interstial microinjury central tendon necrosis frank partial rupture acute complete rupture

Table 1.1 Terminology for tendon disorders and tendon injuries.

Bone

Structure and Function

The skeleton consists of bone, a special type of connective tissue that remodels continuously as a response to a complex interplay between mechanical loading, systemic hormones, and the calcium level in the blood. Bone may be classified as cortical (compact) or trabecular (spongy), and the two types of bone have different functions and properties. The long bones consist primarily of cortical bone, whereas the vertebrae in the spinal column consist of trabecular bone. Bone has many important functions, such as protecting the underlying organs, serving as the body's major calcium store, and providing the environment for hematopoiesis in marrow. However, in relation to injuries, the skeleton's most important function is as a lever in the locomotor apparatus.

Like other connective tissue, bone consists of cells, collagen fibers, and extracellular matrix. Bone cells develop from stem cells in the bone marrow, primarily as osteocytes, osteoblasts, or osteoclasts. The osteoblasts and osteoclasts are responsible for remodeling bone. Located on bone surfaces, osteoblasts are bone-forming cells. When an osteoblast has formed enough bone to be completely surrounded by a mineralized matrix, it is called an osteocyte. Osteoclasts are also found on the surface of bone–their job is to absorb bone. Osteocytes communicate with each other and with osteoblasts and osteoclasts on the surface through channels in the extracellular matrix, and this is an important signaling path from mechanical loading to remodeling. A recommended daily intake of minerals (calcium and magnesium) and vitamin D is necessary for optimum remodeling of bone.

The extracellular bone matrix consists of both organic and inorganic components. The inorganic component constitutes more than half the bone mass and consists primarily of calcium and phosphate as crystals of hydroxyapatite. The inorganic components contribute greatly to the characteristic hardness and strength of bone. Strength increases with increasing bone mineral density, but skeletal architecture is also very important. The main organic component is collagen, which contributes to bone's elastic properties.

The skeletal surface is covered by a thick layer of fibrous connective tissue, called periosteum. Periosteum has a rich supply of nerves and blood. For this reason, direct trauma that causes bleeding in or underneath the periosteum can be very painful. Periosteum is particularly well attached to bone in areas where muscles, tendons, and ligaments attach to the skeleton. In these areas, collagen bundles (Sharpey's fibers) go down from the periosteum and into the underlying osseous tissue.

The longitudinal growth of the skeleton takes place in the growth zones (the physes) (Figure 1.8). The growth zones are subject to injuries: 15% of all acute fractures

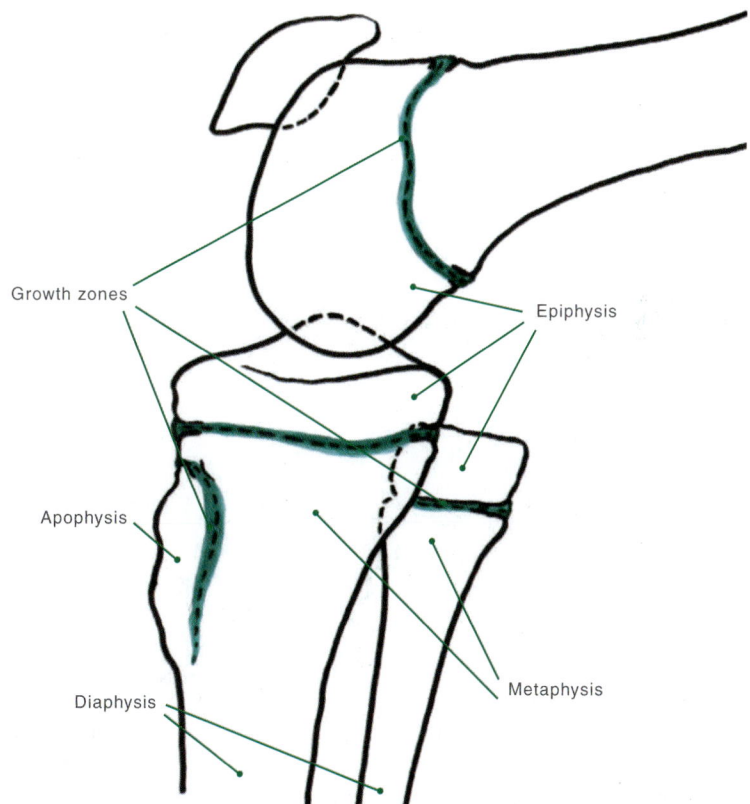

Figure 1.8 Growth zones in the tubular bones, example from the tibia, fibula, and femur. The physes are vulnerable to injuries during the growth spurt. (© Medical Illustrator Tommy Bolic, Sweden.)

Growth zones

Epiphysis

Apophysis

Metaphysis

Diaphysis

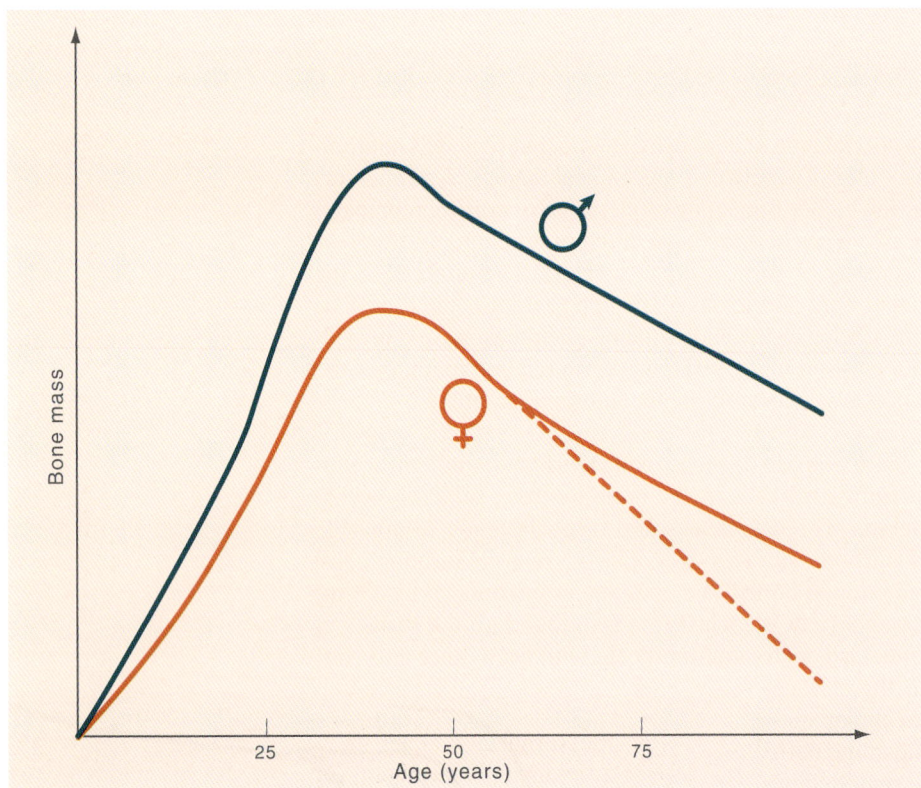

Figure 1.9 The development of bone mass as a function of age and sex. The dotted line shows the potential development in osteoporotic women after menopause. (Reproduced with permission from the Norwegian Sports Medicine Association.)

in children involve the physes. In addition, the apophyses are subject to overuse injuries during the growth spurt. The combination of rapid development of muscle strength and a large amount of training leads to physeal overuse injury (e.g., the quadriceps muscle, as in Osgood–Schlatter disease, and the triceps surae muscle, as in Sever disease insertions). Bone mass also increases during the growth period and peaks when the athlete is in her third decade (Figure 1.9). After a period where bone mineral remains stable at best, density decreases quite rapidly (1% per year or more) in most women after menopause.

Bone has characteristic stress–deformation curves (Figure 1.10). Initially, in the elastic zone, there is a linear relationship between load and deformation. If the load increases into the plastic deformation zone, even small changes in force will cause greater and greater deformation. Greater loading in the deformation zone results in a complete fracture.

Adaptation to Training

When considering the effect of physical training on bone, it is important to consider both the material property of bone ("bone mass") as well as the geometric properties (bone shape and size). Bone is a structure (like a building or a bridge) and its strength depends both on the material it is made of (bone mass in this case) and the shape in which the material is arranged (geometry). That's why there is an emphasis on estimating the effect of physical training on bone strength—the load that a bone can withstand before fracturing. Bone strength includes aspects of both bone mass and bone geometry.

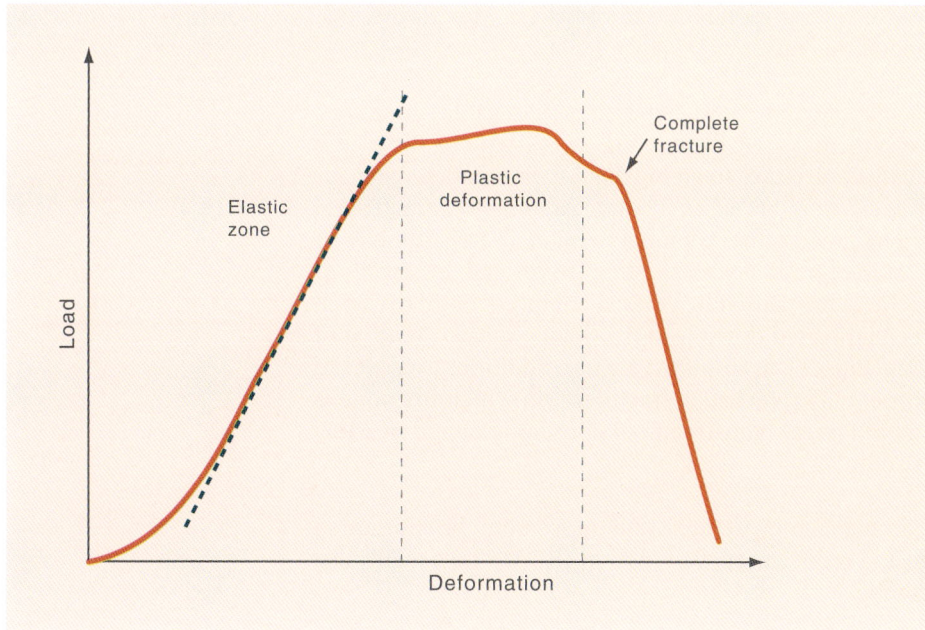

Figure 1.10 Acute stress–deformation curve for bone. (Reproduced with permission from the Norwegian Sports Medicine Association.)

Physical training increases bone mass (which can be measured as bone mineral density using a DXA scanner) and bone geometry (measured using a peripheral CT scanner). Training-related increases in bone strength are site specific to loaded bone. Jumping will not improve upper limb bone strength, tennis increases strength of the dominant arm only. Importantly, not all types of activity increase bone mass. Bone responds to fast signals–rapid deformation–not to slow, gentle loads.

Athletes in power and jumping sports, such as weight lifters, gymnasts, volleyball players, and squash players, have greater bone strength, all other things being equal (e.g., size and sex), than other athletes. Normal weight runners are in the midrange of athletes for bone strength; cyclists and swimmers have no higher bone mineral density than control groups. This pattern emphasizes the need for impact loading to promote bone strength.

With respect to the trajectory of change in bone strength over time, bone responds maximally to physical activity during the growing years. In just two peripubertal years (age 10–12 approximately in girls and 11–13 in boys), the individual can accumulate 25% of adult bone mass.

During the adult years (20s to 40s) intense training leads to preservation of bone strength–bone mass is retained and structural (shape) changes occur to maintain bone strength. In the postmenopausal years, strength training can largely prevent the natural decline in bone strength that occurs in nonexercising women. Thus, compared with women who do not exercise, older exercising women have a *relative* net benefit in bone strength because they avoid the loss that is "physiological" in their nonexercising counterparts.

Fractures

Fractures can be classified in various ways, but the most important difference is between acute fractures and stress fractures. Acute fractures are caused by trauma that exceeds the tissues' ability for tolerance, direct trauma (e.g., a kick to the leg), or indirect trauma (e.g., twisting of the lower leg) (Figure 1.11).

Acute fractures can be broadly classified as transverse fractures, crushing fractures, oblique fractures, and compression fractures, depending on the type of force that caused the fracture, which usually contributes to giving them their characteristic appearance. Transverse fractures are generally caused by direct trauma to a small area, commuted fractures are caused by greater direct trauma to a larger area, oblique or spiral fractures are caused by indirect trauma with twisting (rotational, torsional) of the bone, and compression fractures are caused by vertical compression of the bone (e.g., by the femoral condyle being pressed down into the tibial plateau). Tearing of the tendon or ligament insertion causes avulsion fractures. In addition, two special types of fractures occur in children: (1) "greenstick fractures" (in which the bone is "bent" like a soft twig) and (2) epiphyseal plate fractures (loosening of and possibly a fracture through the growth zone).

Diagnostic signs of fractures are malalignment, abnormal movement, or shortening of an extremity. Pain, swelling, and reduced range of motion (ROM) are usually also present, but are less specific signs.

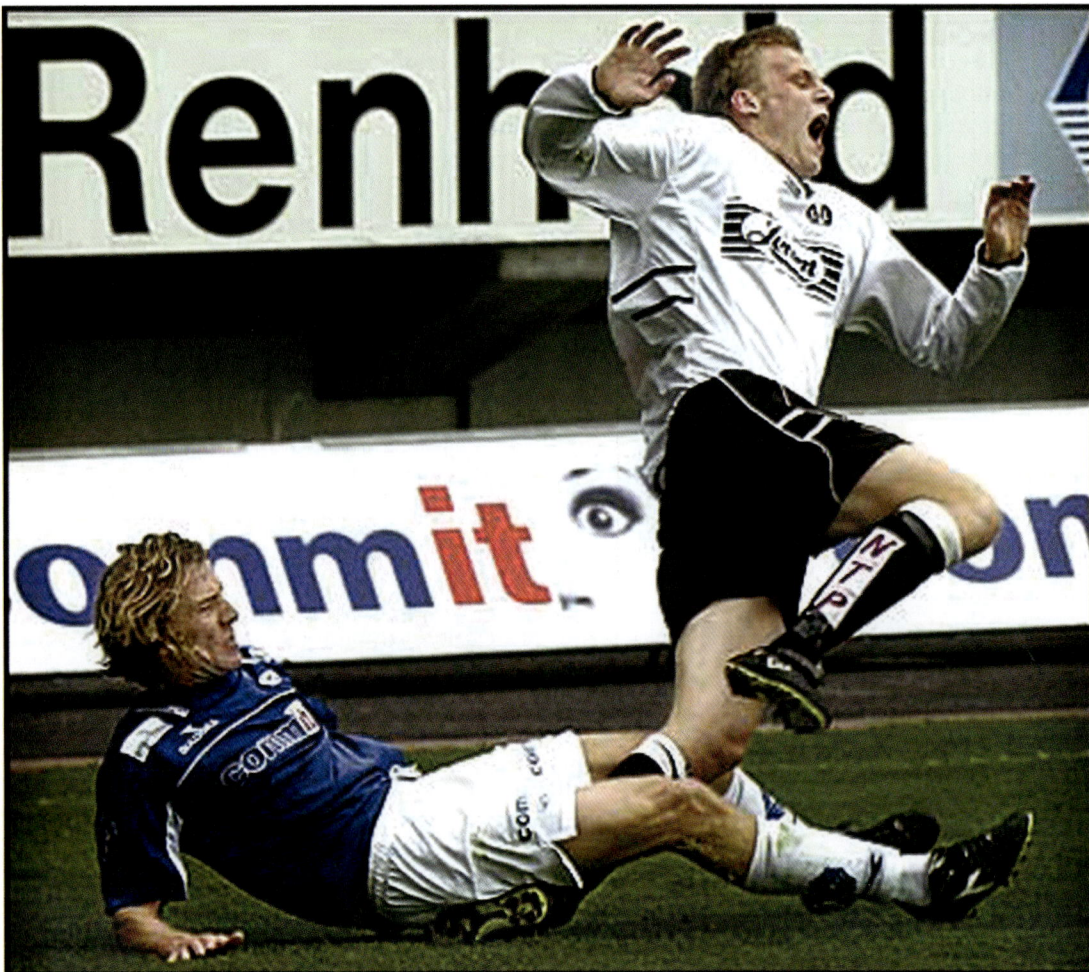

Figure 1.11 Torsional trauma like this can cause a fracture. (© Oslo Sports Trauma Research Center.)

Unlike acute fractures, stress fractures do not necessarily have any specific triggering trauma. In addition, there is a continuum of clinical reactions to loading. As mentioned in the preceding text, bone remodels continuously throughout life. Increased loading results in microinjuries, circulatory injuries, and accelerated remodeling, with increased osteoclast and osteoblast activity. At first, symptoms are absent despite accelerated remodeling. Routine X-rays do not demonstrate any changes, although magnetic resonance imaging (MRI) will demonstrate bone marrow edema, and scintigraphy will demonstrate increased uptake of technetium. If excessive loading continues, mild pain will set in a while after the training session begins, and eventually earlier and earlier into the training session. This is different from pain from soft tissues (such as the tendons), which typically occurs at the beginning of training and usually decreases after warm-up. Continued training will increase the intensity of pain, so that the pain will also be present after training and during other activities such as regular walking. In these cases, both MRI and scintigraphy will usually be positive, whereas plain X-rays often do not show any changes except a subtle periosteal reaction. Positive X-rays will, of course, be seen if there is a complete fracture. The development of stress fractures represents a physiological and clinical continuum from normal remodeling via accelerated remodeling, stress reaction, and stress fractures to complete fractures. Early diagnosis reduces treatment time.

As with other loading injuries, a combination of factors contributes to stress. Key among these are training errors ("too much, too often, and too quickly, and with too little rest"), muscle fatigue (which presumably affects the shock-absorbing ability of the foot when running), and malalignment in the lower extremities, surface, and equipment (particularly footwear). If training is accurately documented, it will usually be seen that the athlete has made significant changes in training during recent weeks. Menstrual and eating disorders can cause reductions in bone mineral density and increase the risk of stress fractures.

Cartilage

Structure and Function

Cartilage consists of the basic elements in connective tissue, cells, and extracellular matrix. There are three types of cartilage—elastic, hyaline, and fibrocartilage—of which hyaline is the most important. Hyaline cartilage consists of several layers characterized by a horizontal organization of cells in the extracellular matrix in the surface layer and a vertical organization in the deeper layers (Figure 1.12).

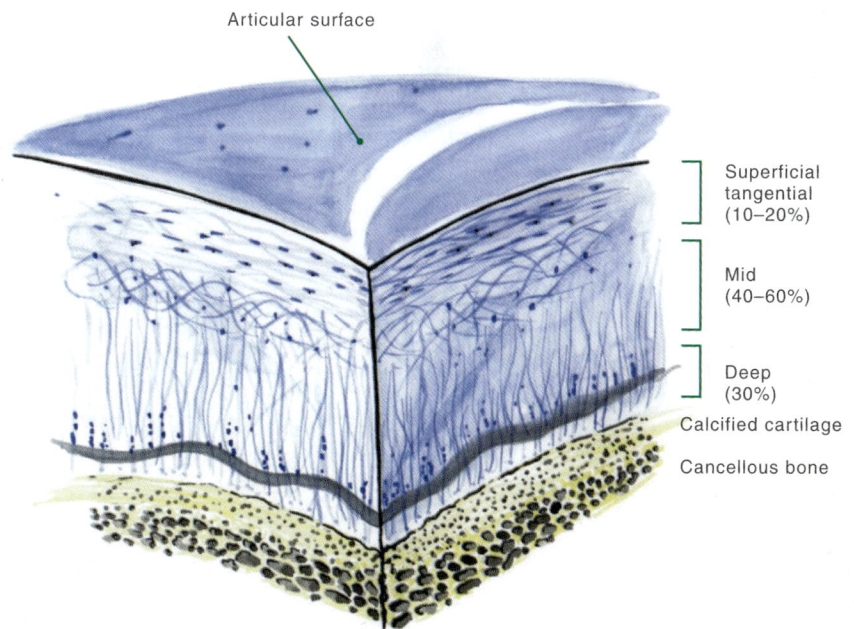

Articular surface

Superficial tangential (10–20%)

Mid (40–60%)

Deep (30%)

Calcified cartilage

Cancellous bone

Figure 1.12 Structure of cartilage. (© Medical Illustrator Tommy Bolic, Sweden.)

The articular surface of most joints is covered by hyaline cartilage that is 1–5 mm thick. Cells constitute less than 10% of the volume of the hyaline cartilage, the remainder consisting of macromolecules

(20%) and water (70%). The macromolecules are primarily collagen fibers and proteoglycan. Cartilage strength is mainly due to collagen–primarily type II, which is organized like a network of long fibrils. The proteoglycans are woven into this network and have two important properties: (1) they bind water and (2) they are negatively charged, so that they repel each other. This causes the cartilage to naturally absorb water and swell up. The amount of proteoglycan and water is greater in younger than in older athletes.

Hyaline cartilage does not have a nerve supply, blood supply, or lymph drainage. The cartilage cells obtain oxygen and nutrients from the surrounding tissue and articular fluid and dispose of waste matter through diffusion. When a joint is loaded so that the cartilage surfaces are pressed against each other, the fluid is pumped out. The cartilage receives its nutrient supply through this process of cyclic loading and unloading. Another key element of joint function is that the filmy synovial fluid between the two hyaline cartilaginous surfaces makes friction very low, as low as wet ice on glass.

To understand the relationship between loading and deformation of hyaline cartilage, it is important to remember that the collagen fibers are organized as a network–horizontally on the surface, more multidirectional in the middle section, and more vertical in the deep layer. When loading begins, the fibers will be organized in a wavy pattern (Figure 1.13). Eventually, the fibers will straighten out, and deformation increases linearly with the increase in load until tearing occurs–initially among individual fibers and later among larger groups of fibers.

Fibrocartilage is strong and flexible; and it is located near joints, tendons, ligaments, and in the intervertebral disks, where it forms a protective surface between the tendons, ligaments, and bone. Therefore, fibrocartilage is primarily found in larger joints, such as the hip, shoulder (glenoid lip), knee (menisci), and wrist (triangular fibrocartilage complex). In the knee, fibrocartilage contributes to improving the articular congruence between the hyaline cartilaginous surfaces and to absorbing shock, whereas in the hip, shoulder, and wrist it contributes to expanding the articular surface, as well, thereby increasing stability. Unlike hyaline cartilage, fibrocartilage can have a blood and a nerve supply. For example, the nucleus fibrosis has a

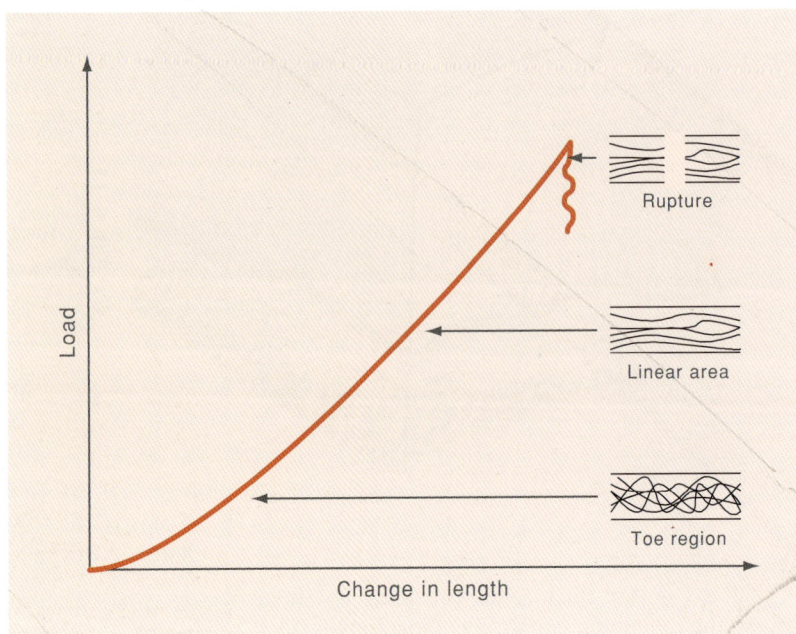

Figure 1.13 The stress–deformation curve for hyaline cartilage shows the relationship between loading and changes in length. (Reproduced with permission from the Norwegian Sports Medicine Association.)

nerve supply in the outer superficial portion, whereas the menisci in the knees have a blood supply in the inner capsular portion.

Adaptation to Training

Active loading of the articular cartilage causes the nutrients to diffuse in and outside of the cartilage. Consequently, regular loading is necessary for normal cartilage function. Cartilage adapts to activity (Figure 1.14). Immobilization, such as in a cast, reduces function. It is also assumed that too much loading reduces biological properties.

Cartilage Injury

In acute injuries, hyaline cartilage can be destroyed through contusion, which causes cracks, or when shearing forces in the joint cause vertical or horizontal rifts. Cartilage injuries occur often in connection with acute joint injuries. Patients with acutely sprained ankles that result in lateral ligament injuries often have macroscopic cartilage injuries. Of patients who have an arthroscopic examination after having sustained an acute knee ligament injury, full-thickness cartilage injuries are common. Some patients have an isolated cartilage injury; others have osteochondral injuries in which the underlying bone is also injured.

Articular cartilage injuries are classified on the basis of the size and depth of the lesion and the cause and accompanying pathology of the injury. The most important is to distinguish between degenerative cartilaginous injuries (osteoarthrosis), where changes are found at several places in the joint, and focal articular cartilage injuries, where localized changes are found in one or two places in the joint. If the patient has osteoarthrosis, hyaline cartilage degeneration, sclerosis of the underlying bone, and the development of ossified cartilage in the outer edges of the joints (osteophytes) occur. Large acute ligament injuries, such as anterior cruciate ligament injuries, increase the risk of secondary osteoarthrosis later on. However, it is not known whether this occurs because the acute injury starts the degenerative processes in

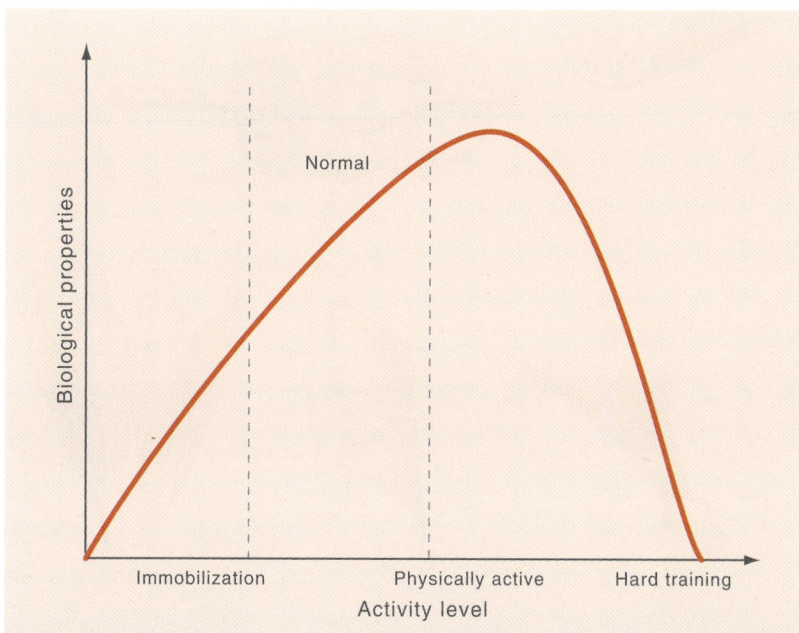

Figure 1.14 Hypothetical relationship between physical loading and the development of biological properties in hyaline cartilage. (Reproduced with permission from the Norwegian Sports Medicine Association.)

the knee joint or because the loading pattern in the knee is changed as a result of increased laxity. The cause of primary osteoarthrosis is still unknown, yet the process may be due to increased loading of a normal joint or to cartilage failure despite normal loading. Even without a recognized injury, it appears that the occurrence of osteoarthrosis is more prevalent in former athletes than in the general public.

The ability of hyaline cartilage to repair is limited after injuries. This is attributed to the lack of blood and nerve supply and the relative lack of cells in the cartilaginous tissue. The inability to regenerate increases the risk that osteoarthrosis will develop after a cartilage injury.

Fibrocartilage is also regularly injured in meniscal injuries and labrum injuries. In most cases, these injuries are acute, but degenerative changes also occur. The blood supply to fibrocartilage varies. In the meniscus of the knee, blood supply is good in the capsular portions ("red meniscus"), where the possibilities for repair are good. However, central portions ("white meniscus") have a less good blood supply and consequently poor potential to repair.

Muscle

Structure and Function

Muscles make up 40–45% of body mass. The structure of the musculature (Figure 1.15) reflects its central function–to generate power. The muscle fibers

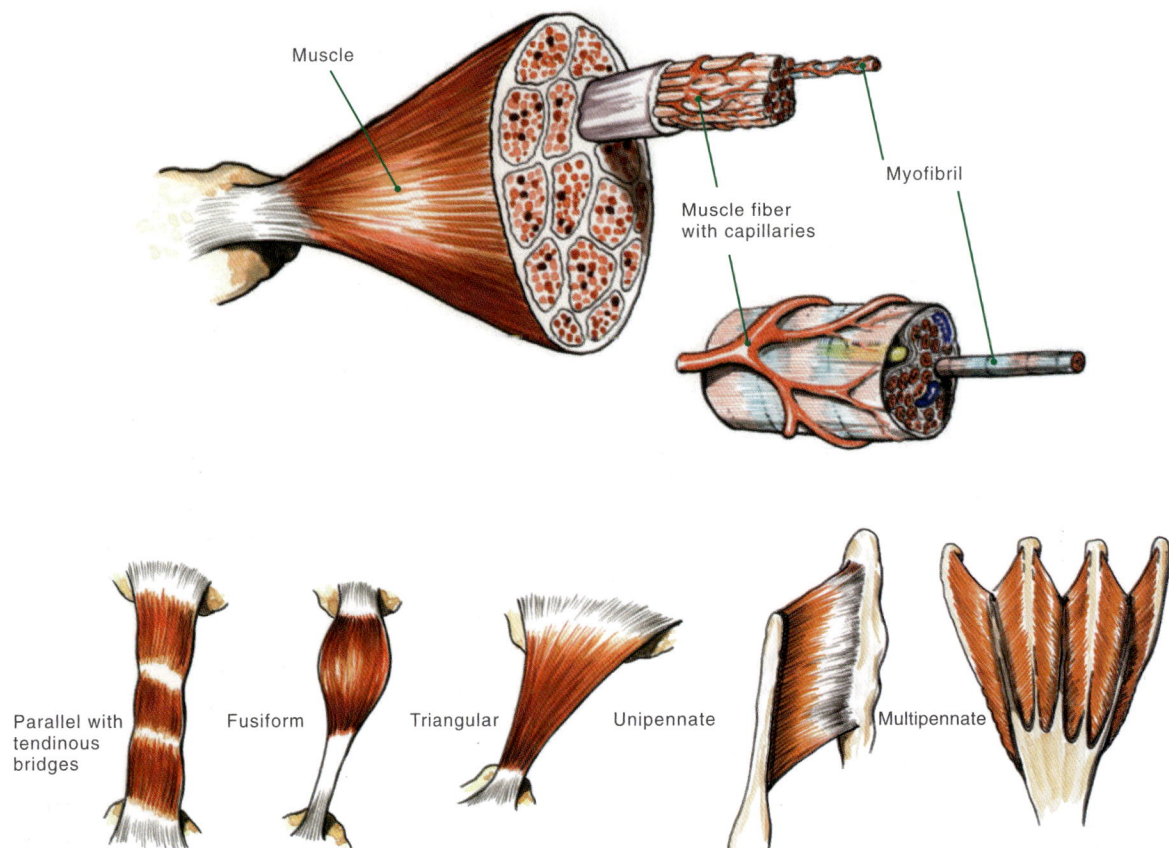

Figure 1.15 Schematic overview of the structure of musculature. (© Medical Illustrator Tommy Bolic, Sweden.)

(muscle cells) are the muscles' central unit, and these can be organized in several ways, such as unipennate, multipennate, or fusiform patterns. Pennate muscles are generally stronger than fusiform muscles, because several muscle fibers can work parallel to each other. However, because they contain shorter fibers, the maximum contraction speed is lower. The striated muscle cell is a fiber with a diameter of 10–100 μm and a length up to 20 cm. The primary elements in the muscle fibers are myofibrils, which are composed of protein filaments (mainly actin and myosin). Capillaries surround the muscle fibers, so that the ability to supply the fibers with oxygen and nutrients is very good.

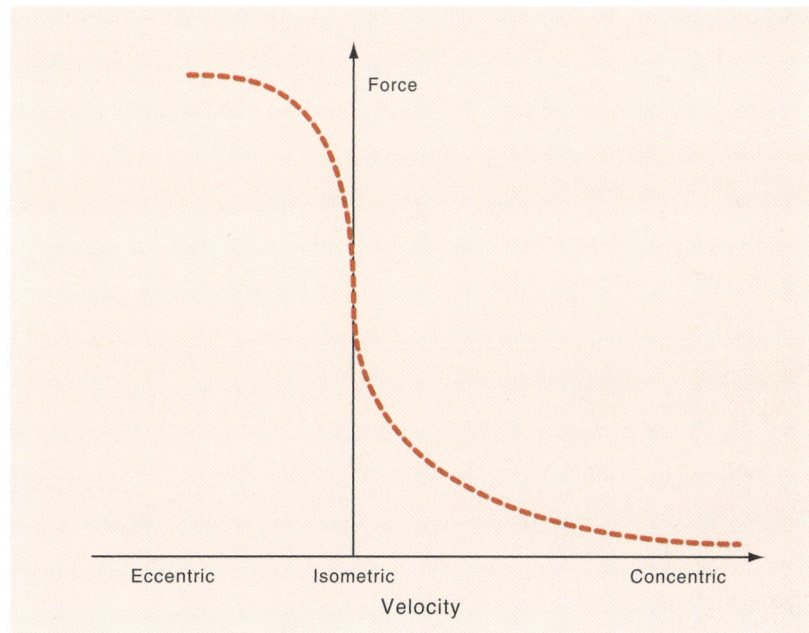

Figure 1.16 The relationship between force and speed in different types of muscular exertion. (Reproduced with permission from the Norwegian Sports Medicine Association.)

Figure 1.17 Force generation in various types of jumps. (Reproduced with permission from the Norwegian Sports Medicine Association.)

The ability to generate force depends on the working conditions, as shown in Figure 1.16. The generation of force without changes in the joint angle is called an "isometric" or "static" muscle action (the length of the muscle is constant, but the tension changes), whereas the muscle contraction where the length changes but tension remains constant is called "isotonic." The generation of power while the muscle is shortened is called "concentric" muscle contraction, whereas the term "eccentric" is used when the muscle is extended while it offers resistance. For concentric muscle action, maximal muscle force is reduced when the speed of contraction increases, whereas in eccentric muscle activity, muscle force increases with increasing speed. This means that the risk of muscle injuries is greater with eccentric than with concentric muscle action.

That working conditions play a decisive role in the generation of force can be illustrated by comparing various types of jumps. Figure 1.17 shows a notable difference between the generation of force against the surface from a squat jump (a strict concentric jump from a 90° knee bend), a countermovement jump (a continuous eccentric–concentric movement), and a drop jump (jumping after dropping down from a height). The greater force generated from a drop jump significantly increases the risk of acute strains, and the risk of overuse injuries is high in sports characterized by this type of muscle action. This is true not only of the muscles but also of other structures, such as tendons, cartilage, and bone.

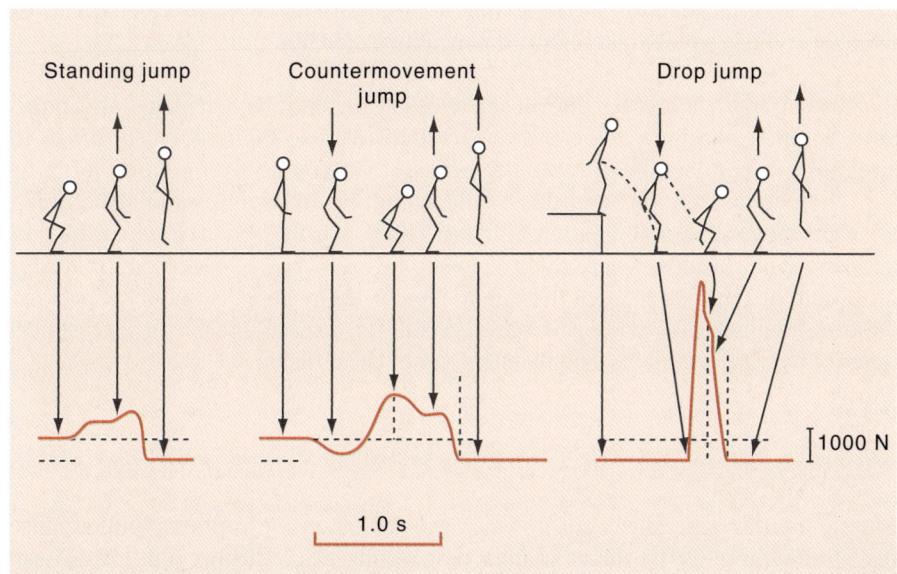

Adaptation to Training

Muscle is the tissue that shows the greatest and most rapid response to training. Muscle volume and strength increase significantly after a short period of specific strength training (Figure 1.18). Two factors contribute to increasing strength: (1) the ability to recruit several muscle fibers at the same time for the contraction (neural factors) and (2) muscle volume (muscular factors). Muscle volume primarily increases as a result of individual muscle fibers increasing their cross-sectional area (hypertrophy), and also by forming new muscle cells (hyperplasia) from stem cells (satellite cells) in the musculature. Neural factors contribute most to the initial strength increase, whereas hypertrophy is primarily responsible for the subsequent strength increase.

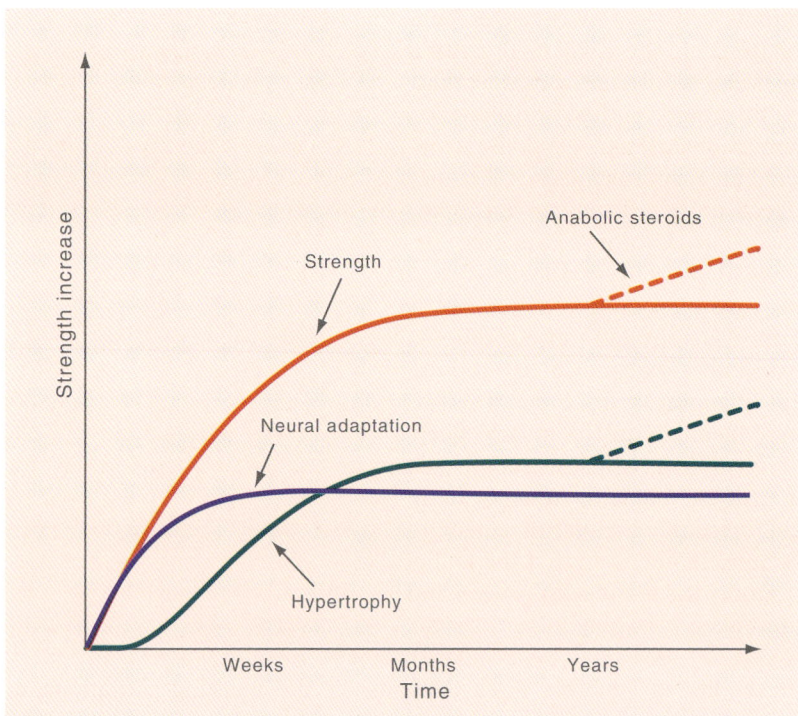

Figure 1.18 Increase in strength as a result of systematic strength training. (Reproduced with permission from the Norwegian Sports Medicine Association.)

The enhancement of endurance capacity of muscles, in turn, involves training-induced increases in the oxidative capacity of the muscles (e.g., increased capillary density and number of mitochondria). Both main types of training, endurance (low-intensity, high volume) and strength (high-intensity, short duration) training, are known to improve the energy status of working muscle, subsequently resulting in the ability to maintain higher muscle force output for longer periods of time. Recent experimental data demonstrate that strength training can also lead to enhanced long-term (>30 min) and short-term (<15 min) endurance capacity in well-trained individuals and elite endurance athletes when high-volume, heavy-resistance strength training protocols are applied. The enhancement in long-term endurance capacity appears to involve training-induced increases in the proportion of type IIA muscle fibers, as well as gains in maximal muscle strength and rapid force characteristics, while also likely involving enhanced neuromuscular function.

Because strength increases after a few weeks but tendons, cartilage, and bone require months to adjust, there is a danger that overuse injuries will occur in these structures in connection with the beginning of systematic strength and jump training. The patellar tendons and the Achilles tendons are examples of structures that are especially vulnerable in adult athletes. This is particularly true when the patient uses anabolic steroids, where there seems to be an increased risk for a total rupture of muscle or tendons (e.g., of the quadriceps or the pectoralis major) is present. In children and adolescents (e.g., Osgood–Schlatter disease and Sever disease), these types of overuse problems usually affect apophyseal disks.

Muscle Injuries

Muscle injuries generally occur in two ways: (1) distension ruptures (pulled muscles, i.e., strains) and (2) by direct trauma that results in contusion ruptures. Muscular lacerations also occur, although they are rare in sport. In addition, the musculature is sometimes injured as a result of unusual and hard training, especially eccentric training. This may cause muscular soreness called delayed onset muscle soreness (DOMS).

Distension ruptures (strains) usually occur close to the myotendinous junction in connection with maximum eccentric muscle action, such as in sprinters. The usual locations are the hamstrings, adductor, and gastrocnemius muscles, but ruptures may affect a large number of muscle groups. The athlete experiences immediate pain from the muscle at the moment of impact, followed by tenderness and reduced contraction strength. The athlete can sometimes feel a bump in the muscle right away. Eventually, this is replaced by swelling due to bleeding.

Contusion ruptures primarily occur in the quadriceps muscles, which are exposed frontally and laterally on the thigh and, therefore, can easily be hit, for example, by an opponent's kneecap. The severity of contusion injuries varies from very mild strain injury like DOMS to "real" strains, shearing type of muscle injuries, in which myofibers and the associated connective tissue structures including blood vessels are ruptured. Muscle injuries involving rupture of blood vessels cause internal bleeding in the musculature. This is because the musculature is well vascularized and the blood flow is usually high when the injury occurs. Therefore, a hematoma will occur almost instantly with this type of injury. Bleeding may be either intramuscular, if there is no injury to the muscle fascia, or intermuscular, if the blood can escape from the muscle compartments through an injured fascia (Figures 11.1 and 11.4). In general, healing time is significantly longer with intramuscular bleeding than it is for intermuscular bleeding.

What distinguishes the healing of injured skeletal muscle as well as the other soft tissues from that of fractured bone is that the skeletal muscle heals by a repair process, whereas the bone heals by a regenerative process. When most of the musculoskeletal tissues are being repaired, they will heal with a scar, which replaces the original tissue, whereas when a bone regenerates, the healing tissue is identical to the tissue that existed there before.

The healing of an injured skeletal muscle follows a fairly constant pattern irrespective of the underlying cause (contusion, strain, or laceration). As described in the preceding text for the soft-tissue injuries in general, three phases have been identified in this process. These are (1) inflammatory (destruction), (2) proliferative (repair), and (3) maturation (remodeling) phases.

In short, the natural course of muscle injury healing takes place as follows. After the initial trauma, the ruptured myofibers contract and a hematoma fills the gap between the myofiber stumps. The injured ends of the myofibers undergo only local necrosis, because the torn sarcolemma is rapidly resealed allowing the rest of the ruptured myofibers to survive. Activated platelets secrete growth factors that function as chemoattractants for the inflammatory cells. Macrophages, having first invaded the injury site from the torn blood vessels, remove the cell debris and secrete growth factors that initiate angiogenesis, that is, blood supply to the injured area and also activate the satellite cells, that is, the regenerative (reserve) stem cells of the muscle tissue. The satellite cells reside between the sarcolemma and the basal lamina of the myofibers and can survive even though the surrounding tissue undergoes necrosis. There are two different populations of satellite cells, *committed* and *stem* satellite cells, with very defined functions: *committed* satellite cells begin to differentiate into myoblasts immediately after injury, whereas *stem* satellite cells begin to proliferate first. After the round of proliferation, *stem* satellite cells contribute one daughter cell to the formation of regenerating myoblasts, at the same time providing new satellite cells by asymmetric cell division for future needs of regeneration. Thus, the regenerating myoblasts arise from both the *committed* and *stem* satellite cells then fuse to form myotubes within a couple of days. The regenerating young myotubes grow in length and size and, finally, mature into myofibers.

Simultaneously with the muscle fiber regeneration, the concomitant production of a connective tissue scar by fibroblasts takes place between the regenerating muscle fibers that try to pierce into connective tissue. Thus, the ends of the regenerating myofibers do not usually reunite, but instead their ends attach to the extracellular matrix of the interposed scar via adhesion molecules at the newly formed myotendinous junctions. Thus, each ruptured myofiber remains divided into two independent fibers bound together by the interposed (small) scar. Finally, the maturation of the regenerated myofibers, retraction and reorganization of the scar tissue, and recovery of the functional capacity of the muscle occur over time during the maturation phase (Figure 1.19).

Tissue injury and bleeding result in an inflammatory reaction with the formation of scar tissue. After this type of injury, there is little muscle tissue regeneration, so that the injured muscle tissue is replaced by fibrous scar tissue without contractile properties. This contributes to the highly increased risk of recurrent injuries, for example, hamstrings strains.

Occasionally, muscle hematomas lead to an unfortunate complication: myositis ossificans (calcification or ossification of the injured tissue). The most common

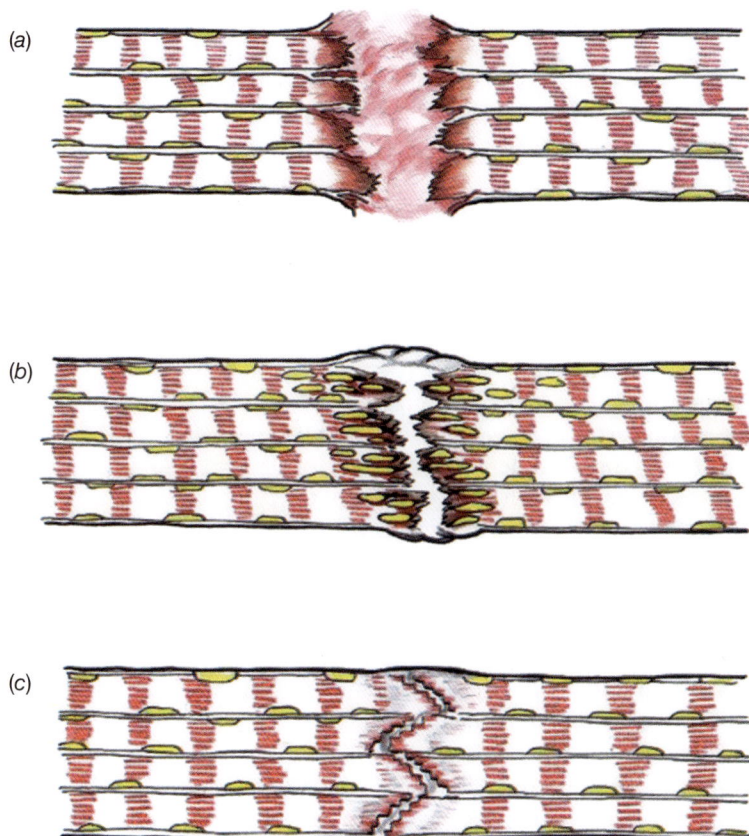

Figure 1.19 In strains not only the myofibers rupture but also their basal lamina as well as mysial sheaths and blood vessels running in the endo- or perimysium are torn (*a*). The ruptured myofibers become necrotized only over a short distance. The injured part of the ruptured myofiber inside the remaining old basal lamina is replaced by the regenerating myofiber, which then begins to penetrate into the connective tissue scar between the stumps of the ruptured myofibers (*b*). The maturation of the regenerating myofibers includes formation of a mature contractile apparatus and attachment of the ends of the regenerated myofibers to the intervening scar by newly formed myotendinous junctions (*c*). The retraction of the scar pulls the ends closer to each other, but they appear to stay separated by a thin layer of connective tissue to which the ends remain attached by newly formed myotendinous junctions. (© Medical Illustrator Tommy Bolic, Sweden.)

location is on the thigh. After quadriceps contusion, it can affect as many as one of five patients. Myositis ossificans is a nonneoplastic proliferation of bone and cartilage within the skeletal muscle at the site of a previous single major trauma or repeated injury or/and hematoma. Being a relatively rare complication of muscle injury, the scientifically valid evidence regarding either the pathogenesis or the most optimal treatment is virtually nonexisting. In sports, myositis ossificans is typically associated with prior sports-related muscle injury (i.e., re-injury to the same location), the incidence being the highest in the high-contact sports in which the use of protective devices is uncommon (e.g., rugby). The most common muscle involved is the quadriceps femoris, where even up to 20% of injuries could lead into myositis ossificans. Increased susceptibility to myositis ossificans has also been described in individuals with hemophilia or other bleeding disorder in conjunction with a soft-tissue injury.

Clinically, myositis ossificans should be suspected if pain and swelling are not clearly subsiding 10–14 days after an injury to a skeletal muscle or if the healing does not seem to progress normally despite the execution of a proper conservative treatment. One should be particularly alert if the symptoms intensify weeks (or months) after the trauma, especially if the site of injury becomes more indurated and the injured extremity displays reduced joint ROM. Although it is sometimes possible to detect the first signs of the ectopic bone in radiographs as early as 18–21 days after the injury, the formation of ectopic bone usually lags behind the symptoms by weeks, and thus, a definite radiographic diagnosis can only be made substantially later, even months after the actual injury. It is important to be aware that the radiographic appearance of the bone mass in the early stage can be confused with osteogenic sarcoma. The conditions can be difficult to distinguish on histology as well.

Due to its rarity, the treatment principles of myositis ossificans are based more on empirical experience than on clinical or experimental evidence than any other type of muscle complaint. The proper first aid of muscle trauma (the prevention of formation of a large hematoma) naturally creates the foundation for the treatment of this complication. However, if the myositis ossificans still occurs despite the best prevention efforts, there is little that can or should be done in the acute phase. Although indomethacin is quite commonly used in orthopedics in preventing heterotopic ossification, it has not been validated for the prevention and/or treatment of myositis ossificans. The surgical excision of the bone mass can be considered at later phases, if the symptoms do not reside despite 12 months of watchful waiting. However, surgery should not be performed until the ectopic bone has fully "matured," which is 12–24 months after the onset of the symptoms, as the excision of immature bone often results in recurrence. Overall, the myositis ossificans could be considered to underscore the importance of proper initial treatment of athletes with muscle injury. Despite the fact that a great majority of muscle injuries heal virtually irrespective of the primary treatment, compromised healing of muscle injury (myositis ossificans) results in a delay in return to sports that is highly comparable–and often even longer–than that associated with the failed treatment of other sports-related major injuries.

Another complication of intramuscular hematomas is compartment syndrome. Bleeding and intracellular and intercellular edema can cause such an increase in pressure that circulation in a muscle compartment is compromised. This affects the muscle primarily on the capillary level, rarely the large vessels. Thus, a good pulse distal to the hematoma does not necessarily exclude the possibility of compartment syndrome. The primary symptom is pain, eventually extreme pain, and the muscle compartment is hard on palpation. Nerve function may be affected so that the patient feels paresthesia distally. If it is untreated, compartment syndrome may result in necrosis of the muscles and major sequelae in the long term.

Muscle lacerations are rare in sport but may occur as a result of cuts from the edge of a skate or a downhill ski. Transverse lacerations cut across the muscle fibers. The wound muscle rupture is repaired as described in the preceding text for contusions and strain, that is, with a fibrous scar tissue without contractile properties. This may have consequences for muscle function.

Muscle stiffness (DOMS) is a troublesome but generally harmless symptom or the mildest type of muscle injury that all active sports people will have experienced at some point. DOMS is commonly a consequence of an overenthusiastic exercise of untrained muscle, which is tolerated while engaged in that activity, but followed by muscle soreness 1–3 days after the exercise. This phenomenon strikes especially if the exercise includes eccentric work, that is, lengthening of contracted muscles like in running downhill or squatting with weights. The symptoms of stiffness, soreness, and tenderness with palpation develop during the first 1–2 days with a peak on days 2 or 3, and they disappear usually with no treatment by days 5–7. The pain is aggravated by passive stretch of the sore muscle and the strength of the muscle is decreased. This is usually associated with a rise in serum creatine kinase (CK), which is usually modest but sometimes up to 20-fold. CK values peak around days 3–6 and usually return to normal during the first week after the eccentric exercise. Inflammatory reaction has been reported in both experimental animals and in humans. The pain in DOMS is mediated by nociceptors, which in DOMS are most likely stimulated by factors (such as bradykinin, prostaglandins, and serotonin) released from the inflammatory cells. Nonsteroidal anti-inflammatory drugs (NSAIDs) have been used to reduce the pain, but the relatively mild inflammation does not actually need any alleviation by treatment with NSAIDs. In humans, DOMS develops after eccentric work excessive for the fitness level of the muscle. Even though DOMS is associated with CK rise, which must indicate some degree of sarcolemmal damage inducing leak of sarcoplasmic proteins, it has been demonstrated that in DOMS usually no frank necrosis of myofibers ensues. The main structural finding has been focal loss of the myofibrillar (sarcomeric) structures.

2 Treating Sports Injuries

Roald Bahr[1], Jill Cook[2], Henning Langberg[3], Domhnall MacAuley[4], Gordon Matheson[5], and Sverre Mæhlum[6]

[1]Norwegian School of Sport Sciences, Oslo, Norway
[2]Monash University, Frankston, VIC, Australia
[3]Bispebjerg Hospital, Copenhagen, Denmark
[4]University of Ulster, Jordanstown, UK
[5]Stanford University, Stanford, CA, USA
[6]Hjelp24 NIMI, Oslo, Norway

Treating Acute Injuries—The PRICE Principle

Acute injury causes local tissue damage with disruption of the blood supply, loss of cellular structure, and possible neurological damage. Damage to even small blood vessels leads to bleeding, which may indeed add to the local tissue damage, but also triggers a clotting cascade and an inflammatory response. The body responds immediately with pain, swelling, and impairment of mobility. The scale of the response varies from the almost imperceptible minor injury to major muscle damage and ligament rupture but the principles are similar.

Most significant acute injuries, whether they affect the muscles, ligaments, tendons, or bone, are characterized by bleeding immediately after the injury. A muscular hematoma can occur as early as 30 seconds after a muscle injury. If the patient sustains an acute ligament rupture and remains untreated, a significant hematoma will be visible within a few minutes.

The goal of treatment for acute soft-tissue injury is to limit immediately internal bleeding as much as possible and prevent or relieve pain, in order to improve conditions for subsequent treatment and healing of the injury. Measures to limit bleeding after an acute injury have traditionally been called ICE therapy, an acronym for *Ice* (cooling), *Compression* (with a pressure bandage), and *Elevation* (of the injured part of the body). This acronym has been expanded to PRICE, with "P" standing for *Protection* and "R" for *Rest*. More recently, a modification suggests substituting *Optimal Loading* for Rest. Rest implies inactivity whereas symptom-limited activity aids recovery rehabilitation. Optimal loading neatly creates a new acronym—POLICE.

It is essential that treatment begins as soon as possible after an injury (Figure 2.1, *a* through *h*). After a preliminary examination to identify the site and nature of the injury, and rule out major dislocations or fractures, treatment should begin. Early cooling may help reduce bleeding and swelling and make later accurate diagnosis easier.

The IOC Manual of Sports Injuries, First Edition. Edited by Roald Bahr.
©2012 International Olympic Committee. Published 2012 by John Wiley & Sons, Ltd.

The PRICE treatment continues after the patient has been transported home or to the hospital for further testing. If treatment continues at home, the patient must be given detailed instructions. Bleeding and plasma exudation will continue for 48 hours after an acute soft-tissue injury occurs. Therefore, to be effective, PRICE treatment must continue for 2 days.

Protection and Rest/Optimal Loading

The goal of protection is to avoid additional injury by reducing the potential for further tissue damage and bleeding. Tissue function is already impaired and more susceptible to further injury. Rest is a relative concept. With significant injury, any immediate activity may stimulate further bleeding. But, after the immediate acute phase, the aim is to begin progressive movement and regain function without tissue damage. Muscle is very vascular and contraction may precipitate further bleeding. Ligaments, such as the ankle or knee ligament are less vascular. Crutches may help reduce weightbearing and the potential for further muscle activity. Early mobilization and accelerated rehabilitation is effective for ankle ligament injury.

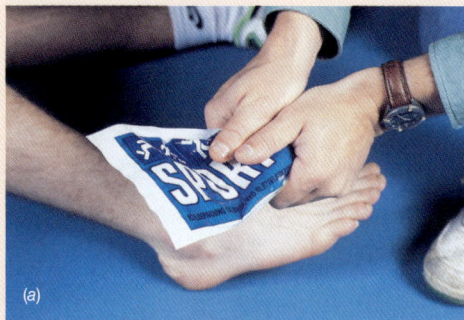

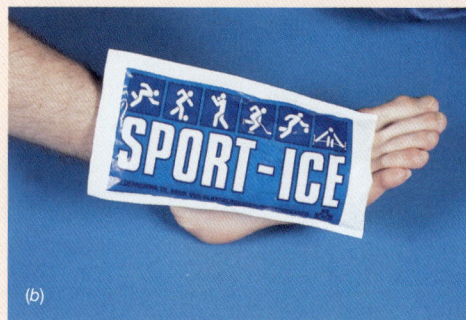

Figure 2.1 Example of PRICE therapy for an acute ankle sprain after inversion trauma, with a suspected lateral ligament injury. The patient must not bear weight on his ankle. Squeeze a hole in the inner bag (a), and place the cold pack over the lateral malleolus (b).

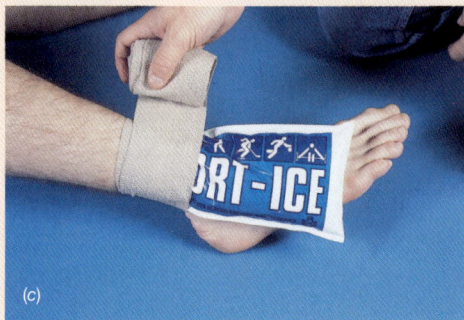

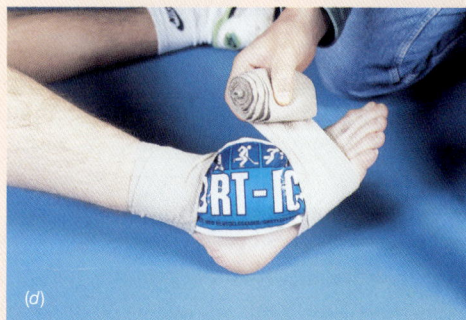

To attach the cold pack, the elastic bandage should be wrapped around the proximal (c) and distal (d) ends of the foot, and then the compression bandage should be applied tightly around the cold pack. When placed properly, the cold pack will augment the compression effect.

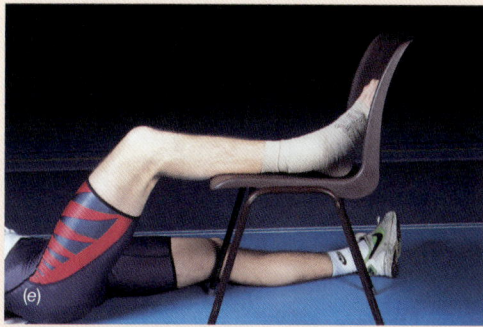

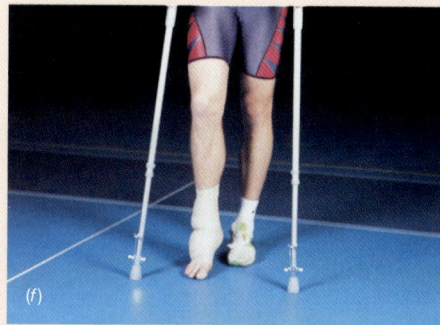

The patient must keep his leg as high above heart level as possible (e) for at least half an hour. The cold effect can be prolonged by shaking the cold pack (the foot) once in a while, to mix the chemicals. If the patient needs to move, he should use crutches and bear absolutely no weight on the injured leg. The cold pack is used to provide maximum compression during transport, even if the effect of the cold treatment has subsided (f).

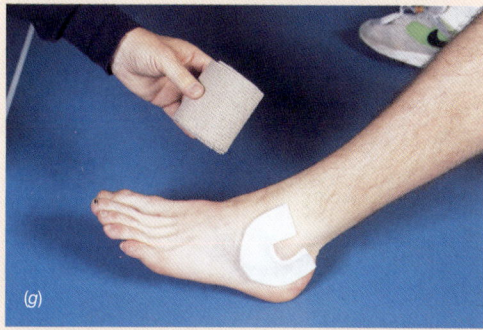

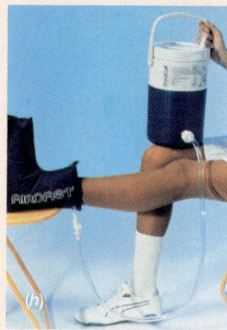

The clinical examination is given after a minimum of 30 minutes of PRICE therapy. At home, the patient continues compression treatment, wearing an elastic bandage continuously for the first 2 days, preferably with a horseshoe-shaped, foam-rubber pad placed around the malleolus (g). Cooling has a good analgesic effect and may be provided without compression by using running cold water from the tap with the plug in. Special equipment for cold treatment (h), available for most joints, can also be used for this purpose. If an ice pack is used, a thin cloth may be placed under the ice to avoid frostbite.

Cold Treatment (Ice)

Cooling has traditionally been used in the management of sports injury. There is little consensus on the mode or duration of cold application and there are many recommended treatments including cold water, sprays, ice (crushed or ice cubes), chemical coolant packs, reusable gel packs, and the cryocuff, which combines compression with cooling. Coolant sprays work by evaporation and, while reducing skin temperature, are unlikely to have an effect in the deeper muscle tissue. The most recent high-quality evidence from systematic reviews recommends intermittent application of ice of 10 minutes (melting iced water at 0°C) for up to 2 hours and this treatment is most effective in the first 48 hours after injury.

The physiological response to ice has not been studied in detail and most of the early work was from animal studies. The potential benefits include limitation of bleeding by vasoconstriction, reduction of swelling, limitation of inflammation, slowing the metabolism of local tissues thus reducing hypoxic damage, a local anesthetic effect and pain reduction, and inhibition of local muscle spasm. If ice is used on the field of play the effects on neuromuscular control could possibly increase the risk of further injury or reinjury.

Ice should be used with caution where there is impaired circulation and should not be used if there is nerve or skin damage. Ice can burn the skin if applied directly, and should not be used if it increases pain.

Compression Treatment

Compression is an integral part of soft-tissue injury management. Empirical evidence and experience supports its use although there are few clinical trials. By increasing resistance, local compression reduces blood extravasation following trauma, and in the absence of major blood loss can reduce bleeding and swelling. Much of the rationale for compression is extrapolated from research relating to deep venous thrombosis (DVT) prophylaxis and lymphedema management and there is little original research. Eccentric exercise producing delayed-onset muscle soreness (DOMS) is often used in experimental work as a proxy for soft-tissue injury. One of the few clinical trials in this area showed that compression reduced elevation of creatine kinase following the eccentric exercise and prevented loss of motion, decreased perceived soreness, reduced swelling, and promoted recovery of force production. It is difficult to apply compression to dynamic joints but, more recently, specially designed compression cuffs that mould to the shape of a joint have become available. In the past, compression was often applied using a cylindrical elastic compression bandage that did not conform to the shape of the injured joint or limb with uneven compression pressures; the most extreme example is the tubular bandage applied to the 90° ankle joint.

Compression treatment may be the most important measure in limiting the development of hematoma. Diastolic pressure in an extremity at rest is about 40–70 mmHg. If compression increases blood pressure under the bandage to about 85 mmHg, it reduces the blood supply by about 95% within a few seconds. After warm-up an athlete has a blood pressure of about 80 mmHg in the vastus lateralis muscle, but with a tight elastic bandage, blood flow under the bandage may be 0–10% of normal. Reduced blood flow increases linearly with pressure underneath the bandage, so that if the elastic bandage is loosely fit, the blood flow is reduced only by about 60%. Applying a firm pad underneath the compression bandage can increase local pressure over the injury site. An ice bag works in the same manner (see Figure 2.1).

Elevation

Elevation is based on the principle that confounding the gravitational effect may reduce blood flow and swelling. Ideally, it should be combined with compression. Elevation inevitably requires immobility and is only useful in distal joints.

Early rehabilitation has become increasingly important in recovery from soft-tissue injury and there is less emphasis on rest. Progressive mechanical loading is more likely to restore the strength and morphological characteristics of collagenous tissue. Indeed, early mobilization with accelerated rehabilitation is very effective after acute ankle strain and functional rehabilitation of an ankle sprain, which involves early weightbearing usually with an external support, is better than cast immobilization for most types of sprain severity. Functional rehabilitation encourages recovery–a type of mechanotherapy–whereby mechanical loading prompts cellular responses that promote tissue structural change. The challenge is in finding the balance between loading and unloading during tissue healing. Optimal Loading means early activity to promote early recovery.

Treating Overuse Injuries—Changing the Loading Pattern

Overuse injuries account for approximately 30–50% of all injuries in sport. Athletes are particularly vulnerable in endurance sports, where they undertake huge training loads (with respect to frequency, duration, and intensity), and where training may be repetitive (as in long-distance running, cycling, and cross-country skiing). Overuse injury is also a problem in technical sports and team sports, where the same movement is repeated numerous times in training and competition (e.g., tennis, golf, javelin, baseball, volleyball). Repetitive movement may, it has been argued, lead to local tissue overload, and possibly to microrupture. This microdamage requires time to heal but without sufficient time for recovery, injury progresses. The normal adaptive response, which would lead to tissue strengthening, does not occur and there is progressive tissue damage with pain and impaired function.

In overuse injury, unlike acute injury, there is no well-defined traumatic event. The precipitating factor is often an acute overload–a rapid increase in training load (volume or intensity). Treatment is not just about managing the injury but it is essential to address the risk factors that contributed to the development of the injury. These risk factors can categorized as internal or external factors (also see Chapter 3). A precise understanding of these factors, how they interact, and their relative contribution to the development of the injury allows the athlete and coach to understand what caused the problem, modify training, and eliminate them in the future (Figure 2.2). Because the injury is the result of overuse, the loading pattern must be altered for treatment to succeed.

Once the internal and external factors are successfully modified, the cause of the overuse is removed and, in many cases, the tissue recovers simply because these trigger factors are altered (Figure 2.2). In other cases, however, it is also necessary to treat the injury. This treatment may include medication or by aiding the healing process by passive or active modalities. The aim is to enable the athlete to return to the previous activity level.

External Risk Factors

External risk factors may include a variety of factors, for example, improper training, new equipment, cold weather, and a slippery or hard surface. A thorough training history may reveal problems in the training load such as "too much," "too often," "too soon," or with "too little rest." In taking a training history, the objective is to record precise details of training and, in particular, to identify any recent changes in the training routine such as an increase in the intensity, frequency, or duration that add to the overall training load. With overuse, an athlete may have increased the volume or intensity of training too quickly. These principles apply to both elite and recreational athletes.

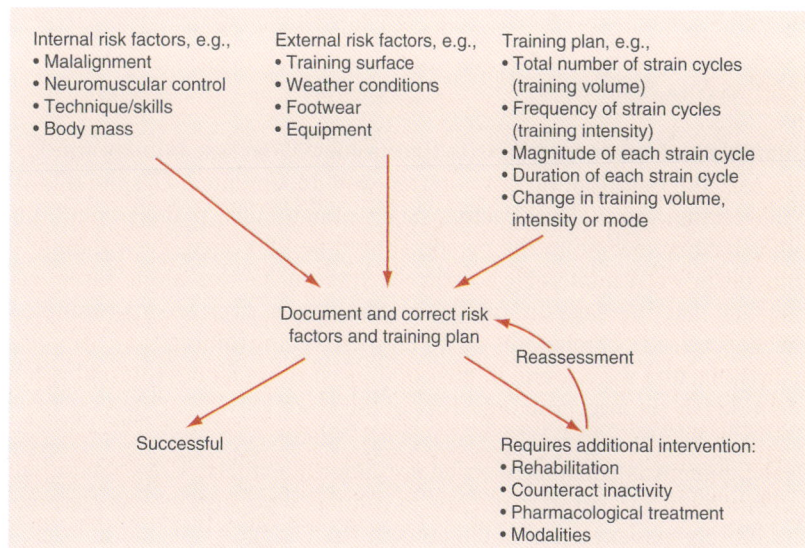

Internal risk factors, e.g.,
• Malalignment
• Neuromuscular control
• Technique/skills
• Body mass

External risk factors, e.g.,
• Training surface
• Weather conditions
• Footwear
• Equipment

Training plan, e.g.,
• Total number of strain cycles (training volume)
• Frequency of strain cycles (training intensity)
• Magnitude of each strain cycle
• Duration of each strain cycle
• Change in training volume, intensity or mode

Document and correct risk factors and training plan

Reassessment

Successful

Requires additional intervention:
• Rehabilitation
• Counteract inactivity
• Pharmacological treatment
• Modalities

Figure 2.2 Treatment strategy for overuse injuries.

People are particularly vulnerable when starting fitness training. If they have not been involved in fitness training before, they often start at too high a level and progress too quickly.

Many experienced athletes train extremely hard and are continually on the verge of overuse. For such elite athletes it is crucial to maintain the correct balance, training sufficiently to optimize performance yet with sufficient variation to allow recovery. Occasionally this goes wrong, leading to overuse. Times when elite athletes are particularly vulnerable include: when athletes intensify their training after a vacation, an illness, an injury, or a pause in training. Constant adjustments are needed.

Injuries are not always caused by increases in training volume but may result from a change in the loading pattern, for example, when new training drills are introduced or when the athlete changes his or her technique. There may be a change in the environment or type of training, for example, when a cross-country skier switches from training in the gym or on roller skis to poling on snow, or when a tennis player shifts from one type of court surface to another.

Factors other than the training itself may increase the training load. Equipment not properly adjusted and fitted to the specific training may alter the loading pattern that, alone or in combination with other factors, may trigger overuse. Changes in equipment such as footwear in patients with injuries to the lower extremities, rackets, golf clubs, skis, bicycles, and oars may also contribute to the development of injuries. For example, the load on a tennis player's elbow is highly dependent on the thickness of the handle, on the size of the racket, and on how tight the strings are. Similarly, changing the size of the golf club grip or oar handle changes load.

Climate and surface are other factors that may trigger injury. Runners, for example, whether they are sprinters or long-distance runners, experience more muscle and tendon problems in cold climates than in warm climates. Volleyball and basketball players sustain overuse injuries to their knees more easily playing and jumping on hard floors than on softer floors. Runners who introduce hill-climbs may also need to change their running style and reduce the training volume to avoid injuries.

Internal Risk Factors

Internal risk factors contribute to the etiology of overuse injuries although their relative role and contribution has not been well documented. Despite this, it is generally believed that internal risk factors such as anatomical malalignment, poor skills, or other factors specific to the person should be identified, even though they may be difficult or even impossible to correct. Internal factors alone rarely cause overuse but they may increase the risk of specific tissues overuse, for example, anatomical malalignment in combination with an increase in training load. In one study, internal risk factors were found in 40% of injured runners, but internal risk factors were identified as the trigger in only 10% of the cases.

Malalignment is considered to be an important internal risk factor. Although malalignment occurs more frequently in runners who sustain overuse injuries, there is little direct evidence that malalignment itself triggers specific injuries. However, it may prevent optimal load distribution and thus overload specific structures or tissues leading to injury. Knowing that the long-distance runner takes about 5000 steps per hour makes it easy to understand how even minor malalignment may cause cumulative abnormal loading of individual structures. A varus position in the knee (Figure 13.11) should, in theory, lead to increased compression forces on the medial structures in the knee, for example, the medial meniscus, and increased distension forces on the lateral side of the ankles and knees, whereas a valgus position (Figure 13.10) should result in the opposite loading pattern.

To assess alignment, the athlete should be examined both at rest and during loading. High-speed camera recording may be required to uncover alignment during activity, for example, to observe running style. However, it is important take into account the malalignment relative to the load. The same degree of malalignment may be of minor importance to a person who runs a few miles for fitness purposes, but apply a significant cumulative load on the tissue of a marathon runner who runs 150–200 km per week.

Poor muscle strength or relative muscle balance around a joint may contribute to the development of injury. Some athletes, for example, have weak hamstring muscles ("H," measured during eccentric contraction) relative to the strength of the quadriceps muscles ("Q," measured during concentric contraction), referred to as a low H/Q ratio. This may cause asymmetric loading of the knee or in the muscles close to the knee, a pattern that predisposes to injury. This may occur in an athlete who was previously injured where, with suboptimal rehabilitation, muscle imbalance persists–the patient may have a deviant movement pattern and potentially develop an overuse injury. Inadequate rehabilitation of previous injuries is probably one of the most important risk factors for the development of new injury. A history of previous injury as part of the routine physical examination or periodic health examination may guide interventions to prevent new injury.

Athletes with particularly good strength or range of movement, or who have rapidly increased their strength or range of movement, may also be at risk of overuse injury. If a talented javelin thrower rapidly increases their throwing distance, or a high jumper their jumping height after a specific strength-training program, the muscles will adapt quickly. Cartilage, tendons, and ligaments adapt more slowly and are more at risk of injury. If a highly skilled long jumper can develop very high forces during the push-off phase, they are more exposed to overuse injury–due to this innate "neuromuscular" talent–than a person with a slower take-off. In such cases, training should be adjusted to the skills, strengths, and weaknesses of each individual.

Joint mobility and laxity potentially increase the risk of injuries. Poor mobility (hypomobility) may result in overuse injuries. Short, stiff hip flexor muscles, for example, may cause the pelvis to tilt forward when an athlete extends his hip during high-speed running. This increases the load on the lower part of the lumbar region, leading to back pain during or after the activity. Stretching and elongating the hip flexors may improve of the range of movements and reduce back pain. Excessive mobility (hypermobility) may also lead to injury. Some have generalized joint laxity, others are hypermobile in a single joint. The athlete should strengthen the muscles around the joint to reduce the direct stress on the joint.

Many internal factors may cause overuse injuries. Some factors, such as age, are impossible to change. Others, such as poor muscle strength, poor mobility, and being overweight, can be changed. In treating an overuse injury, it is important to correct internal factors.

Prevention of Overuse Injuries

Few high-quality prospective studies describe interventions to prevent overuse injury. The most important risk factor in sports injury, in general, is previous injury. Thus, proper rehabilitation is extremely important in the prevention of new injuries.

The rehabilitation of sports injuries will be dealt with in each of the Chapters 4 through 15.

From a practical point of view the most important factor in preventing overuse injury is to correct training errors. The general rules include the following:

- Only increase distance, intensity, surface, new equipment, or types of training one at a time.
- Only increase one aspect of distance, time, or intensity by 10% a week.
- Ensure adequate time for recovery within the training schedule, for example, days off, light days, and cross training.
- Keep a training log and follow the training schedule.
- Monitor heart rate, weight, and sleep quality. An increase in resting heart rate of more than 10% or a sudden change in weight or sleep quality indicates that the body might be stressed and need more recovery time.

Preventing Inactivity

Patients who have an overuse injury often reduce their activity level, either on their own or because they have been told to by health care personnel. An important part of treating any injury is to ensure that the healthy parts of the body are kept in shape to allow the athlete to return to sport as soon as possible after recovery. Immobilized muscle tissue loses approximately 10% of its strength within the first 2 weeks, equivalent to 1% of strength and cross-sectional area of the muscle per day of immobilization. Inactivity affects others tissues too, for example, cartilage and ligaments, so inactivity, particularly complete immobilization, must be avoided.

Muscle atrophy may occur in other situations. Reflex inhibition from pain or joint swelling may cause atrophy. Aerobic muscle fibers (Type I fibers) atrophy quickest, and there may be transition between fiber types. Isometric contractions may help counteract the atrophy but cannot prevent it entirely. Electrical stimulation of the musculature may also reduce atrophy but is primarily reserved for situations where voluntary contractions are not possible.

Articular cartilage (hyaline cartilage) is particularly vulnerable. Histological changes are visible as early as 6 days after immobilization, with reduced proteoglycan synthesis and aggregation. If this continues, it may lead to osteoarthrosis although the point at which this becomes irreversible is unknown. Loading of the joints and physical activity counteracts this deterioration. Early mobilization is key and continuous passive motion is very useful in situations, such as post surgery, where the patient is unable to move the joint on their own. The results seem to be particularly good for small non-weight-bearing joints. When activity is resumed after a period of non-weight bearing, joint loading should begin with caution to avoid tissue overload. Activity that is too intense may further damage the cartilage. Tendons, capsules, and ligaments are also affected by inactivity so that after 8 weeks, 40% of strength, and 30% of stiffness in the tendons is lost.

Principles for Rehabilitation of Sport Injuries

The goal of rehabilitation is to bring the patient back to the desired activity level. Hence, it is necessary to eliminate pain and reestablish range of motion, technique, and coordination, while avoiding the loss of muscle strength and endurance, during the period the athlete cannot train at maximum.

Rehabilitation can be divided into the following three stages:

1. *Acute stage*: lasts a few days to weeks.
2. *Rehabilitation stage*: lasts from weeks to months.
3. *Training stage*: lasts a few weeks to months.

The stages often overlap. What determines when an athlete passes from one stage into another is not the time that has elapsed but the progress the patient has made and the healing of the injury.

Acute Stage

The main goal of the acute stage is to avoid making he injury worse. The athlete often has to reduce or completely stop participating in routine training or competition. The type of injury that the athlete sustains and the sport in which the athlete is involved will determine how long she will have to stay away from sport. For acute injuries, the principles of PRICE therapy (described earlier), often with brief or total immobilization and initial unloading, apply. If the patient has an overuse injury, unloading the injured structure may also be necessary to begin with, even though it often means partial, and in rare cases complete, unloading. Some patients may correct malalignment by using specially adjusted insoles in their running shoes—for example, to provide medial support to correct overpronation. Unloading may also be accomplished by choosing appropriate shoes, by using shock-absorbing soles or heel cups, or possibly by relieving pressure with felt pads or similar devices. Protection against blows or impact can be achieved with the help of specially fitted braces.

When the causes and triggering factors that predispose an athlete to injuries are documented, the athlete will be able to resume all activity that does not contribute to worsening the injury. Then it is necessary to plan a way to eliminate factors that could provoke the symptoms. During this stage, in the cases where the athlete is limited by inflammation or pain, the use of nonsteroidal anti-inflammatory drugs (NSAIDs) or other anti-inflammatory therapy may be called for.

Rehabilitation Stage

During this stage the main goals are to prepare the athlete to train normally and in full. That is, it is necessary to ensure:

• normal range of motion,
• normal strength,
• normal neuromuscular function,
• normal aerobic capacity.

The main tool to determine how much and what types of training to use during rehabilitation is to monitor pain and swelling. The usual rule is to train at a level that does not cause pain. However, this is debatable. Many factors indicate that it is necessary to tolerate some pain, at least as long as pain or swelling does not worsen from one training session to the next. Gradually increasing pain or swelling is a sign that loading for training needs to be reduced and that the patient may need to consider other types of training.

The best way to reestablish normal range of motion is for the patient to use active stretching exercises. This may not succeed at first. If it does not, the patient will need to train passive stretching or stretching with the assistance of equipment or a therapist. Normal range of motion is key, because it is a prerequisite for returning the athlete to normal technique. In addition, reduced range of motion may limit the patient's ability to do strength training. For example, a patient who does not have full extension in her knee may not be able to train her vastus medialis muscle and, consequently, it will not be possible for her to optimize her knee function. Specific stretching of the injured tissue can be completed according to the same principles with frequent light stretching during the early rehabilitation stage and more forceful and longer stretching later in the rehabilitation period.

To maintain general strength and muscular endurance, alternative forms of training are used that do not load the injured area. Examples of this are bicycling, swimming, or running in water (Figure 2.3). Well-performed alternative training will allow the athlete to return to the athletic field sooner. In addition to alternative training, the athlete can engage in the parts of the regular training program that do not load the injured part of the body. For example, a wrestler can train for upper body, abdominal, and back strength, even if he has a knee injury that prevents him from running or training for wrestling. It is often possible for the athlete to train more during this stage than he would have done if he had not been injured.

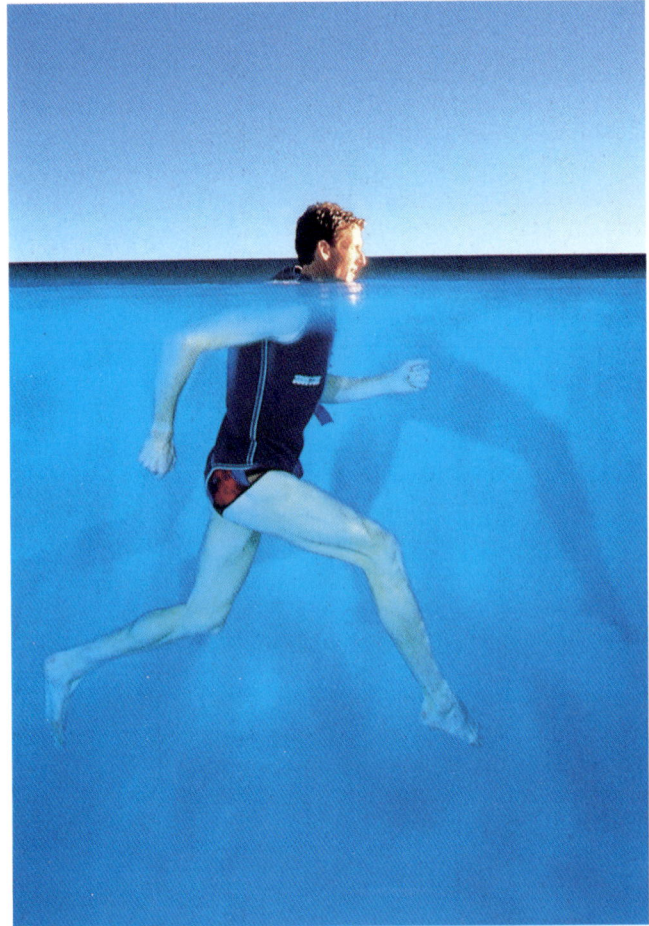

Figure 2.3 Alternative training: running in water while wearing a wet vest.

In addition to alternative training, the athlete must also engage in specific training—that is, training that affects the injured structures. The amount (including intensity, frequency, and duration) of training stimuli will depend on the location of the injury, which tissue is injured, how long the patient has had the injury, and any surgical intervention. Remember that all training is specific. The athlete improves only in what he trains for. When an athlete retrains after an overuse injury, it is necessary to place the greatest emphasis on exercises that train for both the type of strength (concentric, eccentric, or isometric) and for the muscle groups that the athlete requires for his sport. The specific training will be highly repetitive—numerous repetitions of the same movement in several series, several times a day. For example, the athlete may increase the amount of training once a week or every other week, preferably in consultation with a physical therapist. To the extent possible, technique and coordination are monitored and trained parallel to specific training for a particular sport. It is necessary to ensure that an athlete has regained at least 85–90% of his original strength before he is allowed to participate in competition again.

All athletes who must remain completely or partially at rest in connection with an injury will lose endurance. Aerobic capacity needs to be restored for the athlete to return to the level he was at before the injury. It is often necessary to select slightly different types of training, because the injury limits the possibility for customary training. For example, a runner with Achilles tendinosis will not be able to run on the ground, but he or she will often be able to bicycle or to run in water without pain.

Many assume that the rehabilitation is completed when pain is gone; when mobility, strength, and neuromuscular function have been regained; and when lost endurance has been restored. This can be true for nonathletes. The injured body part functions again, and the patient may return to his normal level of activity. This is not necessarily the case for a competitive athlete. The rehabilitation stage has enabled the athlete to train at a nearly normal level, but some work probably still remains before the athlete's ability to perform is back to normal.

Specific exercises to regain normal neuromuscular function are vital to the rehabilitation of patients, whether they have an overuse injury or an acute injury. Painful conditions may result in reflex inhibition. This causes changes in the recruitment pattern of muscles around an injured joint, thereby resulting in a change in technique, which may contribute to maintaining an unfavorable loading pattern. Acute ligament injuries may also result in reduced joint position sense and coordination, which may contribute to the joint being more vulnerable to new injuries. Specific neuromuscular exercises that challenge coordination and the ability to balance, to transfer weight, and to react quickly to changes of position are key elements of training that help an individual avoid new injuries.

Training Stage

The goal of the training stage is to ensure that the athlete regains her normal ability to perform in sport, to tolerate the loading that is unavoidable in competition, and to tolerate normal amounts of training before being allowed to compete again. The training stage is a critical phase for top athletes. A previous injury is the main risk factor for sustaining a new injury, probably because many athletes return to competitive sport before they are completely rehabilitated after previous injuries.

During this stage, it is important for the athlete and the coach to ensure a gradual transition from controlled rehabilitation to exercises that are more and more like the sport itself. The role of the physician and the physical therapist is to ensure that the athlete undergoes practical testing to determine whether he can tolerate the anticipated loading required for competitive activity. This is often difficult, because pressure is only maximal during actual competition. However, the test situation should come as close as possible to emulating a competitive situation. Only after the athlete has completed this type of test, and is mentally prepared to resume competition, should he be allowed to participate again.

An athlete must be highly disciplined, and strong motivation is often required from the athlete, as well as the physician, and physical therapists to achieve the desired result. It is crucial for the athlete to be continuously instructed and, if necessary, to keep a training and pain diary, to record and monitor, his response to training. With injuries that require a prolonged rehabilitation period, health care personnel can be considered more like coaches than caregivers. Some claim that the rehabilitation of overuse injuries is more a matter of instructing than it is of providing treatment.

Methods of Supportive Therapy

Exercises alone can have an effect on inflammation and pain, but a number of adjunct therapies are available that have a more or less well-documented effect, such as medication, heat treatment, cold treatment, and various forms of electrotherapy. Anti-inflammatory and pain-relieving therapy can be important to enable the patient to begin rehabilitation exercises, thus avoiding atrophy, reduced coordination, and reduced muscular endurance and strength. However, anti-inflammatory and pain-relieving therapy is rarely sufficient as the only therapy. Acute injuries usually cause tissue damage that results in bleeding and inflammation. Some patients with overuse injuries experience an acute onset with obvious signs of inflammation; others experience this stage in connection with an acute worsening of the condition. Anti-inflammatory and pain-relieving therapy may be used to minimize inflammation in newly formed, relatively vascular scar tissue after acute injuries, to minimize acute symptoms of inflammation in patients with acute bursitis or paratenonitis, or strictly for the purpose of relieving symptoms of chronic overuse injuries.

Drug Therapy

Pain is almost always a prominent symptom in sport injuries—in both acute and overuse injuries. Pain may be due to chemical irritation of the nerve endings as a result of inflammation of the surrounding tissue or strictly caused by mechanical irritation. Pain is also the prominent symptom of tendinopathies.

Pain can be treated with a number of drugs that have a peripheral analgesic effect, including paracetamol (acetaminophen), acetylsalicylic acid, or other NSAIDs (see Nonsteroidal Anti-inflammatory Drugs), or with analgesics with an effect on the central nervous system such as codeine, dextropropoxyphene, and tramadol. In low doses acetylsalicylic acid has a pain-relieving effect for peripheral pain, in addition to an antipyretic effect, and in high doses it also has an anti-inflammatory effect. However, because acetylsalicylic acid inhibits platelet aggregation and, therefore, may result in an increased bleeding tendency, the drug has limited use for sport injuries. Paracetamol has a pain-relieving effect and is antipyretic, but it does not have an anti-inflammatory effect, and it has no effect on blood platelets. Therefore, paracetamol can be used to relieve pain for acute injuries.

Although pharmacologic agents like NSAIDs, acetaminophen, and topical over-the-counter agents are effective in controlling pain, it should be noted that data regarding their efficacy in expediting healing and time to recovery is less convincing. Also, athletes consume analgesic agents on their own in hopes of alleviating pain and allowing continuation of sports without adequate time for healing, unaware of the potential toxicities of such agents.

A number of different injectable agents have gained popularity lately in sports injury treatment, including autologous blood, platelet-rich plasma (PRP), sclerosants, aprotinin, and various forms of prolotherapy. However, their clinical acceptance in managing tendon and muscle injuries seems to have superseded scientific evidence.

Nonsteroidal anti-inflammatory drugs. Drugs in this class are widely used for treating sport injuries. They are available as tablets, in gel form (for local application), and injections. The preparations have anti-inflammatory, analgesic, and antipyretic properties, and they work by inhibiting the enzyme cyclooxygenase, thus inhibiting the release of prostaglandin, an important mediator in the local inflammatory injuries (Figure 1.6). There is no documentation to indicate that any specific NSAID preparation is more effective or has fewer side effects than others. The choice of a drug seems to be largely dependent on pharmacokinetics. Fast-acting preparations may be preferable for acute injuries.

Cyclooxygenase exists in two isoforms, COX1 (which is expressed in the mucosal membranes of the stomach and kidneys) and COX2 (which is expressed by inflammation). The prostaglandins in the mucosal membranes have a protective effect, and inhibition of these prostaglandins via inhibition of COX1 increases the risk of ulcers. Therefore, NSAIDs that inhibit COX1 as well as COX2 (traditional NSAIDs) increase the risk of gastric ulcers. It must be emphasized that this side effect applies primarily to long-term use. However, it can also occur with short-term use, such as that for acute sport injuries. To avoid this side effect, so-called specific COX2 inhibitors have been developed. These drugs do not inhibit prostaglandin synthesis in the mucosal membranes and therefore, have a lower frequency of gastrointestinal side effects.

NSAID/COX2-inhibitor treatment also seems to contribute to more rapid mobilization of the patient after acute injuries, such as ankle sprains, even though better documentation is desirable. It is also unclear as to whether this is due to their analgesic effect, which allows early mobilization, or if the anti-inflammatory effect is also important. In acute cases, oral treatment should be started as soon as possible using maximal doses, and it should be continued for 4–5 days. For overuse injuries, there is little evidence to indicate that anti-inflammatory treatment provides anything more than temporary relief from symptoms, except possibly for bursitis and tenosynovitis. This is true for oral treatment, local application in gel form, and injections.

It should be noted that NSAIDs should not be used with fractures. Prostaglandins play an important role in bone homeostasis, stimulating both bone resorption through osteoclasts and bone formation through osteoblasts. Numerous animal studies have demonstrated a delay in bone consolidation when NSAIDs are taken, even the selective COX2 inhibitors. Although clinical studies are equivocal for acute bone trauma and after bone surgery, it is recommended to avoid NSAIDs at least during the first weeks after a fracture and in cases of stress fractures.

As COX2 inhibitors have the anti-inflammatory and analgesic properties yet do not inhibit platelet function to the same extent as traditional NSAIDs, some advocate their use with deep muscle injuries. However, there is no clinical evidence to support one class of NSAIDs in favor of the other in muscle injuries. In fact, both classes of NSAIDs may inhibit collagen turnover and muscle regeneration, and therefore, adversely affect the strength of the healing tissue.

Corticosteroids. Since the 1950s, the injection of corticosteroids has been a popular method of treating rheumatoid arthritis. This type of treatment also has a long tradition in sports medicine, even though there is no convincing documentation of a causal effect of the therapy, for both oral and injected corticosteroids. This is primarily because of the lack of placebo-controlled studies. Corticosteroids are usually given in combination with local anesthesia, and the actual cause of the effect is unknown. Despite the lack of satisfactory documentation, injections are often used for overuse injuries, particularly bursitis, synovitis, and peritendinitis.

Cortisone and other corticosteroids block the earliest step in the inflammation cascade (the release of arachidonic acid) and, consequently, have significant effects on the inflammatory process (Figure 1.6). In addition to inhibiting undesired inflammatory effects, corticosteroids can also inhibit and delay the formation and maturation of granulation tissue. In addition, unanticipated effects may occur, such as osteoporosis, weight gain, reduced glucose tolerance, euphoria, local skin atrophy at the site of the injection and an increased risk of infection. The risk of side effects is related primarily to long-term oral treatment, and this type of treatment is rarely indicated for sport injuries. The risk of side effects is considerably lower for single injections or short-term (4–5 days) oral treatment. However, tendon ruptures are a feared side effect from injections into or close to the tendons. Therefore, these types of injections should be avoided.

Autologous blood and platelet-rich plasma injection. Autologous blood and PRP injections are suggested to work through growth factors carried in the blood, acting as humeral mediators to induce a healing cascade and accelerate repair of injured tendons, muscle, and other tissues. Autologous blood is drawn from the patient, and then injected in the injured tissue. PRP is simply a sample of autologous blood with high concentrations of platelets. Firm recommendations on the effectiveness of PRP in the clinical setting to support the healing processes of muscle, tendon, ligament, and cartilage injuries cannot be given and it is recommended to proceed with caution in the use of autologous blood and PRP in athletic injuries.

Sclerosing injections (polidocanol). Based on the hypothesis that the neovascularization and nerve ingrowth observed in tendinopathy are responsible for the pain, ultrasound-guided injection therapy with sclerosing agents such as polidocanol was developed to destroy the vasculoneural ingrowth. Although most studies investigating the effect of sclerosing injections with polidocanol have shown some improvement, the effect is moderate in most patients.

Cold Therapy

Cold treatment is an integrated part of the PRICE therapy for acute injuries, as described earlier. Despite its frequent use the exact physiological responses to therapeutic cooling are not fully known. Also there are very few papers investigating whether cold therapy will enable the athlete to return to play more rapidly. During the acute stage of an injury cold treatment primarily is thought to have a pain-relieving effect. This is accomplished through a slowing of nerve conduction velocity. The effect may last up to 30 min after application.

Later in the course of treatment for acute injuries and for overuse injuries, cold treatment will result in vasoconstriction and thereby reduce the blood flow into the superficial tissue (2–4 cm down). Cold therapy in addition reduces tissue temperature and thus tissue metabolism will decrease due to reduced enzyme function. Therefore, the demand for adenosine triphosphate (ATP) will decrease, which in turn prolongs tissue survival during hypoxia. One theory is that this effect contributes to a reduction in the "secondary injury area" in soft-tissue injuries. In addition, since cold treatment reduces or eliminates the transfer of impulses into peripheral pain fibers, it could also have a favorable effect on muscle spasms.

Cold treatment, therefore, can be used before training to reduce pain and spasms during the early stages of rehabilitation to counteract pain or swelling as a result of training. Cold treatment can be administered in many different ways, such as disposable cold packs, multiuse gel packs, ice or snow packed into a wet cloth, running water, or an ice bath. The optimal cold effect is achieved after 20–30 minutes of treatment; beyond that, the application of cold does not appear to have any additional effect and increases the risk of cold injuries. It is necessary to be especially aware of the danger of cold injuries to the skin or superficial nerves near the joints, such as the ulnar nerve or the peroneal nerve.

Heat Therapy

Heat treatment should be avoided during the acute stage of acute injuries because it increases blood flow. However, it is thought to be a method for improving collagen tissue elasticity, increasing joint mobility, and reducing muscle spasms. However, the scientific rationale behind these treatments is not solid.

In some situations the application of heat minimizes pain. The analgesic effect is assumed to be caused by an increased pain threshold in the peripheral nerve fibers and in the free nerve endings, a positive effect on the muscle spindles, and removal of mediator substances that cause pain. Through a combination of these types of effects, heat treatment suppresses the undesired development of a pain–spasm–pain cycle.

Heat treatment causes peripheral vasodilation and, consequently, increases the local blood flow that may be useful in the later phases of healing. In addition, vein and lymph drainage increases. The supply of oxygen increases, as well as tissue metabolism, and the numbers of leukocytes and phagocytes. An undesired effect of heat treatment may be increased vascular permeability, which causes leakage of intravasal fluid, thereby increasing the tendency for edema.

Heat treatment may be administered in several forms, from hot baths and heat packs to various types of electrotherapy, laser, light, and ultrasound therapy. Because they can be used during training, neoprene and similar heat bandages are useful aids in the rehabilitation and prevention of new injuries.

TREATING SPORTS INJURIES

3 Preventing Sport Injuries

Evert Verhagen[1], Kathrin Steffen[2], Willem Meeuwisse[3], and Roald Bahr[2]

[1]*VU University Medical Center, Amsterdam, The Netherlands*
[2]*Norwegian School of Sport Sciences, Oslo, Norway*
[3]*University of Calgary, Calgary, AB, Canada*

Introduction

A physically active lifestyle and active participation in sport are undoubtedly important for all age groups. The motives for choosing an active lifestyle may vary. These motives include pleasure and well-being, competitiveness, social interaction, and a desire to maintain or improve physical condition and health. However, participation in sport involves the risk of overuse injuries and acute injuries. Although rare, injuries may even result in permanent disability or death. Of course, not all injuries are equally serious, but a disturbing proportion of the "serious" injuries, particularly concussions and anterior cruciate ligament (ACL) injuries, occur in some sports (such as basketball, soccer, team handball, and alpine skiing). Injuries like serious knee injuries result in a long-term absence from work and sport and in an increased risk of early osteoarthritis, which cannot be prevented with our current treatment methods.

For obvious reasons, the focus tends to be on major acute injuries, but the burden of overuse injuries should not escape attention. Although the knowledge and understanding of overuse injuries lags behind compared to acute injuries, overuse injuries represent a significant burden on the athlete, not only in terms of sports time lost, but also, and maybe more importantly, in terms of pain and impaired athletic performance.

Consequently, sport injuries constitute a significant problem for sports, society, and for the affected individuals. Nevertheless, many reports indicate that the health benefits from regular physical activity exceed the risks connected with injuries, even for elite athletes. Studies from Finland show that former national team athletes in endurance and team sports live to an older age, mainly because they have a lower incidence of cancer, lung disease, and heart and vascular disease. Former elite athletes also have a lower risk of hospitalization, although they are at greater risk for musculoskeletal and skeletal problems (primarily osteoarthritis in the knees and hips) than others, in most cases related to injuries sustained during their athletic career.

Although the net health gains from regular physical activity include an increased life expectancy and a lower risk of cardiovascular disease and diabetes, injury prevention in connection with sport and physical activity should be emphasized. This chapter begins with a description of the epidemiology of sport injuries, with an

The IOC Manual of Sports Injuries, First Edition. Edited by Roald Bahr.
©2012 International Olympic Committee. Published 2012 by John Wiley & Sons, Ltd.

emphasis on the occurrence and severity of sport injuries. Next, causes and risk factors are described. Finally, ways to prevent sport injuries are discussed.

One of the main risk factors for injuries is a previous injury of the same type. Measures for avoiding reinjury (secondary prevention) are included in the sections on rehabilitation in Chapters 4–15. While injury prevention measures differ between sports, it is not possible to provide a complete description of all measures for all sports here. Therefore, the principles of prevention are described using examples for the most common types of injuries. For a more in-depth and comprehensive description of prevention opportunities for specific athletic injuries we refer to the "Sports Injury Prevention" handbook that has been published within the same series of IOC Handbooks on Sports Medicine and Science.

Incidence and Severity of Sport Injuries

Athletics, soccer, and ice hockey caused the greatest portion of injuries in the 2008 summer and 2010 winter Olympic Games. Out of all injuries registered during both tournaments, 18% occurred in athletics, 12% in soccer, and 6% in ice hockey (Table 3.1). However, this does not mean that athletes in these sports are at the greatest risk of injury. The explanation is that these disciplines have a large number of participants. A simple measure of injury risk can be given through the percentage of injured athletes in a given discipline. In Table 3.1 one can then see that soccer is the discipline with highest injury risk, followed by field hockey, ice hockey, and team handball, respectively.

	13–17- year-olds	18–24- year-olds	25–64- year-olds	Persons older than 64 years
Soccer	30	36	33	3
Team handball	13	12	11	2
Volleyball	2	3	3	—
Basketball	8	5	1	2
Ball sports (unspecified)	7	6	6	4
Slalom/downhill skiing	5	6	5	1
Cross-country skiing	2	3	20	40
Ski jumping	2	2	4	—
Telemark skiing	3	2	2	1
Other ski sports including snow-boarding	2	1		
Skating	1	1	1	—
Ice hockey	2	2	1	—
Gymnastics/martial arts	8	9	4	9
Track and field/jogging	3	4	6	11
Boating and water sports	2	1	2	3
Horseback riding	3	1	1	1
Other	3	3	6	16
Unspecified	2	2	3	7
Total (%)	100	100	100	100

Table 3.1 Injury distribution at outpatient clinics by sport and sex (n = 244,000). The distribution is based on figures from the Norwegian Public Health Registration at five Norwegian hospitals (1989–1997, Lereim 2000). Totals do not add up to 100 because of rounding off.

However, to compare the risk of injuries between various sports or injury types, the injury rate should ideally be expressed as "incidence" or "prevalence." Incidence is best suited for describing the rate of acute injuries. It can be defined as the number of new injuries within a given time in a given population. It is usually expressed as the number of injuries per 1000 hours of participation. For example, a soccer team with 16 players who train 8 hours a week during a 40-week season will have a combined exposure time of 5120 practice hours. If the team sustains a combined total of 46 injuries during the same period, the incidence is nine injuries per 1000 practice hours (46/5120 × 1000). When two of the sustained injuries are ACL injuries, the incidence of ACL injury is 0.4 per 1000 practice hours (2/5120 × 1000).

Incidence can also be expressed in other ways, such as the number of injuries per 1000 skier days or 1000 runs, which are usually used to describe the incidence of injuries in downhill skiing.

Prevalence is the best way of describing the occurrence of overuse injuries. It can be defined as the percentage of athletes in a given population with an injury at a given time or during a given period. For example, the prevalence is 30% if three out of ten javelin throwers state that they have elbow pain.

Comparing the incidence between different sports or types of injuries presumes that the same definition of injury is used. Usually, only injuries that result in an absence from training or competition are counted. If other injuries that require treatment were included, the incidence would be significantly higher. Limited information is available about some sports, but comparable figures exist for many Olympic sports (Table 3.2). As Table 3.2 shows, for team sports the number of injuries occurring during competition is higher than during training. This is to be expected, because the intensity is higher during competition and because much training time is used for warm-up exercises and technical training, during which the risk of injuries is typically low. The difference in incidence during games versus during training can be substantial, particularly in sports with a high frequency of competition, such as professional ice hockey or basketball.

To fully understand the risk related to participation in sport, one must consider not only the incidence of injuries but also about their severity. The severity of an injury can be described in terms of the type and location of the injury, the type and duration of treatment, absence from sport or work, pain, impaired athletic performance and permanent disability, or direct and indirect costs. For example, the incidence of ankle injuries in volleyball is about the same as for ACL injuries in team handball among women. But because a high risk for future loss of function can be predicted after an ACL injury and a slight risk after an ankle injury, injuries are a greater concern in team handball than in volleyball. The severity of an ACL injury will also be reflected in more comprehensive medical treatment,

Sport	Incidence (number of injuries per 1000 participation hours)	
	In competition	In training
Basketball	2–3	5–6
Soccer	11–35	2–8
Team handball	14	1–2
Ice hockey	29–79	1–3
Volleyball	3–6	1–4

Table 3.2 Incidence of acute injuries during competition and training in selected team sports based on studies of Scandinavian elite sports.

longer absence from sport and work, a greater degree of medical disability, and higher direct and indirect treatment costs. Preventive measures in sports that have a high incidence of serious injuries should therefore be emphasized. Knee injuries have been mentioned, but head and neck injuries may be even more serious.

Causes and Risk Factors

To prevent sport injuries, it is absolutely essential to have a good understanding of the cause(s) of the injuries. Even in cases in which the cause of an injury appears to be very obvious, such as a direct kick on the shin causing a transverse tibial fracture, in reality the cause may be complex. In this example, contributing factors could be leg pads that were too short, a previous subclinical stress fracture in the area, an osteoporotic skeleton (e.g., due to an eating disorder), or simply that the athlete was too tired and did not pay attention toward the end of a tough game.

Because the causes of sport injuries are often complex, more complete models have been developed to describe the multicausal relationships that also take into consideration the chain of events that result in an injury (Figure 3.1). Meeuwisse's multifactorial causal model classifies internal or athlete-related factors as predisposing factors that may be necessary, but are rarely sufficient, to trigger an injury. Examples of internal factors include age, reduced range of motion, previous injuries that reduce neuromuscular function or cause mechanical instability, and osteoporosis. The existence of one or more internal factors may contribute to predisposing an athlete to an injury. External factors affect the athlete from the outside environment. Examples include playing team handball on floors where the friction is too high or too low, playing soccer on an uneven grassy surface, sprint training in cold weather, and running on hard asphalt or with bad shoes. Both internal and external factors are usually separated in time from the moment when the injury occurs and are rarely sufficient to cause injuries alone, but the combination of, and the interaction between, these factors contributes to making the athlete vulnerable to injury.

To be able to both prevent injuries and provide effective treatment advice, the practitioner must understand the causes. This is particularly true of overuse injuries, which often return if the athlete is unable to change his loading pattern.

The inciting event is the last link in the chain that results in an injury, and the athlete can usually describe it quite accurately (e.g., trauma to the lateral side of the knee that results in a medial ligament injury). Because an injury can often be described in simple kinematic terms, there is a danger that the description of the

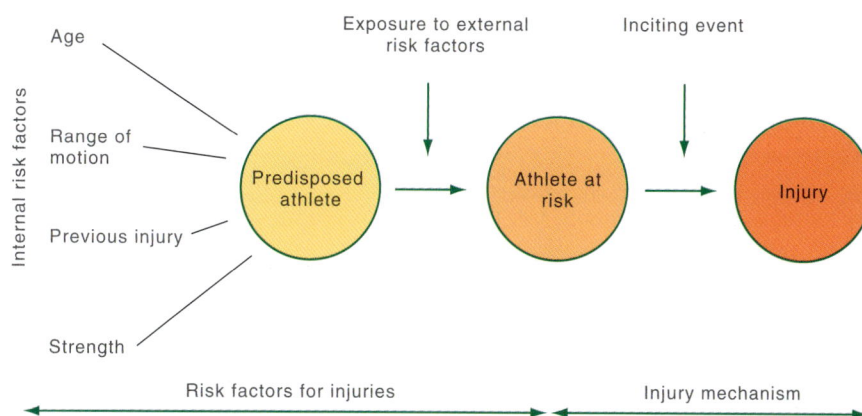

Figure 3.1 Causes of sport injuries. Meeuwisse's dynamic, multifactorial causal model divides the causes into internal and external risk factors and describes the injury mechanism in the inciting event. (Reproduced with permission from the Norwegian Sports Medicine Association.)

injury mechanism may draw attention away from important internal or external risk factors. Even if it is often more difficult, these must also be accurately documented to facilitate successful treatment and prevention of sport injuries. Also, it is important to note that even if the forces or moments acting on a limb or a joint can be described in detail, this is not always sufficient to plan preventive measures. It is necessary to expand the traditional biomechanical approach to describing the inciting event, if the objective is to prevent injuries. A complete description of the mechanisms for a particular injury type in a given sport needs to account for the events leading to the injury situation (playing situation, player and opponent behavior), as well as to include a description of whole body and joint biomechanics at the time of injury. To address the potential for prevention, the information on injury mechanism must be considered in a model that also considers how internal and external risk factors can modify injury risk.

Risk Analysis

It is possible to do a risk analysis to document the parts of the season when athletes are at the greatest risk for sustaining injuries as a result of the training or competitive programs (Figure 3.2). Examples of situations in which risk increases are when athletes switch from one training surface to another (e.g., from grass to gravel) or to new types of training (e.g., at the start of a strength training period). This type of analysis is an important basis for planning preventive measures, particularly for the purpose of avoiding overuse injuries. The analysis is based on the idea that the risk of injuries is greater during transitional periods and that each stage has certain characteristics that may increase risk. The risk profile usually varies from sport to sport. Health care personnel responsible for teams or training groups should do this type of analysis in collaboration with the coaches and athletes and create a plan for relevant preventive measures, based on the risk analysis.

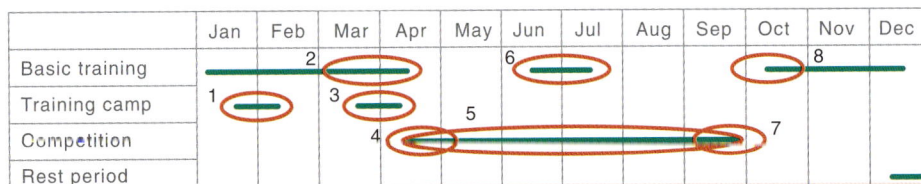

	Jan	Feb	Mar	Apr	May	Jun	Jul	Aug	Sep	Oct	Nov	Dec
Basic training		2				6				8		
Training camp	1		3		5					7		
Competition				4								
Rest period												

1. Change of surface, climate, and running tempo during training camp in Portugal.

2. Transition to greater training loads and high-intensity training, combined with several practice games indoors and on artifi cial turf.

3. Final training camp to polish up on form before beginning the competitive season, including practice games on hard grassy playing fi elds on Cyprus. Competition for a spot on the team increases the intensity during competition and training.

4. Start of the competitive season. A high tempo and packed competitive schedule to which the athlete is unaccustomed. Change of surface to soft grass.

5. High risk of acute injuries during the competitive season, featuring a packed competitive schedule at full intensity.

6. Period of hard basic training, including resistance training to which the athlete is unaccustomed, and more running than normal.

7. The end of the competitive season. Worn out and tired players?

8. Transition to basic training period, with running on gravel.

Figure 3.2 Risk profile. Examples of periods of the season when an increased risk of injuries to a senior-level soccer team exists. Comments concern the risk periods that are circled. (Reproduced with permission from the Norwegian Sports Medicine Association.)

Principles for Preventing Sport Injuries

Ideally, injury prevention measures are developed on the basis of research information about the risk factors and the injury mechanisms in various sports. Because risk factors and injury mechanisms may be extremely different in different sports, it is not possible to describe specific measures for individual sports here. First, Haddon's matrix, a general model that may form the basis for developing preventive measures for various sports, is described. Next, training methods that were developed to prevent some common injury types are described.

Haddon's matrix is an injury prevention model that was developed primarily for motor vehicle accidents but that can be adapted to sport injuries (Table 3.3). The model is two-dimensional. The first dimension divides injury prevention measures into three stages: precrash, crash, and postcrash. When the model is applied to sport, the second dimension can be divided into at least three groups: (1) factors related to the athlete, (2) the equipment, and (3) the environment. Table 3.3 gives examples of how the model can be applied to develop injury prevention measures within various sports. The measures in the model assume good knowledge of the causes, but whereas there is detailed information about the risk factors and injury mechanisms for some sports and types of injuries, the information for other sports and injuries is insufficient.

Measures related to the precrash stage, have been developed to counteract potential injury-causing situations, by preventing accidents altogether. Precrash measures can focus on the athlete; for example, a downhill skier can improve his skiing technique to prevent falls, a soccer player can increase his eccentric hamstring strength to avoid hamstring strains, or a team handball player can develop neuromuscular knee control to prevent landing with the knee in a vulnerable position. Precrash measures related to the surroundings may include changing floor friction (if friction is too high it may result in injuries to the knees and ankles, and if it is too low the athlete may slip and fall) or changing the rules or their enforcement to prevent dangerous play (e.g., penalties for dangerous tackles in ice hockey and soccer). Equipment-related examples of precrash measures may include changing footwear in accordance with the playing surface, for example, shoes should be worn that have cleats with a proper length and style, depending on weather conditions and whether the playing surface is artificial turf or grass.

Measures related to the second stage, the crash stage, have been developed to protect the athlete against injuries if a potentially harmful situation arises. Well-known examples of crash measures from traffic medicine are the use of safety belts and airbags in cars and the wearing of helmets by cyclists. Crash measures for sport injuries place special emphasis on athlete conditioning to train their muscles, ligaments, and

	Precrash	Crash	Postcrash
Athlete	Technique	Training status	Rehabilitation
	Neuromuscular function	Falling techniques	
Surroundings	Floor friction	Safety nets	Emergency medical coverage
	Playing rules		
Equipment	Shoe friction	Tape or brace	First aid equipment
		Ski bindings	Ambulance
		Leg padding	

Table 3.3 Haddon's matrix applied to sport injury prevention: measures effective in preventing sport injuries.

skeleton so that they can tolerate the load resulting from accidents or collisions. Equipment, the area in which most injury prevention measures have been developed, includes release bindings on downhill skis, leg pads for soccer players, helmets for a number of different sports, taping or braces to protect knee and ankle joints, and glasses or visors as eye protection in racket sports and ice hockey.

Postcrash measures focus on reducing the consequences of an injury. These measures deal primarily with the medical treatment sequence, from first-aid measures and equipment to transport to the hospital and rehabilitation of the injury. This is an area in which medical personnel who assume responsibility for acute medical coverage during a sporting event have a special obligation.

General Injury Prevention Measures

Various sports may have widely different injury panoramas, different causes of and risk factors for injuries, and especially different training traditions and requirements for performance. Nevertheless, a few general measures apply to many sports. For a more in-depth and comprehensive description of prevention opportunities for specific injury types we refer to the "Sports Injury Prevention" handbook that has been published within the IOC Handbook on Sports Medicine and Science series.

Warm-up and stretching. Proper warm-up before all training and competition is a prerequisite for good performance and for avoiding injuries. Warm-up should begin with a general exercise at moderate intensity (such as jogging), to increase body temperature, and should be followed by stretching to prepare muscles and joints for maximum exertion. Stretching, including static stretching exercises 10–15 seconds in duration, at least three times for each muscle group, and all central muscle groups for the relevant sport, should be included, at least in explosive sports. Whether stretching is beneficial to prevent injuries in endurance sports, is controversial. This type of stretching (which is for the purpose of preparing the muscle and joint for maximal efforts) should be distinguished from flexibility training (which is for the purpose of increasing the maximum range of motion). Additional specialized exercises adapted to a particular sport should be included to gradually approach the desired intensity.

Preventive programs. A variety of injury- and sport-specific preventive exercise programs exist. Some of these will be discussed later in this chapter. Typically, such programs consist of exercises focusing on core stability, balance, dynamic stabilization, agility and plyometrics, and muscle strength. They are often designed to be used as structured warm-up programs to ensure that all players are exposed to the preventive effects on a regular basis, and studies typically show that they reduce injury risk by approximately 50%. The 11+ program is a good example of a multifaceted preventive program that includes core stability, balance, strength, and running exercises, while emphasizing neuromuscular control as well as hip control and knee alignment that avoids excessive knee valgus during both static and dynamic movements (Figure 3.3). Similar programs exist for other sports such as floorball and team handball, and the same concept can be translated to other sports settings.

Appropriate training progression. One of the most important risk factors for overuse injuries is changing training load too rapidly. However, if an athlete is going to increase his performance, he must increase training loading beyond what he is used to. This may be achieved by increasing the intensity, duration, or frequency of training, or by choosing new types of training. Experience has shown that the risk of injuries is greatest in connection with changing the training program—for

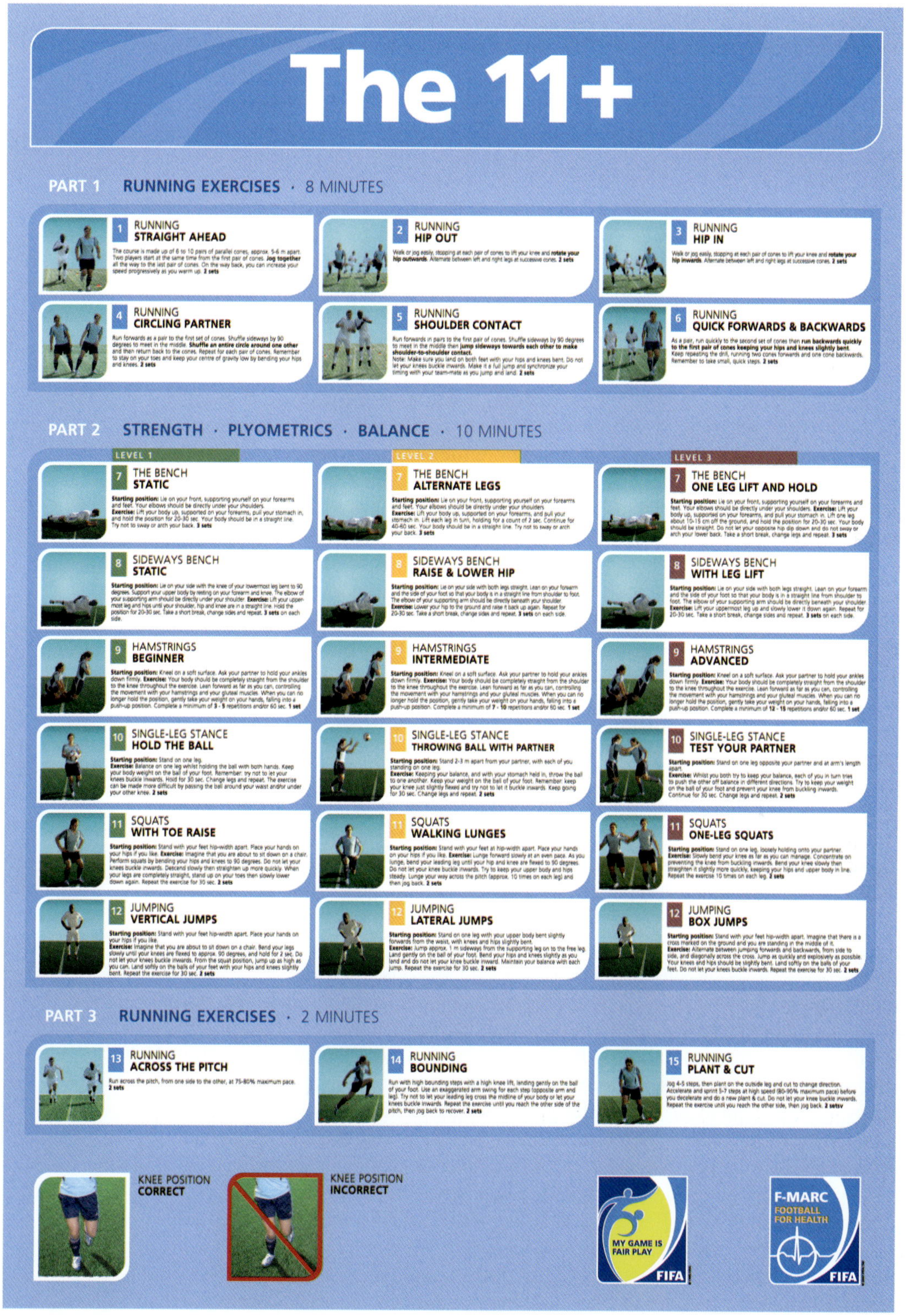

Figure 3.3 The 11+ exercise program used to prevent injury in youth soccer. The 11+ is divided into three parts: it starts off with running exercises (part I), moves on to six exercises with three levels of increasing difficulty to improve strength, balance, muscle control, and core stability (part II), and concludes with further running exercises (part III). The different levels of difficulty increase the program's effectiveness and allow coaches and players to individually adapt the program. The 11+ takes approximately 20 minutes to complete and replaces the usual warm-up before training. Prior to playing a match, only the running exercises (part I and III) are performed, for about 10 minutes. (Reproduced with permission from FIFA/F-MARC.)

example, at training camp, where the total amount of training may reach twice the normal level. Changes in training load should be well planned, and special attention should be paid to the risk of overuse injuries. This is particularly true of teams (such as a soccer team) that are training together, where it may take some athletes more time to adjust to changes in training load than others. Similarly, the practitioner should be aware that a change in surface (e.g., from a soft surface like grass or gravel to a hard field surface) may result in changes in the loading pattern that can lead to injuries.

Protective gear. Protective gear is one of the most well-documented injury prevention measures in sports. When worn by athletes (e.g., glasses, helmets, tooth protectors, mouthguards, braces, and leg or arm padding), it is crucial that it fits properly. Protective gear on the playing field (e.g., the placement of safety nets on a downhill ski trail and padded referee stands in volleyball) must also be closely examined. Playing surfaces need to be evaluated. For example, globs of hand glue on a team handball court may create areas of extremely high friction. A poorly maintained soccer field may have holes or uneven areas that are potentially dangerous. A key job of the team doctor is to ensure that potentially dangerous elements are removed from the competitive field or court and that it is padded in a responsible manner. Worn or damaged protective gear should be replaced.

Fair play. The playing rules in various sports are gradually adjusted to accommodate factors including the development level of the athlete and new equipment. Some changes in playing rules have been made specifically for the purpose of preventing dangerous situations from arising, such as stricter reactions to tackling from behind in soccer and ice hockey, high-sticking and hooking in hockey, and rules against dangerous behavior in a number of sports. In many cases, playing rules may include requirements for wearing safety gear, such as leg padding, visors, or helmets. Enforcement of playing rules is the responsibility of the referees, and safety factors should be a central part of referee training. Nevertheless, it is even more vital for coaches and trainers to be aware of their responsibility and to clearly communicate attitudes toward fair play and respect for the rules of the sport. Fair play also includes being aware of signs of doping among athletes.

Periodic health exams. The IOC has published a number of consensus statements, one of which covers the topic of periodic health examinations. As these consensus documents are based upon the latest scientific and clinical evidence it is recommended to be aware of the most recent available update. Even so, the full consensus document contains specific information on the value and recommendations on the content of periodic health exams for musculoskeletal injury, eating disorders, cardiovascular problems, and so on. At present, the periodic health exam serves other purposes than screening athletes for future health problems. One important goal of a periodic health exam is to ensure that current health problems are managed so the athlete can safely continue or return to play. The periodic health exam also represents an opportunity to screen an athlete for risk of future injury or disease. However, there is limited evidence that a periodic health exam may predict such future outcomes. Nevertheless, for some areas (e.g., injury risk) the exam may closely guide medical overseeing of an athlete. As such the uptake of a regular exam in the medical coverage of an athlete is highly recommended.

Preventing Ankle Injuries

Injury mechanisms and risk factors. Ankle injuries are mainly caused by internal rotation and supination of the ankle when landing in plantar flexion, such as when running or landing on an uneven surface. In team sports such as basketball and volleyball, the injuries often result from one athlete landing on the foot of another, whereas ankle injuries in soccer may be caused by a combination of landing and tackling. The main internal risk factor for ankle injuries is previous injuries, particularly a relatively recent injury. Ankle sprains may result in mechanical instability if the lateral ligaments do not heal, or they may reduce neuromuscular function–that is, the ability to register and correct the position of the foot. Some athletes with previous injuries have both mechanical instability and reduced neuromuscular function. Athletes may be at a higher risk for ankle injuries because of poor basic skills and experiences (beginners) or poor ability to register where teammates and opponents are located on the field. External risk factors may include an uneven surface–which causes numerous ankle injuries in orienteering–or it may be a hard surface, which the athlete is not used to. This may occur, for example, when a soccer player makes the transition from training on grass to training on gravel or when a track and field athlete switches from training on grass and gravel in running shoes to running on a track with spiked shoes.

Preventive measures. Teaching appropriate sports specific basic skills is an important preventive measure. It is crucial to take the athlete's skill level into consideration when introducing risky exercises. There are several sports in which it is worthwhile to take time to do exercises that emphasize basic movement skills, such as lateral movements, takeoffs, and landings, as an addition to more sports-specific training. It is not known how helpful balance exercises, likely with the knee extended, are for improving ankle control to prevent injuries in athletes who have not injured their ankle previously, but for athletes who have had previous ankle injuries and instability problems, neuromuscular training has a significant effect on ankle function and the risk of new injuries. The use of ankle tape or a brace is also a proven effective measure of prevention. Although recent studies do suggest a strong primary preventive effect of braces in basketball, most evidence of external measures points toward an effect primarily for athletes with previous ankle injuries. The reason may be that ankle braces work by stimulating neuromuscular function, not primarily by providing mechanical support. Therefore, there is reason to recommend that athletes with a previous injury and generally reduced neuromuscular function use tape (Figure 3.4a–c) or a brace (Figure 3.5a–b). In any case, ankle support should be used until an appropriate neuromuscular training program is completed.

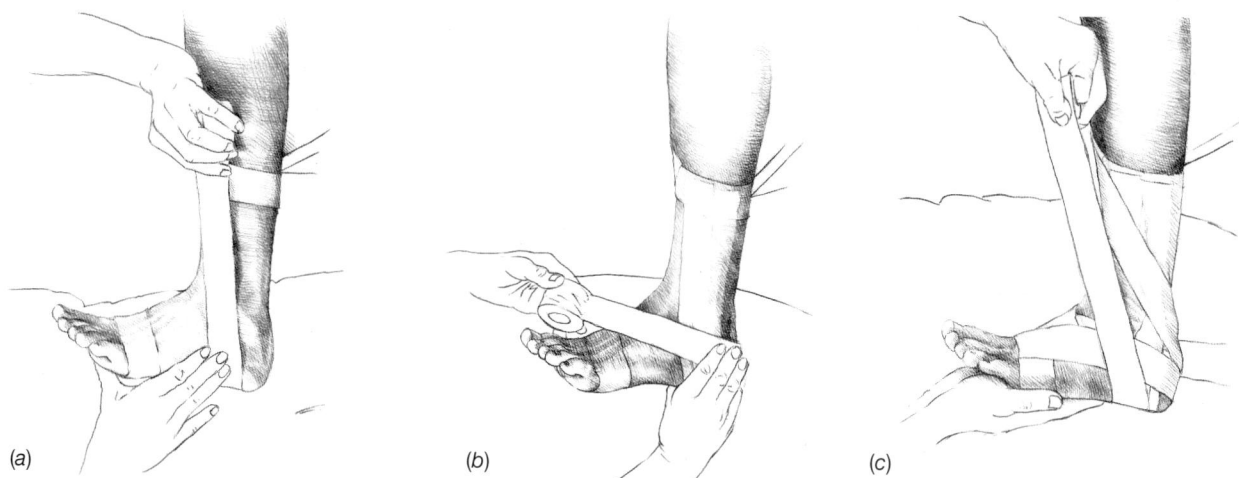

(a) (b) (c)

Figure 3.4 Ankle taping. One of many techniques that can be used. Three alternate turns are made around forefoot (b) and as "stirrups" under the heel (a). Finally, the tape is locked using half (c) or whole figure eights around the heel. (Reproduced with permission from the Norwegian Sports Medicine Association.)

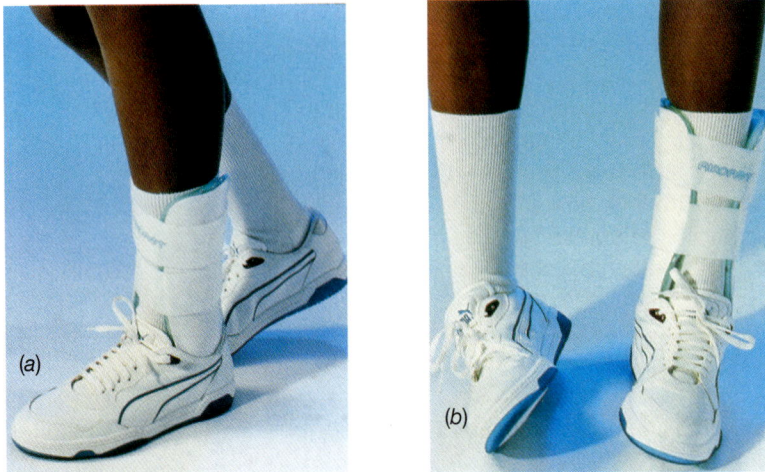

Figure 3.5 Use of the ankle brace. The brace is designed to allow free mobility for plantar/dorsal flexion (*a*) while simultaneously providing support for supination (*b*). (Reproduced with permission from the Norwegian Sports Medicine Association.)

Ankle Program

Athletes with previous ankle injuries should complete a balance training program on a wobble board according to the "10–5–10" rule (i.e., 10 minutes, 5 times a week, for 10 weeks). This type of training may also be useful for preventing injuries in people with "healthy" ankles. In the basic position, the athlete stands on one leg while the other leg is lifted in the air with the knee bent at 90° (Figure 3.6). The arms are crossed in front of the chest, and the goal is primarily to use an "ankle strategy" to maintain balance—that is, to attempt to make all balance correction using the ankle joint only, while using the arms, hips, and knees as little as possible. At first, balancing on the floor may represent an adequate challenge, particularly if the athlete has his/her eyes closed. The difficulty of the exercises can be increased gradually by having the patient stand on an unstable balance mat or a balance board, and ball or partner exercises may be added to make training more challenging and fun.

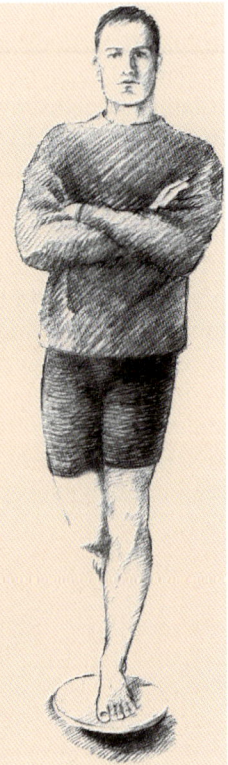

Figure 3.6 Balance exercises—ankle training. The basic position is with the arms crossed over the chest and the knee extended. The goal is to correct balance using the ankle alone. (Reproduced with permission from the Norwegian Sports Medicine Association.)

Preventing Knee Injuries

Injury mechanisms and risk factors. The mechanisms that cause knee injuries are described in detail in Chapter 12, but for the sake of simplicity here they are classified as contact injuries and noncontact injuries. Contact injuries result from collisions with another athlete or an object; noncontact injuries result from landings or cutting maneuvers with the knee in a vulnerable position, where the ligaments, particularly the ACLs, can be torn. The most common situation in which noncontact injuries occur seems to be a powerful stop (with eccentric quadriceps activation) on a nearly extended knee that collapses into a valgus position. However, there is a paucity of evidence linking all potential risk factors to noncontact ACL injuries. With respect to ACL injury risk factors, this type of injury has been proven to be three to five times more common among women than among men in comparable sports. Several theories have been advanced to explain this difference in distribution between the sexes—such as narrower cruciate ligaments, a narrower intercondylar notch, other anatomical differences, hormonal effects on ligaments, poorer neuromuscular control, reduced strength, or inappropriate stopping and landing techniques—but the cause is still unknown. The main external risk factor that has been advanced is the effect of friction between shoes and the surface. Friction that is too high is considered to increase the risk of injuries; the foot can abruptly stop planting to cut, or when landing, causing the knee to twist suddenly.

Preventive measures. Because most injuries occur in a cut & plant or landing situation, it is natural to focus on changing the faking and landing technique. This may be accomplished by teaching the athlete to land on two legs instead of one. Two-legged landings will reduce the forces affecting the knee, thus reducing loading on the ACL. The players can practice faking and landing movements with the knees bent even more. This will distribute the forces that affect the knee over a larger range of motion movement, thus reducing the maximum force that affects the ACL. An individualized program that emphasizes neuromuscular training of the knee joint has been demonstrated to reduce the risk of ACL injuries. This program uses balance exercises to gain better control over, and to make the athlete more aware of, knee positioning during fakes and landings. The goal is to train athletes to avoid having the knees go into valgus. Use of a knee orthosis is known to prevent knee injuries, particularly medial and lateral collateral ligament injuries, especially in contact sports like football. No effect has been proven in noncontact sports in general, or for ACL injuries in particular.

Knee Program

Balance Exercises

The main exercise is a balance exercise that emphasizes knee control, "knee over toe" (Figure 3.7). The goal is primarily to use a "knee strategy" to maintain balance—that is, to attempt to correct balance in the knee joint as much as possible and to minimize the use of arms, hips, and ankles. The exercises are normally done standing on a balance board or on an unstable balance pad, with the knee slightly flexed. Ball or partner exercises may also be included to make the training more challenging and fun. The exercises can be adjusted to the relevant sport, with faking and landing exercises that imitate the requirements of the sport, while always emphasizing knee control. The exercises are well suited for use as part of a warm-up program. During an initial training period of at least 5 weeks, the exercise should be done at least three times per week, training 10–15 minutes each time. Training of these exercises should be maintained once or twice a week throughout the competitive season.

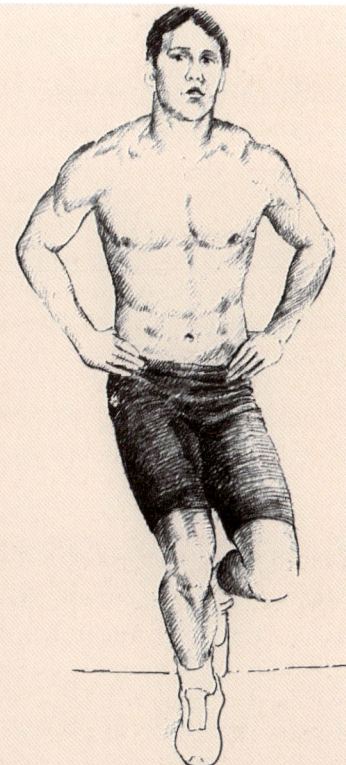

Figure 3.7 Balance exercises—knee control. The basic position is with the hands on the hips and the knee slightly bent. The goal is to make all balance corrections using the knee. (Reproduced with permission from the Norwegian Sports Medicine Association.)

Preventing Hamstring Strain

Injury mechanisms and risk factors. Hamstring muscle ruptures (ruptures of the semi-membranosus, the semitendinosus, and the biceps femoris muscles) occur in the myo-tendinous junction deep within the muscles. The hamstring muscles are two joint muscles that extend the hip joint and flex the knee joint. The injuries usually occur during maximum sprinting, when resisting knee extension, or at foot strike, when the muscle is close to maximum length and eccentric power generation is at its maximum. Hamstring strain is the most common injury among soccer players and sprinters. An important risk factor is poor warm-up. For example, a soccer player may begin training with maximum sprints or shooting at the goal. Two less-well-documented risk factors for hamstring strain are reduced range of motion and poor strength. In some individuals, a previous strain that caused scar tissue to form in the musculature may result in reduced range of motion. If the quadriceps musculature is strong but the hamstring muscles are weak in relation, the risk of hamstring strain is increased.

Preventive measures. The most important step in preventing hamstring strain is to warm up thoroughly—in particular, to stretch out the posterior side of the thigh before maximal sprinting—so that the muscles are prepared for maximum loads. This is especially true if the weather is cold. In cold weather, athletes should be warmly dressed, and perhaps it may not even be advisable to do maximal sprint training. This type of stretching is not for the purpose of increasing range of motion, it is only to prepare for maximal effort. This type of stretching before training is not sufficient if the athlete wants to increase range of motion. Then the athlete must also engage in separate systematic stretching sessions, preferably at the end of the regular training session. In addition, athletes should strengthen the posterior musculature, particularly during the eccentric muscle action. Figures 3.8 through 3.10 show an exercise program for preventing hamstring injuries.

Hamstrings Program

Warm-up Exercises

During warm-up before every single training session and game, stretch your hamstring musculature *before* beginning sprinting or shooting exercises (Figure 3.8). Use support, preferably from another athlete. Allow your ankle to relax. Press your heel against the ground for 5–10 seconds, to activate the hamstring muscles, then relax and use your hand to straighten out your knee. Hold the stretch for about 20 seconds. If necessary, bend forward slightly at your hip until you feel the stretch in the hamstrings, but be sure to keep your back straight. Stretch each leg three times.

Figure 3.8 Warm-up exercises—hamstring stretching. The goal is to prepare for maximal effort. (Reproduced with permission from the Norwegian Sports Medicine Association.)

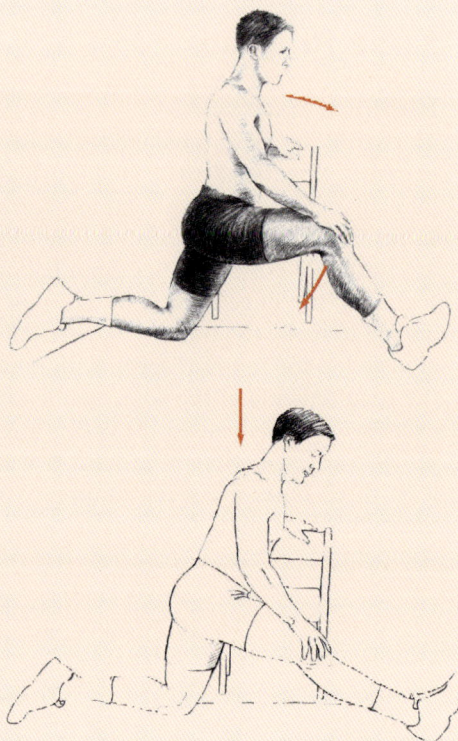

Hamstring Flexibility Training

Do 5–10 minutes of hamstring muscle stretching regularly if your range of motion is limited, at least three times a week during the preseason period and twice a week during the competitive season (Figure 3.9). Your partner lifts your leg with the knee slightly bent, until you feel stretching on the posterior side of your thigh. Hold this position for a while before actively pressing your leg against your partner's shoulder, so that your knee straightens out. Hold for 10 seconds. Then relax completely while your partner carefully stretches, by leaning forward. Hold that position for at least 45 seconds. It is important to relax your ankle, so you stretch the posterior side of the thigh, not the lower leg. Stretch each leg three times.

Figure 3.9 Flexibility training—hamstring stretching. The goal is to increase range of motion in the hip joint. (Reproduced with permission from the Norwegian Sports Medicine Association.)

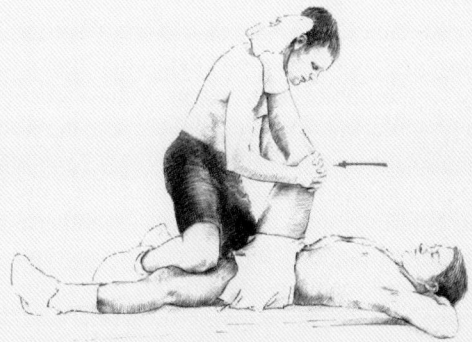

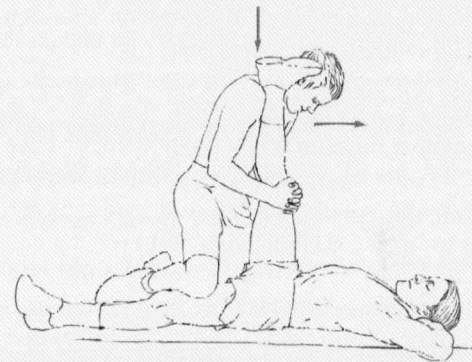

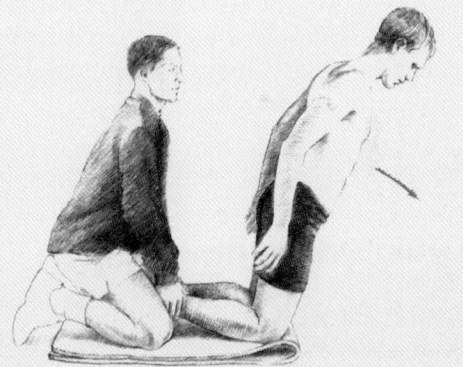

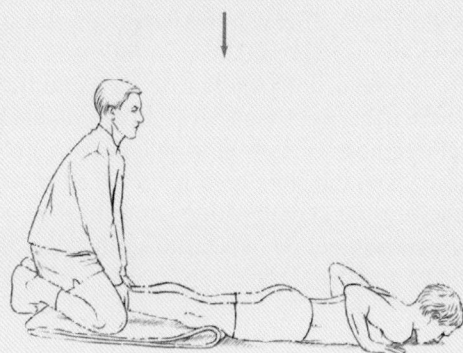

Hamstring Strength Training

Do eccentric strength training for the hamstring group regularly, at least three times a week during the preseason period and twice a week during the competitive season (Figure 3.10). Some American football and European soccer teams have successfully used this type of eccentric strength training exercises. The strength exercises are partner exercises, in which your partner stabilizes your legs. Lean forward in a smooth movement, keep your back and hips extended, and work at resisting the forward fall with your hamstring muscles as long as possible until you land on your hands. Go all the way down so that your chest touches the ground and push off immediately with your arms until the hamstring muscles can take over and you can straighten up into a kneeling position again.

Figure 3.10 Eccentric strength training for the hamstrings. The goal is to hold the descent as long as possible, to achieve maximum loading of the hamstrings during the eccentric stage. (Reproduced with permission from the Norwegian Sports Medicine Association.)

Preventing Groin Injuries

Injury mechanisms and risk factors. Groin injuries are among the most commonly encountered injuries in the Olympic sports of ice hockey, speed skating, soccer, swimming, and athletics. Yet they are often difficult to diagnose and treat. Groin injuries may be acute, but often become chronic in nature. One of the issues with groin injuries is that the injury mechanism is difficult to identify as these injuries often have the characteristics of an overuse injury. Even when the injury mechanism is known, depending upon different injury mechanisms several structures can be damaged. The three most commonly described injured groin structures are the abdominal muscles, adductor muscles, and the iliopsoas muscles (see Chapter 10). Overall this makes it difficult to describe causal risk factors. However, a few well-established modifiable risk factors for groin injury have been distinguished. These are a decreased hip abduction range of motion, a low level of preseason sport-specific training, and abdominal muscle recruitment. Although previous groin injury is considered a nonmodifiable risk factor, it is an important factor that can be targeted in preventive programs.

Preventive measures. To prevent recurrence of previous groin injuries treatment of the damaged structures should be combined with an exercise program to reestablish the pelvic stability and a rehabilitation program gradually including the demands and skills needed to participate in the particular sport before allowing the athlete to return to full participation. Although a decreased hip range of motion is suggested to be a risk factor for injury, there is no evidence that stretching or flexibility training can prevent groin injuries. Even so, there are indications that a normal range of motion is important and stretching of the hip muscles should be encouraged. Finally, strengthening the adductors and the abductors with low back and abdominal muscle recruitment, plus sport-specific exercises, are strongly advised as an integral part of the preseason program. Figures 3.11 and 3.12 show examples of static and dynamic exercises. A comprehensive groin program, as also described in "Sports Injury Prevention" handbook, includes a series of static as well as functional exercises.

Groin Program

Static Exercise

Ensure that the pelvic floor, deep transversus abdominus, and deep multifidus muscles are recruited while the athlete is breathing quietly with his abdominals. This will help maintain the spine in the neutral position (not lordotic or kyphotic or bent into side flexion). With both hips in a neutral posture, both knees extended and the tubing around the right ankle, abduct the right leg to 15° while maintaining the spine posture and the left leg posture as well as maintaining an elevated medial arch of the left foot. Maintain this hold for 5–10 slow and gentle breaths. Slowly return back to the start position (both hips in a neutral posture). Do not force the movement or move into or through pain with this movement. Repeat 5–20 times each side.

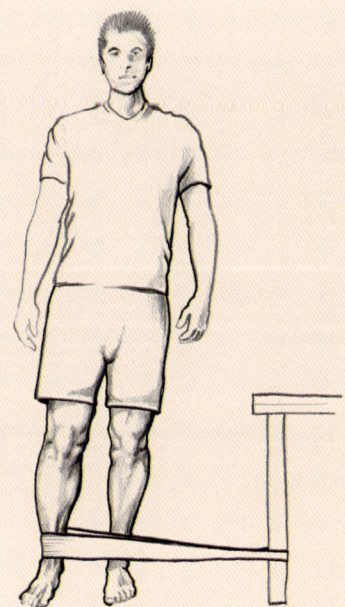

Figure 3.11 Standing with a unstable pelvis with good torso control using tubing and performing concentric abduction or eccentric adduction. (© Medical Illustrator Tommy Bolic, Sweden.)

Functional Exercise

Ensure that the pelvic floor, deep transversus abdominus, and deep multifidus muscles are recruited while the athlete is breathing quietly using his abdominals. This will help stabilize the spine. Arms behind your back, resting lightly on the back. With the hips and knees flexed approximately 20°, squeeze a soccer ball between your knees while maintaining an elevated medial arch of the left foot. Maintain this hold for 5–10 slow and gentle breaths. Slowly return back to the start position. Note this can be made more difficult by squatting deeper squat on your left leg. Do not force the movement or move into or through pain with this movement. Repeat 5–20 times each side.

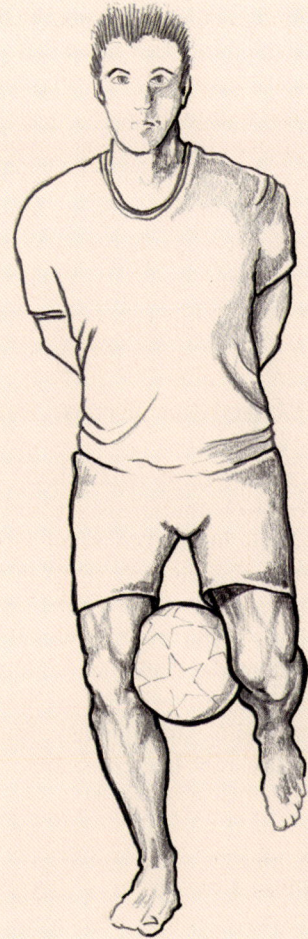

Figure 3.12 Isometric adduction with or without superimposed squats on the left leg. (© Medical Illustrator Tommy Bolic, Sweden.)

Preventing Shoulder Injuries

Injury mechanisms and risk factors. Little is known about the risk factors contributing to shoulder injury, but previous injury, gender, and weakness of the scapular stabilizers have been suggested. Stronger evidence for a causal relationship is available for some anatomical factors (e.g., posterior capsular tightness, ligamentous laxity, and crowding of the coracoacromial space) and exposure-related factors (e.g., age, number of pitches thrown, or hours of swimming). Shoulder injuries can be either traumatic or overuse in nature. The risk factors mentioned contribute mostly to the onset of overuse injuries and to a limited extent to acute injuries. Mechanisms for acute injury can be either direct or indirect in nature. Direct injuries are falls or blows directly on the shoulder, most often on the lateral side or the front. The resulting injury depends upon the direction of the force and the anatomical structure that is subject to the trauma. Indirect injuries are due to a transmission of force through the arm, for example, a fall on an outstretched arm. Overuse injuries to the shoulder are primarily caused through repeated forces on the soft tissue structures about the shoulder, for example, pitching or swimming.

Preventive measures. Although scientific evidence is lacking, a common-sense strategy to prevent acute injuries includes protective equipment (e.g., shoulder pads in

American football, breakaway bases in baseball), rule changes, and rules enforcement (e.g., rules on head-first sliding techniques in baseball), as well as better coaching, education, and risk awareness. The shoulder's stabilizing muscles can be trained trough a prophylactic program (see examples in Figures 3.13, 3.14, and 3.15). A standard shoulder-training program should always address the strength of the stabilizing muscles, coordination of the kinetic chain, and stretching to prevent tightness of the posterior capsule, the rhomboid muscles, the latissimus dorsi muscle, and the pectoralis minor muscle. Some exemplary exercises are given; for a full program, refer to the "Sports Injury Prevention" handbook.

Shoulder Program

Stabilizing Muscles

In the standing position the athlete ties a rubber band around the left foot and holds the other end in the right hand. By elevating his right shoulder, he trains the upper part of the trapezius (also called Trapezius 1). When flexing the right arm further posterior, he trains the middle and lower parts of the trapezius (also called Trapezius 2 and 3). At the same time the left arm and shoulder can grab the rubber band and be pushed forward, in order to train the left serratus anterior muscle. During these exercises, thoracic extension can also be trained by lifting the sternum. The lumbar spine must be kept stable.

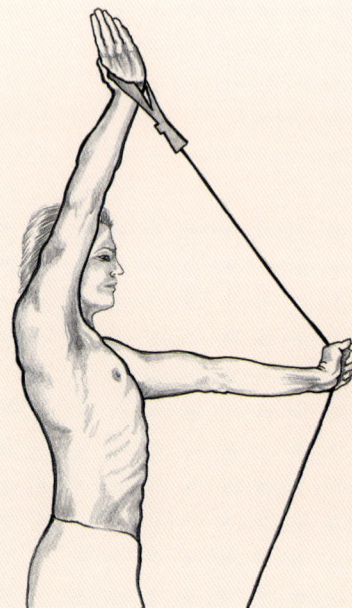

Figure 3.13 Training of the trapezius and the opposite serratus anterior muscles. (© Medical Illustrator Tommy Bolic, Sweden.)

Coordination

The athlete lays on the floor balancing a fit-ball on his hand while changing position of the arm into flexion/extension and abduction/adduction. The exercise should be performed for 3 minutes.

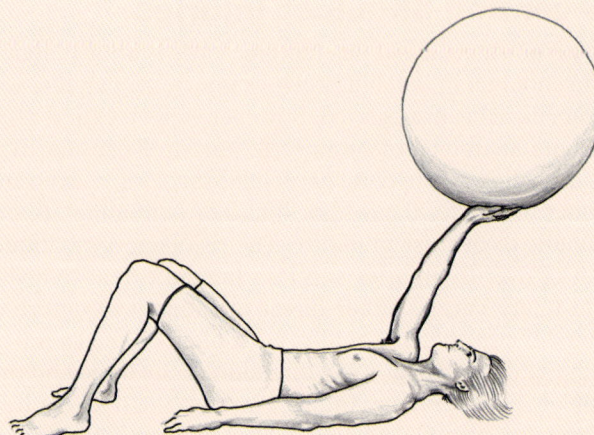

Figure 3.14 Training of coordination with a fit-ball. (© Medical Illustrator Tommy Bolic, Sweden.)

Stretching

The athlete is side-laying with his right arm in 90° of flexion. The left arm presses the humeral head posterior and inwardly (medially) rotates the right arm at the same time. Each position should be kept for 40 seconds.

Figure 3.15 Stretching of the posterior capsule and outward (lateral) rotators.
(© Medical Illustrator Tommy Bolic, Sweden.)

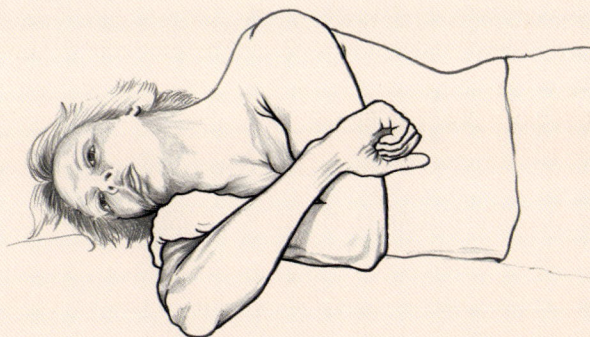

4 Head and Face

Head Injuries

Paul McCrory[1,2], Peter D. le Roux[3], Michael Turner[4], Ingunn R. Kirkeby[5], and Karen M. Johnston[6]

[1]*University of Melbourne, Melbourne, VIC, Australia*
[2]*Monash University, Frankston, VIC, Australia*
[3]*University of Pennsylvania, Philadelphia, PA, USA*
[4]*British Horseracing Authority, London, UK*
[5]*Oslo University Hospital, Rikshospitalet, Oslo, Norway*
[6]*University of Toronto, Toronto, ON, Canada*

Clinicians have to recognize and manage a spectrum of head injury ranging from mild concussion through to fatal penetrating brain trauma. The most common form of brain injury is concussion. Sports medicine physicians, trainers, and others involved in athletic care need to have a thorough understanding of the early management of the concussed athlete and the potential sequelae of such injuries that may impact upon the athlete's ability to return to sport. This chapter primarily deals with sport-related head injury.

Definition

Head trauma is the broad description applied to injuries to the brain or its coverings, skull, soft tissues, and vascular structures of the head and neck. In this chapter, when considering such injuries, the term traumatic brain injury (TBI) will be applied to the injuries of the brain or central nervous system and head injury to incorporate injuries to other structures of the head including the skull and craniofacial bones. Both forms of injury can occur in the same patient. For example, a depressed skull fracture may be associated with a scalp injury, lacerate the dura mater and cause a contusion in the brain.

Occurrence

TBI is one of the leading causes of morbidity and mortality worldwide. Because of differing injury definitions and methodology, the precise incidence of TBI is

Most common	Less common	Must not be overlooked !
Brain concussion, p. 65	Post-traumatic epilepsy, p. 76	Diffuse cerebral swelling second impact syndrome, p. 71
	Post-traumatic headache, p. 76	Cranial fracture, p. 72
		Acute subdural hematoma, p. 72
		Extradural hematoma, p. 73
		Traumatic intracranial hematoma/contusion, p. 74
		Traumatic subarachnoid hemorrhage, p. 75

Table 4.1 Overview of differential diagnoses for acute head injuries. (Reproduced with permission from the Norwegian Sports Medicine Association.)

The IOC Manual of Sports Injuries, First Edition. Edited by Roald Bahr.
©2012 International Olympic Committee. Published 2012 by John Wiley & Sons, Ltd.

problematic. The crude incidence for all traumatic brain injuries is estimated at approximately 300 per 100,000 inhabitants per year with the majority of those suffering a mild TBI. High-risk groups for sport-related TBI include males and those with a previous history of TBI. Males are more than twice as likely to suffer a TBI than females with a peak incidence among the 15–24-year-old population. However, in the nonsporting context, TBI demographics are changing. There now is trifocal age-specific TBI incidence—young children, young adults, and the elderly.

In hospital-based surveys of brain trauma, sporting injuries contribute approximately 10–15% of all cases and the sports most commonly associated with severe brain injuries are golf, equestrian sports and mountain climbing. Sporting-related deaths due to brain injury are fortunately rare, although these injuries have not been rigorously studied outside American and Australian football. The Center for Disease Control now estimates that 1.6–3.8 million sports-related concussions occur each year in the United States.

Differential Diagnoses

In moderate to severe brain injury, the differential diagnosis is limited and the fact that an athlete has sustained a significant brain injury usually is obvious (see Table 4.1). The critical diagnostic problem in this situation is to sort out the different types of intracranial injury (e.g., subdural hematoma and extradural hematoma) that may present with similar clinical features initially and then determine the most appropriate management priorities.

In mild brain injury and in particular, the subset of concussion, the diagnosis is often missed because the symptoms are subtle, the athlete does not seek medical attention or the athlete recovers rapidly before a full assessment can be made. Most sport-related head injuries occur without loss of consciousness. In this situation, the most common differential diagnosis is that of post-traumatic migraine that may manifest similar early symptoms. The key clinical symptom of concussion used to establish the presence of this injury is cognitive disturbance that may include altered memory, reaction time, or judgment.

Diagnostic Thinking

The key objectives when assessing any athlete who has sustained a TBI is to:

1. institute an appropriate first aid sideline assessment of the injured athlete;
2. make an accurate diagnosis;
3. manage the injury appropriately, minimizing the risk of any "secondary" injury, such as might be seen with coexistent hypoxia or hypotension;
4. remove safely the athlete from the field of play to an appropriate medical facility for further investigation and assessment;
5. determine subsequently when it is safe for the athlete to return to play.

Although a number of general classification schemes for TBI have been proposed, the most widely used system is the Glasgow Coma Scale (GCS). The GCS is incorporated in the SCAT2 tool (see Figure 4.2, pp. 67). However, the GCS does not provide specific information about the pathophysiologic mechanisms of the injury. The GCS has two distinct and separate uses (a) for serial measurement of brain injury status and (b) to separate TBI into a clinically and prognostically useful injury severity grading. In the former role, an immediate GCS is performed at the time of the initial or baseline assessment of an injured patient and then serially to monitor progress. In the second role, the separation of mild (GCS 13–15), moderate (GCS 9–12) and severe (GCS ≤8) TBI is based upon a scoring system that uses eye opening, verbal response and motor response to standard stimuli and should be measured at 6-hour postinjury after resuscitation has been completed. It is important to note that the term concussion (or commotio cerebri) refers to a different injury construct and is not synonymous with the term "mild TBI," that is, a concussed athlete may have a normal GCS. The GCS also provides useful information about expected outcome after TBI (see www.tbi-impact.org/ for an online tool to help with predicting prognosis) but not for concussion.

The treating clinician at a sporting event also must decide who should be referred to a hospital emergency facility or neurosurgical center. There are a number of urgent indications that are listed in Table 4.2. While it is acknowledged that a number of these indications are based on anecdotal rather than evidence-based information, these are widely accepted. The overall approach should be *when in doubt, refer.* Where no physician is present and the initial management is in the hands of an athletic trainer, physical therapist or paramedic, then an urgent medical referral should be considered mandatory in all cases of head injury.

Case History

Usually the fact that an athlete has suffered a head injury is obvious to the team medical staff. Head injuries in collision sports are usually the result of direct trauma to the athlete's head but should also be considered when there has been a rapid acceleration and deceleration type injury but no direct head contact. Eyewitness information or where available, videotape of the episode, is vital to help understand the nature of the injury especially if the athlete is unconscious or incapable of providing a lucid history. Information about the event and about the immediate clinical findings must be directly conveyed to the hospital staff. Key elements of the assessment of a head injured athlete are set out in Table 4.3.

The specific symptoms of acute concussion are outlined in the Pocket SCAT2 tool and the SCAT2 (see Figures 4.1 and 4.2). For practical purposes, the *Pocket SCAT2* can be utilized on-field or on the sideline to screen for concussion and once

Any player who has or develops the following:

- Fractured skull
- Penetrating skull trauma
- Deterioration in conscious state following injury
- Focal neurological signs
- Confusion or impairment of consciousness >30 minutes
- Loss of consciousness >5 minutes
- Persistent vomiting or increasing headache postinjury
- Any convulsive movements
- More than one episode of concussive injury in a session
- Where there is assessment difficulty (e.g., an intoxicated patient)
- Children with head injuries
- High-risk patients (e.g., hemophilia, anticoagulant use)
- Inadequate postinjury supervision
- High-risk injury mechanism (e.g., high-velocity impact)

Table 4.2 Indications for urgent hospital referral and neuroimaging. (Reproduced with permission from the Norwegian Sports Medicine Association.)

- Time and place of injury
- Mechanism of injury (eyewitness or video)
- Presence or duration of loss of consciousness
- Postinjury symptoms
- Postinjury behavior
- Presence of convulsions postinjury
- Past medical history
- Medication use

Table 4.3 Early assessment of head injury—history. (Reproduced with permission from the Norwegian Sports Medicine Association.)

concussion diagnosed then the player removed to the medical room and the full SCAT2 assessment tool then used by a physician. If the diagnosis of concussion is confirmed following assessment, then the player should not be returned to play on the day. In addition to postinjury assessment, it is recommended that the SCAT2 be baseline tested in the preseason. This is helpful for interpreting the postconcussion test score as it provides an objective record for possible change.

Sideline or First-aid Management

It is essential that all team physicians who have an on-field injury management role in their sport have formal training and certification in both first aid and trauma management. Depending upon the country concerned there may be regional differences

Pocket SCAT2

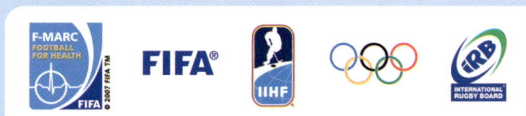

Concussion should be suspected in the presence of **any one or more** of the following: symptoms (such as headache), or physical signs (such as unsteadiness), or impaired brain function (e.g. confusion) or abnormal behaviour.

1. Symptoms

Presence of any of the following signs & symptoms may suggest a concussion.

- Loss of consciousness
- Seizure or convulsion
- Amnesia
- Headache
- "Pressure in head"
- Neck Pain
- Nausea or vomiting
- Dizziness
- Blurred vision
- Balance problems
- Sensitivity to light
- Sensitivity to noise
- Feeling slowed down
- Feeling like "in a fog"
- "Don't feel right"
- Difficulty concentrating
- Difficulty remembering
- Fatigue or low energy
- Confusion
- Drowsiness
- More emotional
- Irritability
- Sadness
- Nervous or anxious

2. Memory function

Failure to answer all questions correctly may suggest a concussion.

"At what venue are we at today?"
"Which half is it now?"
"Who scored last in this game?"
"What team did you play last week/game?"
"Did your team win the last game?"

3. Balance testing

Instructions for tandem stance
*"Now stand heel-to-toe with your **non-dominant** foot in back. Your weight should be evenly distributed across both feet. You should try to maintain stability for 20 seconds with your hands on your hips and your eyes closed. I will be counting the number of times you move out of this position. If you stumble out of this position, open your eyes and return to the start position and continue balancing. I will start timing when you are set and have closed your eyes."*

Observe the athlete for 20 seconds. If they make more than 5 errors (such as lift their hands off their hips; open their eyes; lift their forefoot or heel; step, stumble, or fall; or remain out of the start position for more that 5 seconds) then this may suggest a concussion.

Any athlete with a suspected concussion should be IMMEDIATELY REMOVED FROM PLAY, urgently assessed medically, should not be left alone and should not drive a motor vehicle.

Figure 4.1 Pocket SCAT2 instrument is designed for rapid on-field assessment of concussed athletes.

in certification and accreditation courses; some of the best known include Advanced Trauma Life Support (ATLS); Emergency Management of Severe Trauma (EMST); Pre-Hospital Emergency Care Course (PHECC); Pre-Hospital Trauma Life Support (PHTLS) and the British Association of Immediate Care Course (BASICS). This list is not exhaustive; however, they all deliver the skill set required to appropriately and safely manage acute injuries.

The major priorities at this early stage are the basic principles of first aid. The simple mnemonic DR ABC may be a useful aide-memoire (Table 4.4). When a patient is transferred to an emergency room this same approach in management is taken, that is, ensure a secure airway with proper oxygenation and circulation.

Once these basic aspects of first aid care have been achieved and the patient stabilized, then consideration of removal of the patient from the field to an appropriate facility is necessary. Only trained individuals should remove helmets or neck protective equipment.

At this time, careful assessment for the presence of a cervical spine or other injury is necessary. If an alert patient complains of neck pain, has evidence of neck tenderness or deformity or has neurological signs suggestive of a spinal injury, then neck bracing and transport on a suitable spinal frame is required (see Chapter 5). If the patient is unconscious, then a cervical injury should be assumed until proven otherwise. Airway protection takes precedence over any potential spinal injury.

The clinical management may involve the treatment of a disorientated, confused, unconscious, uncooperative or convulsing patient. The immediate treatment priorities remain the basic first aid principles of ABC–airway, breathing and circulation. Once this has been established and the patient stabilized, a full medical and neurological assessment exam should follow. On site physicians are in an ideal position to initiate the critical early steps in medical care to ensure optimal recovery from a head injury.

Clinical Examination

When examining a head injured athlete, a structured and focused neurological examination is important. Because the major management priorities at this stage are to establish an accurate diagnosis and exclude a catastrophic intracranial injury, this part of the examination should focus on key clinical findings such as

1. level of consciousness (measured using the GCS);
2. pupil response and conjugate eye movement;
3. motor function.

D	Danger	Ensuring that there are no immediate environmental dangers that may potentially injure the patient or treatment team. This may involve stopping play in a football match or marshalling cars on a motor racetrack.
R	Response	Is the patient conscious? Can he/she talk?
A	Airway	Ensuring a clear and unobstructed airway. Removing any mouthguard or dental device that may be present.
B	Breathing	Ensure the patient is breathing adequately
C	Circulation	Ensure an adequate circulation

Table 4.4 Initial on-field assessment of concussion. (Reproduced with permission from the Norwegian Sports Medicine Association.)

During the evaluation, one should determine whether the pupils are in the normal position, that is, not deviated to one side and are equal and reactive to light and if all extremities are moving and moving symmetrically in a normal manner. A dilated pupil that does not react to light should be considered an emergency since it may indicate incipient herniation of the brain due to raised intracranial pressure (ICP). In these patients, immediate decompressive surgery may be lifesaving.

A baseline measurement of the Glasgow Coma Score, preferably after initial resuscitation but before additional medications such as sedatives or paralytics are given should be performed in all head-injured patients. The importance of this initial neurologic exam is that it serves as a reference to which other repeated neurologic examinations may be compared and there is little interobserver variability. A GCS of ≤8 indicates coma and airway intubation and ventilation should be considered urgently. It is necessary to record all clinical findings so that an overall trend in improving or deteriorating mental function can be clearly and objectively documented. In addition, the head and face should be inspected and palpated carefully to look for lacerations, fractures and to check for cerebrospinal fluid (CSF) leak from the nose or ears. Fluid that runs from the nose or ears can be clear or mixed with blood. Bloody CSF when it drips onto a gauze sponge will form a halo. A positive glucose stick test suggests that the fluid is CSF and this can be confirmed in the hospital with B-transferrin analysis. The assessment of cognitive function in this situation is covered on p. 66.

Vital signs must be recorded following an injury. Although head injury produces several types of respiratory patterns, an acute rise in ICP with central herniation can lead to an increase in blood pressure and falling pulse rate (the Cushing response). Hypotension is rarely due to brain injury, except as a terminal event, and alternate sources for the decrease in blood pressure should be aggressively sought and treated. This includes major scalp lacerations especially in young children or a cervical spinal cord injury. Restlessness is a frequent accompaniment of brain injury and can be an early indicator of increased ICP, intracranial bleeding or hypoxia, all of which can aggravate any underlying brain injury. If the patient is unconscious but restless, attention should be given to the possibility of increasing hypoxia, a distended bladder or painful injuries elsewhere. Only when these causes have been ruled out, should drug sedation be considered. This point cannot be overstated since hypotension and hypoxia adversely influence outcome following brain injury and are easily treatable factors.

When time permits, a more thorough physical exam should be performed to exclude coexistent injuries elsewhere in the body, a sensory evaluation and to detect the late developing signs of skull injury. This includes Battle's sign (subcutaneous hematoma over the mastoid bone) and hemotympanum (blood in the middle ear) that often suggest petrous temporal bone fractures or raccoon eyes (bilateral periorbital hematomas) that are common with other skull base fractures. Injury to cranial nerves, for example, the 7th (facial) and 8th (vestibulocochlear) nerve, is common after skull base fractures.

In recent times, the application of simple neuropsychological tests has created considerable interest as a means to objectively assess the mental status of concussed athletes. The standard approach of asking the orientation items (e.g., day, date, year, time, and date of birth) has been shown to be unreliable in following concussive brain injury. More useful are questions of recent or working memory. These are included in the Maddock's questions (Table 4.5) and in the Pocket SCAT2 (Figure 4.1) and SCAT2 (Figure 4.2).

- Which ground are we at?
- Which team are we playing today?
- Who is your opponent at present?
- Which quarter is it?
- How far into the quarter is it?
- Which side scored the last goal?
- Which team did we play last week?
- Did we win last week?

Table 4.5 Postconcussion memory assessment (Maddock's questions). (Reproduced with permission from the Norwegian Sports Medicine Association.)

Having determined the presence of a concussive injury, the patient needs to be serially monitored until full recovery ensues. If the concussed player is discharged home after recovery, then he should be in the care of a responsible adult. Each patient and his attendant must be given a head injury advice card upon discharge. An example of a head injury card is included in the SCAT2 (Figure 4.2, p. 67).

Supplemental Examinations

Computerized tomography (CT). A brain CT scan is the most useful diagnostic test after head injury. CT evaluation should proceed as soon as the patient is hemodynamically stable and all immediately life-threatening injuries have been addressed. Even if a first CT scan is normal, repeat imaging should be considered when there is patient deterioration since delayed hematomas, evolution of a small contusion or cerebral edema may evolve over time. There may be practical difficulties especially in children when attempting to perform a CT scan and often children, especially if young, may need to be sedated or anaethetized to achieve an optimum scan.

Indications for emergent cranial CT imaging in the initial evaluation of the head-injured patient are similar to the points already outlined in Table 4.2. The primary goal of imaging is to establish whether there is a surgical lesion, that is, intracranial hemorrhage. A depressed level of consciousness and in particular a GCS ≤8, are the strongest predictors of intracranial hemorrhage. Other signs that suggest surgical pathology include focal motor weakness and an asymmetrical pupil exam. There may be situations however where the clinical examination is obscured by alcohol, drugs, metabolic derangement or postictal state or where the ability to access the patient for serial neurologic examinations is problematic. In such cases, early CT scanning is recommended to enable accurate decision-making. An important question is who needs a head CT scan when their level of consciousness is normal (i.e., GCS is 15)? Guidelines such as the Canadian Head CT Rules and the New Orleans Criteria suggest that factors such as age >60 years, headache, vomiting, intoxication, retrograde amnesia, confusion, loss of consciousness, seizures, visible trauma above the clavicles and injury mechanism indicate a need for a head CT. Acute blood is hyperdense on a noncontrast head CT scan. The head CT also is examined for "mass effect," for example, the amount of midline shift of the third ventricle and the condition of the perimesencephalic cisterns. These can help guide surgical decision-making.

However, a normal head CT scan does not always exclude a TBI or the need for neurosurgical consultation. About 20% of patients admitted to hospital after even mild TBI may develop posttraumatic abnormalities on subsequent imaging even after the initial head CT scan was normal.

Magnetic resonance imaging (MRI). The role of MRI in the evaluation of acute head trauma is limited, in part because it is time-consuming, expensive, and less sensitive to acute hemorrhage than CT. In addition, access to critically ill or unconscious patients is restricted during the time of image acquisition that is much longer than CT, and the strong magnetic fields generated by the scanner necessitate the use of nonferromagnetic resuscitative equipment. However, MRI can be useful in the subacute or chronic phases after injury to help explain failure to improve in the days following injury. Advanced MRI, for example, functional MRI, Diffusion Tensor Imaging or spectroscopy, can be useful in research studies or assessment of long term recovery.

Skull X-ray examination. Skull X-ray series (AP, Caldwell, Waters, and lateral views) have been replaced by the use of CT scans and are very rarely obtained. However, plain skull radiographs are inexpensive and can easily obtained in an emergency room and if a fracture is present particularly when there is a focal finding or depressed level of consciousness, suggest an extradural hemorrhage. The overall predictive value of skull X-rays is low.

Neck imaging. Cervical spine injury is common in patients with head injury. Consequently plain cervical X-rays, CT and even MRI are indicated where appropriate.

Vascular imaging. Blood vessels in the neck and head can be examined using several tests including Doppler ultrasound, CT angiography, MR angiography or venography and, if necessary, digital subtraction angiography. Vascular studies should be considered when there is penetrating injury, a neurologic deficit that is not explained by head CT scan, fractures over the venous sinus, some neck injuries, for example, fractures through the foramen transversarium or certain craniofacial injuries such as Lefort II or III fractures. Early identification of vascular injuries can help reduce the incidence of stroke.

Neuropsychological testing. Neuropsychological testing to determine recovery from TBI is accepted worldwide. In recent decades, sports such as Australian football, American professional football and ice hockey (NHL) have followed similar strategies. More detail is included in the section Rehabilitation of Acute Head and Facial Injuries on p. 96.

Specific Diagnoses—Common Injuries

Brain Concussion—*Commotio Cerebri*

Concussion is defined as a complex pathophysiological process affecting the brain, induced by traumatic biomechanical forces, either by a direct blow to the head, face, neck or elsewhere on the body with an "impulsive" force transmitted to the head. Research suggests that linear acceleration or rotational shearing forces may result in short-lived neurochemical, metabolic or gene-expression changes. Concussion typically results in the rapid onset of short-lived impairment of neurologic function that resolves spontaneously. Although concussion may result in neuropathological changes, the acute clinical symptoms largely reflect a functional disturbance rather than a structural injury, although the athlete may have sustained a significant impact to the brain. Per definition, no abnormality is seen on standard structural neuroimaging studies. Concussion results in a graded set of clinical symptoms that may or may not involve loss of consciousness. Resolution of the clinical and cognitive symptoms typically follows a sequential course; however, it is important to note that in a small percentage of cases postconcussive symptoms may be prolonged.

HEAD AND FACE

Frequently, in episodes of mild concussion ("bell ringers"), the athlete will be dazed or stunned for a period of seconds only and continue playing. Alert medical and training staff should closely observe the actions of a player who has received a knock to the head for any signs of impaired performance.

- Symptoms and signs: Common symptoms of concussion include headache, nausea, dizziness and balance problems, blurred vision, memory loss, a feeling of slowness or fatigue. A more complete list of symptoms is shown in Figure 4.2 (p. 67). These symptoms are not specific to concussion and in some cases may present in a delayed fashion. Clinical features that are more specific to a diagnosis of concussion include: loss of consciousness/impaired conscious state, concussive convulsions/impact seizures, confusion or attention deficit, memory disturbance (unaware of period, opposition, game score) and balance disturbance. These features however may not be present in all cases and in some cases may present in a delayed fashion. Other physical signs with concussion include poor coordination, slow to answer questions or follow directions, easily distracted, poor concentration, displaying unusual or inappropriate emotions, vomiting, vacant stare/glassy eyed, personality changes, slurred speech, double/blurred vision.

- Diagnosis: The Pocket SCAT2 (Figure 4.1) can be utilized on the sideline to screen for concussion and once concussion is diagnosed then the player can be removed to the medical room. The full SCAT2 assessment tool (Figure 4.2) is then used by a physician. The diagnosis is made by having any new concussion symptoms or by failing either of the cognition or balance components of the Pocket SCAT2. The full SCAT2 is a more detailed medical assessment form that also incorporates additional cognitive questions and physical examination findings. This tool also incorporates the Maddock's questions and the SAC. Any abnormality on any component of this test would indicate a concussive injury. Generally, an uncomplicated concussion does not need routine neuroimaging. However, imaging has a role in the exclusion of suspected intracranial injury (Table 4.2). There is no reliable or scientifically validated system of grading the severity of sports-related concussion. At the present time, there are at least 45 published anecdotal severity scales. The danger is that athletes and/or their coaches may "shop around" for a scale that is not in their best medical interests. At the end of the day, good clinical judgment should prevail over published anecdotal grading scales.

- Treatment: Once concussion is diagnosed, then the player should be removed from the game or training and not return to play on that day. A variety of immediate motor phenomena (e.g., tonic posturing) or convulsive movements may accompany a concussion. Although dramatic, these are a nonepileptic manifestation of concussion, are generally benign and require no specific management beyond the standard treatment of the underlying concussive injury. The principal concern of premature return to play of a concussed athlete is that due to the impaired cognitive function (e.g., slowed information processing, reduced attention) the athlete will sustain further injury (both concussive and other) when returning to a dangerous playing environment. Furthermore, if a player recommences playing while symptomatic, postconcussive symptoms may be prolonged. This may also increase the chance of developing the "postconcussive syndrome," in which fatigue, difficulty in concentration and headaches persist for some time, often months, following the original injury. This syndrome is uncommon in sport. These patients should undergo formal neuropsychological testing as well as an MRI brain scan. If these tests are normal, there is no specific treatment other than rest and reassurance. Following a concussive injury, players should be returned to play in a graduated fashion once clinical features have resolved and cognitive function returned to "baseline." When considering return to play, the athlete should be off all medications at the time of considering commencement of the rehabilitation phase or at

SCAT2

Sport Concussion Assessment Tool 2

F-MARC FIFA · *FIFA®* · *IIHF* · Olympic Rings · *IRB INTERNATIONAL RUGBY BOARD*

Name _____

Sport/team _____

Date/time of injury _____

Date/time of assessment _____

Age _____ Gender ☐ M ☐ F

Years of education completed _____

Examiner _____

What is the SCAT2?[1]

This tool represents a standardized method of evaluating injured athletes for concussion and can be used in athletes aged from 10 years and older. It supersedes the original SCAT published in 2005[2]. This tool also enables the calculation of the Standardized Assessment of Concussion (SAC)[3,4] score and the Maddocks questions[5] for sideline concussion assessment.

Instructions for using the SCAT2

The SCAT2 is designed for the use of medical and health professionals. Preseason baseline testing with the SCAT2 can be helpful for interpreting post-injury test scores. Words in Italics throughout the SCAT2 are the instructions given to the athlete by the tester.

This tool may be freely copied for distribution to individuals, teams, groups and organizations.

What is a concussion?

A concussion is a disturbance in brain function caused by a direct or indirect force to the head. It results in a variety of non-specific symptoms (like those listed below) and often does not involve loss of consciousness. Concussion should be suspected in the presence of **any one or more** of the following:

- Symptoms (such as headache), or
- Physical signs (such as unsteadiness), or
- Impaired brain function (e.g. confusion) or
- Abnormal behaviour.

Any athlete with a suspected concussion should be REMOVED FROM PLAY, medically assessed, monitored for deterioration (i.e., should not be left alone) and should not drive a motor vehicle.

Symptom Evaluation

How do you feel?

You should score yourself on the following symptoms, based on how you feel now.

	none	mild		moderate		severe	
Headache	0	1	2	3	4	5	6
"Pressure in head"	0	1	2	3	4	5	6
Neck Pain	0	1	2	3	4	5	6
Nausea or vomiting	0	1	2	3	4	5	6
Dizziness	0	1	2	3	4	5	6
Blurred vision	0	1	2	3	4	5	6
Balance problems	0	1	2	3	4	5	6
Sensitivity to light	0	1	2	3	4	5	6
Sensitivity to noise	0	1	2	3	4	5	6
Feeling slowed down	0	1	2	3	4	5	6
Feeling like "in a fog"	0	1	2	3	4	5	6
"Don't feel right"	0	1	2	3	4	5	6
Difficulty concentrating	0	1	2	3	4	5	6
Difficulty remembering	0	1	2	3	4	5	6
Fatigue or low energy	0	1	2	3	4	5	6
Confusion	0	1	2	3	4	5	6
Drowsiness	0	1	2	3	4	5	6
Trouble falling asleep (if applicable)	0	1	2	3	4	5	6
More emotional	0	1	2	3	4	5	6
Irritability	0	1	2	3	4	5	6
Sadness	0	1	2	3	4	5	6
Nervous or Anxious	0	1	2	3	4	5	6

Total number of symptoms (Maximum possible 22) ▢

Symptom severity score ▢
(Add all scores in table, maximum possible: 22 x 6 = 132)

Do the symptoms get worse with physical activity? ☐ Y ☐ N
Do the symptoms get worse with mental activity? ☐ Y ☐ N

Overall rating

If you know the athlete well prior to the injury, how different is the athlete acting compared to his / her usual self? Please circle one response.

no different	very different	unsure

Figure 4.2 SCAT2 instrument is designed for full medical assessment of concussed athletes.

Cognitive & Physical Evaluation

1 **Symptom score** (from page 1)

22 **minus** number of symptoms | of 22

2 **Physical signs score**

Was there loss of consciousness or unresponsiveness? | Y | N
If yes, how long? | minutes
Was there a balance problem/unsteadiness? | Y | N

Physical signs score (1 point for each negative response) | of 2

3 **Glasgow coma scale (GCS)**

Best eye response (E)

No eye opening	1
Eye opening in response to pain	2
Eye opening to speech	3
Eyes opening spontaneously	4

Best verbal response (V)

No verbal response	1
Incomprehensible sounds	2
Inappropriate words	3
Confused	4
Oriented	5

Best motor response (M)

No motor response	1
Extension to pain	2
Abnormal flexion to pain	3
Flexion/Withdrawal to pain	4
Localizes to pain	5
Obeys commands	6

Glasgow Coma score (E + V + M) | of 15

GCS should be recorded for all athletes in case of subsequent deterioration.

4 **Sideline Assessment – Maddocks Score**

"I am going to ask you a few questions, please listen carefully and give your best effort."

Modified Maddocks questions (1 point for each correct answer)

At what venue are we at today?	0	1
Which half is it now?	0	1
Who scored last in this match?	0	1
What team did you play last week/game?	0	1
Did your team win the last game?	0	1

Maddocks score | of 5

Maddocks score is validated for sideline diagnosis of concussion only and is not included in SCAT 2 summary score for serial testing.

5 **Cognitive assessment**

Standardized Assessment of Concussion (SAC)

Orientation (1 point for each correct answer)

What month is it?	0	1
What is the date today?	0	1
What is the day of the week?	0	1
What year is it?	0	1
What time is it right now? (within 1 hour)	0	1

Orientation score | of 5

Immediate memory

"I am going to test your memory. I will read you a list of words and when I am done, repeat back as many words as you can remember, in any order."

Trials 2 & 3:

"I am going to repeat the same list again. Repeat back as many words as you can remember in any order, even if you said the word before."

Complete all 3 trials regardless of score on trial 1 & 2. Read the words at a rate of one per second. Score 1 pt. for each correct response. Total score equals sum across all 3 trials. Do not inform the athlete that delayed recall will be tested.

List	Trial 1	Trial 2	Trial 3	Alternative word list		
elbow	0 1	0 1	0 1	candle	baby	finger
apple	0 1	0 1	0 1	paper	monkey	penny
carpet	0 1	0 1	0 1	sugar	perfume	blanket
saddle	0 1	0 1	0 1	sandwich	sunset	lemon
bubble	0 1	0 1	0 1	wagon	iron	insect
Total						

Immediate memory score | of 15

Concentration

Digits Backward:

"I am going to read you a string of numbers and when I am done, you repeat them back to me backwards, in reverse order of how I read them to you. For example, if I say 7-1-9, you would say 9-1-7."

If correct, go to next string length. If incorrect, read trial 2. One point possible for each string length. Stop after incorrect on both trials. The digits should be read at the rate of one per second.

		Alternative digit lists		
4-9-3	0 1	6-2-9	5-2-6	4-1-5
3-8-1-4	0 1	3-2-7-9	1-7-9-5	4-9-6-8
6-2-9-7-1	0 1	1-5-2-8-6	3-8-5-2-7	6-1-8-4-3
7-1-8-4-6-2	0 1	5-3-9-1-4-8	8-3-1-9-6-4	7-2-4-8 5 6

Months in Reverse Order:

"Now tell me the months of the year in reverse order. Start with the last month and go backward. So you'll say December, November ... Go ahead"

1 pt. for entire sequence correct

Dec-Nov-Oct-Sept-Aug-Jul-Jun-May-Apr-Mar-Feb-Jan | 0 | 1

Concentration score | of 5

[1] This tool has been developed by a group of international experts at the 3rd International Consensus meeting on Concussion in Sport held in Zurich, Switzerland in November 2008. The full details of the conference outcomes and the authors of the tool are published in British Journal of Sports Medicine, 2009, volume 43, supplement 1.
The outcome paper will also be simultaneously co-published in the May 2009 issues of Clinical Journal of Sports Medicine, Physical Medicine & Rehabilitation, Journal of Athletic Training, Journal of Clinical Neuroscience, Journal of Science & Medicine in Sport, Neurosurgery, Scandinavian Journal of Science & Medicine in Sport and the Journal of Clinical Sports Medicine.

[2] McCrory P et al. Summary and agreement statement of the 2nd International Conference on Concussion in Sport, Prague 2004. British Journal of Sports Medicine. 2005; 39: 196-204

[3] McCrea M. Standardized mental status testing of acute concussion. Clinical Journal of Sports Medicine. 2001; 11: 176-181

[4] McCrea M, Randolph C, Kelly J. Standardized Assessment of Concussion: Manual for administration, scoring and interpretation. Waukesha, Wisconsin, USA.

[5] Maddocks, DL; Dicker, GD; Saling, MM. The assessment of orientation following concussion in athletes. Clin J Sport Med. 1995;5(1):32–3

[6] Guskiewicz KM. Assessment of postural stability following sport-related concussion. Current Sports Medicine Reports. 2003; 2: 24-30

Figure 4.2 Continued

6 Balance examination

This balance testing is based on a modified version of the Balance Error Scoring System (BESS)[6]. A stopwatch or watch with a second hand is required for this testing.

Balance testing

"I am now going to test your balance. Please take your shoes off, roll up your pant legs above ankle (if applicable), and remove any ankle taping (if applicable). This test will consist of three twenty second tests with different stances."

(a) Double leg stance:

"The first stance is standing with your feet together with your hands on your hips and with your eyes closed. You should try to maintain stability in that position for 20 seconds. I will be counting the number of times you move out of this position. I will start timing when you are set and have closed your eyes."

(b) Single leg stance:

"If you were to kick a ball, which foot would you use? [This will be the dominant foot] *Now stand on your non-dominant foot. The dominant leg should be held in approximately 30 degrees of hip flexion and 45 degrees of knee flexion. Again, you should try to maintain stability for 20 seconds with your hands on your hips and your eyes closed. I will be counting the number of times you move out of this position. If you stumble out of this position, open your eyes and return to the start position and continue balancing. I will start timing when you are set and have closed your eyes."*

(c) Tandem stance:

*"Now stand heel-to-toe with your **non-dominant foot** in back. Your weight should be evenly distributed across both feet. Again, you should try to maintain stability for 20 seconds with your hands on your hips and your eyes closed. I will be counting the number of times you move out of this position. If you stumble out of this position, open your eyes and return to the start position and continue balancing. I will start timing when you are set and have closed your eyes."*

Balance testing – types of errors
1. Hands lifted off iliac crest
2. Opening eyes
3. Step, stumble, or fall
4. Moving hip into > 30 degrees abduction
5. Lifting forefoot or heel
6. Remaining out of test position > 5 sec

Each of the 20-second trials is scored by counting the errors, or deviations from the proper stance, accumulated by the athlete. The examiner will begin counting errors only after the individual has assumed the proper start position. **The modified BESS is calculated by adding one error point for each error during the three 20-second tests. The maximum total number of errors for any single condition is 10.** If an athlete commits multiple errors simultaneously, only one error is recorded but the athlete should quickly return to the testing position, and counting should resume once subject is set. Subjects that are unable to maintain the testing procedure for a minimum of **five seconds** at the start are assigned the highest possible score, ten, for that testing condition.

Which foot was tested: ☐ Left ☐ Right
(i.e. which is the **non-dominant** foot)

Condition	Total errors
Double Leg Stance (feet together)	of 10
Single leg stance (non-dominant foot)	of 10
Tandem stance (non-dominant foot at back)	of 10
Balance examination score (30 minus total errors)	of 30

7 Coordination examination

Upper limb coordination

Finger-to-nose (FTN) task: *"I am going to test your coordination now. Please sit comfortably on the chair with your eyes open and your arm (either right or left) outstretched (shoulder flexed to 90 degrees and elbow and fingers extended). When I give a start signal, I would like you to perform five successive finger to nose repetitions using your index finger to touch the tip of the nose as quickly and as accurately as possible."*

Which arm was tested: ☐ Left ☐ Right

Scoring: 5 correct repetitions in < 4 seconds = 1

Note for testers: Athletes fail the test if they do not touch their nose, do not fully extend their elbow or do not perform five repetitions. Failure should be scored as 0.

Coordination score	of 1

8 Cognitive assessment

Standardized Assessment of Concussion (SAC)

Delayed recall

"Do you remember that list of words I read a few times earlier? Tell me as many words from the list as you can remember in any order."

Circle each word correctly recalled. Total score equals number of words recalled.

List		Alternative word list	
elbow	candle	baby	finger
apple	paper	monkey	penny
carpet	sugar	perfume	blanket
saddle	sandwich	sunset	lemon
bubble	wagon	iron	insect

Delayed recall score	of 5

Overall score

Test domain	Score
Symptom score	of 22
Physical signs score	of 2
Glasgow Coma score (E + V + M)	of 15
Balance examination score	of 30
Coordination score	of 1
Subtotal	**of 70**
Orientation score	of 5
Immediate memory score	of 15
Concentration score	of 5
Delayed recall score	of 5
SAC subtotal	**of 30**
SCAT2 total	**of 100**
Maddocks Score	**of 5**

Definitive normative data for a SCAT2 "cut-off" score is not available at this time and will be developed in prospective studies. Embedded within the SCAT2 is the SAC score that can be utilized separately in concussion management. The scoring system also takes on particular clinical significance during serial assessment where it can be used to document either a decline or an improvement in neurological functioning.

Scoring data from the SCAT2 or SAC should not be used as a stand alone method to diagnose concussion, measure recovery or make decisions about an athlete's readiness to return to competition after concussion.

Figure 4.2 Continued

HEAD AND FACE

Athlete Information

Any athlete suspected of having a concussion should be removed from play, and then seek medical evaluation.

Signs to watch for

Problems could arise over the first 24-48 hours. You should not be left alone and must go to a hospital at once if you:
- Have a headache that gets worse
- Are very drowsy or can't be awakened (woken up)
- Can't recognize people or places
- Have repeated vomiting
- Behave unusually or seem confused; are very irritable
- Have seizures (arms and legs jerk uncontrollably)
- Have weak or numb arms or legs
- Are unsteady on your feet; have slurred speech

Remember, it is better to be safe.
Consult your doctor after a suspected concussion.

Return to play

Athletes should not be returned to play the same day of injury. When returning athletes to play, they should follow a stepwise symptom-limited program, with stages of progression. For example:
1. rest until asymptomatic (physical and mental rest)
2. light aerobic exercise (e.g. stationary cycle)
3. sport-specific exercise
4. non-contact training drills (start light resistance training)
5. full contact training after medical clearance
6. return to competition (game play)

There should be approximately 24 hours (or longer) for each stage and the athlete should drop back to the previous asymptomatic level if any post-concussive symptoms recur. Resistance training should only be added in the later stages.
Medical clearance should be given before return to play.

Tool	Test domain	Time	Score			
		Date tested				
		Days post injury				
	Symptom score					
	Physical signs score					
	Glasgow Coma score (E + V + M)					
SCAT2	Balance examination score					
	Coordination score					
	Orientation score					
	Immediate memory score					
SAC	Concentration score					
	Delayed recall score					
	SAC Score					
Total	SCAT2					
Symptom severity score (max possible 132)						
Return to play			☐Y ☐N	☐Y ☐N	☐Y ☐N	☐Y ☐N

Additional comments

- -

Concussion injury advice (To be given to concussed athlete)

This patient has received an injury to the head. A careful medical examination has been carried out and no sign of any serious complications has been found. It is expected that recovery will be rapid, but the patient will need monitoring for a further period by a responsible adult. Your treating physician will provide guidance as to this timeframe.

If you notice any change in behaviour, vomiting, dizziness, worsening headache, double vision or excessive drowsiness, please telephone the clinic or the nearest hospital emergency department immediately.

Other important points:
- **Rest and avoid strenuous activity for at least 24 hours**
- **No alcohol**
- **No sleeping tablets**
- **Use paracetamol or codeine for headache. Do not use aspirin or anti-inflammatory medication**
- **Do not drive until medically cleared**
- **Do not train or play sport until medically cleared**

Clinic phone number

Patient's name

Date/time of injury

Date/time of medical review

Treating physician

Contact details or stamp

Figure 4.2 Continued

the final medical assessment. Return to sport is not advisable while symptoms are present as exercise appears to prolong the condition. More detail of the rehabilitation process and return to sport following concussion are included in the section Rehabilitation of Acute Head and Facial Injuries on pp. 96–97.

- Prognosis: Most sports-related concussive injuries are uncomplicated and recover fully over 1–3 weeks. However, it is worth noting that detailed neuropsychological testing shows that 20% of athletes will still have unrecognized cognitive deficits 10 days after concussion. For this reason, reliance on nonscientific nostrums ("miss a week") or symptoms alone to guide return to play is not recommended as best practice care. This fact highlights the important role of neuropsychological testing to inform clinical decision-making and as one of the cornerstones of management. In postconcussive athletes with persistent symptoms or cognitive deficits (>14 days) consideration of referral to a multidisciplinary concussion program may be worthwhile. One of the key problems to consider in this setting is mental health issues (such as depression, anxiety and suicide) that have been reported as consequence of TBI including sports concussion. Neuroimaging studies using functional MRI suggest that a chronic symptoms and depressed mood following concussion may reflect an underlying pathophysiological abnormality consistent with a limbic-frontal model of depression. All players with ongoing symptoms or a prolonged clinical course should be screened for depression using standard clinical tools, for example, Hospital Anxiety and Depression Scale, Beck Depression Inventory.

Other Specific Diagnoses

Diffuse Cerebral Swelling and Second Impact Syndrome !

Second impact syndrome is frequently mentioned in the concussion literature but, surprisingly, has little scientific evidence for its existence. It is a term used to describe the potential catastrophic consequences resulting from a second concussive blow to the head before an individual has fully recovered from the symptoms of a previous concussion. The second head injury is believed to result in loss of cerebrovascular auto-regulation, which in turn leads to brain swelling secondary to increased cerebral blood flow (Figure 4.3). There is a lack of evidence to support the claim that the second impact is a risk factor for diffuse cerebral swelling. However, there is evidence that acute (and delayed) brain swelling may occur following a single blow to the head, in association with a structural injury such as a subdural hematoma and also in disorders of calcium channels, suggesting a possible genetic basis for some of these cases. Such events are virtually only seen in children and adolescents.

- Symptoms and signs: Anecdotal reports usually record an athlete collapsing on a sporting field or after practice. A blow to the head may be witnessed but typically is not. The clinical features are those of an unconscious athlete.
- Diagnosis: Diagnosis is usually made with a urgent CT brain scan or MRI. Clinical examination, for example, papilledema on fundoscopy, decerebrate posturing, may also provide a clue to the diagnosis.
- Treatment: If cerebral swelling is suspected or noted on imaging studies an urgent neurosurgical consultation is required. Elevated ICP requires a variety of

Figure 4.3 Axial CT images of the brain that demonstrate diffuse cerebral swelling with sulcus effacement and loss of ventricular and cisternal spaces. (Reproduced with permission from the Norwegian Sports Medicine Association.)

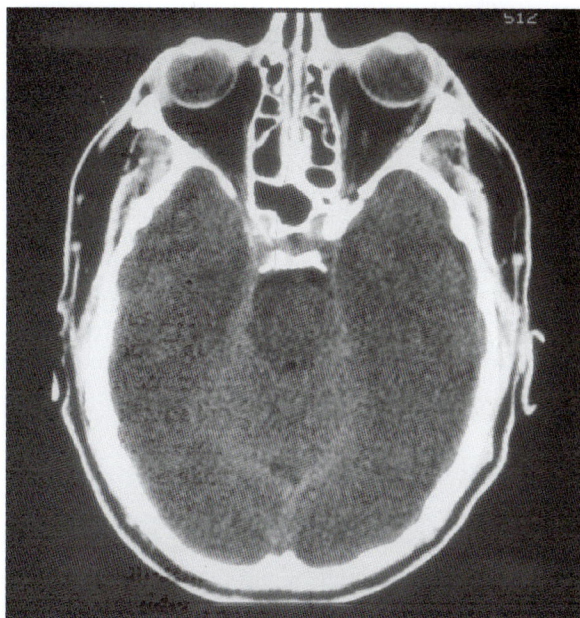

treatments. Adequate analgesia, sedation, correction of physiologic derangements and mild head elevation (15° to 30°) are the initial treatments when elevated ICP is suspected. Specific treatments that should be guided by an ICP monitor include: sedation and mechanical ventilation, hyperventilation in select patients, ventricular CSF drainage, osmotherapy (e.g., mannitol or hypertonic saline), blood pressure control, induced coma or surgery when indicated.
- Prognosis: Mortality in this condition approaches 100%.

Cranial Fracture—*Skull Fracture* !

All types of athletic activity in which trauma to the head occurs have the potential to cause a cranial fracture. Cranial fractures can be divided into three broad categories: linear fractures, skull base fractures and depressed fractures. Skull fractures can be further classified as open (associated with an overlying scalp laceration) or closed and as simple or comminuted. Most linear fractures are uncomplicated and occur over the lateral convexities of the skull. However the presence of a linear fracture in the temporal region often can be associated with an acute extradural hematoma. Fractures that involve air sinuses or overlie venous sinuses in the skull require special consideration. A depressed fracture caused by a blow to the head from even a relatively small object may cause the bone fragments to impact or tear the dura mater or the brain. These fractures can be associated with brain contusions, CSF leaks and seizures. Basal skull fractures involve the floor of the anterior and middle cranial fossas. These fractures may be associated with cranial nerve and vascular injuries.

- Symptoms and signs: Athletes with a cranial fracture usually have a headache and may or may not have symptoms of an underlying brain injury. Local soft tissue swelling may also indicate an underlying fracture. The scalp should be carefully inspected and palpated to establish whether the skull fracture is open or closed. A Battle's sign or raccoon eyes suggest a basal skull fracture. Rhinorrhea and otorrhea indicate that skull fracture is associated with torn dural membranes.
- Diagnosis: The diagnosis is usually made with a plain skull X-ray or CT scan of the brain.
- Management: In all cases of skull fracture, especially if a CSF leak is present, an urgent neurosurgical consultation is required. When a skull fracture is suspected, the patient should always be hospitalized for observation and neurosurgical evaluation. The physician should cover the injured area of an open cranial fracture with a sterile dressing. Fractures that are depressed beyond the thickness of the inner cranial table often require surgical treatment as do fractures that involve the posterior table of the frontal sinus particularly when there is pneumocephalus. CSF leaks usually will respond to bed rest and head elevation but some may require CSF drainage through a lumbar or ventricular drain and rarely direct repair. Prophylactic antibiotic treatment is not recommended for CSF leaks.
- Prognosis: Linear fractures heal in a few months to a year, and if no additional injury occurs, the athlete can often return to her sport. The grade of brain injury will usually determine the outcome. The prognosis is often good when the brain and membranes are uninjured. Patients who require a craniotomy to repair a frontal sinus fracture or depressed skull fracture may not be able to participate further in collision or contact sports.

Acute Subdural Hematoma !

Subdural hematomas (Figure 4.4) may result from either nonpenetrating or penetrating trauma to the head but typically are associated with rapid acceleration and deceleration that tear small bridging veins between the brain and dura. Extravasation of blood into the subdural space causes hematoma formation. In addition, subdural hematomas frequently are associated with underlying brain injury, for example, contusions. These injuries are typically seen following falls on hard surfaces or assaults with nondeformable objects rather than low velocity injuries. They are also more common in elderly subjects and should be considered into those taking medications such as anticoagulants. Acute subdural hematomas are the most common traumatic mass lesions and occur in 30% of severely head-injured patients. Chronic subdural hematomas may occur in individuals with brain atrophy and evolve over several weeks even after very mild head injury.

- Symptoms and signs: Clinical signs and symptoms depend on the size and location of the subdural hematoma and how quickly it developed. In general, the more severe the head injury the more likely the presence of an acute subdural hematoma. There may be a brief period of confusion or loss of consciousness but many patients are in coma from the onset. Few patients remain lucid throughout their course. Impaired alertness and cognitive function are found frequently on initial examination. Soft tissue injuries may be seen at the site of impact but their absence does not mean there is no intracranial injury. Enlargement of the hematoma or an increase in edema surrounding the hematoma produces additional mass effect, with further depression of the patient's level of consciousness, increases in motor or speech deficit, and eventually ipsilateral compression of the third nerve and midbrain (i.e., herniation).
- Diagnosis: In the acute phase, the diagnosis is usually made with a CT scan of the brain.
- Treatment: A patient with a subdural hematoma requires urgent neurosurgical consultation. Initial management depends on the clinical condition but is aimed at controlling ICP (see the preceding text). In a patient with a depressed level of consciousness, focal findings or elevated ICP surgical evacuation through a craniotomy is necessary. In addition, subdural hematomas that on CT are thicker than 1 cm and associated with >5 mm of midline shift should be removed. Operative treatment is directed toward evacuation of the entire subdural hematoma; control of the bleeding source; resection of contused, nonviable brain or intracerebral hematoma in select patients; and in some patients a decompressive craniotomy. This may performed at the time of initial surgery or in a delayed fashion if further cerebral swelling develops. A chronic subdural hematoma may be removed through only a burrhole in many patients.
- Prognosis: Acute subdural hematoma usually are associated with underlying injury to the cerebral parenchyma and consequently the prognosis is poor. Patients who require a craniotomy for evacuation of subdural hematoma may not be able to participate further in collision or contact sports.

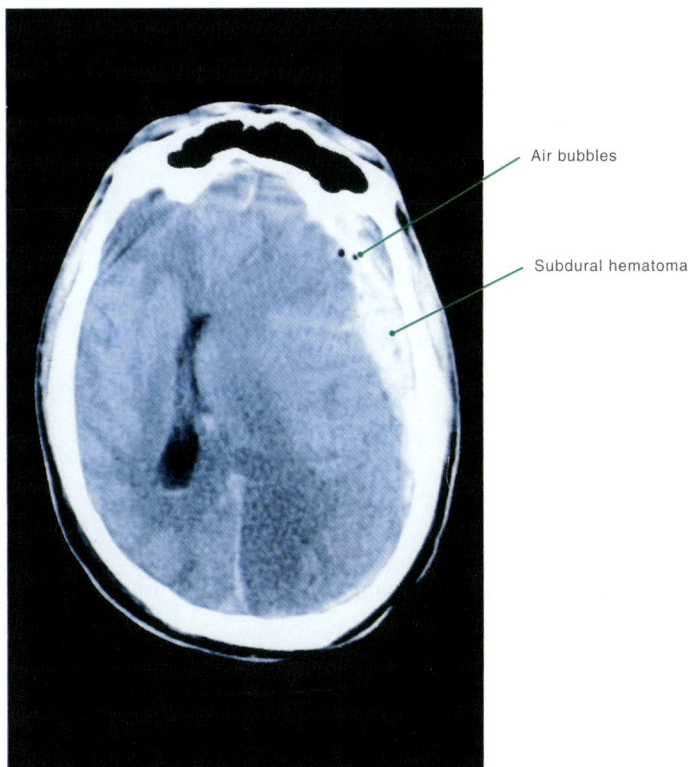

Figure 4.4 Subdural hematoma with cerebral edema. Left-side subdural hematoma with air bubbles as a sign of skull fracture and torn dura, cerebral edema, and midline shift. (Reproduced with permission from the Norwegian Sports Medicine Association.)

Extradural Hematoma !

Extradural hematomas are found in 10% of comatose TBI patients. They generally result from head impact in the temporal region that deforms or fractures the skull.

The adherent dura is forcefully detached and hemorrhage occurs (Figure 4.5), arterial (the middle meningeal artery), venous, or both sources. Hemorrhage may also be seen under a fracture line in other regions of the skull. Injury to the brain under an extradural hematoma is rare.

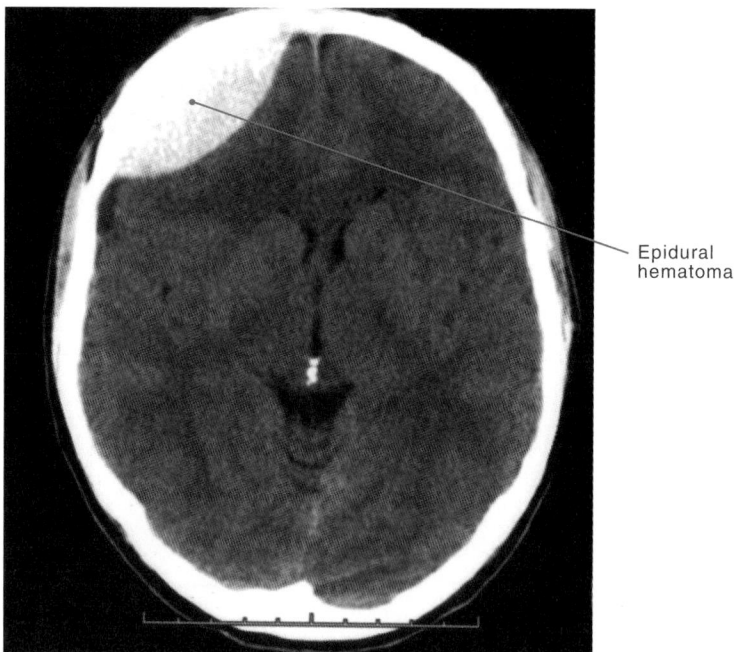

Epidural hematoma

Figure 4.5 Epidural hematoma. (Reproduced with permission from the Norwegian Sports Medicine Association.)

- Symptoms and signs: Extradural hematomas may have a varied clinical presentation. The classic presentation is considered a loss of consciousness, recovery of consciousness (lucid interval) then a decline in consciousness. The presentation depends on the size and site of the hematoma, the rate of expansion, and the presence of associated intradural pathology. Extradural hematomas that involve the middle fossa (i.e., after temporal bone fracture) can cause precipitous decline in neurologic function since the mass effect has an early impact on the brainstem. In these patients contralateral weakness and ipsilateral pupil dilatation are common. Alteration in consciousness is the hallmark of extradural hematomas.
- Diagnosis: On brain CT scan acute extradural hematomas are hyperdense and lenticular or biconvex in shape.
- Treatment: Urgent neurosurgical consultation is required when an extradural hematoma is suspected. Rapid diagnosis and prompt surgical evacuation through a craniotomy are indicated when there are neurologic findings and depressed consciousness. Some surgeons advocate hematoma removal even in patients with only a headache when the blood clot is thicker than ≥15 mm or 30 ml in volume and associated with ≥5 mm of midline shift.
- Prognosis: When rapidly treated, the chances of a full functional recovery are excellent even in patients with profoundly abnormal neurological findings before surgery. Generally, patients who require a craniotomy for drainage of an extradural hematoma would not necessarily be precluded from further sports participation assuming full clinical and cognitive recovery.

Traumatic Intracerebral Hematoma/Contusion !

Intracerebral hematomas and contusions are bleeding within the brain substance that appear as mass lesions. They may be divided into acute or delayed subtypes. Acute traumatic intracerebral hematoma occurs at the time of the initial head injury. Delayed traumatic intracerebral hematomas, which are more common, may develop in the hours or days (and even weeks) after initial injury particularly severe TBI. Brain tissue can be seen interspersed with hemorrhage on head CT scan in contusions but forms a coalesced hyperdense mass in an intracerebral hematoma on CT scan. Contusions are frequent in the frontal and temporal lobes since this tissue "slides" over the underlying rough bony surface of the skull base during acceleration/deceleration of the head. Contusions also may be seen under a depressed skull fracture. Penetrating head injury is also associated with intracerebral hematomas and contusions (Figure 4.6).

- Symptoms and signs: Intracerebral hematomas are more likely in more severe TBI but the clinical signs and symptoms depend on the size and location of the intracerebral hematoma as well as the rapidity of its development. In many cases, there is a period of confusion or loss of consciousness but only one third of the patients remain lucid throughout their course. Impaired alertness and cognitive function are found frequently on initial examination. Focal findings are frequent and depend on lesion location.

- Diagnosis: In the acute phase, the diagnosis is usually made with a CT scan of the brain.
- Treatment: When this condition is suspected or diagnosed on imaging studies, an urgent neurosurgical consultation is required. Initial management is directed to control of ICP (see cerebral edema in the preceding text) and correction of any coagulation abnormalities. Intracerebral hematomas of >30 ml in volume, >3 cm in diameter, or associated with >5 mm of midline shift should be evacuated. However, the decision to operate depends on many factors, for example, hematoma location, patient age and coagulation status among others. For example, a 20 mL intracerebral hematoma in the temporal lobe may require surgical evacuation. The alert patient with a focal neurologic deficit and a small intracerebral hematoma (<3 cm) particularly those that are in a deep location can be observed closely. Occasionally an intracerebral hematoma may spread into the ventricles and cause intraventricular hemorrhage and hydrocephalus. These patients may benefit from a ventriculostomy. Patients with an intracerebral hematoma should receive seizure prophylaxis for 7 days unless seizures occur when a longer course is required. There is no role for corticosteroids.
- Prognosis: The overall recovery depends on what other injuries there are but when there is a small intracerebral hematoma in isolation, particularly in young individuals, recovery is generally good. However, overall mortality after traumatic intracerebral hematoma is about 30%. Patients who require a craniotomy for evacuation of intracerebral hematoma may not be able to participate further in collision or contact sports.

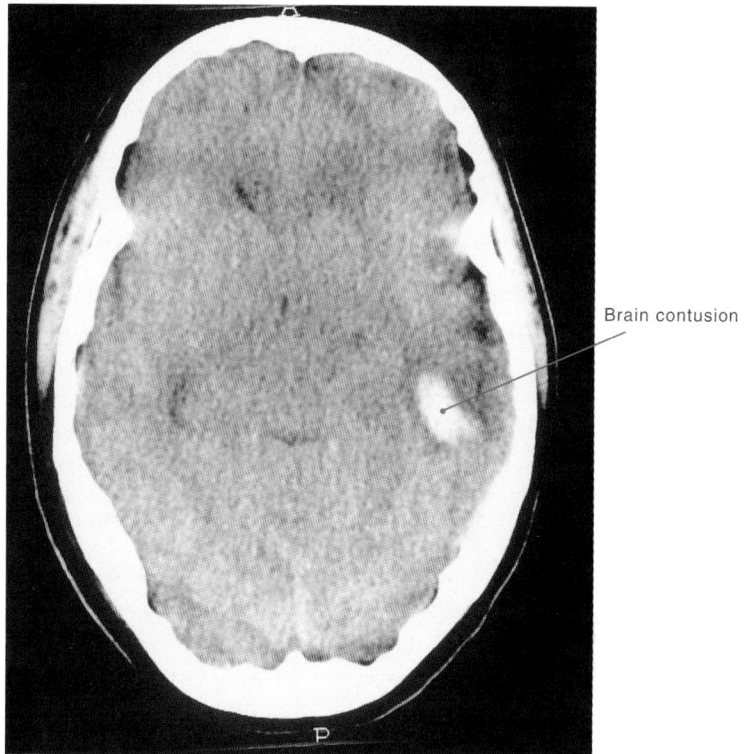

Brain contusion

Figure 4.6 Brain contusion. Left-side brain contusion in the temporal lobe, following a fall from a bicycle. (Reproduced with permission from the Norwegian Sports Medicine Association.)

Traumatic Subarachnoid Hemorrhage !

Subarachnoid hemorrhage often is found following severe or moderate head injury. Traumatic subarachnoid hemorrhage may occur in isolation but often occurs with other intracranial pathology, in particular subdural hematomas or intracerebral hematoma. In addition traumatic subarachnoid hemorrhage may result from blood vessel injury, for example, a vertebral artery dissection.

- Symptoms and signs: Subarachnoid hemorrhage typically presents with meningeal symptoms such as headache, neck stiffness and photophobia. The most common initial symptoms of vertebral artery injury causing subarachnoid hemorrhage are neck pain and occipital headache that may precede the onset of neurological symptoms. Traumatic subarachnoid hemorrhage usually is found in a diffuse pattern over the convexities and in the subarachnoid space. It is hyperdense on head

CT scan and unlike subarachnoid hemorrhage associated with a ruptured cerebral aneurysm is not usually observed in the basal cisterns.

- Diagnosis: When traumatic subarachnoid hemorrhage is suspected or diagnosed on imaging studies, an urgent neurosurgical consultation is required. Vascular imaging may be necessary to exclude a vascular injury particularly when there is penetrating injury or suspected vessel dissection that involves either the carotid or vertebral arteries.
- Treatment: There is no specific treatment of traumatic subarachnoid hemorrhage although there is some suggestion that calcium channel antagonists may be useful in some patients. Subarachnoid hemorrhage is associated with the development of vasospasm (delayed narrowing of cerebral vessels) that can contribute to delayed cerebral ischemia. These patients therefore require very careful fluid management. In addition, hydrocephalus may occur and require ventricular drainage or a shunt.
- Prognosis: The presence of traumatic subarachnoid hemorrhage is a factor associated with poor outcome after TBI. Patients who require a craniotomy for evacuation of hematoma or aneurysmal clipping may not be able to participate further in collision or contact sports.

Post-traumatic Epilepsy

Post-traumatic epilepsy may occur and is more common with increasing severity of brain injury and in particular intracranial pathology such as hemorrhage or a depressed skull fracture. A convulsing patient is at increased risk of hypoxia that can exacerbate the underlying brain injury. Airway management in these patients is important as is control of oxygenation and blood pressure. Management of post-traumatic seizures is determined by the timing of their occurrence in relation to the head injury. Since seizures may increase ICP or contribute to secondary brain injury, intense efforts should be made to prevent seizures during the recovery phase of the acute head injury. Prophylactic anticonvulsant medication is indicated when there is (1) an altered level of consciousness for a protracted time, (2) severe TBI (GCS ≤8), (3) focal lesions on CT, (4) depressed skull fractures, and (5) penetrating head trauma. Benzodiazepines (e.g., lorazepam, clonazepam, diazepam) can be used for the acute treatment of post-traumatic seizures, but they will produce at least transient impairment of consciousness. In the absence of a seizure, prophylactic medication can be stopped 7 days after injury since these medications do not prevent the development of post-traumatic epilepsy. If a patient develops further seizures, that is, post-traumatic epilepsy he or she should be managed in the same manner as symptomatic focal epilepsy from any etiology.

Post-traumatic Headache

Trauma to the head and neck in sport may lead to the development of headache. The initiating traumatic event may not necessarily be severe. The International Headache Society has published diagnostic criteria for post-traumatic headache and these include (a) the presence of significant head trauma as documented by loss of consciousness and/or post-traumatic amnesia >10 minutes; (b) at least two abnormalities of the following: clinical examination, skull X-ray, neuroimaging, evoked potentials, CSF examination, vestibular function test, neuropsychological testing; (c) headache onset <14 days post-trauma; and (d) the headache disappears within 8 weeks after trauma. There are a number of specific subtypes of post-traumatic headaches and these include post-traumatic migraine, extra-cranial vascular headache, and dysautonomic cephalalgia.

Post-traumatic migraine may resemble a typical migraine headache and is commonly seen in sports such as soccer, where repetitive heading of the ball gives rise to the term "footballer's migraine." One particular syndrome that is recognized in the setting of minor head blows is migrainous cortical blindness. This disturbing condition often raises fear of serious cerebral injury but tends to resolve over 1–2 hours. These are treated pharmacologically as for typical migraine. *Extracranial vascular headache* is periodic headaches at the site of head or scalp trauma. These headaches may share a number of migrainous features, although at times they can be described as "jabbing" pains. These are treated pharmacologically as for typical migraine. *Dysautonomic cephalalgia* occurs in association with trauma to the anterior triangle of the neck, resulting in injury to the sympathetic fibers alongside the carotid artery. This results in autonomic symptoms such as Horner's syndrome and excessive sweating associated with a unilateral headache. Propranolol has been used with some success in the management of this condition.

Facial Injuries

Per Skjelbred[1], Glenn Maron[2], and Robert Gassner[3]

[1]*Oslo University Hospital, Oslo, Norway*
[2]*Emory University School of Medicine, Atlanta, GA, USA*
[3]*Medical University of Innsbruck, Maximilianstrasse, Innsbruck, Austria*

Occurrence

Sport activities, traffic accidents, and violence are the three most prevalent causes of facial injuries. Injuries to the maxillofacial complex account for 3–29% of all sports-related injuries. Approximately 60–90% of these injuries occur in males between the ages of 10–29 years. The incidence of this type of injury varies and is difficult to establish due to the variety of environments and lack of reports. Facial injuries are caused by direct contact between athletes or sport equipment, such as hockey sticks, shoe spikes, goal posts, or railings. The shoulder and upper limb and the head of an opponent are the body parts that most frequently cause injuries to the face.

In amateur boxing, ice hockey, bandy, horseback riding, motorcycle sports, martial arts, and American football, mandatory protective equipment has indirectly reduced the number of facial injuries. Athletes in several sports wear mouthguards to prevent dental and orofacial injuries.

Differential Diagnoses

Soft-tissue injuries including abrasions, lacerations and contusions are the most common sports-related maxillofacial injuries. In this setting, the practitioner must have a high suspicion for facial fractures and dental injuries. Often concomitant facial fractures accompany soft tissue injuries (see Table 4.6) and it is essential to arrange for appropriate clinical and radiographic investigations.

Most common	Less common	Must not be overlooked ❗
Grazes, p. 82	Tooth fractures, p. 86	"White eye syndrome", p. 89
Soft tissue contusions, p. 83	Soft-tissue loss, p. 87	Maxillary fracture, p. 90
Lacerations/cuts, p. 83	Intraoral soft-tissue injuries, p. 88	Retrobulbar hematoma, p. 90
Nasal fractures, p. 83	Frontal bone fracture, p. 88	Nasoorbitoethmoid fracture, p. 91
Mandibular fractures, p. 84	Orbital fracture, p. 89	Panfacial fractures, p. 91
Zygomatic fractures, p. 84	Alveolar ridge fracture, p. 92	Corneal erosion, p. 93
Tooth luxation, p. 86	Foreign object in the eye, p. 92	Contusion of the eyeball, p. 93
		Perforation of the eyeball, p. 94
		Septum hematoma

Table 4.6 Overview of differential diagnoses for facial injuries. (Reproduced with permission from the Norwegian Sports Medicine Association.)

Diagnostic Thinking

Sport-related facial injuries are seldom life threatening. However, the expanding use of new sport equipment, such as in-line skates, snowboards, and all-terrain bicycles, has increased the complexity of the injury pattern. The result is that primary caregivers are more frequently confronted with serious injuries. After the initial assessment of airways, breathing and circulation and an evaluation of cervical spine injuries, the examination of the maxillofacial complex may begin. If facial injuries are not treated properly, they may have functional or aesthetic sequelae. Referral to the appropriate specialist and thorough clinical examination is necessary to determine whether a patient with a facial injury needs to be sent for diagnostic imaging to exclude fractures.

If the patient has a severe facial injury, the airway may be obstructed by a foreign body, a blood clot, loose teeth, bone or a dislodged mouthguard. On-site treatment includes securing the airway and hemostasis. If this is difficult, the patient must be intubated. A cricothyreotomy may be necessary as an emergency procedure.

Direct pressure to a wound is a simple initial management of bleeding. It may be difficult to control bleeding from the throat, nose and mouth. Various methods, including nasal tamponade, an epistaxis catheter and compresses in the mouth may be used. Profuse facial bleeding may require intubation, epistaxis catheter, packing of throat and mouth with compresses, compresses over the face and circumfacial elastics to compress the entire maxillofacial complex. Imaging with angiography may be indicated followed by surgery or interventional radiography to control bleeding.

The goal of the clinical examination during the acute phase is to evaluate whether there is a soft-tissue injury or a more complex injury that requires treatment by a specialist. Patients with suspected fractures must be sent to the emergency room for imaging. A dentist must treat all patients with dentoalveolar injuries immediately. If the most important differential diagnoses can be excluded by means of a clinical evaluation, additional examinations for this purpose are unnecessary.

The injury mechanism is used as a basis for making the proper diagnosis and for determining the extent of the injury (see Figure 4.7). In most cases of facial injuries, the injured athlete is able to account for the injury mechanism. Most case histories

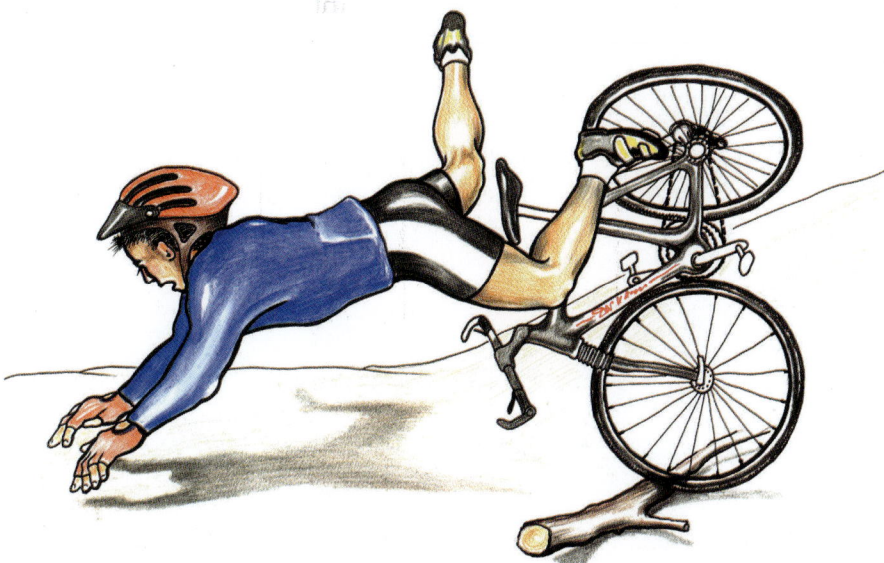

Figure 4.7 Injury mechanisms for facial injuries. Falls from bicycles often result in soft-tissue injuries, tooth injuries, and facial fractures. (© Medical Illustrator Tommy Bolic, Sweden.)

are one of two types: either the patient hit himself in the face or he got hit. The observations of fellow players may be important in making a proper diagnosis. Injuries to the oral cavity are often caused by direct trauma to the lips or teeth, caused by a blow or kick from an opposing player or by sport equipment, such as hockey stick, ice hockey puck, bandy ball or a ski pole.

Clinical Examination

Inspection. The examination should take place as soon as possible after the injury. However, often the patient is not examined until several hours after the event. Swelling and pain may make the examination difficult. Double vision and/or occlusal bite changes are hallmarks of significant facial trauma. All wounds should be washed and cleaned. Then the patient's face is systematically examined. Depression fractures may be visible in the forehead. The bridge of the nose and the nasal septum are checked for deviation. Fractures in the nasoethmoidal area increase the distance between medial corners of the eyes (telecanthus), cause the tip of the nose to turn upward, and change the palpebral aperture (round doll's eye) on the affected side. A depressed zygomatic complex causes the contour of the cheekbone to become flattened. Injuries in the orbital area may cause changes in the position of the eyeball, such as proptosis (protrusion of the eyeball), hypophthalmos (inferiorly positioned eyeball) and enophthalmos (recessed eyeball), double vision, and reduced ocular movement. A depressed, elongated, widened midface indicates a fracture with dislocation (see Figure 4.8). Open bite often occurs. Malocclusion may be caused by fractures to both the upper and the lower jaw. Injuries to the lacrimal canal cause annoying tearing. Zygomatic arch fractures often interfere with jaw movement, hindering either opening or closure.

Palpation. If the patient has hematoma and a swollen face, thorough palpation of the underlying structures and the surrounding areas is necessary to exclude fractures in the area (see Figure 4.9). The facial skeleton is palpated for "depressions" or discontinuity. A depression in the middle lower section of the forehead, a loose nasal

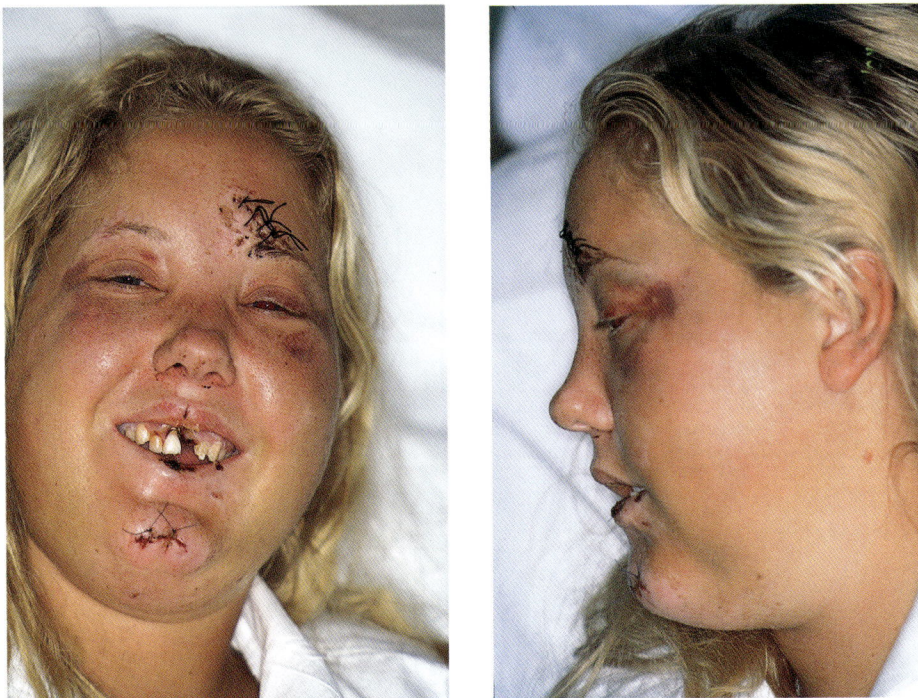

Figure 4.8 Midface fracture. Note that the midface is depressed and widened.

pyramid, and steps in the orbital margin are typical signs of fractures. In case of a zygomatic arch fracture, the arch may show a V-shaped depression between the zygoma and ear. Levels I–III Le Fort fractures cause the upper jaw or midface to be mobile. The temporomandibular joint spaces can be palpated, and an injury will usually cause pain here. In addition, the patient's mouth-opening range will be conspicuously reduced. Pathological movement when the lower jaw is bimanually palpated is an indication of fractures in the area. Irregularities in occlusion and in the dental arch are findings that require follow-up.

Jaw movement. The normal mouth-opening range of an adult is between 35 and 50 mm, measured between the incisive teeth in the upper and lower jaws.

The distance that the lower jaw can be moved forward varies from 2 to 6 mm in adults (measured in the area of the incisive teeth). Lateral movements range between 3 and 7 mm (measured in the canine-tooth region). If the patient has an acute injury, the mouth-opening range and the distance it can be moved forward and laterally may be conspicuously reduced. If there is a temporomandibular joint dislocation, the patient is unable to close the mouth. These dislocations also cause the lower jaw to deviate toward the contralateral side of the dislocation. Inability to open the mouth following an impact to the side of the head is often due to zygomatic arch trauma in a closed-mouth position, while inability to close an open mouth can be related to a broken zygomatic arch in an open-mouth position.

Neuromuscular function. Facial fractures can cause deficit in three sensory nerve branches of the trigeminal nerve. Injuries to the supraorbital nerve reduce sensation in the forehead. Injuries to the infraorbital nerve reduce sensation in the midface, whereas injuries to the inferior alveolar nerve and the mental nerve reduce feeling in the lower jaw and lower lip. Traumatic facial paresis rarely occurs in isolation although may be a complication of an underlying skull fracture. Deep facial cuts may cause damage to the nerve.

Supplemental Examinations

Radiographic examinations. Plain radiographs for diagnosis of facial fractures are mostly limited to the nasal bone, mandible and teeth. An orthopantogram (OPG) can show mandibular fractures. If tooth fractures, tooth luxation, or fractures of the alveolar process are suspected, an OPG should be supplemented with dental X-rays. Nasal fractures are diagnosed using lateral X-rays, but decisions regarding the need

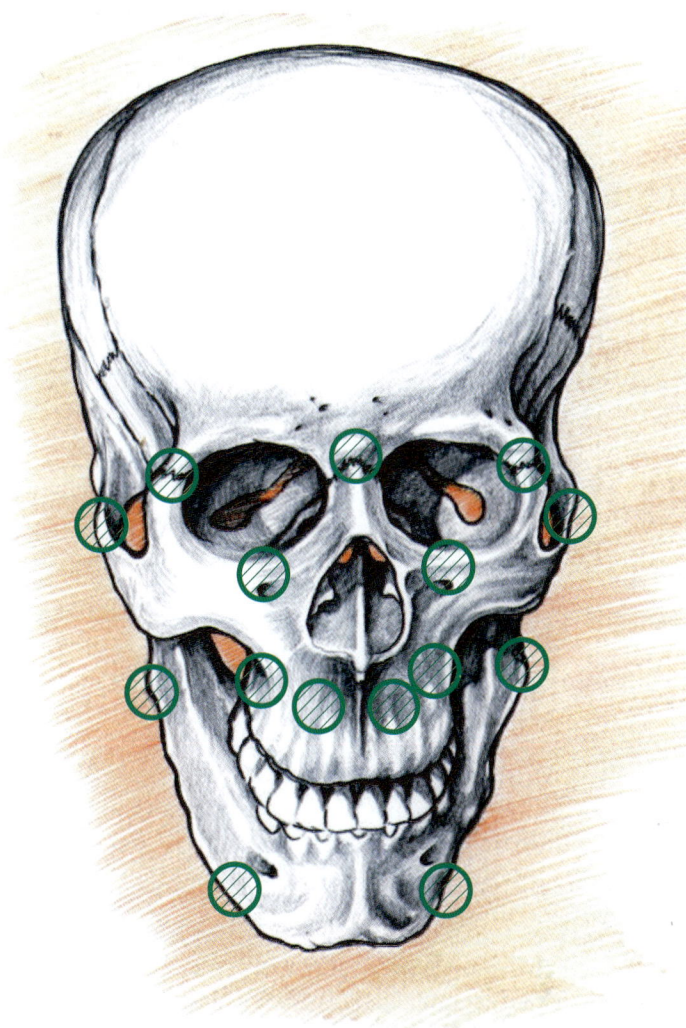

Figure 4.9 Common midface fractures. Key palpation points are marked. (© Medical Illustrator Tommy Bolic, Sweden.)

HEAD AND FACE

for surgery on a nasal fracture depend on the clinical evaluation. Institutions that have DVT (digital volume tomography) devices can provide three-dimensional (3D) information based on dentofacial radiology. If fractures are found, additional CT scans are often indicated.

CT scans. CT scans with axial, coronal, sagittal and 3D images are mandatory if facial fractures are suspected, but should be ordered by a specialist, if possible. Coronal and sagittal images are necessary to demonstrate the extent of isolated orbital floor fractures. For Le Fort-type midface fractures, all possible types of CT scan projections (i.e., axial, coronal, and sagittal, as well as 3D reconstruction) should be used in the preoperative work, to obtain the best possible overview of the extent of the fractures. Newer CT machines may completely replace conventional radiographic examinations, because both OPG and dental X-rays are possible.

MRI. An MRI is not used for standard facial injury examinations. It may however, provide useful information about injuries to the eye and the surrounding soft tissue as well as in evaluation of temporomandibular joint trauma.

Specific Diagnoses—Common Injuries

Grazes

Grazes occur frequently.

- Symptoms and signs: Superficial wounds limited to the epidermis and dermis are caused by falls on a rough surface (see Figure 4.10).
- Diagnosis: The diagnosis is made clinically by inspection (and palpation) of the injured area after dirt has been removed.
- Treatment by physician: Abrasions are partial damage to the skin. Abrasions heal by re-epithelialization. Wounds that are penetrated by dirt particles often heal with permanent tattooing if the particles are not removed. If the graze has much dirt, cleaning is a painful procedure, and sometimes it must be done under general anesthesia.
- Prognosis: Healing is usually uncomplicated if the wound is protected by a thin layer of antibiotic ointment and cleaned daily, to remove exudative residue. Occlusive dressings have been shown to improve healing of skin lesions rather than the traditional approach of open or "dry" wound dressing.

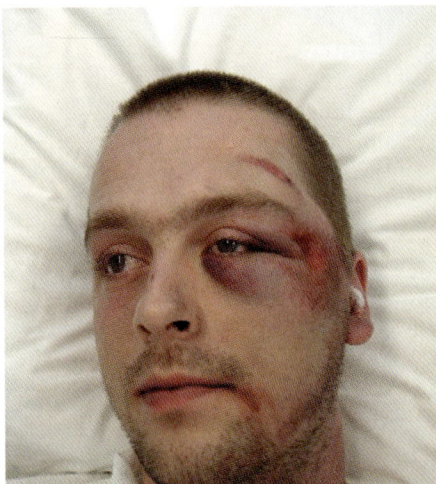

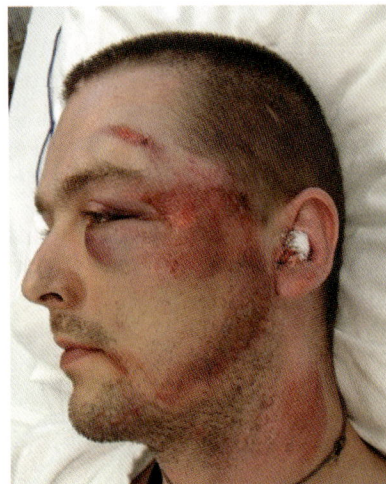

Figure 4.10 Abrasion. Facial grazes after falling while rollerblading.

Soft Tissue Contusions

Blows and pinching injuries are among the most frequent soft-tissue injuries in sport.

- Symptoms and signs: Ruptures of small veins, with bleeding in the skin, cause redness and variable degrees of hematoma formation in the affected area.
- Diagnosis: The diagnosis is made clinically by inspection and palpation of the injured area, after dirt has been removed.
- Treatment by physician: After underlying fractures have been excluded, the most important task is to reduce inflammatory reactions. Elevation of the head and ice packs during the first 2–4 hours will counteract swelling and discomfort. After 48 hours, the acute inflammatory phase begins to subside. Paracetamol and glucocorticoids have been documented to reduce swelling and pain in the facial area.
- Prognosis: Most contusion injuries require no further treatment after 48 hours and heal spontaneously in 1–2 weeks.

Lacerations/Cuts

Cuts include tears and puncture wounds that are often caused by sport equipment penetrating the skin. For example, cuts are often caused by knobs on soccer shoes, spiked shoes, and sharp edges on ski equipment.

- Symptoms and signs: Less complicated cuts and punctures are usually superficial.
- Diagnosis: If the wound is deep, a neurological examination must be performed, so that nerve damage can be ruled out.
- Treatment by physician: Superficial tears and puncture wounds are treated with skin sutures and taping. The use of 5.0 sutures is recommended.
- Prognosis: The patient must be informed that it takes several months before facial scars are finally mature. Martial arts practitioners, in particular, must be informed that resuming the sport too soon after the injury may lead to complications during the healing period. For the first 6 months, scars must be protected from the sun by applying sun block or bandages to prevent hyperpigmentation.

Nasal Fractures

Fractures of the nasal skeleton are among the most frequent types of sport injuries to the face:

- Symptoms and signs: Symptoms and signs of nasal fractures are malalignment of the nasal skeleton, hematoma, and soft-tissue swelling.
- Diagnosis: For a proper diagnosis, the practitioner must evaluate the following: blows to the nasal area, mobility and crepitation of the nasal skeleton, bleeding, swelling, hematoma, and reduced airflow in the nose. Nasal fractures are diagnosed radiographically, using lateral images, but the need to surgically treat a nasal injury depends on the clinical evaluation (see Figures 4.11a, 4.11b, 4.11c).
- Treatment by physician: The patient should be referred to an ear, nose, and throat specialist. Septum hematoma must be evacuated. Closed nasal bone reposition is the most common treatment. This should be done either immediately after the injury or 3–7 days later, when the swelling is reduced.
- Prognosis: The prognosis is good. The patient should wear a protective splint or face mask for 4 weeks when participating in training or competition.

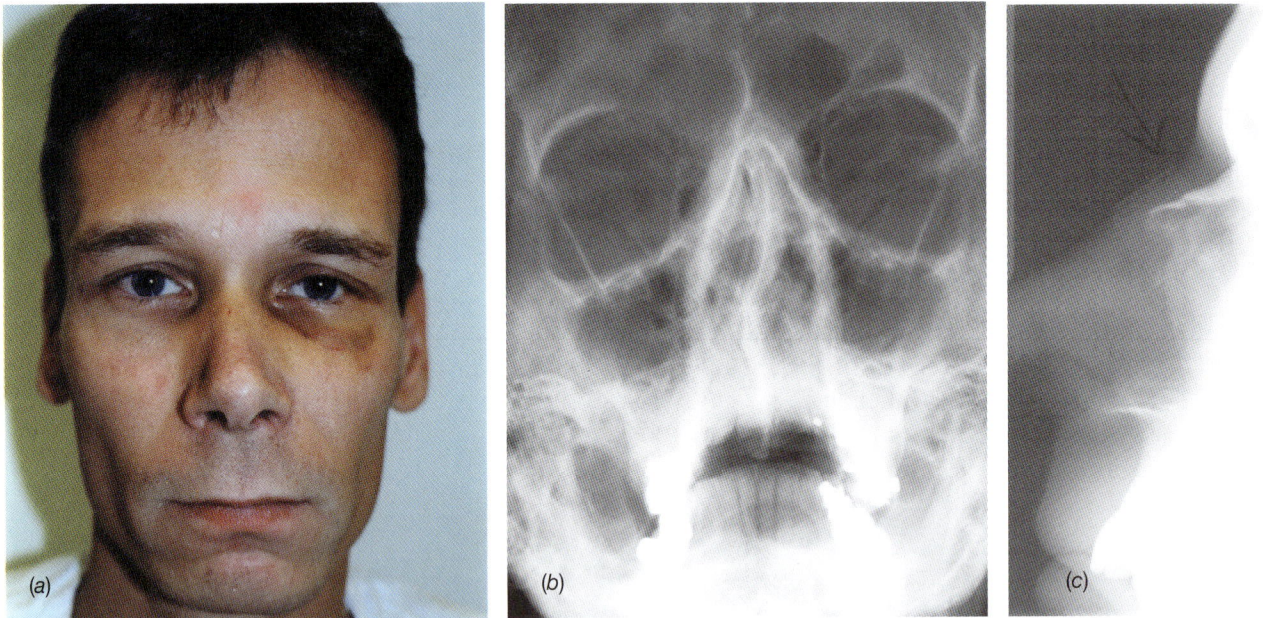

Figure 4.11 Nasal fracture with deviation of the bridge of the nose. The sagittal view shows a nasal bone fracture (a). The frontal view demonstrates traumatic septum deviation (b). Nasal fracture with deviation (c).

Mandibular Fractures

Mandibular fractures are the second most common group (13–45%) of sport-related facial injuries. They are usually caused by a blow to the lower jaw, such as may occur in fighting and team sports. Falls in which the lower jaw or the chin hits a hard surface are another common injury mechanism.

- Symptoms and signs: Symptoms and signs of mandibular fractures are malocclusion, pathological mobility and anesthesia of the inferior alveolar nerve. Fractures of the joint may cause laceration and bleeding from the ears.
- Diagnosis: Definite signs of a fracture are changes in occlusion resulting from differences in the level of the tooth row and mobility in the area of the fracture. The standard radiographic examination is an OPG (see Figures 4.12a and 4.12b) or CT scans. Fractures of the joint causes deviation of the chin when opening the mouth.
- Treatment by physician: Most mandibular fractures should be treated by a specialist. To achieve proper occlusion, the fractured fragments must be anatomically reduced and then fixed using mini titanium plates. Mandibular fixation is always used intraoperatively but is seldom needed after surgery. Soft food is recommended for 4 weeks. Temporomandibular joint fractures with fracture lines in the joint area are difficult to operate on and are treated conservatively with intermaxillary fixation for 3–6 weeks.
- Prognosis: The prognosis depends on the extent and the location of the fracture. If proper occlusion is achieved after the operation, the prognosis is good. Fractures in the joint may cause permanent malocclusion and reduced mouth opening ability.

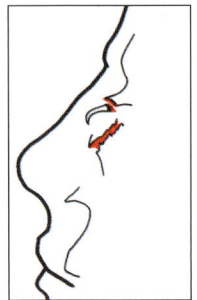

Zygomatic Fracture

Typical cheekbone fractures involve fractures in the suture lines between the zygoma and the adjacent bones (sphenoid, frontal, maxilla, and temporal bone) (see Figures 4.13a and 4.13b). Cheekbone fractures are the third most common sport

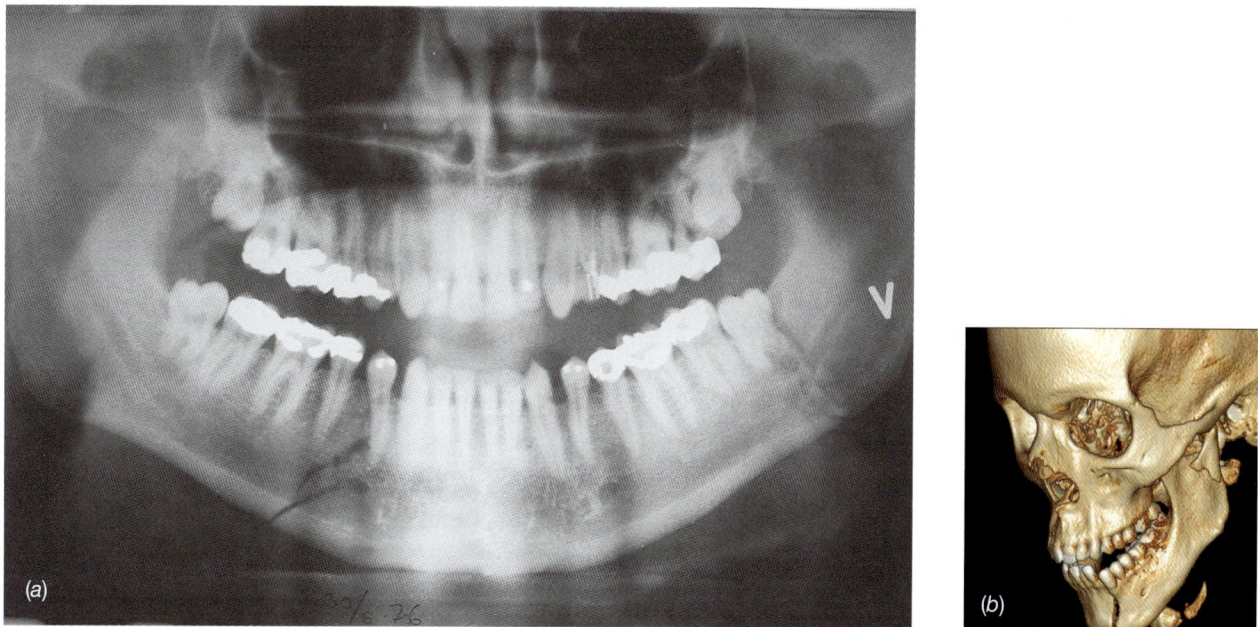

Figure 4.12 Mandibular fracture. The orthopanthomogram (OPG) demonstrates a right-side subcondylar fracture, a right-side angulus fracture, and a left-side body fracture (*a*). The three-dimensional reconstructed CT image illustrates a paramedial mandibular fracture and a subcondylar fracture (*b*). (Reproduced with permission from the Norwegian Sports Medicine Association.)

injury to the face. In case of an impending injury, the athlete will often turn the head to the side, making the cheekbone more vulnerable to injury.

• Symptoms and signs: The clinical presentation of a cheekbone fracture is a flattening of the prominence of the cheekbone. If the cheekbone is pressed inward, it may be difficult for the patient to open the mouth wide. Double vision and nerve injury corresponding to the infraorbital nerve are symptoms of a fracture in the orbital floor. Isolated fractures of the zygomatic arch can be palpated.

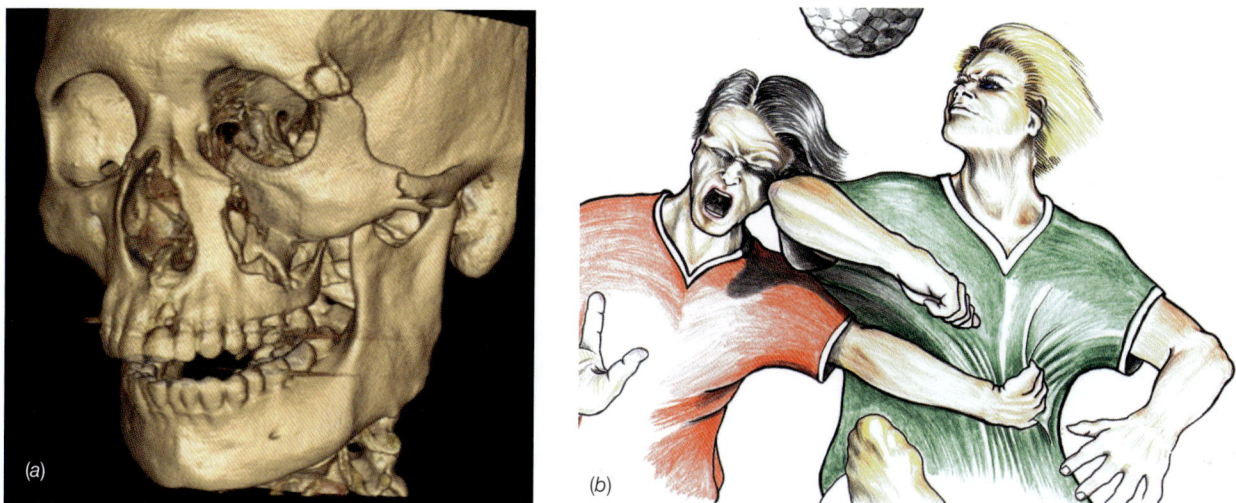

Figure 4.13 Zygomatic fracture. Dislocated left-side zygomatic fracture (*a*). A common injury mechanism is trauma to the cheekbone (*b*). (© Medical Illustrator Tommy Bolic, Sweden.)

- Diagnosis: Dislocations and broken edges that can be palpated on the infraorbital rim, the intraoral zygomaticomaxillary buttresses, and the lateral orbital rim are definite signs of a fracture. A CT scan (with axial and coronal views) provides the best imaging.
- Treatment by physician: Treatment consists of open reposition and plate osteosynthesis. If the lateral orbital floor is fractured, the herniated orbital content is reduced and the orbital floor is reconstructed. A facial injury specialist should treat these injuries.
- Prognosis: The extent of the fracture and the possibility for surgery immediately after the injury determine the result. Secondary corrections are generally considered difficult, as they require a more extensive approach for reconstruction with several osteotomies prior to reduction and refixation.

Tooth Luxation

Tooth luxations (dislocations) are divided into subtotal and total luxations. Subluxation often occurs when the alveolus is fractured, causing the tooth to be luxated out of normal position. Total luxation is complete avulsion of the tooth. In these cases the alveolus is often without fractures.

- Symptoms and signs: The tooth is subluxated or completely knocked out of the alveolus.
- Diagnosis: Diagnosis is made through a clinical examination.
- Treatment by dentist: The treatment of subtotal luxations consists of reposition in the proper anatomic position and fixation with the help of an arch bar. The fixation period is 4 weeks. For total luxation, vital tissue on the root surface must be treated carefully. The outcome of the treatment depends on how long the tooth is outside the alveolus and in which medium it is stored. Ideally, the tooth should be put back in the alveolus immediately and held in place with the patient's mouthguard or a foil splint until an urgent dental consultation is achieved. The ultimate prognosis of tooth replantation depends upon its time out of the mouth. In general, once a tooth has been out for more than 20 minutes, the chances of a successful replantation are reduced substantially.

If the tooth is contaminated, it should be carefully cleaned in sterile saline. It must not be scrubbed as the periodontal cells critical for healing may be damaged. The best temporary storage media are sterile saline, saliva or milk. The tooth is reimplanted as quickly as possible and fixed using an arch bar for 1–2 weeks, if the alveolus is intact. In case of total luxations and alveolar fractures, fixation time is 4 weeks. Prophylactic antibiotic treatment is recommended.

- Prognosis: Teeth that have not completed root growth may be revitalized. If root growth is complete, root canal treatment should be undertaken 7–10 days after luxation. Even after successful replantation the root may be resorbed after some time. While replantation of permanent frontal teeth should be the prime goal in children and adolescents due to facial growth patterns, a dental implant should always be considered as an alternative to replantation in adults.

Tooth Fracture

Tooth fractures are divided into crown fractures and root fractures (see Figures 4.14a and 14.4b).

• Symptoms and signs: Crown fractures may occur without or with pulp exposure. If the crown of the tooth is bleeding, the pulp is exposed. Malalignment of the entire crown of the tooth is another sign.
• Diagnosis: Diagnosis is made by clinical examination and (radiography) dental X-rays.
• Treatment by dentist: Normally, crown fractures are reconstructed with dental materials. If the pulp is open, root canal filling is usually necessary. In children, however, because the growth of the root of the tooth is not complete, only the upper portion of the pulp is removed. Split or longitudinal fractures result in extraction of the tooth. Root fractures are treated by exact repositioning of the crown of the tooth using a stable arch bar. The brace should be worn for 2–3 months.
• Prognosis: The esthetic result is often very good for crown fractures without opening of the pulp. Pulp opening and subsequent root filling may cause varying degrees of discoloration of the tooth. The prognosis for root fractures is good if the fracture ends are slightly displaced. If dislocation of the crown fragments is substantial, fracture healing is not very likely. Root filling of these teeth must be done early.

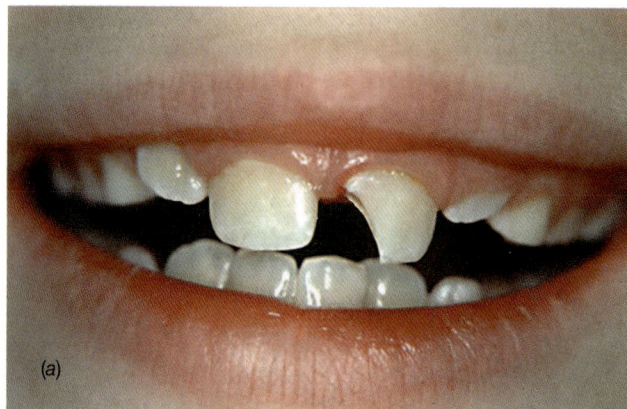

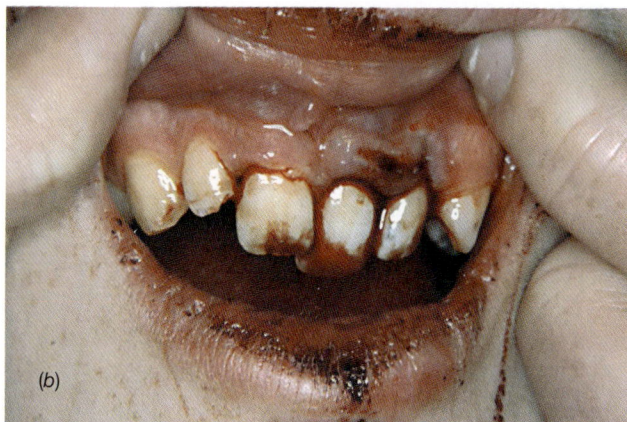

Other Specific Diagnoses

Soft-Tissue Loss

Extensive facial injuries with tissue loss are rare in sport. They occasionally occur as a result of horseback riding, skiing, and bicycling accidents (see Figures 4.15).

• Symptoms and signs: Extensive soft-tissue injuries are often combinations of lacerations, abrasions, and contusions.

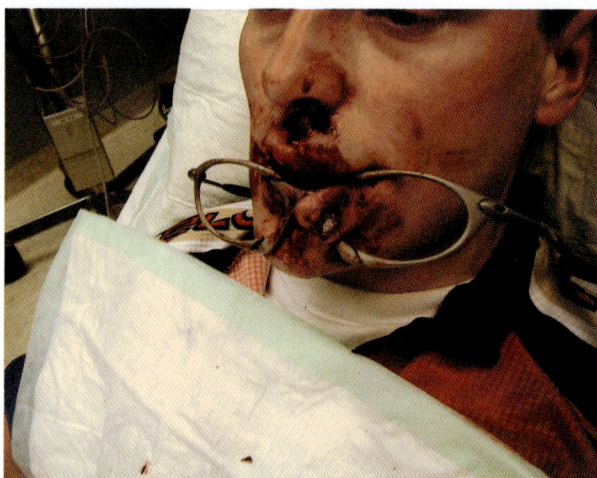

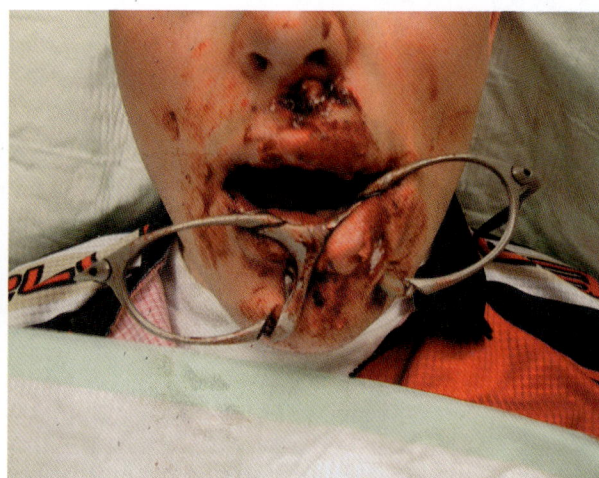

(a)

(b)

Figure 4.14 Crown and root fractures. Crown fracture with exposed pulp (a). Root fracture with a dislocated crown fragment (b). (Reproduced with permission from the Norwegian Sports Medicine Association.)

Figure 4.15 Soft-tissue injury. A bicyclist who got his own glasses stuck in his lower lip. (Reproduced with permission from the Norwegian Sports Medicine Association.)

HEAD AND FACE

- Diagnosis: Initially, this type of injury is examined carefully after a thorough cleaning. If palpation indicates an injury to the underlying bone structure, the athlete must be sent for radiographic clarification. The trigeminal nerve and facial nerve must be tested for skin sensation and motor innervation.
- Treatment by physician: Debridement must be conservative for star-shaped wounds, so that enough tissue is kept to allow closing, thus preventing displacement of neighboring structures. Major defects require plastic reconstructive techniques.
- Prognosis: This treatment often has a surprisingly good outcome, with few disfiguring scars.

Intraoral Soft-tissue Injuries—*Soft-tissue Injuries in the Oral Cavity*

The most frequent injuries occur to the lips and the anterior part of the mucous membrane of the mouth. Injuries to the buccal mucosa and to the palate are rare:

- Symptoms and signs: Symptoms and signs are bleeding from the oral cavity and lips and, frequently, hematoma and swelling shortly after the injury occurs.
- Diagnosis: The physician must thoroughly inspect and palpate the injured area. This requires good light and suction.
- Treatment by physician: The principles that apply for extraoral soft-tissue injuries also apply for intraoral injuries. The use of ointments and bandages is unnecessary. Suturing with 3.0 resorbable sutures is recommended. In the lip area, single 5.0 nonresorbable sutures are recommended. Precise suturing of the red-white lip line is key. The sutures are removed after 7 days. Good oral hygiene is maintained by rinsing with chlorhexidine gluconate, because it may be difficult for the patient to brush the teeth.
- Prognosis: Normally, wounds in the oral cavity heal without complications.

Frontal Bone Fracture

Fractures of the forehead are often caused by a blow to the lower portion of the forehead and are typically the result of (being kicked by a horse or of) head duels in soccer. These fractures are rare: They represent only 2% of sport-related injuries to the face.

- Symptoms and signs: Visible or palpable depressions in the area above the frontal sinus indicate frontal bone fracture (see Figure 4.16).
- Diagnosis: A definite sign of a fracture is a palpable depression with crepitation in the anterior wall of the frontal sinus. Sensory deficit in the area of innervation of the supraorbital nerve is also considered a sign of a fracture in this area. To exclude a frontobasal injury, the doctor must always order a CT scan.
- Treatment by physician: Fractures with depression of the anterior wall of the frontal sinus may cause

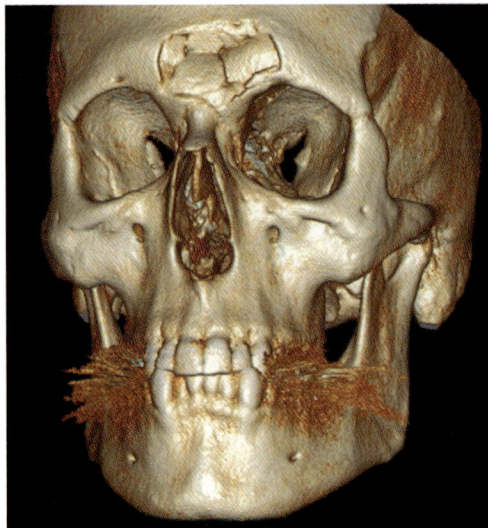

Figure 4.16 The three-dimensional reconstructed CT image illustrates an impression fracture of the forehead. (Reproduced with permission from the Norwegian Sports Medicine Association.)

aesthetic and functional sinus problems. Surgery is often recommended. If there are fractures of both the anterior and the posterior wall of the frontal sinus, with air intracranially and liquorrhea as signs of dura damage, further treatment must be given, in collaboration with a neurosurgeon.

• Prognosis: The prognosis is good. For larger injuries, the prognosis depends on additional intracranial injuries.

Orbital Fracture—*Eye Socket Fracture*

Fractures of the orbit includes the floor, medial wall, roof and lateral wall. Lateral wall dislocation indicates that there is a zygomatic fracture. Roof fractures are seen in frontal fractures. Blunt trauma to the orbital region results in fractures of the floor and medial wall (blow-out fractures). Blow-out fractures are among the least common sport injuries. The classic causes are tennis or squash balls hitting the eye. The most common orbital floor fractures seen are those caused by running into elbows or fists during team sports. Fractures of the infraorbital rim are a relatively common result of this type of injury:

• Symptoms and signs: Findings that indicate fractures are periorbital swelling, monocle hematomas, lateral subconjunctival bleeding, recessed eyeball (enophthalmos), inferiorly positioned eyeball (hypophthalmos), sensory deficit in the area of the infraorbital nerve, limited ocular movements, and double vision.
• Diagnosis: A CT scan of the orbit with coronal, axial and sagittal sections provides a good overview of fractures in the orbit (see Figure 4.17).
• Treatment by physician: Indications for surgical intervention are mainly diplopia caused by enlargement of the orbit with hypophthalmos and enophthalmos.
• Prognosis: The extent of the fracture and the possibility of surgery immediately after the injury determine the outcome. Secondary corrections are often difficult, and the results are not as good as they are for immediate surgery.

"The White Eye Syndrome" *!*

In young persons, trauma to the orbital region may cause a green-stick fracture in the floor that traps the inferior rectus muscle:

• Symptoms and signs: Upward rotation of the eye is restricted (Figure 4.18).

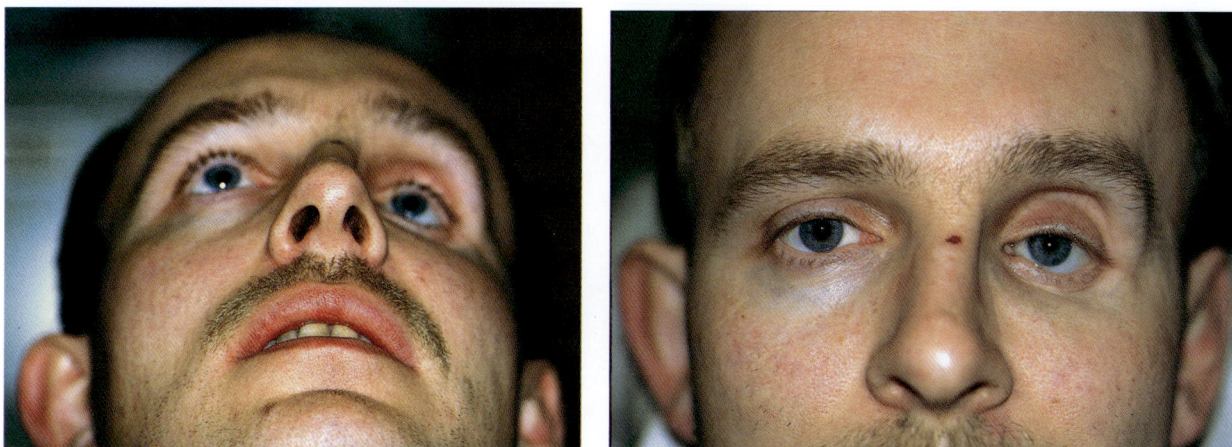

Figure 4.17 Orbital fracture with enophthalmos and hypophthalmos. Injury to the orbital floor may lower the position of the bulb, whereas fractures in the floor and walls increase the volume of the orbit and causes a recessed eyeball. (Reproduced with permission from the Norwegian Sports Medicine Association.)

- **Diagnosis:** Diagnosis is based on recent trauma and restricted upward rotation. CT is not necessary and delays treatment.
- **Treatment by physician:** This is an emergency that needs surgical intervention within 24 hours to avoid permanent damage to the muscle.

Retrobulbar Hematoma !

Trauma to the orbital region may cause retrobulbar bleeding (Figure 4.19). This may cause an orbital compartment syndrome that affects circulation and nerve function:

- **Symptoms and signs:** Elevated, protruded, red eye. Gradual loss of vision and eye movement (the ability to move the eye).
- **Diagnosis:** A history of trauma and the findings described in the preceding text is sufficient for diagnosis. CT or MRI scans may verify the diagnosis, but valuable time is lost.
- **Treatment by physician:** A lateral canthotomy should be performed as fast as possible to save vision. This procedure can be done in local anesthesia.

Maxillary Fracture—*Midface Fracture* !

Maxillary fractures result from trauma to the midface. The result is a loosening of (1) the upper jaw (Le Fort I); (2) the upper jaw with the nasal bone (Le Fort II); or (3) the entire midface with the upper jaw, cheekbone, and nasal bones (Le Fort III) (see Figure 4.20). Sport-related Le Fort fractures are rare and make up only 1–3% of all sport injuries to the face. The most common injury mechanisms are falls from great heights, high-speed trauma, winter sport trauma, and bicycling and climbing accidents:

- **Symptoms and signs:** Malocclusion combined with(problems involving mobility of the upper jaw or the central or entire midface and bleeding are characteristics of all Le Fort fractures. Typical symptoms are periorbital hematoma (raccoon eyes), rhinorrhea, and backward and downward dislocation of the midface (dish face) with anterior open bite.
- **Diagnosis:** Definite signs of fracture are changes in occlusion combined with mobility in the upper jaw or midface. A CT scan provides the best overview.

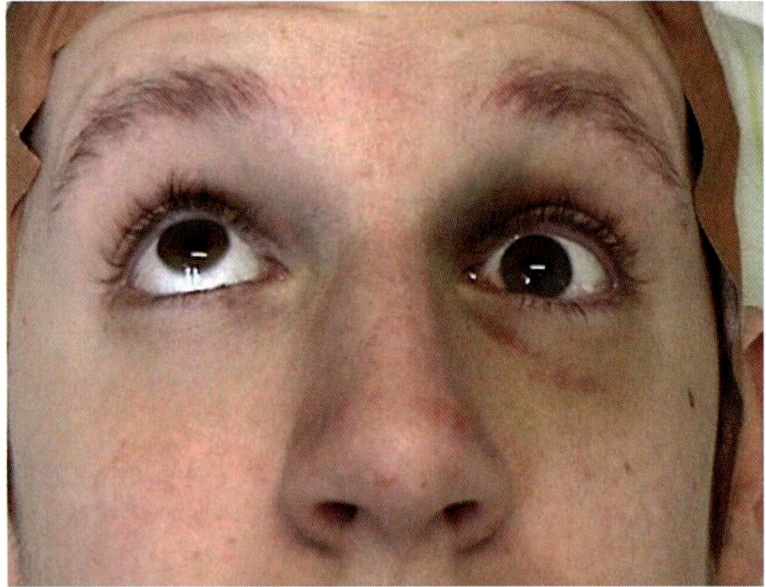

Figure 4.18 Youth with white eye syndrome after trampoline accident. (Reproduced with permission from the Norwegian Sports Medicine Association.)

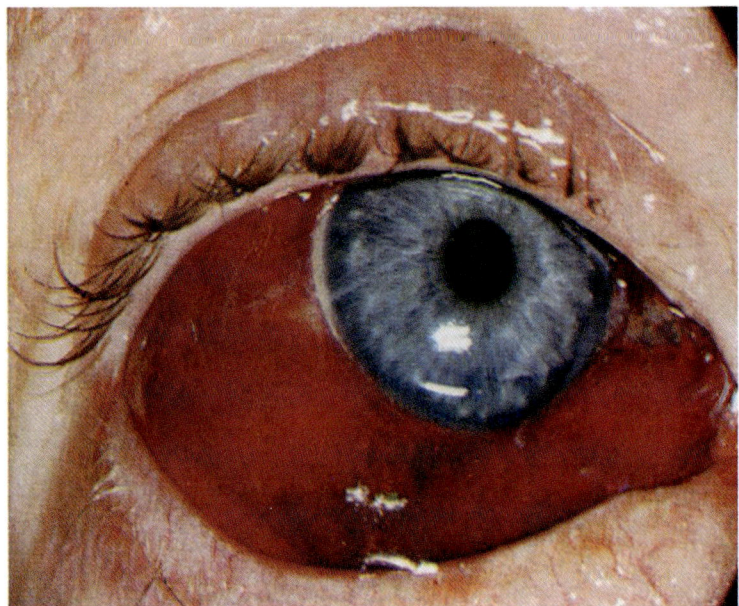

Figure 4.19 Retrobulbar hematoma. (Reproduced with permission from the Norwegian Sports Medicine Association.)

- Treatment by physician: Maxillary injuries should be treated by a facial injury specialist. Dislocated fragments are reduced and fixed using titanium plates.
- Prognosis: The extent of the fracture and the possibility for surgical intervention immediately after the injury determine the result. Secondary corrections are difficult to make, and the results are not as good as the results of immediate correction.

Nasoorbitoethmoid Fracture—*Combined Nose and Lacrimal Bone Fractures* !

Nasoorbitoethmoid fractures are localized to the area between the eyes, consisting of the nasal bone (and), the frontal process of maxilla, the lacrimal bone and the ethmoid bone. (see Figure 4.21). These bones are thin and fracture easily. Therefore, parts of the nasal complex can be pushed posteriorly and laterally. This may cause damage to the lacrimal canal and the medial attachment of the eyelids (canthal ligament). The medial attachment of the eyelids may become loose and displaced laterally.

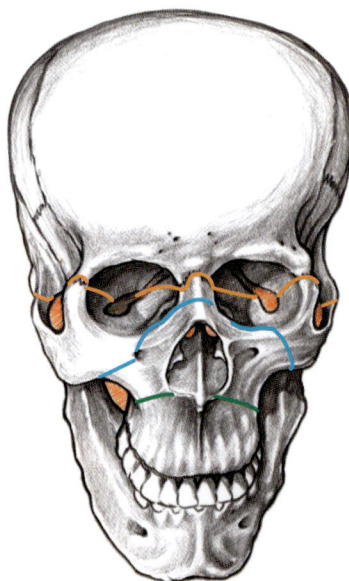

Figure 4.20 Le Fort I–III fractures. The most common fracture lines in the midface. (© Medical Illustrator Tommy Bolic, Sweden.)

- Symptoms and signs: Symptoms and signs include the depressed bridge of the nose, an increased distance between the medial canthi (telecanthus), a changed palpebral aperture (doll's eye), and a turned-up apex of the nose.
- Diagnosis: Diagnosis is made using a CT scan and is indicated by an increased distance between the canthi combined with a fractures in the area.
- Treatment by physician: A specialist in facial injuries should treat this type of injury.
- Prognosis: The prognosis depends on the complexity of the fracture. A good outcome depends on surgery immediately after the injury occurs, with exact repositioning of the bone fragments and canthal ligaments (canthopexy). Secondary corrections are very difficult, and the results are not as good as the results of immediate correction.

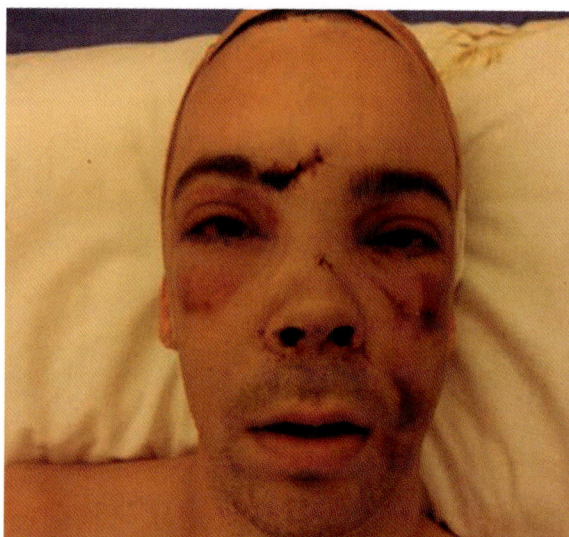

Figure 4.21 Nasoorbitoethmoid fracture. The typically depressed root of the nose, turned up apex and telecanthus.

Panfacial Fractures—*Multiple Fractures in the Facial Skeleton* !

Panfacial fractures are caused by major trauma to the face. They include multiple fractures in the facial skeleton (i.e., the forehead, cheekbone, nose, upper jaw, and lower jaw):

- Symptoms and signs: Symptoms and signs are total crushing of the face, with pathological movement of the fragments; and flattened, widened, and lengthened midface, combined with occlusion problems.
- Diagnosis: Clinical examination and CT scan.
- Treatment by physician: A facial injury specialist must treat this type of fracture. Extensive exposure of the facial skeleton combined with careful repositioning and plate fixation in a given sequence is required. Lost bone is replaced with calvary bone grafts.
- Prognosis: Prognosis is good when the fragments are properly reduced.

Alveolar Ridge Fracture

Alveolar ridge fractures are segment jaw fractures with two or more teeth (see Figure 4.22):

- Symptoms and signs: Symptoms and signs are abnormal mobility of the tooth segment, changes in occlusion, differences in the level of the tooth row, bleeding, and injuries to the mucous membrane.
- Diagnosis: The diagnosis is made radiologically, with OPG and dental X-rays; and clinically, by mobility of the tooth segment.
- Treatment by physician: The physician performs repositioning and fixation of the fractured fragment with the help of arch bars. The bars are used for 4 weeks. If insufficient stability is achieved using labial arches, the patient must have intermaxillary fixation for a few weeks. Open reposition using plates may cause healing problems in the form of poor circulation to the reduced fragments and is seldom used.

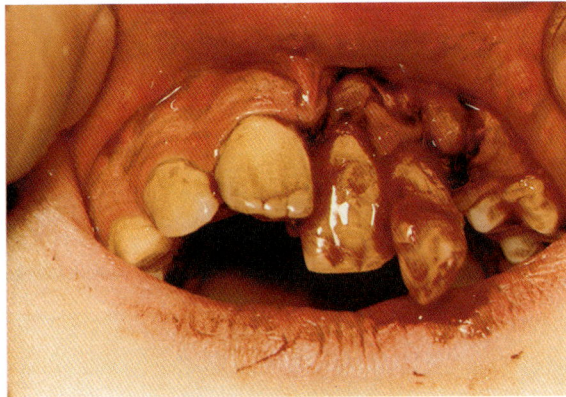

Figure 4.22 Alveolar ridge fracture. Fracture of the tooth alveolus with subluxation of the teeth. (Reproduced with permission from the Norwegian Sports Medicine Association.)

- Prognosis: The result depends on reduction of the injured fragments. If this is done correctly, permanent changes in bite are avoided. A dentist must evaluate the teeth with respect to the need for root canal treatment.

Foreign Object in the Eye

Specks of dust often get stuck in the tarsal sulcus on the inside of the upper eyelid.

Blinking is painful and may cause epithelium damage on the cornea:

- Symptoms and signs: Symptoms and signs are pain, red eye, and tearing.
- Diagnosis: The foreign object is visible when the eyelid is examined by turning it inside out.
- Treatment by physician: Foreign objects are removed, possibly after anesthetization with oxybuprocaine eye drops. Antibiotic ointment for 3 or 4 days is recommended as an infection prophylactic.

Corneal Erosion !

Contact with branches, fingernails, or other objects often cause wounds on the cornea (see Figure 4.23):

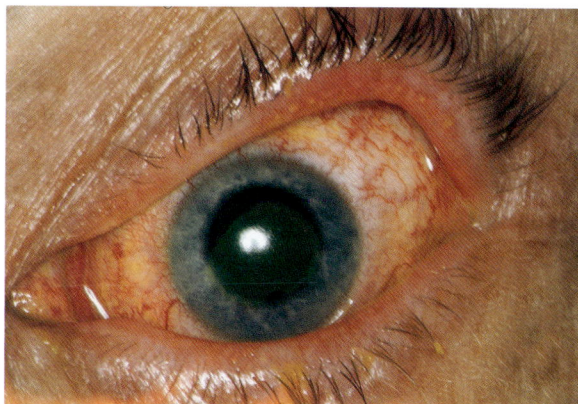

Figure 4.23 Corneal erosion. Fluorescein-colored corneal erosion. (Reproduced with permission from the Norwegian Sports Medicine Association.)

- Symptoms and signs: Strong pain, tearing, eyelid cramps (blepharospasm), sensitivity to light, and blurred vision are symptoms and signs of corneal erosion.
- Diagnosis: Diagnosis is made by fluorescein solution, which colors erosion.
- Treatment by physician: Local antibiotics, such as chloramphenicol ointment overnight, and perioral analgesics are used. Diclofenac eye drops may be tried.
- Prognosis: In most cases, healing occurs within 24 hours.

Contusion of the Eyeball !

Contusion of the eyeball (see Figure 4.24) may be caused by direct blows to the eye (boxing), a ball in the eye (squash), crashing into a hard object, and falling accidents.

- Symptoms and signs: Tearing, light sensitivity, and blepharospasm (cramps of the eyelid) are signs and symptoms of contusion of the eyeball.
- Diagnosis: Diagnosis is made if any of the following have occurred: swelling and bleeding in the eyelid, subconjunctival bleeding, corneal edema, corneal damage, bleeding in the anterior chamber

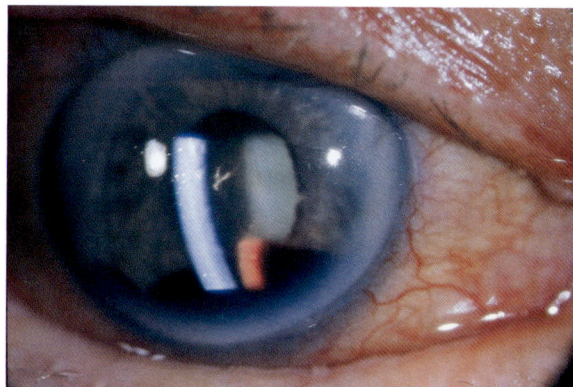

Figure 4.24 Contusion of the eyeball. Bleeding in the anterior chamber and the iris. (Reproduced with permission from the Norwegian Sports Medicine Association.)

(hyphema), separation of the iris (iridodialysis), traumatic paresis of the pupil (mydriasis, oval pupil), accommodation paresis, lens damage or dislocation, bleeding in the vitreous, retinal damage (bleeding or edema), or damage to the optic nerve.
- Treatment by physician: The physician should examine the eye while it is under surface anesthesia, and refer the patient to an ophthalmologist. Blunt trauma to the eyeball may have serious consequences. The diagnosis may be difficult to make, because several areas of the eye may be injured. For this reason, the threshold for referral to an ophthalmologist should be low.
- Prognosis: Prognosis depends on the extent of the injury and the possibility of treatment by an ophthalmologist.

Perforation of the Eyeball !

Ski poles in the eye, bow and arrow shooting accidents, and accidents with other sharp objects frequently cause eye perforation (see Figure 4.25). Ruptures of the eye may also be caused by powerful blunt contusion trauma. In that case, the eye ruptures at the weak points (along the limbus and the optic nerve):

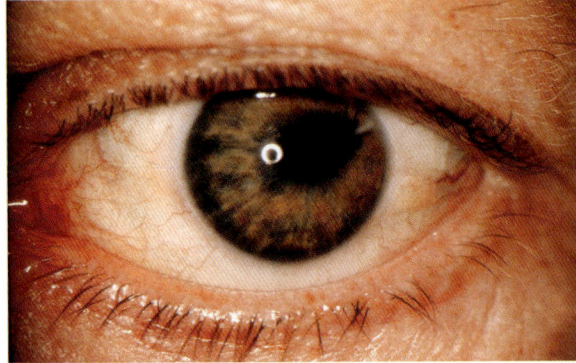

Figure 4.25 Perforation of the eyeball. Perforated eye that is not circular. Contusion changes of the pupil. (Reproduced with permission from the Norwegian Sports Medicine Association.)

• Symptoms and signs: The case history is crucial. Perforation may be difficult to see. If perforation is suspected, the patient should be sent to the nearest ophthalmology department. The parenteral use of an antibiotic prophylactic (e.g., benzylpenicillin) may be necessary if transport will take a long time. It is critical that the patient avoids straining or coughing otherwise extrusion of the intraocular contents may result. Consideration of the use of a parenteral antiemetic during transport is recommended.

• Diagnosis: A specialist confirms the diagnosis.

• Treatment by physician: Treatment of a perforated eyeball must be done by a specialist.

• Prognosis: Prognosis depends on the extent of the injury.

Rehabilitation of Acute Head and Facial Injuries

Paul McCrory[1,2], Peter D. le Roux[3], Michael Turner[4], Ingunn R. Kirkeby[5], and Karen M. Johnston[6]

[1]University of Melbourne, Melbourne, VIC, Australia
[2]Monash University, Frankston, VIC, Australia
[3]University of Pennsylvania, Philadelphia, PA, USA
[4]British Horseracing Authority, London, UK
[5]Oslo University Hospital, Rikshospitalet, Sognsveien, Oslo, Norway
[6]University of Toronto, Toronto, ON, Canada

Goals and Principles

Table 4.7 lists the goals for rehabilitation of acute head and facial injuries.

The functional outcome in patients who have sustained an acute head injury varies greatly. Fortunately in sport most injuries are mild and recover rapidly without any lasting sequelae. In contrast, moderate and severe traumatic brain injuries have a variable and unpredictable outcome. Lasting problems include both mental (such as personality changes and memory deficit) and physical (such as hemiparesis and speech disturbance).

The goal of rehabilitation of patients with severe head injuries is to get the patient back to a level of function in which he is as independent of others as possible. In the best case, the patient will return to the level he was at before the injury. In principle, rehabilitation of patients with serious head injuries begins at the hospital immediately after the injury or operation. Most rehabilitation occurs during the first 6 months after the injury, but it is not until a year later that there is any degree of certainty about which level the patient will attain. However, the rehabilitation potential of many patients extends beyond one year. Physical therapy and occupational therapy are not only vital in reducing contractures and improving strength in the extremities, but also for stimulating the patient's own motivation.

	Goals	Measures
Phase 1	Prevent secondary brain damage	Acute treatment at the proper level of care
Phase 2	Mobilization and regaining primary functions	Practical help from physical and occupational therapists
Phase 3	Complete recovery of lost functions	Specialized rehabilitation program

Table 4.7 Goals and measures for rehabilitation of head injuries. (Reproduced with permission from the Norwegian Sports Medicine Association.)

Return to Sport

Concussion

Return to play decisions remains difficult. Expert consensus guidelines recommend that players should *not* be returned to competition until they have recovered *completely* from their concussive injury. Currently, however there is no single gold standard measure of brain disturbance and recovery following concussion. Instead, clinicians must rely on indirect measures to inform clinical judgment. In practical terms, this involves a multifaceted clinical approach, which includes assessment of symptoms, physical signs (such as balance) and cognitive function.

The general management principle is that no return to play on the day should be contemplated for a concussed athlete. It is not within the scope or expertise of a physiotherapist, trainer or non-medical person to manage a concussive injury or determine the timing of return to play. A player should never return to play while symptomatic. "When in doubt, sit them out!"

The cornerstone of concussion management is physical and cognitive rest until symptoms resolve and then a graded program of exertion prior to medical clearance and return to play (see "Concussion injury advice" page 4 of SCAT2 form; Figure 4.2). Similarly, the use of alcohol, narcotic analgesics, anti-inflammatory medication or sedatives can exacerbate symptoms following head trauma, delay recovery or mask deterioration and should also be avoided. Specific advice should also be given on avoidance of activities that place the individual at risk of further injury (e.g., driving).

Following a concussive injury, players should be returned to play in a graduated fashion once clinical features have resolved and cognitive function returned to "baseline." When considering return to play, the athlete should be off all medications at the time of considering commencement of the rehabilitation phase or at the final medical assessment. There is no mandatory period of time that a player must be withheld from play following a concussion. However, at the very minimum, a player must be symptom free at rest and with exertion, and determined to have returned to baseline level of cognitive performance. A stepwise Graduated Return to Play Protocol is recommended (Table 4.8).

Rehabilitation stage	Functional exercise at each stage of rehabilitation	Objective at each stage
1. No activity	Complete physical and cognitive rest	Recovery
2. Light aerobic exercise	Walking, swimming or stationary cycling keeping intensity <70% HR max. No resistance training.	Increase heart rate
3. Sport-specific exercise	Skating drills in ice hockey, running drills in soccer. No head impact activities.	Add movement.
4. Noncontact training drills	Progression to more complex training drills, for example, passing drills in hockey and football.	Exercise, coordination and cognitive load
5. Full contact practice	Following medical clearance participate in normal training activities	Restore confidence and assess functional skills by coaching staff
6. Return to play	Normal game play	

Table 4.8 Graduated return to play protocol. (Reproduced with permission from the Norwegian Sports Medicine Association.)

If a player remains asymptomatic for 24 hours at level 1, they may progress to level 2. They are allowed to advance provided that they remain asymptomatic. Using this protocol, an athlete should take approximately a week before returning to normal game play. If any symptoms surface during the progression, players should drop back to the previous level in which they were asymptomatic for a further 24 hours before attempting to progress.

A player who has suffered from a concussive injury must not be allowed to return to play before having a medical clearance. In every case, the decision regarding the timing of return to training should be made by a medical doctor with experience in concussive injuries.

Children younger than 10-year-old report different symptoms, so age and developmentally appropriate evaluation is recommended. An additional consideration in assessing the child or adolescent athlete with a concussion is that in the clinical evaluation by the healthcare professional there may be the need to include both patient and parent input as well as teacher and school input when appropriate. Children should not be returned to practice or play until clinically completely symptom free, which may require a longer time frame than for adults. In addition, the concept of "cognitive rest" is highlighted with special reference to a child's need to limit exertion with activities of daily living and to limit scholastic and other cognitive stressors (e.g., text messaging, videogames) while symptomatic. School attendance and activities may also need to be modified to avoid provocation of symptoms.

Screening computerized cognitive tests are strongly encouraged in the routine management of concussion in sport. Computerized tests provide a quick, valid and reliable measure of cognitive recovery following a concussive injury. These include test platforms such as Axon CCST (www.axonsports.com), ImPACT (www.impact-test.com), Headminders (www.headminders.com), and a tool developed by the US military–Automated Neuropsychological Assessment Metrics (www.armymedicine.army.mil/prr/anam.html). Overall, it is important to remember that neuropsychological testing is only one component of assessment, and, therefore, should not be the sole basis of management decisions.

Catastrophic or Severe Head Injury

Return to sport following a severe or potentially life threatening brain injury is controversial and few guidelines exist for the clinician to follow. There are some situations where the athlete could place himself at an unacceptably high risk of sustaining further injury and hence should be counseled against participation in collision sport (Table 4.9). In such situations, common sense should prevail.

- Persistent postconcussional or postinjury symptoms
- Permanent neurological sequelae—hemiplegia, visual deficit, dementia or cognitive impairment
- Hydrocephalus with or without shunting
- Spontaneous subarachnoid hemorrhage from any cause
- Symptomatic neurologic or pain producing abnormalities about the foramen magnum
- Craniotomy for evacuation of intracerebral or subdural hematoma

Table 4.9 Conditions contraindicating return to contact sport. (Reproduced with permission from the Norwegian Sports Medicine Association.)

HEAD AND FACE

Although sports physicians should keep an open mind when assessing neurological recovery from severe brain injuries nevertheless it is recommended that at least 12 months pass before such a decision is contemplated.

Thoughtful deliberation and analysis of all the available medical evidence should occur when making such a decision. It is also recommended that the counsel of a neurologist or neurosurgeon experienced in sport head injury management be sought. This is an important point because a number of individuals who suffer a moderate to severe TBI may be left with a lack of insight and impaired judgment over and above their other neurological injuries. This in turn may make such an individual unreliable in gauging recovery. The use of neuropsychological assessment as well as information from family and friends may assist the clinician in his deliberation. The assessment of cognitive performance and/or clinical symptoms when fatigued is often useful.

Return to collision sport is relatively contraindicated in almost any situation where surgical craniotomy is performed. In such situations, the subarachnoid space is traumatized thus setting up scarring of the pia-arachnoid of the brain to the dura with both loss of the normal cushioning effect of the CSF and vascular adhesions that may subsequently bleed if torn during head impact. Even if neurologic recovery is complete, a craniotomy for anything other than an extradural hematoma effectively precludes return to collision sport.

With an extradural hematoma without brain injury or other condition where surgery is not required, return to sport may be contemplated in selected cases as per the discussion in the preceding text after a minimum of 12 months assuming neurologic recover is complete.

Soft-tissue Injuries

In most cases, athletes with grazes and contusions may begin training and participate in competition shortly after the injury occurs. For cuts and extensive soft-tissue injuries with tissue loss, the practitioner must tape sutured wounds for support or protection, so that healing is not interfered with to avoid scarring. In some cases this means that the athlete must continue to take it easy until after the sutures have been removed, normally 7 days postoperatively.

Abrations should be treated with sterile ointment during the healing period, which may be for several weeks. Compression of lacerations for several weeks may reduce scarring. Meticulous initial reconstructive soft tissue surgery reduces scar formation. Revision procedures should be delayed for at least 3 months, as scars usually (may) improve over time.

Dentoalveolar Injuries

All tooth injuries that result in loosening of one or more teeth or tooth-bearing fragments require dental fixation with an arch bar. The bar is used for 1 week for luxated teeth without alveolar fractures, for 4 weeks for subluxated teeth with alveolar fractures, and for 8 weeks for root fractures. During that period, the athlete may train and compete in sports, except for martial arts and other sports where blows to the mouth and face occur. Consideration of the use of a mouthguard with improved dental protection is worthwhile. An example of this would be a custom-moulded laminated guard with or without a hard inset anteriorly depending upon the sport involved.

Fractures of the Facial Skeleton

All facial fractures take 4–6 weeks to heal. The question of whether the athlete may train or compete depends entirely on the extent of the injury and must be evaluated in every single case. In most cases, light training is possible as early as 1 week after the injury. In some cases, the athlete may participate in the sport only if he wears a special protective face mask. In most cases, the athlete is not able to compete until 3–4 weeks later.

Preventing Reinjury

It has become a widely held belief that having sustained a concussive injury, that one is then more prone to future concussive injury. The evidence for this contention is limited at best. It would seem obvious that in any collision or contact sport the risk of concussion is directly proportional to the amount of time playing the sport. Therefore the likelihood of repeat injury may simply reflect the level of exposure to injury risk. The association of an increased risk of subsequent concussions reported in players with a past history of concussion is thought to reflect a player's style of play where his risk of injury may be increased by utilizing dangerous game strategies and illegal tackling techniques.

When assessing an injured player, details regarding protective equipment employed at time of injury should be sought. The benefit of this approach allows for modification and optimization of protective behavior and an opportunity for head injury education. There are relatively few methods by which brain injury may be minimized in sport. The brain is not an organ that can be conditioned to withstand injury. Thus, extrinsic mechanisms of injury prevention must be sought.

There is no good clinical evidence that currently available protective equipment will prevent concussion although mouthguards have a definite role in preventing dental and oro-facial injury. Biomechanical studies have shown a reduction in impact forces to the brain with the use of head gear and helmets. For skiing and snowboarding there are a number of studies to suggest that helmets provide protection against head and facial injury and hence should be recommended for participants in alpine sports. In specific sports such as cycling, motor and equestrian sports, protective helmets may prevent other forms of head injury (e.g., skull fracture) that are related to falling on hard road surfaces and these may be an important injury prevention issue for those sports.

Neck muscle conditioning may be of value in reducing impact forces transmitted to the brain. Biomechanical concepts dictate that the energy from an impacting object is dispersed over the greater mass of an athlete if the head is held rigidly. Although attractive from a theoretical standpoint, there is little scientific evidence to demonstrate the effectiveness of such measures.

The major concern with the recommendation for helmet use in sport is the phenomenon known as "risk compensation," whereby helmeted athletes change their playing behavior in the misguided belief that the protective equipment will stop all injury. This is where the use of protective equipment results in behavioral change such as the adoption of more dangerous playing techniques, which can result in a paradoxical increase in injury rates. This may be a particular concern in child and adolescent athletes where head injury rates are often higher than in adult athletes.

HEAD AND FACE

As the ability to treat or reduce the effects of concussive injury after the event is minimal, education of athletes, colleagues and those working with them as well as the general public is a mainstay of progress in this field. Athletes and their health care providers must be educated regarding the detection of concussion, its clinical features, assessment techniques and principles of safe return to play. Methods to improve education including various web-based resources (e.g., www.concussionsafety.com), educational videos, outreach programs, concussion working groups and the support and endorsement of enlightened sport groups must be pursued vigorously.

5 Neck and Back

Acute Neck and Back Injuries

Jens Ivar Brox[1], Mike Wilkinson[2], Robert G. Watkins III[3], Robert G. Watkins IV[3], and Roger Sørensen[1]

[1]Oslo University Hospital, Rikshospitalet, Sognsveien, Oslo, Norway
[2]Allan McGavin Sports Medicine Center, Vancouver, BC, Canada
[3]Marina Spine Center, Marina del Rey, California, CA, USA

Occurrence

In North America, the annual incidence of spinal cord injuries resulting from sport accidents is about 30 for every million inhabitants. Sport activity is the fourth most common cause of spinal column fractures, and, after traffic accidents, it is the most common cause of spinal cord injuries. About half of all sport-related spinal cord injuries result in complete quadriplegia. Therefore, the consequences for those who are affected, and for society as a whole, are significant. More than 30% of all vertebral column fractures and more than 50% of all fractures/dislocations of the cervical spine are caused by diving accidents during unorganized sport activity. Serious back injuries also occur in sports, including horseback riding, motorized sports (especially snowmobiling), parachuting, hang gliding, paragliding, climbing, ice hockey, bicycling, snowboarding, downhill skiing, and ski jumping. A recent Canadian study stated that the incidence of fractures to the spinal column was 0.01 and 0.04, per 1000 ski days, for downhill skiers and snowboarders, respectively. Most snowboarding injuries occurred in connection with jumps. Most skiing injuries occurred as a result of falls. Compression or crushing injuries total more than 70% of the fractures, with T11 and L1 as the most frequent locations. Nine percent of the snowboarders and 24% of the downhill skiers had neurological deficits. About half of those with neurological deficits had spinal cord injuries.

Annually, a reported 0.7 per 100,000 football players and 2.6 per 100,000 hockey players in American high schools sustain serious neck and back injuries. Neck injuries in youth rugby in Australia were observed in 0.7 players per 1000 hours. Forty spinal injuries were registered in Canadian ice hockey from 2000 to 2005; there were five spinal cord injuries. The most common mechanism of injury was impact with the boards (65%) and the most common cause was check/push from behind (35%). A decline was observed compared with a previous registration. This was attributed to improved education about injury prevention and/or specific rules against

Most common	Less common	Must not be overlooked ❗
Muscle contusion and rupture, p. 108	Stable thoracolumbar vertebral body fractures, p. 111	Spinal cord injuries, p. 108
	Fractures of the processus transversus or the processus spinosus, p. 112	Unstable fractures, p. 110
		Inner organ injuries (see Chapter 6)

Table 5.1 Overview of differential diagnoses of acute neck and back injuries. (Reproduced with permission from the Norwegian Sports Medicine Association.)

The IOC Manual of Sports Injuries, First Edition. Edited by Roald Bahr.
©2012 International Olympic Committee. Published 2012 by John Wiley & Sons, Ltd.

pushing/checking from behind. Helmets protect the head, but do not prevent the neck from compression or bending forward, and that is the position in which the individual is most vulnerable to neck injuries. There is no empirical basis for maintaining that the mandatory wearing of helmets reduces the occurrence of serious neck injuries. Stricter enforcement of the regulations regarding tackling or hitting from behind as put in place by the International Ice Hockey Federation and multiple hockey federations would probably be a more effective preventive measure.

In a Finnish study, 9% of all soccer injuries were found to be neck and head injuries. Most of these injuries involved neck pain that did not require specific treatment. However, the prevalence of neck pain in retired soccer players is higher than in the rest of the population, but the number with radiating symptoms or neurological signs is not known.

Differential Diagnoses

Table 5.1 contains an overview of current differential diagnoses. Direct trauma to the back may cause intense pain, which is commonly related to relatively insignificant muscle contusions. Falling with or without twisting may cause muscle ruptures, ligament damage, and/or fractures, and, less frequently, disk injuries.

Apart from following the well-accepted Advanced Trauma Life Support protocols, in sports medicine the practitioner is often in a unique position on the sideline to observe and understand the mechanism of injury and thus the forces that may cause a specific injury and the possible consequences of that injury. Most significantly spinal trauma may cause spinal cord injury. To avoid catastrophic worsening of a back injury, the athlete must be moved in the proper manner whenever there is any suspicion of a possible significant injury either through symptoms or mechanism of injury (e.g., a fall from a jump in ski or boarder cross events).

If the patient has an injury that was caused by a collision, the physician must examine the parenchymal organs (kidneys and spleen [see Chapter 6]), to exclude damage there. Such an injury may be acutely life threatening because of major internal bleeding and hypovolemic shock.

Diagnostic Process

About 80% of all spinal cord injuries occur in connection with multitrauma. Therefore, multitrauma patients must have both an initial neurological examination and repeated and extended evaluations to exclude spinal cord injuries. Many patients who sustain spinal cord injuries due to accidents have no neurological deficit when examined at the site of the accident. It is tragic when a patient is paraplegic on arrival at the hospital and initial examination findings indicated that the patient was able to move both his arms and legs before being transported to the hospital. Good knowledge of, and practical training in, emergency care and spine stabilization is the only way to avoid this type of *unnecessary* catastrophe.

A patient with a possible neck injury must not be moved from the sport facility before a competent examiner has completed a neurological examination that can demonstrate or exclude spinal cord injury or an unstable fracture where spinal cord injury may occur. If serious injuries of this type cannot be excluded, the patient's neck must be stabilized before he is moved—often under intense pressure from officials, spectators, and television (Figures 5.1a–5.1f). A recent study has demonstrated that the "lift and slide" technique for transfer combined with the Trapezius Squeeze technique for head stabilization is the most reliable method to achieve safe stabilization at the scene.

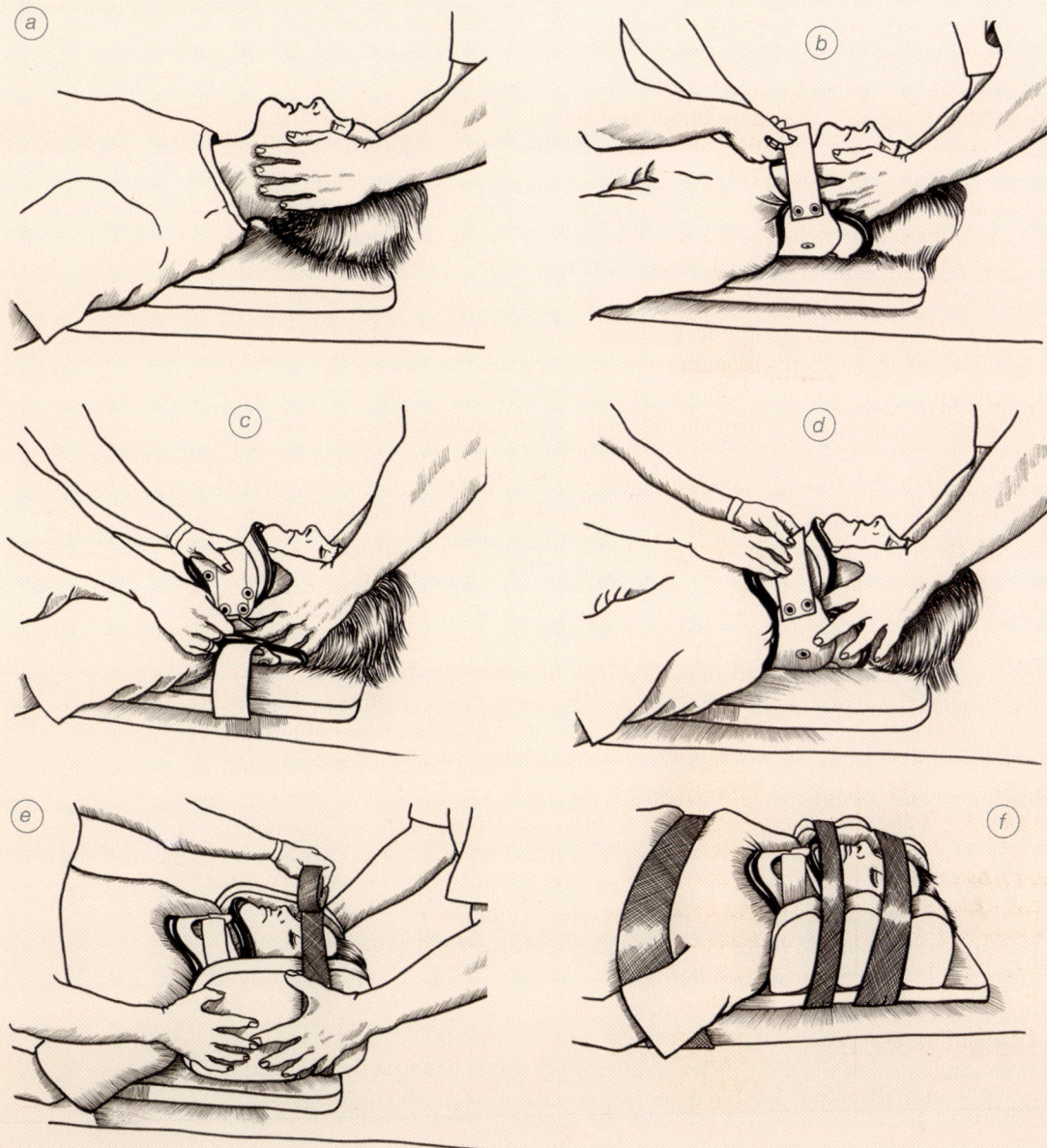

Figure 5.1 Stabilization of patients with a suspected unstable fracture.

- Stabilize the head and neck (*a*)
- Put on the back part of the collar (*b*)
- Put on the front part of the collar (*c*)
- Secure the collar (*d*)
- Roll or lift the patient onto a stiff board or stretcher
- Center the patient on the board
- Place two blanket rolls or foam blocks on the board
- Anchor the blocks around the patientís head (*e*)
- Anchor the blocks to the board (*f*)

(© Medical Illustrator Tommy Bolic, Sweden.)

Presence of or history of dysesthesia and numbness in the legs, in connection with a neck injury, should be treated as signs of a possible spinal cord injury until the contrary has been demonstrated. Awkward positioning or reflex tension in the neck may be the only protection a patient who is awake has against spinal cord injury, and no attempt should be made to correct it. An unconscious patient must not be moved until she is appropriately positioned and stabilized. Unanticipated dislocation of an unstable neck may cause a permanent spinal cord injury to a patient who has no symptoms or signs of this type of injury during the initial examination. Table 5.2 outlines the guidelines for emergency care of a patient with a suspected vertebral column fracture. The most experienced person on site must take charge of the situation when this type of injury occurs.

Patients with history, signs, or symptoms of neurologic injury vertebral column fractures/dislocations must be referred for appropriate orthopedic or neurosurgical care, evaluated in detail, and treated accordingly. The patient's primary health care provider can treat less serious injuries after the evaluation at the hospital has been completed.

Most patients who come to the emergency room with neck pain have been rear-ended in a car accident. Skeletal X-rays are usually negative but may be necessary for insurance purposes. If the case history and clinical examination point to nerve root affection, a magnetic resonance imaging (MRI) of the neck is indicated. A person who goes to the emergency room with neck pain resulting from a sport-related accident, such as a fall while bicycling or skiing, did not have much neck protection at the time of the accident. The forces involved in sliding headfirst into the boards during ice hockey may exceed those present during a low-speed rear-end motor vehicle collision. Therefore, that person's neck may have been subjected to significant forces. Immediate referral for appropriate care is indicated if the patient has neurological damage and/or numbness and paresthesia in the legs.

Case History

Knowledge of the individual sport should make it easier to understand the injury mechanism. The practitioner should determine whether there was sudden strong rotation in connection with an injury sustained during a collision with the ground or with an opponent. Acute back pain triggered by a throwing motion may result from an avulsion fracture of the transverse processes and/or muscle ruptures with hematoma in the quadratus lumborum muscle and/or the iliopsoas muscle. The pain will usually project out toward the iliac crest, the groin, and the thigh (hematoma or referred patterns of pain).

The actual mechanism of a neck injury may be compression of the head or neck, such as that caused by hitting a sideboard in ice hockey (Figure 5.2), being fallen on by another

Stabilize the head; do not correct the position of a patient who is conscious

Establish an open airway and control any bleeding

Perform an initial neurological examination

Call an ambulance

Put the patient in a stable side position; the neck of an unconscious patient must be stabilized

Repeat the initial examination

Make sure that the patient is adequately stabilized

Direct the ambulance driver to drive carefully

Table 5.2 Emergency care of patients with possible spinal cord injury. (Reproduced with permission from the Norwegian Sports Medicine Association.)

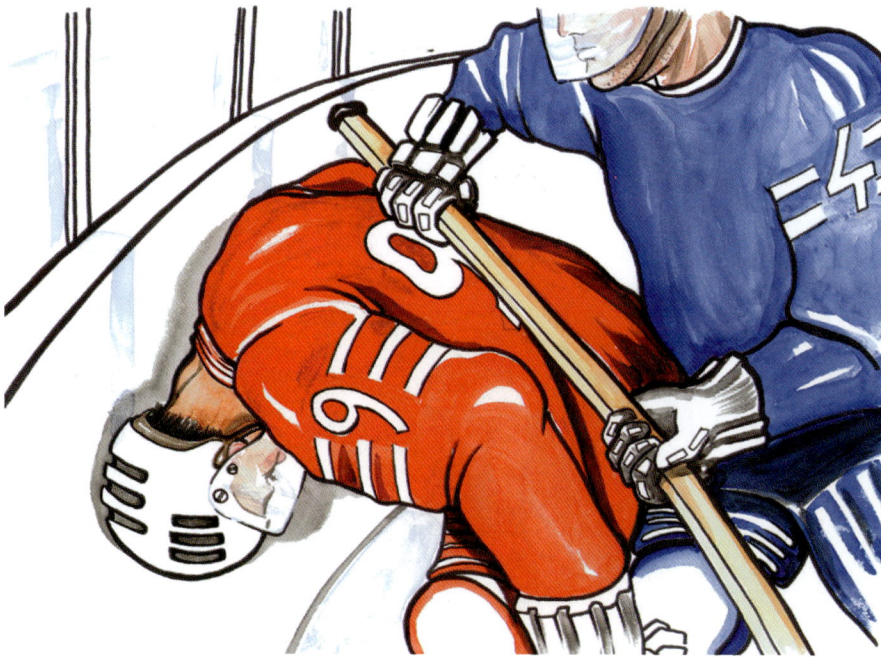

Figure 5.2 Injury mechanism. Serious neck injury may be caused by crashing into the sideboard after being tackled from behind. The helmet protects the head but does not prevent the neck from bending forward slightly. Stricter enforcement of the rules or changing the rules such as the International Rugby Board did for rugby can prevent fatal injuries. (© Medical Illustrator Tommy Bolic, Sweden.)

player during collision sports, falling from a great height when jumping on a snowboard, direct force to the neck in contact sports, or strong forced movement of the neck in a motor vehicle accident. Risk factors for injuries are equipment failure, violation of regulations (such as tackling from behind in ice hockey), or a lack of skill (e.g., when jumping on a snowboard or trampoline). Bending backward may be a consequence of a hard blow to the forehead and may cause a rupture of the anterior longitudinal ligament, forward avulsion of a bone fragment on a vertebral body, or spondylolysis.

Classification systems for both cervical and thoracolumbar fractures are based on the case history and the injury mechanism and may improve the understanding of the consequences of various types of injuries (Figure 5.3). The sagittal section of the vertebral column is divided into three columns. The anterior column consists of the anterior longitudinal ligament, the anterior half of the intervertebral disk, and the vertebral body. The middle column consists of the posterior longitudinal ligament, the posterior half of the intervertebral disk, and the vertebral body. The posterior column consists of the posterior arch with the lamina, the back's transverse processes, the facet joints, the ligamentum flavum, the supraspinal ligament (from C7 nuchal ligament), and the interspinal ligament. If the injury is unstable, it is assumed that at least two columns are involved.

Compression fractures usually involve only one column and are stable. Combined diskoligamentous injuries caused by flexion and extension forces are usually unstable two-column injuries. Rotational trauma (Figure 5.4) causes the highest proportion of neurological injuries. Table 5.3 shows injuries divided according to the degree of severity based on case history and the radiographically evaluated injury mechanism.

Clinical Examination

When a serious injury/fracture to the vertebral column is indicated, the physician must first evaluate the patient's circulation, respiration, and level of consciousness. Next, the patient's neurological status must be evaluated. Can the patient move his hands and feet? Fractures, dislocations, and diskoligamentous injuries, with

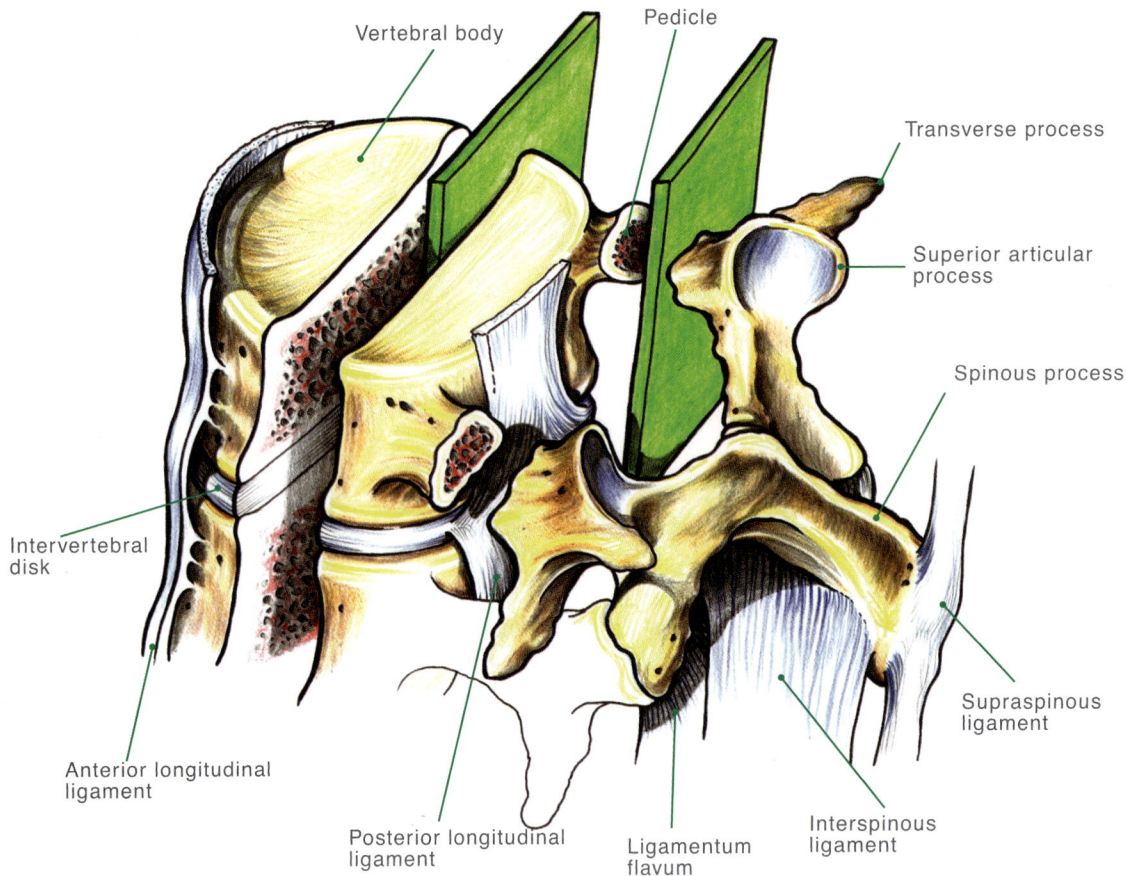

Figure 5.3 Fracture classification. The spine can be divided into three columns; an unstable injury involves at least two columns. (© Medical Illustrator Tommy Bolic, Sweden.)

significant deformity and/or instability, may be present without initial neurological deficit. A careful search by palpation of the spinous processes may indicate a rupture of the interspinal ligament. Numbness and dysesthesia in the legs may be the only symptoms that point toward spinal cord affection. Hyperreflexia is often masked by spinal shock. The level diagnostics are described in Figure 5.5.

Supplemental Examinations

Radiographic examination. The X-ray exam starts with a lateral view from occiput to T1. Frontal and lateral X-rays should be taken of the indicated area. If the patient

Type	Injury mechanism	Neurological damage (%)
A	Compressive forces alone (compression fractures without ligament damage, such as falls on the buttocks or landing on the feet after parachute jumping or using a paraglider)	14
B	Stretching forces in flexion or extension (purely diskoligamentous injuries, or like A, or posterior ligament rupture)	32
C	Rotational injuries alone or in combination with A or B	55

Table 5.3 Classification of fractures according to the AO group. Each type can be divided into a hierarchy of groups and subgroups according to the increasing degree of seriousness (i.e., the degree of neurological damage). (Reproduced with permission from the Norwegian Sports Medicine Association.)

Figure 5.4 Injury mechanism involving rotation. Example of rotational injury causing dislocation, ligament rupture, fracture, and disk injury. Rotational injuries often result in nerve root or spinal cord affection. (© Medical Illustrator Tommy Bolic, Sweden.)

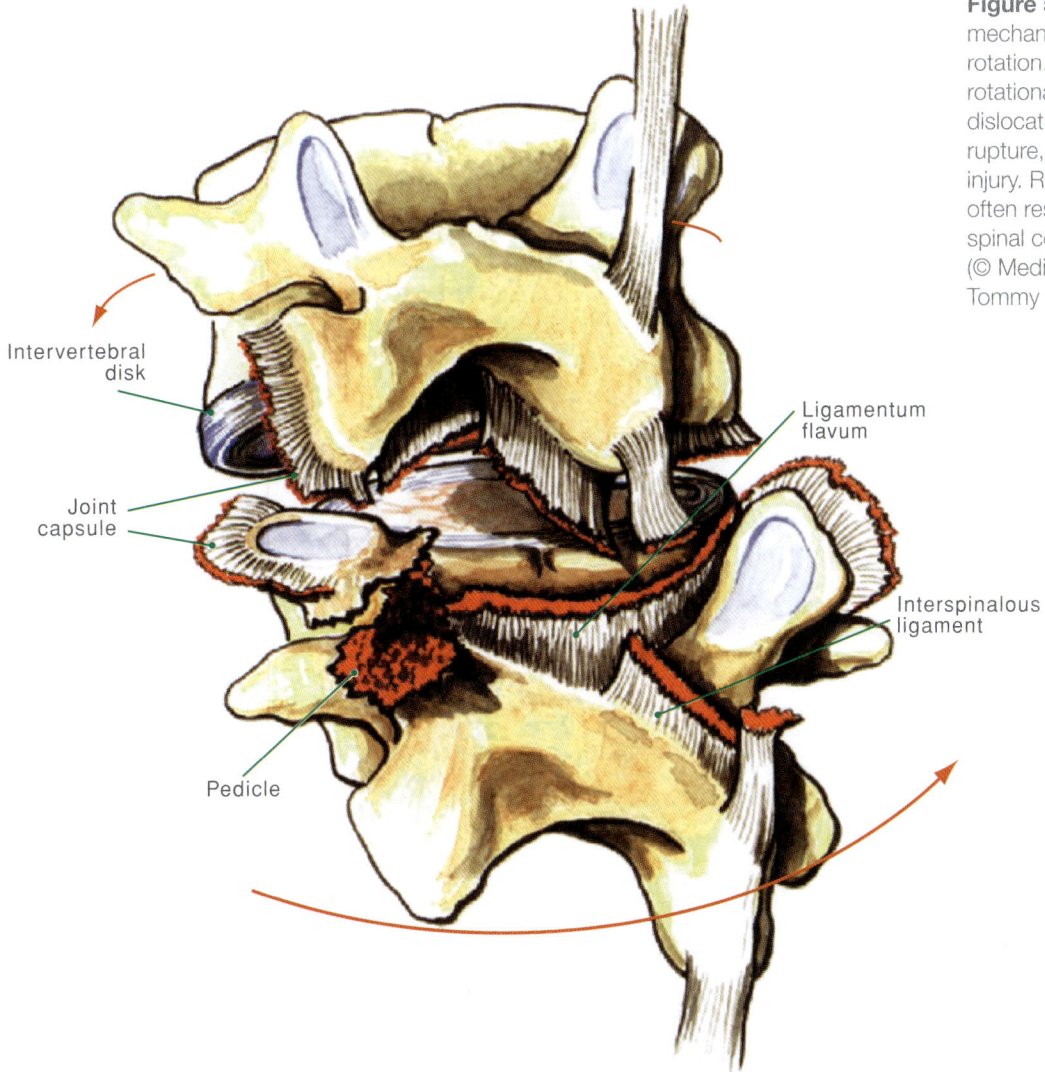

Intervertebral disk

Joint capsule

Pedicle

Ligamentum flavum

Interspinalous ligament

Level	Function	Reflex	Sensation
C3-5	Respiration (diaphragm)		
C5	Shoulder abduction (deltoid muscle)	Biceps	Lateral upper arm
C6	Elbow flexion	Brachioradialis	Lateral forearm
C7	Elbow extension	Triceps	Middle finger
C8	Finger flexion		Small and ring fingers
T1	Finger spreading		Medial forearm
L1-2	Hip flexion		
L3-4	Knee extension	Patellar	Medial thigh
L5	Big toe extension	Medial hamstring	Base, big toe
S1	Plantar flexion and toe flexion	Achilles	Lateral foot
S2-4	Sphincter function on rectal examination	Bulbocavernosus	

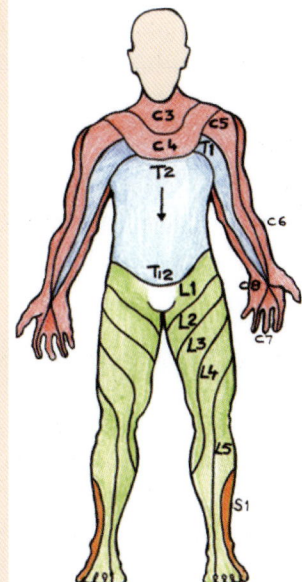

Figure 5.5 Segmental diagnostics, including dermatome charts. (© Medical Illustrator Tommy Bolic, Sweden.)

is unconscious, the neck must be examined, to exclude neck injuries. Because of overprojection of the shoulder section, it is difficult to obtain sufficient information about the cervicothoracic transition (C7/T1) using this examination. *A negative radiographic examination does not exclude an unstable neck injury.* Therefore, extension and flexion images may be necessary, but a skilled professional must perform this examination *after a lateral X-ray from C1 to T1 is evaluated.*

Magnetic resonance imaging (MRI). MRI is the most sensitive means of examining for soft-tissue structures and the medulla. It is also the only test that can demonstrate, in detail, combined injuries of the intervertebral disk and ligament (diskoligamentous injuries). Instability is evaluated by extension and flexion images on a plain X-ray. If the MRI reveals ruptures of the interspinal ligament, the neck is potentially unstable and may be stabilized by surgery.

Computerized tomography (CT). CT is an excellent method for examining the reduction of the spinal canal and the degree of crushing when the patient has a compression fracture. An isolated compression fracture with minor to moderate crushing is stable. *Fractures of the posterior elements may be best seen on the CT scan.*

Common Injuries

Muscle Contusion and Rupture—*Back Muscle Injury*

Muscle contusion occurs frequently in various contact sports. Muscle ruptures are rare and occur most frequently in explosive sports. The injury is often localized to the erector muscles of the spine.

- Symptoms and signs: Palpation causes distinct pain that is usually unilateral. If the patient has a ruptured muscle, he often has cramping when bending forward and when rising. If isometric contraction does not provoke pain, the patient may have an isolated ligament injury.
- Diagnosis: Case history plus exclusion of other causes of pain after a clinical examination and possibly diagnostic imaging for a suspected fracture.
- Treatment by physician: Drug treatment is the same as for acute strain. If the patient has muscle contusion, inform her that the prognosis is good and that she will probably be able to resume full activity in a few days. However, a rupture may prevent her from participating in sport activity for a relatively long time. Mobilization may be indicated if the examination seems to reveal an isolated ligament injury and the injury becomes chronic with limited segmental movement.
- Treatment by physical therapist or self-treatment: Ice and information are the first treatments offered. If the patient has a muscle rupture, he should undergo alternative training after a few days. Gradual progression to a more competitive type of activity during a 3–8-week period is recommended.

Other Injuries

Spinal Cord Injuries !

Spinal cord injuries may be divided into complete and partial injuries (Figure 5.6). A complete injury is defined as a complete loss of sensation and motor function, more than two levels distal to the level of the injury, which lasts longer than 48 hours. Partial injuries are divided according to the long pathways that are affected. Depending on its location, the injury may be classified as anterior, lateral, dorsal longitudinal fasciculus, central, or conus (T12–L1), or as cauda equina syndrome (below L1). An unstable neck

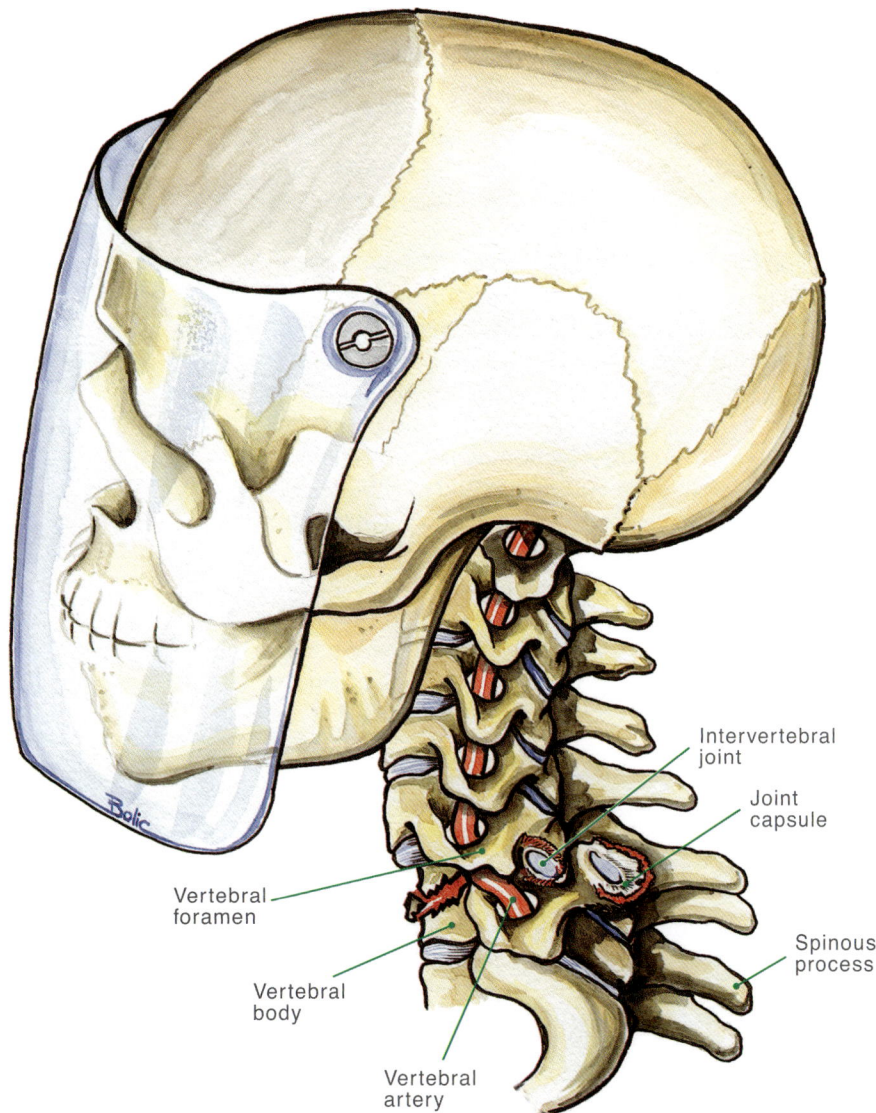

Figure 5.6 Unstable cervical fracture, which may cause a partial anterior spinal cord injury. The symptoms may be caused by direct pressure on the spinal column or compression of the vertebral artery. (© Medical Illustrator Tommy Bolic, Sweden.)

fracture may place direct pressure on the spinal cord or compress the vertebral artery. This can primarily affect the pyramidal tracts and can cause an anterior syndrome with flaccid paralysis, as well as decreasing sensitivity to pain and temperature distal to the site of the injury. Joint sensation in the dorsal longitudinal fasciculus is well preserved.

- Symptoms and signs: Symptoms and signs of spinal cord injuries are neck pain, numbness, dysesthesia, and inability to move the hands and feet. An examination of sensation must include sensitivity to touch and pain (anterior spinothalamic tract), joint sensation, and sensitivity to touch (lateral corticospinal tract). Motor function should be graded from 0 (no contraction) to 5 (normal muscle strength). If the patient has neurological deficits, she should be assigned to the lowest level (Figure 5.5). Shallow respiration, hypotension with bradycardia, areflexia, lack of anal sphincter tone, and loss of sensitivity to pain distal to the injury are signs of spinal cord damage in an unconscious patient.
- Diagnosis: The diagnosis is primarily clinical. The patient must not be moved before being properly stabilized. The patient must be referred to a neurosurgeon for further evaluation and treatment. *The surgeons and the facility must have the capability of providing a high level of specialized care.* This applies regardless of whether the

athlete is examined at the sport facility or in the emergency room. A complete neurological examination and a diagnostic imaging examination using a skeletal X-ray (and MRI) are necessary to exclude the diagnosis. *Spinal cord injured patients are frequently polytrauma patients and should be treated as such.* A patient without symptoms and signs that indicate spinal cord injury may have an unstable fracture.

- Treatment: The patient must be transported to the hospital (Figure 5.1). Abnormal positioning of the head caused by neck muscle contractions or reflectory muscle spasm of the neck may be secondary to spinal cord fractures or injuries and may be the only protection a conscious patient has against medulla damage. Therefore, no attempt should be made to correct the position of the patient. The patient should be transported to the hospital (Figure 5.1). If neurological deficit is present, treatment includes skull traction or surgery for unstable cervical fractures. Eventual surgery consists of decompression and possibly fusion of two or more levels of the joint.

- Prognosis: Signs of spinal activity during the first 72 hours after the injury predict walking function 1 year after a partial injury. Walking function can be expected in about 50% of patients who have partially intact sensory function and in about 85% of those who show signs of motor activity. Lack of motor and sensory activity in the first 72 hours indicates that the patient will not achieve walking function later. If the CT shows compression of the medulla when the patient has a partial spinal cord injury, the medulla must be decompressed, even if the paresis is not progressive, because decompression may reduce the degree of paresis. Performing surgery on patients with complete spinal cord injuries after the hyperacute phase does not improve the prognosis.

Unstable Fractures—*Unstable Fracture in the Neck* !

A fracture is stable if controlled movements do not cause neurological deficit. If the fracture is unstable, controlled movements may result in, or may worsen a nerve root or spinal cord injury. The fracture may be classified according to the number of columns involved. If two or more columns are involved, the injury is unstable (Figures 5.3, 5.7a and 5.7b).

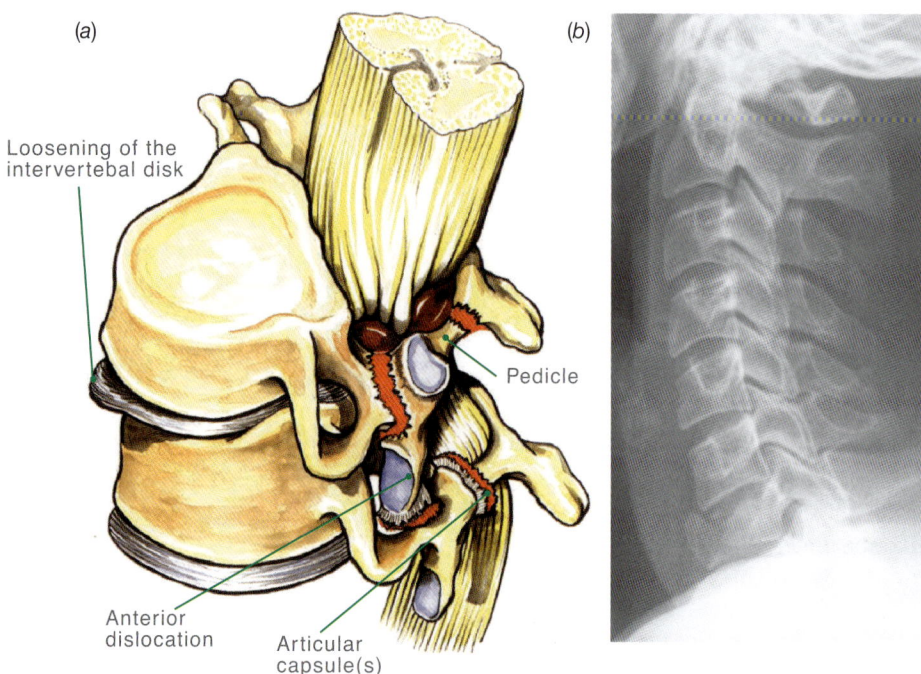

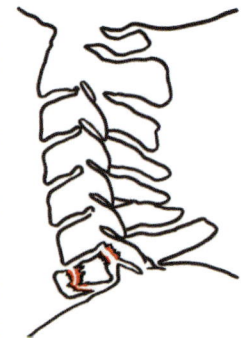

(a)

Loosening of the
intervertebal disk

Pedicle

Anterior
dislocation

Articular
capsule(s)

(b)

Figure 5.7 Unstable cervical fracture. The drawing (a) shows that all three columns are injured with a rupture of the ligamentum flavum, anterior dislocation, fracture of the vertebral arch, loosening of the intervertebral disk, and spinal cord affection. The sagittal X-ray view (b) demonstrates an injury of the anterior column and middle column, with a fracture of the vertebral body and arch.
(© Medical Illustrator Tommy Bolic, Sweden.)

- Symptoms and signs: A combination of high-energy trauma, abnormal positioning of the head caused by neck muscle contractions or reflectory muscle spasm of the neck, or the inability of the patient to stand on her feet are signs of an unstable fracture.
- Diagnosis: The patient must be referred for appropriate neurosurgical or orthopedic care and should be treated as if he has an unstable fracture until the contrary has been proven. This applies regardless of whether the athlete is examined at the sport facility or in the emergency room. A complete neurological examination and a diagnostic imaging examination using a skeletal X-ray (and MRI or CT) are necessary to exclude the diagnosis.
- Treatment: Abnormal positioning of the head caused by neck muscle contractions or reflectory muscle spasm of the neck may be secondary to spinal cord fractures or injuries and may be the only protection a conscious patient has against medulla damage. Therefore, no attempt should be made to correct the position of the patient. The patient should be transported to the hospital (Figure 5.1). If neurological deficit is present, treatment includes skull traction or surgery for unstable cervical fractures. The patient should wear a stiff cervical collar if a slight degree of axial deviation and no neurological deficit are present. Surgery is used to treat unstable thoracolumbar fractures.
- Prognosis: The prognosis is good if an injury is suspected before complications (spinal cord damage) occur and the patient receives adequate transport and treatment.

Stable Thoracolumbar Vertebral Body Fractures—*Crushing Fractures of the Thoracic Vertebrae*

Stable thoracolumbar vertebral body fractures (Figures 5.8a–5.8c) include epiphyseal plate fractures and collapse or crushing of the vertebral body. These are stable if the posterior column is not affected. Fractures that affect the epiphyseal plate are common among young people and the elderly and occur primarily in the thoracic and lumbar sections.

- Symptoms and signs: Symptoms depend on the injury mechanism and the location of the injury. Pain at the fracture site, possibly radiating to the dermatome that corresponds to the fracture, is the most common symptom. The patient has distinct sensitivity to pressure on the spinous process of the injured vertebra, and local muscle spasm is common.
- Treatment: Surgery is commonly performed if the front part of the vertebra is reduced by more than 40% of the average of the vertebrae above and below it. The basis for this strategy is that surgical fixation provides primary stabilization. This is the most secure method of preventing further collapse of the vertebra, and the fracture is stable for training within a few days.

  However, recent reports maintain that there is no indication for surgery on isolated thoracolumbar compression fractures, because the prognosis is similar without surgery. The relationship between the degree of kyphotic angulation caused by the fracture and symptoms is not definite. There is a need for more randomized studies to evaluate the effect of thoracolumbar compression fracture treatment.
- Treatment by physical therapist: The most important step is to mobilize the patient gradually, beginning on the 1st day. Early mobilization reduces the risk of deep venous thrombosis and apparently does not increase kyphosis. Specific back and abdominal muscle exercises have not been shown to be more effective than early mobilization, so no restrictions are placed on the patient's level of activity. Nevertheless, the athlete should wait until healing of the fracture is radiographically verified before returning to full competitive sport activity. Treatment with a brace limits large movements of the trunk but not intervertebral movement. Hyperextension orthosis does not appear to affect the progression of the collapse of a

(a) Spinal cord

Vertebral body

(b)

(c)

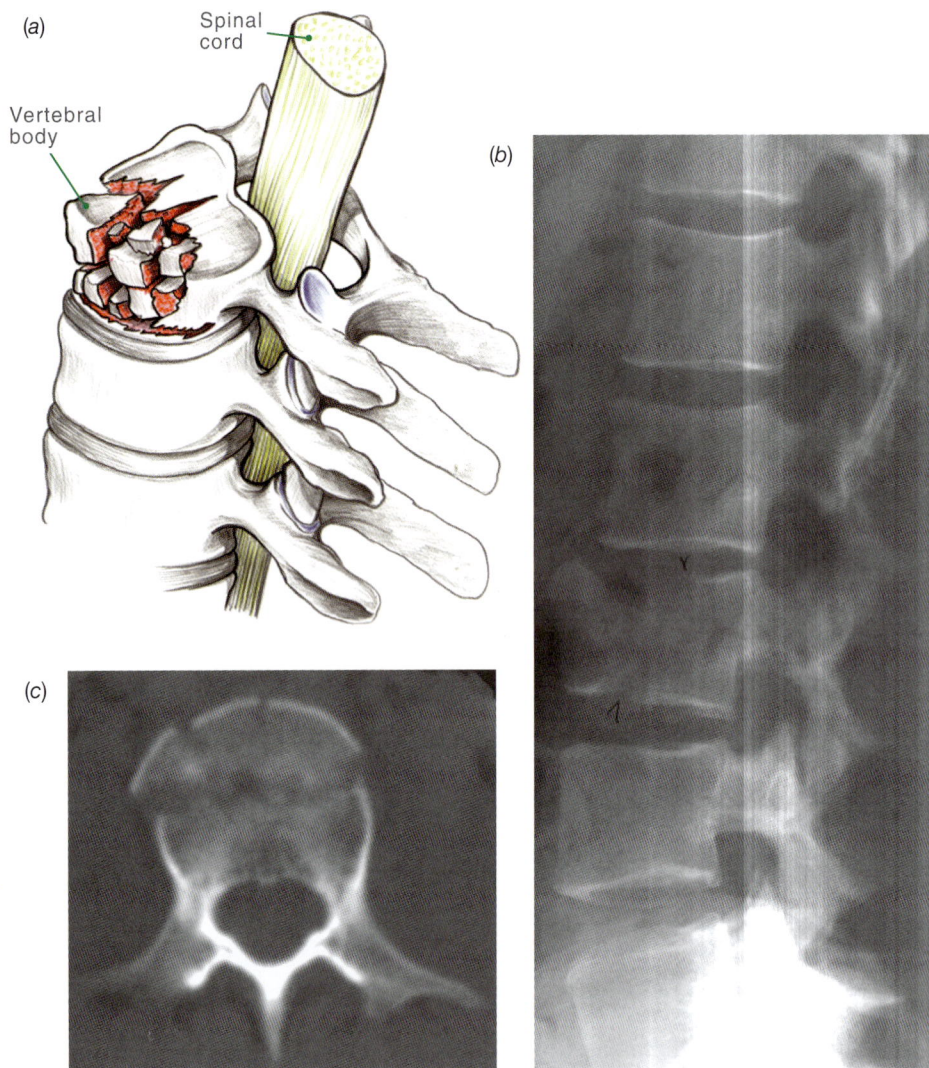

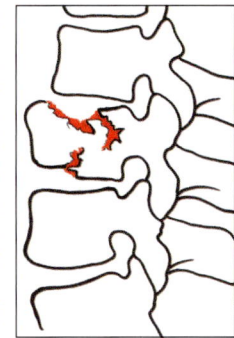

Figure 5.8 Stable compression fracture. Fractures of the end plates, collapse, and crushing of the vertebral body are stable if the posterior column is not affected. Stable compression fractures may occur in the cervical, thoracic, and lumbar regions. The illustration (a) shows a stable cervical compression fracture, whereas the sagittal X-ray view (b) shows a stable lumbar fracture, and the CT image (c) shows a stable thoracic compression fracture. (© Medical Illustrator Tommy Bolic, Sweden.)

compression fracture. Thus, the use of a brace has not been shown to stabilize the fracture. Therefore, a brace should be used only if pain prevents the patient from being mobilized without it.

• Prognosis: Most patients recover or experience only minor pain. Some patients develop chronic pain and do not return to full competitive activity.

Fractures of the Processus Transversus or the Processus Spinosus—*Fractures of the Transverse or Spinous Processes*

Fractures occur in the spinous process and transverse processes (Figure 5.9). Isolated fractures of the spinous process are rare but may be one of several injuries in flexion trauma. Fractures of the spinous process do not require any special treatment, but the physician must exclude any large injury that occurs at the same time. Fractures of the transverse processes are far more common. Usually the fracture occurs in the lumbar section and affects the iliopsoas muscle and the quadratus lumborum muscle.

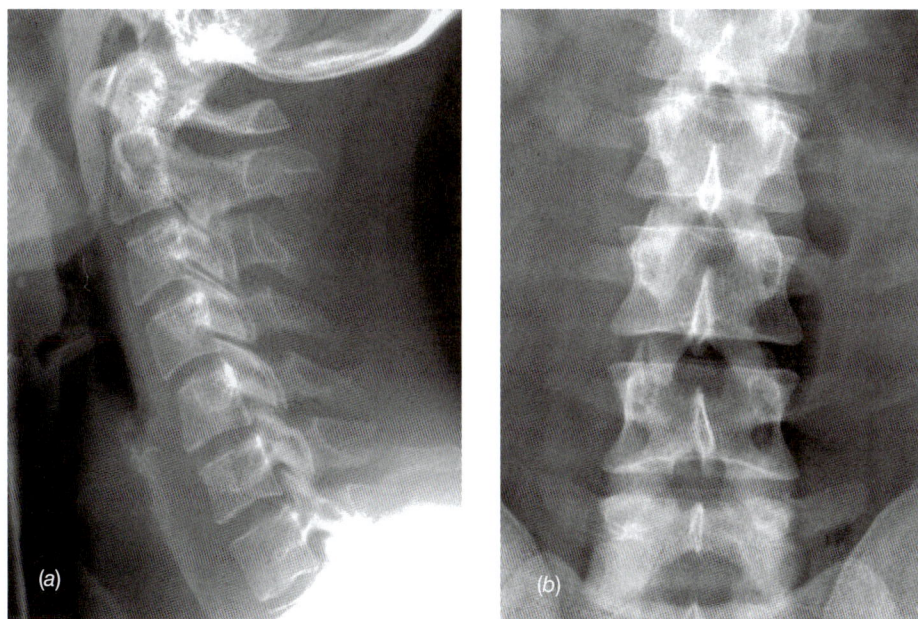

Figure 5.9 Fractures of the spinous process and the transverse process. Fracture of a cervical spinous process (a). A simultaneous major injury must be excluded. Fracture of a lumbar transverse process (b). Simultaneous affection of the psoas muscle, which has its origin on the transverse processes, should be watched for. (© Medical Illustrator Tommy Bolic, Sweden.)

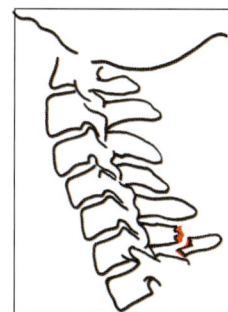

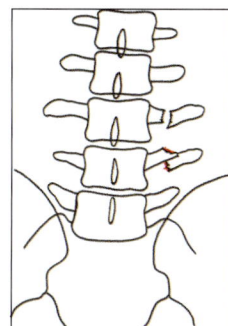

- Symptoms and signs: The patient usually has severe pain in connection with the trauma. If the patient has a fracture of the transverse processes in the lumbar spine, hip flexion and torsion make the pain worse. The patient will be sensitive to palpation: both paravertebrally and in the abdomen. Bleeding from the fracture site and musculature may decrease hemoglobin. Pain is often provoked by hip flexion (iliopsoas muscle) and by lateral flexion (quadratus lumborum muscle).
- Diagnosis: A radiographic examination shows the torn-off processes. A CT scan provides the best overview and is indicated if the X-ray is negative and the case history and clinical examination seem to indicate a fracture.
- Treatment by physician: The patient should be referred immediately for appropriate orthopedic or neurosurgical care if a combined large injury is suspected. Treatment of isolated fractures is conservative. Therefore, a primary care provider can evaluate and treat the patient. If pain does not allow rapid mobilization, the use of a brace may be helpful.
- Treatment by physical therapist: Functional training is recommended.
- Self-treatment: The patient can self-treat by gradually increasing activity.
- Prognosis: The prognosis is good. Healing usually takes place in 6–8 weeks, but an additional 3–4 weeks of gradually increasing training is usually recommended before full activity in contact sports is allowed.

Neck Pain

Jens Ivar Brox[1], Mike Wilkinson[2], Robert G. Watkins III[3], and Robert G. Watkins IV[3]

[1]Oslo University Hospital, Rikshospitalet, Sognsveien, Oslo, Norway
[2]Allan McGavin Sports Medicine Center, Vancouver, BC, Canada
[3]Marina Spine Center, Marina del Rey, California, CA, USA

Occurrence

Neck pain is a common symptom that occurs about as often as back pain, which affects almost 50% of the adult population each year. There are approximately 40–80 new cases of nerve root pain from the neck per 100,000 persons per year.

Thirty percent of the retired Norwegian national soccer players suffer from chronic neck symptoms and limited neck movement. In a study of soccer players and a control group, disk degeneration was found to be significantly more common, and occurred 10–20 years earlier, in the soccer players than in the controls. The causes are apparently (1) the combination of repeated compression and hyperextension loading when making contact with the ball and (2) collisions with other players.

In Western countries, neck pain that results from being rear-ended in a car accident occurs so frequently that it seems to be epidemic. The epidemic is difficult to explain from a biomechanical perspective. The patient seldom has definite pathophysiological changes or specific clinical signs. This type of complaints occurs to a small percentage of athletes who are frequently subjected to corresponding biomechanical forces. The way we focus on this type of complaints seems to have created a culture of disease that contributes to unnecessary anxiety about physical activity being harmful to the neck.

Differential Diagnoses

Neck pain may be classified in various manners. It is common to distinguish between neck pain that radiates (cervicobrachialgia) and pain that does not radiate to the upper extremities. The radiating pain may follow a nerve root pattern (cervical radiculopathy) or worsen by elevation of the arm and palpation of the brachial plexus (thoracic outlet syndrome). It may also be caused by entrapment of the peripheral nerves. A more common differential diagnostic approach to the problem is to distinguish between pain that radiates from the neck down into the shoulder and arm, and

Most common	Less common	Must not be overlooked !
Cervicobrachialgia, p. 118	Acute torticollis, p. 118	Unstable fracture
	Cervical radiculopathy, p. 119	Infection
	Thoracic outlet syndrome, p. 119	Tumor
	Transient pain and paresthesia, p. 120	

Table 5.4 Overview of differential diagnoses of neck injuries. (Reproduced with permission from the Norwegian Sports Medicine Association.)

primary shoulder pain with secondary neck pain. Table 5.4 provides an overview of the most relevant differential diagnoses. Neck pain may also represent referred pain, such as when the patient has a throat infection or a cervical tumor. In the elderly, dizziness and neck pain may be caused by stenosis in the vertebral artery.

Diagnostic Thinking

The examiner must determine whether the pain is coming from the neck or originates elsewhere, whether there are neurological symptoms and signs, and whether the pain is due to a specific neck disorder or is nonspecific (Figure 5.10). Acute neck pain can be very intense, accompanied by improper positioning (torticollis) and stiffness. This pain may make the patient anxious and the situation worse. Therefore, instilling confidence during the initial consultation has a good therapeutic effect. The natural course in patients with acute neck pain is good, so comprehensive treatment is not recommended.

To understand, diagnose, and treat painful conditions in the neck, it is advisable to determine whether the patient has a condition that can be medically alleviated but has no specific medical treatment or if the patient has a condition with obvious diagnostic characteristics and an anticipated course, irrespective of medical treatment. An example of the latter type of condition is radiating neck pain and neurological deficit. Neck pain and stiffness without specific signs is defined as an illness. Degenerative changes revealed by radiographic or MRI examinations occur about as frequently in healthy people as in patients, and the findings are of little diagnostic value. If the pain continues, the physician should determine whether the pain has a significant organic characteristic or whether the symptoms may indicate somatization. In individual cases, the case history and clinical examination may suggest that the patient's symptoms and dysfunction are motivated by the desire for a possible secondary gain in the form of insurance compensation. In this case, it may be useful to observe the patient outside the examining room. Diagnostic imaging is indicated if nerve root affection is suspected or if there is atypical pain.

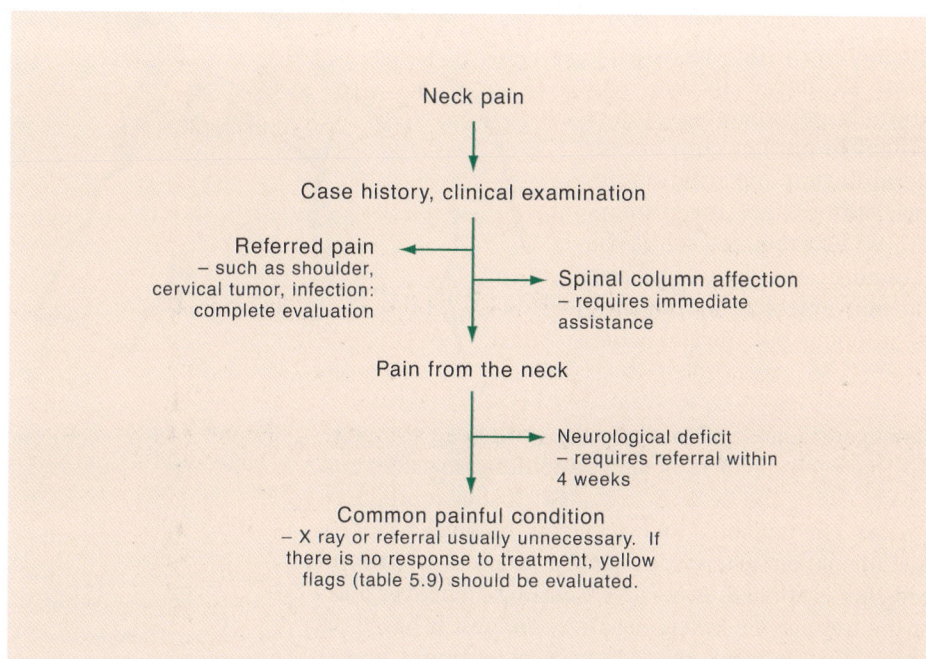

Figure 5.10 Algorithm for evaluating patients with acute neck pain. (Reproduced with permission from the Norwegian Sports Medicine Association.)

Case History

The case history must describe how the pain originated and what the patient's main symptoms are. Did the pain originate in connection with an acute event or has it been developing gradually?

The most essential part of taking the case history is to obtain an accurate description of the location of the pain and any accompanying symptoms, such as headache, a lapse in concentration, dizziness, nausea, and vision or hearing disturbances.

Is the pain diffusely spread or distinctly localized? Is the pain provoked by coughing and sneezing? Does it radiate only to the upper extremities, and if so, does the radiation have a radicular characteristic? Muscle weakness may indicate nerve root affection, but primary shoulder affection and peripheral nerve entrapment must be excluded by means of a clinical examination. To make a differential diagnosis, the practitioner must ask whether the patient has bladder dysfunction. If a change in walking or balance has occurred, this may be a sign of myelopathy.

Clinical Examination

Inspection. Torticollis is the tilting of the head to one side, caused by contraction of the muscles on that side of the neck. The condition may be congenital, or it may be due to a serious injury, reflex muscle activity caused by herniation or facet joint affection, or primarily involve the muscles like a muscle strain. The practitioner must evaluate the patient's muscle tension. Does the patient unconsciously shrug the shoulders? The patient should also be checked for a cervical tumor.

Neurological examination. If the patient has pain that radiates beyond the shoulders, he should be given a neurological examination (Figure 5.5).

Movement. Active and passive movement should be examined. The normal range of motion in the neck is 55° extension, 45° forward flexion, 45° lateral flexion, and 70° rotation. Normal variation is considerable, and a simple check is to ask the patient to put her chin on her chest and to see whether lateral flexion and rotation are symmetrical. If pain and neck stiffness are the primary problems, neck movement should be examined while the patient is sitting, standing, stooping, and lying. If muscle pain and stiffness are present, movement is significantly reduced when the patient is stooping but normal when the patient is supine.

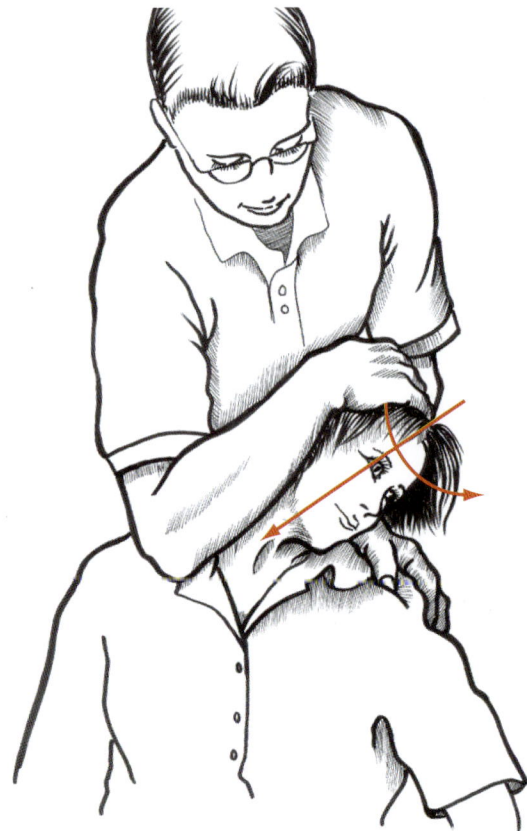

Figure 5.11 Spurling maneuver. The space for the nerve root is reduced when the examiner combines side flexion, extension and rotation with axial compression. (© Medical Illustrator Tommy Bolic, Sweden.)

Spurling test. The Spurling maneuver (Figure 5.11) is first done with head compression in the neutral position (if that reproduces radicular symptoms, one does not need to check the full maneuver). Next, the head is extended (if that reproduces the symptoms, one may stop there). The patient is told to extend the head and look toward the painful arm. Finally, the patient extends the head and looks toward the painful arm while head compression is applied. A positive Spurling maneuver indicates nerve root affection, but the test may be falsely negative. The test is based on the examiner narrowing the space for the nerve root via neck extension, coupled with rotation and bending the head toward the affected side. If this reproduces the pain in the upper extremities, the test is positive.

Shoulder abduction test. If abducting the arm, putting the hand behind the head produces relief of arm pain (Figure 5.12), it is an excellent sign that relief of tension on the nerve root has relieved the arm pain and the findings are positive, indicating cervical radiculopathy. If elevating the shoulder and placing the hand behind the head produces a severe increase in shoulder pain, then shoulder pathology is present.

Roos test. This test (Figure 5.13) is positive if the patient has a thoracic outlet syndrome. For this test the patient repeatedly clenches the fist for 3 minutes while the arm is in an abducted, externally rotated position. If the symptoms are provoked on the affected side, or if the patient has problems clenching the fist, the test is positive.

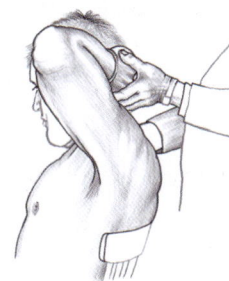

Figure 5.12 Shoulder abduction test. This test can be used to distinguish between cervical radiculopathy and shoulder pathology. (© Medical Illustrator Tommy Bolic, Sweden.)

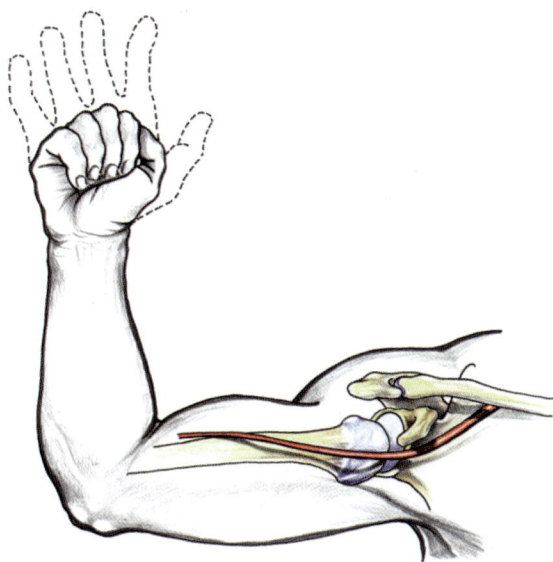

Figure 5.13 Roos test. Have the patient repeatedly clench and open his fist, as shown in the illustration. Impingement of nerves or vascular structures in the scalene port is assumed to be the cause of the symptoms. (© Medical Illustrator Tommy Bolic, Sweden.)

Palpation. The practitioner should palpate the spinous process and the transverse processes, the suboccipital muscles, the trapezius muscle, the levator scapulae, the scalene, and the sternocleidomastoid muscles bilaterally and supraclavicularly. Palpation findings are often difficult to interpret but may be important if the tenderness is unilateral or localized.

Supplemental Examinations

X-rays of the cervical spine with oblique views are indicated for atypical pain and to evaluate the intervertebral foramina when there is radicular pain.

MRI. This is the first choice for clinical symptoms and signs that suggest nerve root affection. The examination is not indicated during the acute phase if drug therapy has an adequate effect on the patient.

Electromyography (EMG) and neurography. These are seldom used but may be helpful (1) in cases in which the patient may have peripheral or central affection, (2) when differentiating between radiculopathy and entrapment, or (3) when differentiating between neurogenic and myogenic disorders. These examinations should normally be ordered by a specialist.

NECK AND BACK

Common Painful Conditions

Cervicalgia/Cervicobrachialgia—*Neck Pain With or Without Radiation*

It is common to classify neck pain that does not radiate to the upper extremities as cervicalgia, and neck pain with diffusely disseminating radiation as cervicobrachialgia. A distinction must be made between cervicobrachialgia and cervical radiculopathy (a condition in which the radiating pain follows a nerve root pattern). Unilateral monotonous loading and psychosocial conditions are contributing factors. Pain may be vertebrogenic, diskogenic, or muscular. Often more than one structure is involved.

- Symptoms and signs: Symptoms and signs are neck pain that may or may not radiate to the shoulder and upper arm, difficulty moving the neck, and normal or slightly reduced passive movement. Accompanying symptoms, such as fatigue, concentration lapses, dizziness, tinnitus, and nausea, indicate stress-related neck pain.
- Diagnosis: A diagnosis is made clinically by excluding nerve root pain and pain referred from other organs. A simple clinical examination, without supplemental diagnostic imaging, is sufficient for the initial examination.
- Treatment by physician: Over-the-counter analgesics or nonsteroidal anti-inflammatory drugs (NSAIDs) for 3–7 days reduce the duration of the acute pain. More potent analgesics may be necessary for sleeping problems. Treatment for chronic pain depends on whether the pain seems to be organic or is mostly stress related. The periodic use of a stiff cervical collar may provide relief and alleviate symptoms of organic pain in elderly patients.
- Treatment by physical therapist: The effects of the various forms of available treatment are not well documented. Mobilization and manipulation appear to be better than no treatment. Manipulation of the neck is not recommended because the effect is minor compared with a few serious complications that have been reported. Several studies indicate that electromagnetic therapy may have an analgesic effect. Active exercises are recommended for chronic pain. If treatment is not effective, the status of the indication should be reevaluated. The patient should continue with general training.
- Prognosis: The prognosis is usually good, but repeated injuries with progressive unrelenting symptoms in patients who participate in contact sports may make it necessary to recommend that the athlete end his sport career.

Other Painful Conditions

Acute Torticollis—*Kink in the Neck*

Torticollis is acute neck pain caused by improper positioning of the neck, usually combined with lateral flexion and rotation.

- Symptoms and signs: The patient often states that the pain began after a sudden movement—for example, while sleeping—after which the neck gradually became stiffer and more painful. Generally, movement is significantly reduced, particularly in the neck, which is stiff and tilts to one side. When movement is tested, pain is often asymmetrical.
- Diagnosis: Diagnosis is based on the case history. A clinical examination should check for other causes of acute torticollis, such as trauma, prolapse (radiculopathy), throat infection, and tumors. The physician should perform diagnostic imaging if the pain has lasted more than 14 days.

- Treatment by physician: Recommended treatments are muscle relaxants, NSAIDs, or paracetamol. The prognosis is good and patients are normally able to resume full activity after a few days.
- Treatment by physical therapist or self-treatment: Ice, information, and mobilization of the neck.

Cervical Radiculopathy—*Nerve Root Pain From the Neck*

Radiculopathy is most common caused by a herniated disk in patients 40 years or younger. In the elderly, pain is more often caused by reduced height of the intervertebral disk and facet joint exostosis that contribute to foraminal stenosis. The prevalence of disk herniation and degenerative changes shown by diagnostic imaging is high in asymptomatic people. Therefore, a cervical prolapse is usually not associated with nerve root pain.

- Symptoms and signs: Common symptoms are neck pain and unilateral shoulder and/or arm pain; numbness or tingling in the fingers; and reduced shoulder, arm, and/or finger muscle strength that follows a nerve root pattern. The diagnosis is strengthened if sensation and muscle strength are reduced and reflexes are abnormal in a nerve root pattern. Manual muscle testing has higher specificity than examining sensitivity and reflexes, and a diagnosis can be made at the proper level in 75–80% (Figure 5.5) of patients. The Spurling maneuver (Figure 5.11) may reproduce the symptoms. In terms of differential diagnoses, the practitioner should ask whether the patient has bladder dysfunction and whether walking or balance has changed (which might indicate myelopathy).
- Diagnosis: The diagnosis is first and foremost clinical. It is based on radiating pain, paresthesia, hyperesthesia and dysesthesia, and weakened muscle strength and reflexes in a nerve root (diminution) pattern. If the diagnosis is in doubt, MRI and X-rays of the cervical spine with oblique images are useful. EMG is not positive acutely, but the nerve conduction study may identify a peripheral nerve compression.
- Treatment by physician: The physician should inform the patient that the natural course is generally good without surgery. Peroral corticosteroids have the best anti-inflammatory effect and are the first choice for drug therapy. Stronger analgesics are indicated for sleep difficulties caused by pain. A stiff cervical collar limits extension and may bring relief during the first phase. Bladder paresis and progressive paralysis in the legs are indications for immediate hospitalization in a neurological or neurosurgical department.
- Treatment by physical therapist: Traction may be indicated if information, drugs, and a stiff cervical collar do not provide sufficient pain relief. Active exercises may counteract stiffness in the neck. Manipulation is contraindicated.
- Self-treatment: The patient should maintain daily activities and seek alternative training that does not make the pain worse.
- Prognosis: The prognosis varies greatly among individuals. Improvement may be marked the first 14 days; still the condition may be long term and result in the athlete having to discontinue participation in competitive sports for several months.

Thoracic Outlet Syndrome

A diagnosis of a thoracic outlet syndrome is made if symptoms are related to compression of nerve or vessel structures between the neck and the axilla. The symptoms are rarely directly related to a cervical rib. They are more often related to muscular dysfunction that includes tense scalene musculature.

- Symptoms and signs: Symptoms worsen when the arm is elevated, with paresthesia corresponding to segments C8–T1, with tenderness over the brachial plexus or above the clavicle, and with a positive Roos test.
- Diagnosis: A diagnosis can be made when at least three of the symptoms and signs are found.
- Treatment by physician: The outcome of surgery is good in less than 40% of the patients, and some patients suffer from disabling complications. Therefore, the physician must diligently evaluate the symptoms and the function level in order to initiate proper treatment. This includes a thorough differential diagnostic evaluation, measuring range of motion in the neck, evaluating muscle strength in the upper extremities, and checking for symptoms of somatization. Hence, a physical medicine & rehabilitation or neurology specialist should evaluate the patient.
- Treatment by physical therapist: Supervised exercise seems to normalize the condition in most patients. The purpose of the exercises is to normalize the pattern of movement in the neck and shoulder girdle to create more space for the neurovascular structures.
- Prognosis: The prognosis is good with nonsurgical treatment, poor with surgery.

Transient Pain and Paresthesia in the Upper Extremities— *Transient Pain and Numbness in the Arms or Trunk and Legs*

The occurrence of transient neck pain with radiation and numbness (burning and stinging) is high in contact sports such as football and rugby. It is believed that repeated hard tackles with lateral flexion of the neck and depression of the shoulder increases the risk of chronic neck pain in this type of sport. The symptoms may be the result of a traction injury of the brachial plexus or affection of one or more nerve roots. Often, the symptoms last only a few seconds, but some patients suffer from chronic disorders. Transitory quadraparesis or quadraparesthesias may result from cervical axial loading injury.

- Symptoms and signs: Symptoms and signs are burning pain and numbness in the upper extremity. The symptoms are localized more circularly than in dermatomes. The symptoms may last a few seconds or have the characteristics of chronic paresthesia and muscle weakness.
- Diagnosis: The diagnosis should be made to exclude cervical radiculopathy and thoracic outlet syndrome. The degree of spinal stenosis or instability should be carefully diagnosed.
- Treatment: To prevent problems, the practitioner should advise an athlete as to what is the risk of continuing to play and what factors can increase or decrease that risk.

Back Pain

Jens Ivar Brox[1], Robert G. Watkins III[2], Robert G. Watkins IV[2], and Mike Wilkinson[3]

[1]*Oslo University Hospital, Rikshospitalet, Sognsveien, Oslo, Norway*
[2]*Marina Spine Center, Marina del Rey, California, CA, USA*
[3]*Allan McGavin Sports Medicine Center, Vancouver, BC, Canada*

Occurrence

Acute back pain is common among athletes. The prognosis is good without comprehensive evaluation and treatment. Most athletes may resume their normal sport activity within 1–2 weeks. Ninety percent of athletes who have acute lumbago for the first time are asymptomatic within 1–2 weeks.

The prevalence of back pain varies from sport to sport. In weightlifting, nearly every elite athlete is affected annually, whereas other athletes, such as runners, rarely have back trouble. It has been reported that 30–40% of elite swimmers and more than 60% of elite cross-country skiers have back pain that periodically affects their activity level. Problems in cross-country skiers are more often related to the classical technique than to skating. A Swedish epidemiological study that included soccer and tennis players, wrestlers, and gymnasts revealed that 50–85% of the athletes had experienced back pain.

Radiographic changes were found in 36–55% of the athletes depending on the sport. The prevalence of spondylolysis among wrestlers was five times as high as in the general population. Former wrestlers have nearly twice the prevalence of back pain as the general population, but lower absence due to illness! The back is the second most common location for injuries in dancers, but there is disagreement about causes of the pain. The prevalence of isthmic spondylolysis or spondylolisthesis is high among dancers and in bowlers in cricket–both among those who have back pain and those who do not.

Most common	Less common	Must not be overlooked !
Acute strain, p. 130	Acute sciatica, p. 135	Tumor
Chronic strain, p. 131	Chronic sciatica, p. 137	Diskitis
Spondylolysis or spondylolisthesis, p. 133	Spinal stenosis, p.138	
	Scoliosis, p.139	
	Morbus Scheuermann, p. 140	
	Morbus Bekhterev, p. 140	

Table 5.5 Overview of differential diagnoses of acute and chronic back pain. (Reproduced with permission from the Norwegian Sports Medicine Association.)

Differential Diagnoses

An overview of the most current differential diagnoses is listed in Table 5.5. Back pain is usually due to affection of the muscles, intervertebral disks, or facet joints. Often several structures are involved. Reflex interplay between the structures makes it difficult to make an exact diagnosis during the acute stage. MRI often provides a specific diagnosis (e.g., protrusion, prolapse, spinal stenosis, recess stenosis, facet joint arthrosis, degeneration of the intervertebral disk, osteochondritis, and spondylolisthesis). If a corresponding evaluation of people with healthy backs were made, the proportion of diagnoses would have been nearly as high as in those patients with back pain. Therefore, the physician must relate findings from diagnostic imaging to clinical findings before giving the patient a specific diagnosis. For example, in adults there is no statistical relationship between radiographic spondylolysis or spondylolisthesis and pain. Spondylolysis or spondylolisthesis should be excluded in young athletes who have back pain.

If the patient has chronic sciatica caused by disk herniation or recess stenosis, a decision must be made about whether or not to perform surgery on the patient and what consequences surgery would have for sport activity in the long and short terms. In the elderly, pain and walking difficulties that improve when the patient bends forward may be caused by spinal stenosis (spinal claudication). In terms of differential diagnoses, cardiovascular diseases should be considered.

In downhill and cross-country skiing, in weightlifting, and in sports that involve throwing (including ball sports), the tendon insertions may become inflamed or may rupture because of sudden or repeated loading. (An example is pain referred from the quadratus lumborum muscle.) Then pain projects toward the groin, thigh, and iliac crest and becomes worse with lateral flexion, extension, and rotation. Repeated loading during martial arts, such as judo and karate, may cause muscle and ligament damage.

Diagnostic Thinking

If the patient has chronic pain, the diagnosis should include a functional evaluation relating to the individual sport. In addition to the examination based on pathological anatomy, psychological, and social factors should be evaluated.

First, the practitioner should determine whether the pain derives from the back or from some other area or cause (e.g., from the abdomen, genitalia, or systemic disease). The practitioner should then determine whether the condition requires immediate attention or referral (spinal cord affection or cauda equina lesion); whether symptoms and signs indicate serious back disease (red flags are noted in Table 5.6), nerve root affection, or specific disorders of the spine; or whether the patient has common back pain. We prefer to use these terms rather than specific or nonspecific back pain. If red flags are uncovered during the examination, it is the physician's job to communicate this without causing unnecessary anxiety. If a supplemental

Pain that does not worsen with activity
Case history: doping, cancer, HIV
Impaired general condition, weight loss
Neurological abnormalities without obvious radicular characteristics
Structural deformity

Table 5.6 Red flags for back pain. The patient should be referred within 4 weeks. (Reproduced with permission from the Norwegian Sports Medicine Association.)

examination is necessary, the patient should be informed that these examinations are often negative, that the specialist will provide additional advice, and that it may be advisable for the patient to reduce his activity level somewhat until after he has been examined by the specialist.

Most patients with acute back pain become asymptomatic within 1–2 weeks without treatment. The pain is often strong and accompanied by significant dysfunction. A patient seeks medical assistance because she wants pain relief and advice about what to do. The patient should be informed that the prognosis for acute back pain is good. A complete examination is not always necessary. Because it is difficult to make a specific diagnosis during the acute stage, the patient should be given an opportunity to return for a complete new examination within 2 weeks. Surgery is indicated during the acute stage if the patient has lost control of urination or defecation or has increasing leg paralysis. In the latter case, the patient should be referred for appropriate orthopedic or neurosurgical care immediately. The prognosis for acute bladder or rectal paresis is worse if it lasts more than 11 hours. Patients with kyphosis or structural scoliosis should be referred for orthopedic evaluation. If Bekhterev disease or another inflammatory disease is present, a rheumatologist should evaluate the patient.

The diagnosis and clinical course are used to determine when to refer a patient to a department or specialist in physical medicine, neurology, orthopedics, or rheumatology. If the condition lasts less than 2 weeks, the patient is usually examined and treated by a primary physician. If it lasts more than 8 weeks, a specialist should evaluate the patient.

If the pain persists, the practitioner should take the time to listen to the patient's case history and do a thorough clinical examination again. Diagnostic imaging is usually not a shortcut to proper diagnosis and treatment but can be a useful supplement to the clinical examination.

Patients in different age groups normally have back pain from different causes. Table 5.7 indicates the conditions that should be given primary consideration for each age group. Back pain during childhood, puberty, and adolescence is fairly common. Most patients do not seek a physician or physical therapist, nor do they need to do so. The challenge lies in figuring out which patients need regular checkups and/or treatment.

Case History

Quantitate the morbidity. Use a scale value of pain, function, and occupation to better estimate the intensity of symptoms. The pain drawing is a major help in accomplishing the objectives of the physical examination. Eliminate (red flags) the possibility of tumors, infections, and neurologic crisis—these diseases have a certain urgency that requires immediate attention.

Delineate the psychosocial factors (yellow flags) like anxiety, depression, fear-avoidance, and self-efficacy beliefs. Know what psychological effect the pain has had on the patient. Know the social, economic, and legal results of the patient's disability. Understand what can be gained by his or her being sick or well. Derive an understanding of what role these factors are playing in the patient's complaints.

Some key factors in the history are: the cause of the injury; the time of day when the pain is worse; a comparison of pain levels during walking, sitting, and standing; the effects of Valsalva maneuver, coughing and sneezing on pain; the type of injury and duration of the problem; the percentage of back versus leg pain.

NECK AND BACK

Children

Congenital (structural) abnormalities, such as hemivertebra or lack of segmentation of the vertebra, accompanied by potentially progressive, unbalanced growth

By the age of 8 years, the prevalence of spondylolysis is comparable to the prevalence in adults

In case of strong back pain that does not subside, a tumor/diskitis, or juvenile prolapse should be ruled out (primary tumors also occur in patients in other age groups)

Puberty

Structural abnormalities that manifest during a growth spurt, such as idiopathic scoliosis, Scheuermann disease, and spondylolysis

Extreme loading during the growth spurt (e.g., in gymnastics or weightlifting)

Adolescence

Fractures in risk sports

Soft-tissue injuries

Anorexia or hormone imbalance as the cause of a stress fracture

Adults

Soft-tissue injuries

Degeneration of intervertebral disk and facet joints contributing to lumbago or sciatica

Fractures in risk sports

Anorexia or hormone imbalance as the cause of a stress fracture

Bekhterev disease or another rheumatic disorder

Elderly

Degenerative changes contributing to lumbago, sciatica, or spinal stenosis

If the patient has nonspecific back pain that begins at a late adult age, a tumor/metastasis should be ruled out, especially if the patient is older than 60 years

Osteoporosis causing a compression fracture

Table 5.7 Diagnoses of the back for various age groups. (Reproduced with permission from the Norwegian Sports Medicine Association.)

Distinguishing between disk-related (diskogenic) and muscular pain is difficult. The practitioner should consider why the patient has chronic pain. Was it undiagnosed during the acute phase? Following a natural course, would the patient be unlikely to recover within 2 weeks? Has treatment been adequate? Did the athlete participate in competition too soon after the worst acute pain wore off? Are complaints related to the patient's activity level or lack of activity? Are other factors contributing to the development of chronic pain?

Athletes are like other patients with back pain—often feeling helpless and afraid that they will have a serious diagnosis or that the pain may prevent planned training and competitive activity, or worse, even end their sport career. Therefore, the way the practitioner handles the patient during the initial consultation is of major importance. The practitioner must instill confidence in the patient and develop a mutual understanding of the disease to create a basis for providing individual treatment advice.

Acute Pain

The origins of pain, as well as the patient's main symptoms and dysfunction, must be described in the case history. The physician must determine what the patient's primary symptom is. Is the pain localized in the back or in the lower extremities? Patients with an acute disk herniation and pain in the lower extremities do not always have back pain. Conversely, a patient with pain referring from the deep muscles in the hip may have pain in both the back and in the lower extremities. Is the pain alleviated at rest or does it get worse when the patient coughs or sneezes? If hyperextension increases the pain but flexion does not, the cause may be spondylolysis or spondylolisthesis.

Classic radiculopathy causes radicular pain radiating into a specific dermatomal pattern, with paresis, loss of sensation, and reflex loss. The radicular pattern of the pain and neurological examination determines the nerve involved. The classic history for radiculopathy resulting from a disk herniation is back pain that progresses to predominantly leg pain. It is made worse by increases in intraspinal pressure such as coughing, sneezing, and sitting. Leg pain predominates over back pain and mechanical factors increase the pain. Physical examination shows positive nerve stretch signs. A dermatomal distribution leg pain that is made worse by straight leg raising, sitting or supine, leg-straight foot dorsal flexion, neck flexion, jugular compression, and by direct palpation of the popliteal nerve or sciatic notch is characteristic of radiculopathy. A source of radicular pain not found in this description is that caused by spinal stenosis. Spinal stenosis usually lacks positive nerve stretch signs, but has the characteristic history of neurogenic claudication (i.e., leg and calf pain produced by ambulation). Pain that does not go away immediately upon stopping is made worse with spinal extension and is relieved by flexion. The pain progresses from proximal to distal.

Distinct back pain accompanied by fever may indicate purulent diskitis. In that case, the erythrocyte sedimentation rate (ESR), C-reactive protein (CRP) and the white blood cell count will be raised. MRI is positive the first days if the patient has diskitis.

If the patient has intense pain and is bedridden, anxiety and fears often contribute to the dysfunction. Therefore, the practitioner should have the patient explain what she thinks is causing her pain. Rapid exclusion of red flags (Table 5.6) is good therapy. If the patient has had similar complaints in the past, the physician must find out what type of treatment she was given and whether it was effective. The patient's expectations about treatment are vital to the outcome of the treatment.

Knowledge of the individual sport may make it easier to understand the injury mechanism. In soccer, the injury mechanism may be extension (throwing), hyperflexion (deflection), compression (falls or collisions), or torsion (dribbling or kicking). In golf, repeated twisting may cause a stress fracture in one or more ribs and trigger pain in the middle or upper section of the back. Dancers compensate for increased external rotation of the hips by increasing lumbar lordosis. In addition, lifting above the head and large numbers of jumps make them susceptible to injuries. Frequently occurring injury mechanisms are listed in Table 5.8.

Injury mechanism	Sports
Repeated loading	Cross-country skiing, rowing, paddling
Repeated loading in contact sports	Soccer, handball, ice hockey, wrestling, judo, karate
Lifting partners	Ballet, dance
Loading during growth period	Weightlifting, gymnastics
Sudden strong muscle contraction	Throwing sports
Hyperextension or torsion	Throwing sports, gymnastics

Table 5.8 Frequently occurring injury mechanisms related to back pain. (Reproduced with permission from the Norwegian Sports Medicine Association.)

Chronic Pain

The transition from normal complaints to prolonged illness and disability is poorly understood, but there are new studies suggesting augmented central pain processing. This transition has recently been attributed to neurobiological and psychobiological sensitization mechanisms. If the patient has chronic pain, the practitioner must review the entire case history. Information is often available from diagnostic imaging or from a specialist when the complaints are chronic. Psychosocial yellow flags should be clarified if the patient does not respond to treatment (Table 5.9). The patient should be allowed to tell his story in his own words. A tentative diagnosis should be made independent of previous examinations. Allowing enough time for the examination provides a good basis for further treatment.

The case history must reveal the nature of the patient's primary complaints. For most patients with low back pain, a precise pathoanatomical diagnosis is difficult to obtain due to weak associations between symptoms and anatomical findings. A high degree of comorbidity, which may influence prognosis, has been described in patients with nonspecific low back pain. To locate the pain, the patient may point to, or make marks on, a pain drawing of the entire body. A substantial proportion of the patients report a number of other subjective health complaints, including widespread pain that suggests somatization. Radiating pain that worsens when the patient sneezes and that follows a dermatome indicates nerve root affection. Pain and dysfunction that increase only in connection with sport activity indicate a need to evaluate technique and physical capacity. Reduced strength in the lower extremities experienced during sport activity suggests mild paresis caused by nerve root affection. The gradual onset of pain and morning stiffness tends to indicate a rheumatic (inflammatory) disease. If no treatment has helped and the patient dramatizes the irritation verbally and with body language, this more often suggests abnormal illness behavior than a serious back disorder. A useful clinical tool to assist in distinguishing anatomic and psychosocial factors for the pain is the Waddell score. The physician should determine whether the patient actually wants to return to his sport career.

Clinical Examination

Acute Pain

The physical examination should address: maneuvers during the examination that reproduce the pain; the presence of sciatic stretch signs; the neurologic deficit; back and lower extremity stiffness and loss of range of motion; the exact location of tenderness and radiation of pain or paresthesias.

The purpose of the clinical examination is to evaluate whether the symptoms are consistent with the clinical signs. Is there an indication for hospitalization or for a quick evaluation by a specialist? Is the patient apprehensive with major dysfunction, although clinical findings are otherwise normal? The physician should evaluate red flags (Table 5.6). If possible, he should make a tentative diagnosis as to whether the pain originates from the nerve root, a specific spinal disorder, the spinal segment and the superficial musculature, the pelvis, or the hips, or is referred from other organs. Diagnostic imaging is usually not indicated as part of the initial examination by the primary health care provider. The following points should be evaluated during the initial examination of a patient with acute back pain:

(a)

(b)

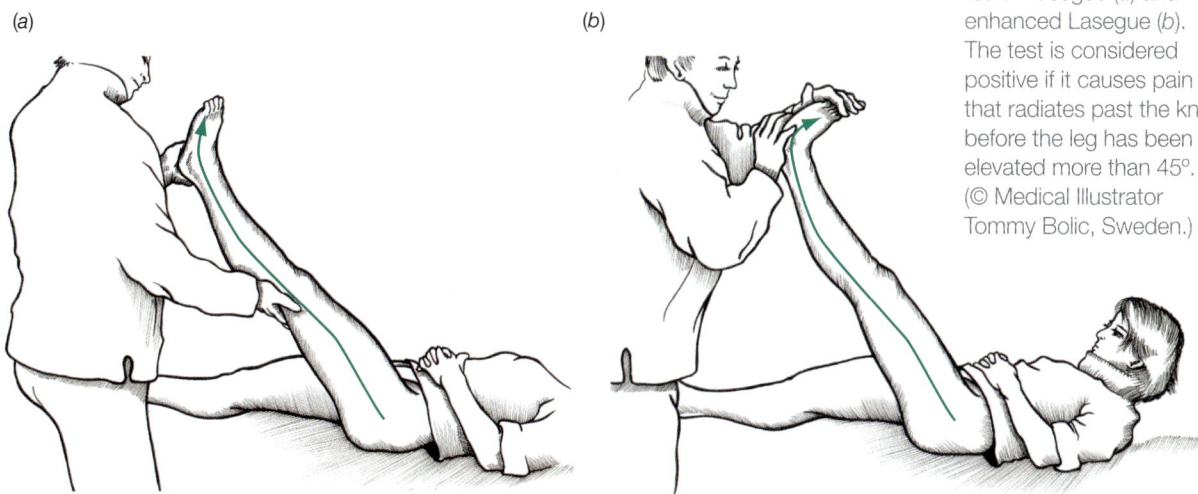

Figure 5.14 Nerve stretch tests: Lasegue (*a*) and enhanced Lasegue (*b*). The test is considered positive if it causes pain that radiates past the knee before the leg has been elevated more than 45°. (© Medical Illustrator Tommy Bolic, Sweden.)

NECK AND BACK

- If the patient has bladder and bowel disturbance, he should be examined for saddle anesthesia and for sphincter function by rectal exploration. To confirm good sphincter control, the patient should be asked to squeeze.
- If there is radiating pain or reported muscle weakness in the extremities, the patient should be asked to walk on his toes (S1) and heels (L5) and to do knee bends (L4). The distal sensation of the calves and feet should also be examined. If this is not possible because the patient is bedridden, motor function should be tested with the patient in a supine position.
- If there is radiating pain or reported muscle weakness in the extremities, the patient should be given nerve tension tests (Figures 5.14a and 5.14b). Nerve tension should be tested first sitting as supine testing avoids pelvic and spine rotation that can be painful and misleading. Nerve tension can be tested with the patient in a supine position. For the Lasegue test, the patient's lower extremity is lifted with the knee extended. The test is positive if the patient's radiating pain is reproduced distal to the knee at an elevation of less than 45°. The test can be strengthened by dorsal flexion of the foot. Short hamstring musculature may contribute to a falsely positive test. In case of doubt, the knee may be slightly flexed and the foot flexed dorsally. The Lasegue test is considered crossed positive when elevation of the contralateral lower extremity reproduces radiating pain. The test is falsely positive if the radiating pain is not reproduced when the examiner does a diversionary maneuver (such as testing plantar flexion) while administering the test. The Cram test or bowstring test is thumb pressure on the sciatic nerve in the popliteal fossa during a supine straight leg raise that produces radiating pain in the leg is an important sign of nerve root tension.
- In terms of differential diagnostics, movement in the hip joint and in the soft tissues in the hips and pelvis are examined.
- Axial deviation suggests leg length discrepancy, a divergent posture that affects the intervertebral disk, or idiopathic scoliosis. Reduced active movement when bending forward and to the side may be due to pain, shortened musculature, or rheumatic disease. Pain triggered by extension of spine while standing on one leg only indicates spondylolysis or spondylolisthesis (Figure 5.15), because movement compromises the posterior structures in the spinal column.

Chronic Pain

Although the main goal of examining patients with acute back pain is to uncover red flags that should lead to an expanded evaluation, patients with chronic back pain must be thoroughly examined for the purpose of making a pathoanatomical diagnosis based on the case history. The examination must take place with the patient dressed in underwear only.

- How does the patient walk? Does he roll the hips? Does he limp (which could indicate trouble with the back or sciatica)?
- Does the patient walk differently when she is asked to walk than she does when she walks spontaneously? Are there signs of a functional walking pattern?
- Is there paresis when he walks on his heels or toes or when he is doing knee bends?
- Is there muscle atrophy?

Inspection of the patient from behind

- Determine whether the patient has scoliosis and/or pelvic deviation. Is the scoliosis structural (Figure 5.16)? The best way to observe scoliosis is to have the patient bend forward, because the torsional component in scoliosis makes the costal arch prominent (gibbus) on the convex side. Scoliosis that is caused by leg length discrepancy disappears when the patient uses an orthotic device, usually a buildup in her shoe.
- Can the patient touch the floor with straight legs? What limits movement? Tight hamstring muscles or back pain? If the patient needs to push off with his hands when he stands up again, this indicates muscular dysfunction.
- Is lateral flexion symmetrical? Unilaterally reduced lateral flexion may indicate that the facet joint is affected. Pain that is provoked by combined rotation of the upper body and pelvis indicates that the pain does not derive from the back
- Single leg hyperextension that causes pain (Figure 5.15) suggests spondylolysis or spondylolisthesis.

Supine position

- In the supine position, the patient should be tested for passive flexion and external rotation of the of the hip with flexed knee. Pain during the FABER test (Flexion, ABduction, and hip External Rotation) (Figure 10.14). To perform this test, place the lateral malleolus on the contralateral knee–push down on the ipsilateral knee. Anterior groin pain is hip joint pathology; posterior pain with the maneuver is nonspecific.
- The Lasegue test is positive when pain radiates distal to the knee at less than 45° elevation of the extended leg. If necessary, the practitioner should examine crossed Lasegue, and with the patient in a sitting position by testing the plantar reflex and distracting the patient at the same time.
- Strength in the anterior tibial muscle, toe extensors, long peroneal muscle, short peroneal muscle, toe flexors, and the triceps muscle of the calf are examined with the knees flexed. Strength of knee extension and hip flexion should be tested. Is the display of strength jerky?

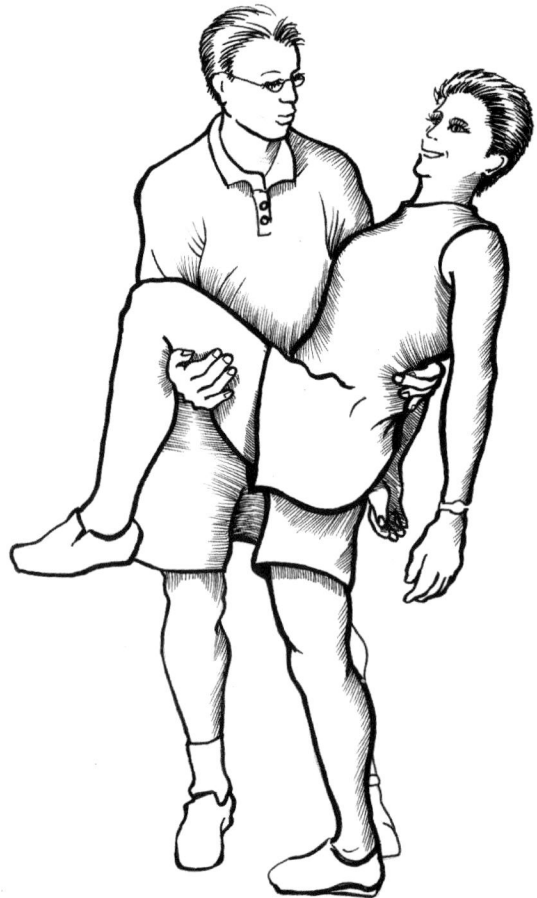

Figure 5.15 Single-leg hyperextension test. The test can also be done with the examiner standing behind the patient and providing support of the leg and pelvis. The goal is to provoke hyperextension in the lumbar column. Recent research suggests that this test should be regarded as supplementary and not diagnostic for spondylolysis/spondylolisthesis. (© Medical Illustrator Tommy Bolic, Sweden.)

- The patellar, Achilles, and plantar reflexes are tested at 90°-knee flexion.
- If the patient has pain in the hip or gluteal region, the practitioner should examine combined hip flexion, external rotation, and adduction (piriform muscle, quadriceps coxae syndrome).
- If the quadratus lumborum muscle seems to be affected, the practitioner should palpate the muscle at the same time that the patient is abducting and pulling his hip toward his body.
- The physician should perform an examination of skin sensation in the L4, L5, and S1 dermatomes and possibly for saddle anesthesia.

Prone position

- The patient's hip rotation should be examined in the prone position, and the differences between the sides should be noted.
- The Lasegue test should be reversed (extension of the hip joint with increasing flexion in the knee causes nerve root pain on the anterior side of the thigh with L4 root affection).
- The practitioner should palpate for pain in the gluteal musculature, over the ischial tuberosity, the greater trochanter, and the external rotators of the hip joint.
- The practitioner should palpate for pain paravertebrally and in the midline above and between the spinous processes. Is the pain localized or widespread? Is pain provoked by light touching or by strong, distinct pressure?

Waddell signs

- If at least three of the five tests are positive, the patient may have abnormal illness behavior. The five tests are the Lasegue test with distraction, combined rotation of the upper body and pelvis, nonphysiological signs (loss of sensitivity in a stocking distribution and jerky paresis), tenderness caused by palpation of both the skin and of the deeper structures, and exaggerated pain behavior.

Supplemental Examinations

Ordering diagnostic imaging examinations during the first consultation is usually unnecessary. Skeletal X-rays are indicated if a fracture or tumor is suspected or if the patient is elderly and has back pain without radicular characteristics. If the patient has a neurological disorder, an MRI is the initial examination. A CT is indicated if spondylolysis is suspected. This must be specified on the order form so that the image sections can be taken at the proper levels. Scintigraphy is used if the case history and clinical findings indicate spondylolysis but the CT is negative or the patient has a history <3 months. The primary health care provider normally should not order an MRI during the first consultation for back pain, but it may be indicated if pain has persisted for more than 4 weeks and is indicated preoperatively if the patient is hospitalized. An immediate MRI is also indicated to exclude hematoma that requires quick evacuation if neurological deficit increases postoperatively. Skeletal X-rays, scintigraphy, MRI, and biopsy are indicated for differential diagnostic evaluation of malignancy and infection. MRI is the first choice for evaluating infection.

When ordering supplemental examinations, the order form should be carefully completed. Case history, the patient's main symptoms, and clinical findings can be described in three sentences. If images were taken earlier, what is the indication for taking new images? Because of cost considerations and the radiation hazard, the need for repeated images to be taken must be unequivocal.

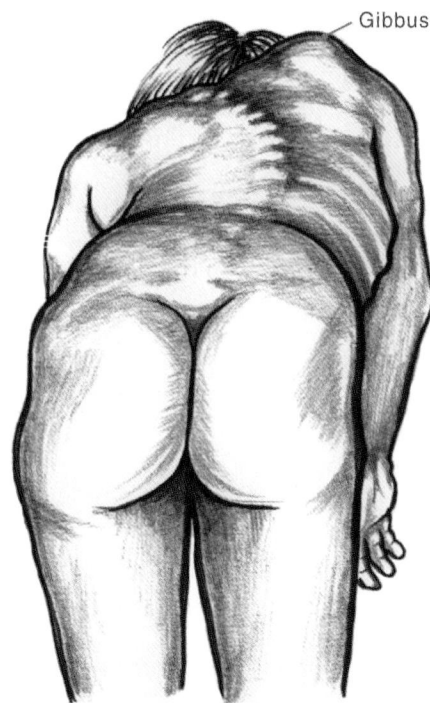

Gibbus

Figure 5.16 Structural scoliosis. The scoliosis is most easily seen when the patient bends forward, because the torsional component in the scoliosis causes the costal arch to become prominent on the convex side. (© Medical Illustrator Tommy Bolic, Sweden.)

NECK AND BACK

X-ray of the lumbosacral spine. A routine X-ray provides information about degenerative changes, spondylolisthesis, previous fractures, or compression fractures. If the primary physician finds structural scoliosis during a clinical examination, standing images of the entire spine can be ordered or the patient may be referred to the orthopedic department without ordering the imaging first. If Scheuermann disease is suspected, lateral images are taken of the thoracolumbar spine.

Lumbar CT. MRI has replaced lumbar CT as a first-choice test for radicular pain. CT is used for evaluation of fractures, spondylolysis, and for specific preoperative indications.

MRI. An MRI is the first choice for suspected malignancy and diskitis and usually replaces myelography for evaluating spinal stenosis or recess stenosis. The examination is sensitive: It shows early degeneration in the intervertebral disk (black disks) or disk protrusion. These findings are nonspecific and should not carry too much weight when choosing treatment, although the relevance of vertebral endplate degeneration or inflammation (Modic changes) is discussed. MRI with contrast is better than CT for distinguishing between scar tissue and a new disk herniation.

Skeletal scintigraphy. Scintigraphy (SPECT) is used if a stress fracture (spondylolysis) or malignancy is suspected. Degeneration, tendonitis, and aseptic necrosis of bone may also generate a positive scan.

Diskography. This procedure is used preoperatively for matters regarding disk-related pain. The patient's pain description on injection is more important than the morphological picture of the intervertebral disk (rupture of the annulus fibrosis). Contrast leakage will almost always occur after prolapse extirpation. To make the diagnosis of diskogenic lumbago, the patient's pain must be reproduced in the affected disk while the disk above it is pain free. The prognostic value of this procedure is questionable. Diskography may only be ordered for differential diagnostic evaluation of selected patients by specialists, but is not an evidence-based procedure to select patients for spinal fusion or artificial disk replacement.

Facet joint anesthesia. The examination must be done using transillumination and must produce at least 50% pain reduction to be positive. In addition, there should be a negative saline injection for a diagnosis of a facet joint syndrome. Isolated facet blocks are not accurate in diagnosing the spinal level causing the back pain because of branching cephalad and caudad of the posterior primary ramus innervating the facet joints.

Common Painful Conditions

Acute strain—*Acute Low Back Pain*

Acute strain is most common in the 20–55-year age group. The cause may be vertebrogenic, diskogenic, or muscular. Often several structures are involved. Because it may be difficult to make an exact diagnosis, the syndrome is described using the collective term "acute lumbago."

- Symptoms and signs: Pain in the lumbar region may or may not radiate to the hip, groin, or posterior side of the thigh. The patient often has difficulty moving in a normal manner and may have sciatic scoliosis. Often all movements are painful and limited. The Lasegue test may be positive but is usually negative when given at the same time as the distraction maneuver.

- Diagnosis: The diagnosis is made clinically, based on the description in the preceding text and by simultaneously excluding other causes of acute back pain. An X-ray is not necessary.
- Treatment by physician: The patient should be informed that the best treatment is to maintain a normal activity level. Not bearing weight and using crutches are not recommended. Over-the-counter analgesics or NSAIDs for 3–7 days decrease the duration of the painful period. Stronger (narcotic) analgesics are seldom needed. The athlete should not participate in competition before he can complete a normal training routine.
- Treatment by physical therapist: During the acute phase, treatment by a physical therapist is unnecessary, but the patient may benefit just as much from an initial examination by a physical therapist as from one by a physician. There is no purpose in starting abdominal and back muscle exercises during the first painful phase, but alternative training to maintain general endurance and strength in the extremities may be started soon after the injury. It is important to be positive when giving advice and not to place unnecessary restrictions on specific movements. The evidence for manipulation is under debate. It may be indicated if the patient has great expectations for this type of treatment or needs supplemental pain therapy.
- Self-treatment: The patient should be advised to keep the activity level as normal as possible, to remain ambulatory, and to resume training within a few days.
- Prognosis: The prognosis is good. Most patients are asymptomatic within a week, but nearly half experience a recurrence within the year. Therefore, a wait and see attitude toward treatment should be taken. Patients who do not have red flags should be informed that back pain is normal and not harmful, but may return just like the common cold. New back pain is not the same as a new injury. The patient should be advised that gradually increasing his level of activity and restricting competitive activity until he is able to train normally may contribute to reducing the frequency of recurrence.

Chronic strain—*Chronic Low Back Pain*

The starting point for the pain may be muscular insufficiency, degeneration of the intervertebral disk, centrally positioned disk herniation, or facet joint arthrosis. The diagnosis of segmental instability is also used. There is no specific clinical or diagnostic imaging examination that serves as the basis for this diagnosis. The criteria for diskogenic pain or facet joint syndrome are specified in the section on supplemental examinations. Muscular insufficiency may also occur in very well-trained athletes. In a study that included elite rowers, increased fatigability in the multifidus musculature verified by EMG was associated with persisting low back pain. Degeneration of the intervertebral disks is not necessarily associated with pain, but occurs frequently in young athletes (Figure 5.17) in a few sports.

The practitioner should evaluate psychosocial yellow flags if the patient has not responded to treatment (Table 5.9). Psychosocial factors, thoughts about the consequences of back pain (fear-avoidance beliefs) and "doctor shopping" are more important risk factors than biomedical symptoms or signs. The high number of different subjective health complaints in chronic low back pain and evidence of the effectiveness of psychological treatments, such as cognitive behavioral treatment, suggest that there are common psychobiological elements in patients with chronic pain and less specificity than the diagnostic labels suggest. Sustained avoidance of movement, social interactions, leisure activities, and work, may increase pain and disability. Interventions to reduce avoidance and attention towards pain, and to increase physical activity should therefore be encouraged by the physician, the physical therapist, and eventually other members of the treatment team.

- **Symptoms and signs:** Pain that gets worse during monotonous activity, in which the patient often changes position while standing or sitting, is a symptom of chronic lumbago. Unilateral pain with morning stiffness that is relieved by NSAIDs may point toward arthrosis, whereas more diffuse pain that gets worse, particularly when working in a stooping position, may suggest predominating muscular pain. Typical symptoms and signs include reduced range of motion during flexion and lateral flexion, an abnormal position off and on, and short hamstring and psoas muscles. Waddell signs are part of the examination.
- **Diagnosis:** The diagnosis is clinical, according to the symptoms and signs described previously. The criteria for diskogenic pain or facet joint syndrome are listed in the section on supplemental examinations. They should be used with caution because of indefinite treatment and prognostic consequences. Diagnostic imaging criteria are described previously, in the section on supplemental examinations.
- **Treatment by physician:** NSAIDs or paracetamol is the first choice. Stronger analgesics are indicated for pain-related sleeping problems. Surgery is rarely indicated.
- **Treatment by physical therapist:** Group exercise is the first choice. The quota principle may apply if it is hard to get started. In some studies, the effectiveness of manual therapy has been documented.
- **Prognosis:** Patients who learn to live with the pain often have a high level of function with brief bad spells. The athlete may need to change his short- or long-term goals. Psychological and social factors are of greater significance than diagnostic imaging and clinical factors. Because the prognosis is generally worse than for other back problems, a comprehensive evaluation is a prerequisite for any surgery.

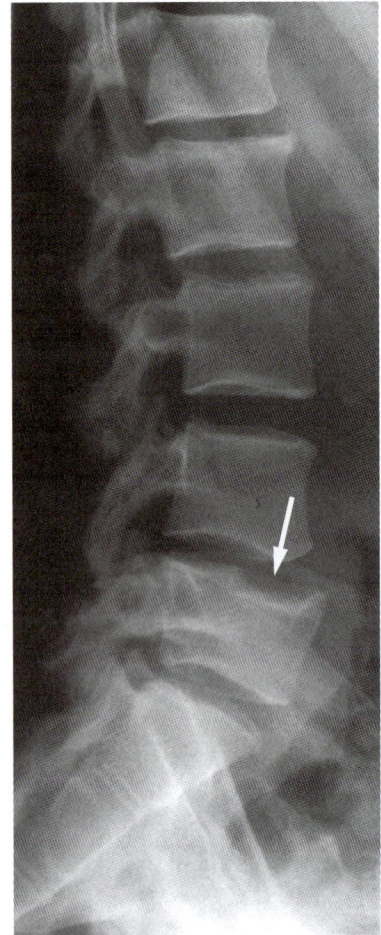

Figure 5.17
Degenerative changes in the lumbar column of a former gymnast. Reduced disk height and mild exostoses in L1–L2. Injury to the upper endplate and deformation of L5.

Previous back pain
Long time away from sports or work
Radicular pain
Reduced muscle strength and endurance in the abdominal and back muscles in relation to the requirements of the individual sports
Reduced range of motion in relation to the requirements of the individual sport
Atypical illness behavior and somatization
Psychological stress and depression, difficulty in sleeping, social isolation
Dissatisfaction
Personal problems: alcohol, cohabitation, finances
Insurance claims
Belief that back pain is harmful and may cause disability
Fear avoidance beliefs about physical activity
Expectation of passive treatment modalities like drugs, electrotherapy, massage

Table 5.9 Yellow flags or risk factors for chronic back pain. (Reproduced with permission from the Norwegian Sports Medicine Association.)

Spondylolysis and Spondylolisthesis—*Stress Fracture in the Vertebral Arch (possibly with slippage)*

In these conditions, a defect (lysis) exists in the vertebral arch (interarticular portion). This defect is caused in various ways, although in athletes the cause is usually a stress fracture. It is prevalent in about 7% of the adult population of the western world. A large epidemiological study of elite Spanish athletes revealed 8% prevalence. The highest prevalence was in throwing sports (27%), in dance sports and acrobatic sports it ranged from 10% to 30%, and in rowing it was 17%. While the incidence of stress fractures is higher in certain types of athletes compared to others, any athlete is potentially subjected to the repetitive twisting and extension motion that is identified with the etiology of spondylolysis. The typical spondylolytic lesion occurs in the pars interarticularis, but may be present in the pedicle or articular process. The sports frequently associated with a significantly increased incidence are diving, gymnastics, wrestling, handball, and weight lifting. The incidence of isthmic defects in female gymnasts is four times that of the general female Caucasian population. The incidence of isthmic defects is approximately 4.5% during the first year of school and is more common in boys than in girls. There are certain familial predispositions in young children and there is an increased incidence of spina bifida in young athletes who have spondylolysis. Spondylolysis rarely leads to progressive high-grade spondylolisthesis.

Spondylolysis in sports is associated with hyperextension, rotation, and torsion with resistance, such as in throwing sports. Because of the increasing use of weightlifting as a training technique in all varieties of sports, many athletes suffer a fatigue fracture in the weight room as opposed to directly on the athletic field. There are certain maneuvers in specific sports such as hyperextension in gymnasts, extension in anterior alignment in weight lifters and extension with rotation in baseball pitchers that can lead to the repetitive loading that produces the fracture.

It was previously reported that about 80% of the athletes have olisthesis between two vertebrae (usually L5 and S1), but only 30% of the athletes in the Spanish study had olisthesis. Slippage is usually low grade. *Spondylolisthesis* can be graded from I to V (Figure 5.18), where grade I is defined as slippage of up to 25% of the sagittal diameter and grade V as the vertebra lying in front of the vertebra underneath it. The location can be at any level of the spine. It is certainly more common at L5, because L5 is a transitional area between the fixed sacrum and the mobile lumbar spine. There is an abnormal distribution of forces at this level, and rotational forces may be inappropriately directed to the pars interarticularis at L5. Increased lordosis can increase the stress at L5. Shear forces at the lumbosacral junction have been shown to predispose the pars to fracture. There is no statistical relationship between radiographic spondylolysis and symptoms in adults. It is estimated that about 10% of the people who have spondylolysis have symptoms.

Spondylolysis is probably to be the most common source for persistent low back pain in adolescent athletes. Slippage may increase during the childhood years and in adolescence, but it almost never increases during adulthood (after puberty).

• Symptoms and signs: Pain in the lumbar region that radiates to the gluteal musculature and to the thighs is a symptom of spondylolysis and spondylolisthesis. Patients are often asymptomatic in the morning but get worse with activity during the day and symptoms improves with rest. Sciatica due to degeneration of the intervertebral disk, facet joint, or hypertrophic tissue in the pseudoarthrosis fissure may occur. The patient may experience distinct pain when one leg is extended

Sacrum

Coccyx

(c)

(d)

(e)

(f)

(g)

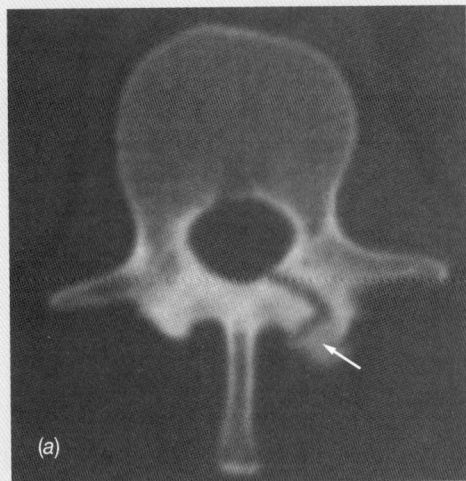

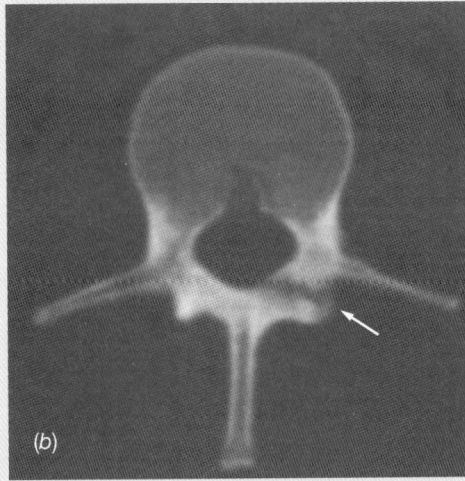

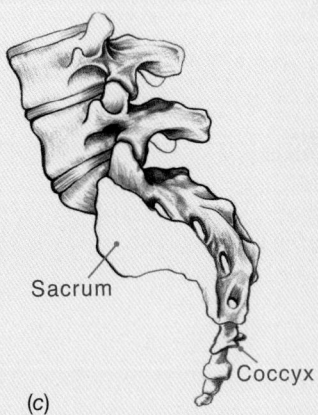

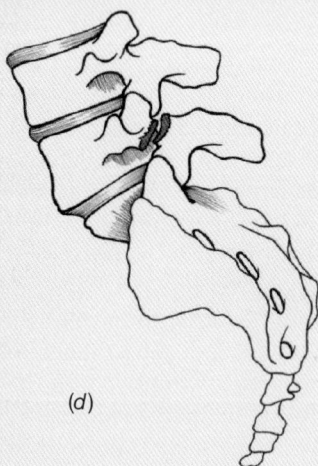

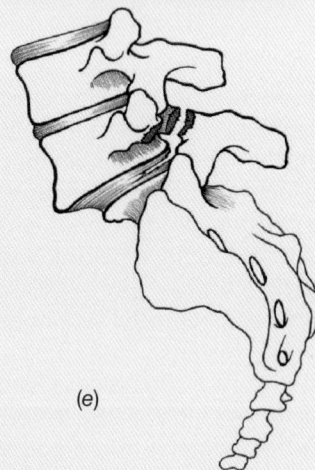

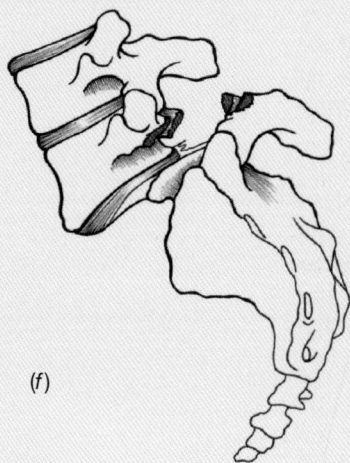

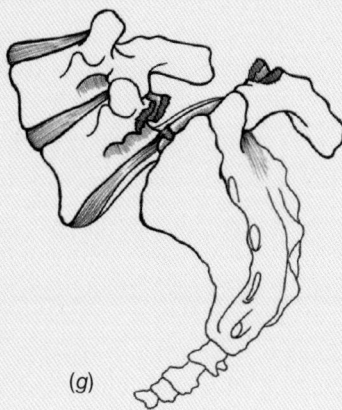

Figure 5.18 Spondylolysis/ spondylolisthesis. CT images demonstrate spondylolysis in levels L1 (*a*) and L2 (*b*) in an internationally competitive javelin thrower. The patient achieved normal throwing function without surgery. The drawings show the grading of spondylolysis (*c*) and spondylolisthesis, grade I (*d*), grade II (*e*), grade III (*f*), and grade IV (*g*). (© Medical Illustrator Tommy Bolic, Sweden.)

while she is standing or lying prone (Figure 5.13), but a negative test does not rule out the diagnosis in adolescent athletes. Spondylolysis is more common in young athletes than spondylolisthesis. If there is a great deal of slippage, it may be possible to palpate a depression above the spinous process of the slipped vertebra. A recent study showed that spondylolisthesis did not significantly reduce the chance of playing in the National Football League for any position, while a history of spondylolysis had a significant effect for running backs. Other studies suggest that spondylolysis is not a significant finding in collegiate American football athletes. Spondylolysis and spondylolisthesis do not necessarily shorten an athletic career.

- Diagnosis: Diagnosis is made by clinical examination of the symptoms and by spondylolysis or spondylolisthesis that was confirmed by radiography. X-rays of the lumbosacral column in frontal and lateral planes are the first choice and will usually demonstrate spondylolisthesis and the degree of slippage. Flexion and stretching images can be used to examine instability. Nuclear imaging (SPECT) is the best method for early diagnosis and a positive SPECT is associated with a painful pars lesion. Studies suggest that up to 35% of young athletes presenting with significant lumbar pain of 6-week duration have a positive bone scan. A CT provides bony details but may rarely be normal in cases with an abnormal SPECT scan. A CT is the best method of demonstrating defects in the vertebral arch. CT may reveal rare differential diagnoses such as osteoid osteoma, osteoblastoma, injured facet joint, or stress fracture in the pedicle, pars, or articular facet. MRI is indicated if tumor or infection is suspected.
- Treatment by physician: It has not been documented whether the use of a brace improves the prognosis and contributes to healing a recent stress fracture. Biomechanical studies do not particularly support their use because it is not documented that the intersegmental motion is restricted. The main effect of bracing is therefore most likely to limit physical activity. A rigid brace may be recommended for 2 months if symptoms do not resolve. One study evaluated the pars defects in 185 spondylolytic adolescent athletes. The patients wore a lumbosacral support corset for periods as long as 6 months, a control group was not included. The defect healed in 73% of the early cases, but only 38.5% of the progressive cases, and none of the terminal cases. The subject of pain relief was not addressed in that study. Paracetamol or NSAIDs are the first choice if drug therapy is necessary. Surgery is indicated for grades III–V if slippage increases, and if conservative treatment does not help with pain.
- Treatment by physical therapist: Instructions to improve activation of the deep trunk musculature should be given to the patient. Progress is not made by increasing the number of repetitions but by integrating increasingly complex activities into the activity pattern. The effectiveness of this treatment strategy has been documented in a recently published randomized study. If rest is advocated in a patient with a positive SPECT, the physiotherapist should initially focus on cardiovascular training, thereafter early core stability before gradually progress to sport-specific exercises. The rehabilitation period may require 2–4 months after a period of rest.
- Self-treatment: Treatment begins with identification of the etiology of the problem. If the etiology of the problem is one specific maneuver in a sport, the athlete is advised not to participate in that sport for a period. The patient with a negative SPECT should be advised to keep the activity level as normal as possible.

Other Painful Conditions

Acute Sciatica

Sciatica is a symptom rather than a specific diagnosis. The most important symptom is leg pain radiating below the knee to the foot. The prognosis is favorable in most

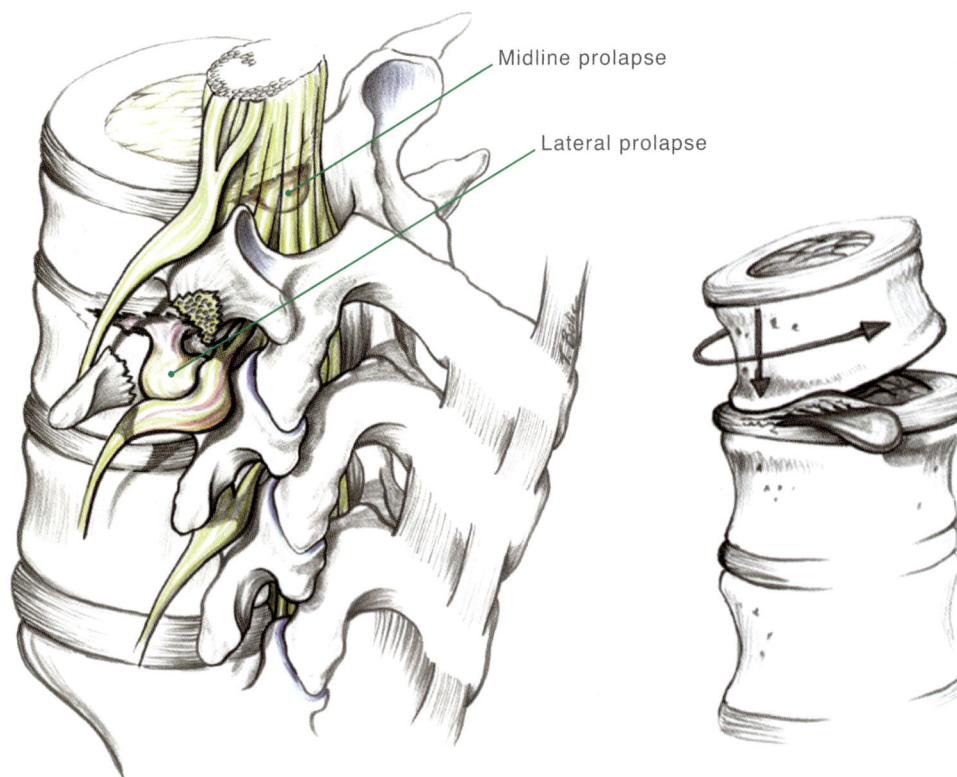

Midline prolapse

Lateral prolapse

Figure 5.19 A midline prolapse and a lateral prolapse with herniation. (© Medical Illustrator Tommy Bolic, Sweden.)

patients and symptoms usually improve within 4 weeks. Disk herniation (Figure 5.19) is the most common cause of sciatica. Recent research suggests that immunological factors contribute to the pain. An autoimmune reaction may occur with the formation of antigen–antibody complexes when the nucleus pulposus ruptures out into the spinal canal. Therefore, inflammation from an immunological source may cause sciatica. Neurological deficit is more likely related to compression of the nerve root. No clear relationship exists between a positive Lasegue test and pressure around the nerve root. A herniated disk may be asymptomatic or cause back pain with or without root symptoms but is not, in itself, an indication for surgery.

• Symptoms and signs: The radiating pain is normally worse than the back pain. Radiating pain distal to the knee and to the foot and toes and pain that worsens when the patient coughs suggest radicular pain. Numbness and paresthesia can also be present. During an examination, the athlete may walk with a limp and with the upper body stooping. This is often due to sciatic scoliosis. If the patient has radiating pain and reports muscle weakness in the extremities, he must be tested by walking on his toes (S1) and heels (L5) and by doing knee bends (L4). The practitioner should also examine the patient for sensory disturbances distally in the calves and in the feet. If this is not possible because the patient is bedridden, motor disturbance is examined with the patient in a supine position. If the patient's bladder and bowel functions are affected, he must be examined for saddle anesthesia. In addition, sphincter function must be examined by rectal exploration. The physician should ask the patient to squeeze, to confirm good sphincter control. The Lasegue test is positive when hip flexion more than 45° with an extended knee causes the patient to experience pain \distal to the knee. The test may be falsely positive, so the patient must also be examined while a distraction maneuver is being used.

- Diagnosis: If the patient reports radiating pain in one leg combined with one or more tests indicating nerve root tension or neurological deficit the diagnosis seems justified. The clinical diagnosis is definite if the patient has sensory deficit, muscle weakness, and weakened reflexes in a nerve root pattern (Figure 5.5). The physician must exclude conditions that require immediate treatment (e.g., fractures, bladder paralysis, or progressive paresis in the lower extremities), for which the patient should be referred to a specialist. It may be sufficient to make a referral based on symptoms and findings of a clinical examination. Imaging is unnecessary if primary treatment is effective. MRI visualizes the vertebral disks, ligaments, and muscles, and the presence of infection or tumors and should be recommended if the condition do not improve within 4 weeks.
- Treatment by physician: Nonoperative treatment primarily aims at pain reduction, either by analgesics or by reducing the pressure on the nerve root. A Cochrane review found little difference in effect on pain and functional status between bed rest and staying active. Corticosteroid injections are probably not more effective than placebo in the short term, and in the long term there is no difference. In most guidelines NSAIDs or paracetamol is recommended as the first-choice treatment, although the effect is moderate. Nerve root pain is usually not a cause for alarm. Inform the patient that most patients recover well without surgery and that normal activity does not delay healing. Referral to a specialist is usually unnecessary until 4 weeks have passed.
- Treatment by physical therapist: Manipulation is contraindicated. Lifting and repeated twisting should be avoided. The patient should adjust to alternative training and the most important role for the physiotherapist is to reassure and motivate the patient. Traction has been compared to placebo in at least seven trials and no consistently superior effect has been shown. The effect of traction is usually short term and does not have a documented effect on the natural course. When the condition improves, sport-specific exercises for the transverse muscles may be added.
- Self-treatment: The patient should be advised to maintain daily activities rather than staying in bed and to find alternative exercises that do not increase the pain.
- Prognosis: Individual variation is great. Off and on improvement the first 14 days is to be expected, in most patients pain and disability is expected to resolve within 4 weeks. The course may be long term, and the athlete usually needs to adjust goals and prepare for the next season.

Chronic Sciatica

Chronic sciatica is usually due to a prolapse of the 4th or 5th lumbar intervertebral disk or lateral recess stenosis. Intraspinal tumors are rare but may make their first appearance with nerve root pain. Irritation of the sciatic nerve (e.g., where it passes the piriformis muscle in the pelvis or where its peroneal branch passes the head of the fibula) may produce a convincing representation of nerve root affection (pseudosciatica).

- Symptoms, signs, and diagnosis: The diagnosis of chronic sciatica can be made if there is neurological deficit. Lumbar MRI is indicated with the clinical likelihood of sciatica after a 4-week case history, if there are no signs of improvement.
- Treatment by physician: NSAIDs or paracetamol are the first-choice treatments. The patient should be informed that most patients recover without surgery and that normal activity does not delay healing. Participation in competition will depend on the type of sport, personal characteristics, degree of pain and paresis, and the possibility for treatment. Progressive or persistent muscle weakness in the lower extremities, in addition to radiating pain after 3 months, is an indication for surgical treatment. Extirpation of a herniated disk using minimal access (Caspar instruments), flavectomy, or partial or full laminectomy, all have a documented

effect. If the surgeon uses a microscope, it is called microsurgery. Recently introduced surgical methods such as tubular prolapse extirpation or laser surgery have been evaluated in clinical trials and have not produced superior results concerning pain, disability, and complications. Numerous studies have reported that surgery is effective for reduction or eliminating radiating pain in most patients, but that back pain may continue after surgery. Consequently, the effectiveness of surgery for disk herniation and for back pain without radiating pain is uncertain. Percutaneous nucleotomy has no documented effect on disk herniation.

- Treatment by physical therapist: For progressing symptoms, the activity level should be reduced or changed. Ballet dancers and others who lift a partner may be able to maintain their activity level by wearing a brace or weightlifter's belt. A consensus has not been reached regarding rehabilitation after disk surgery. A Cochrane review recommends intensive rehabilitation, but recent studies suggest that a normal level of activity should be resumed as soon as the surgical wound is healed and that the strategies applied 20–30 years ago including immobilization with a brace for 6 weeks and thereafter 6–12 weeks rehabilitation before resuming ordinary activity are not necessary. Core strengthening is often advised for athletes, but the evidence that this is better than other exercises before resuming sports activity is sparse.
- Self-treatment: The patient should be advised to find alternative training that does not make the radiating pain worse. Pain is a signal for the athlete to change his activity and should not be considered a relapse. There is no reason for restrictions, with the exception of heavy lifting.
- Prognosis: If sciatica without neurological deficit is likely, the athlete should plan to resume normal sport activity in 6–12 weeks. If neurological deficit is present, the course is usually longer, in the range of 12–24 weeks. Therefore, the caregiver or care giving team should work with the athlete to create a long-term plan to get him back to his former level of sport activity. If the patient does not follow the anticipated course, it is necessary to make a diagnostic evaluation so that his goals can be adjusted.

Spinal Stenosis (Spinal Claudication)

Symptoms of spinal stenosis usually occur in the elderly (average age at onset is 65 years) because degeneration of intervertebral disks and facet joints with calcification contributes to reducing the size of the spinal canal (Figure 5.20). Disk degeneration, facet joint arthrosis, spondylolysis, previous fractures, or back surgery may contribute to spinal stenosis.

- Symptoms and signs: Symptoms and signs are back pain and morning stiffness, radiating pain, paresthesia, and muscle weakness related to activity. Reduced gait distance is the key symptom. Bending forward usually relieves the pain. The Lasegue test is usually negative, and motor disturbance and nonresponse of the patellar reflex are common.
- Diagnosis: The diagnosis is made in patients with characteristic symptoms and a reduced sagittal diameter of the spinal canal. The practitioner must exclude vascular claudication gait distance, reduced distal pulse, and diffuse sensory disturbance).
- Treatment by physician: NSAIDs or paracetamol is the treatment of choice. Lumbar epidural or nerve root steroid injection or peroral steroids may be effective and decrease the need for surgery, but the effectiveness is not documented in clinical trials. Progressive walking difficulties are an indication for referral to a specialist.
- Treatment by physical therapist: The physical therapist may advise active individual or group exercises to improve back function.

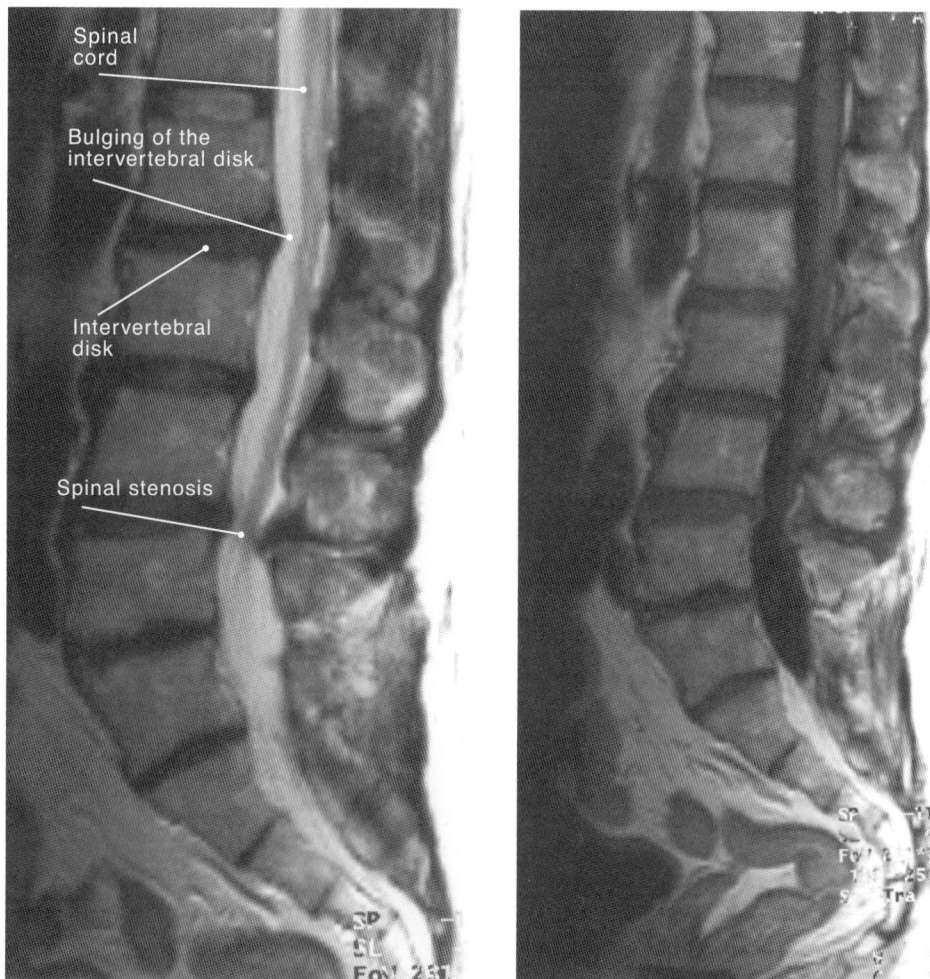

Figure 5.20 Spinal stenosis in levels L4–L5. Moderate degenerative changes with protrusions. (Reproduced with permission from the Norwegian Sports Medicine Association.)

- Self-treatment: The patient should be advised to maintain daily activities rather than stay in bed.
- Prognosis: Surgery has a good effect on lower extremity pain, but its effect on back pain is less certain.

Scoliosis—*Back Curvature*

Curvature of the frontal plane is called scoliosis. Structural scoliosis differs from nonstructural scoliosis in that the latter includes functional or postural scoliosis that disappears when the patient bends forward and a compensatory scoliosis that is present when the patient's legs are different lengths. The five categories of structural scoliosis are (1) idiopathic, (2) neuromuscular, (3) congenital, (4) iatrogenic, and (5) rare syndromes. The prevalence of all scoliosis is about 3% in the general population. Idiopathic scoliosis occurs about seven times more frequently in girls than in boys. Scoliosis tends to increase as long as the individual is growing. The condition is hereditary, and it is presumed that the inheritance is multifactorial or dominant with reduced penetrance.

- Symptoms and signs: The average patient with structural scoliosis generally has only slightly more pain and disability than their peers. Activity of the musculature will be different on the concave and convex side of a scoliosis, and this may explain why patients with scoliosis may report muscle fatigue. It is debated whether grade school students should undergo an annual screening for scoliosis. The screening involves having the students bend forward. If structural scoliosis is suspected, pronounced asymmetry, which resembles the keel of a boat, is evident, corresponding to the costal arch on the convex side (Figure 5.16). The degree of rotation may be measured by a scoliometer.

- Diagnosis: The patient should be referred to an orthopedic department for further evaluation. The diagnosis is confirmed, and the deformity is measured and classified by X-rays.
- Treatment: The disease may take a natural course, or a stiff brace or surgery may be prescribed. The patient must be checked regularly until she is fully grown.
- Self-treatment: The patient should participate in physical activity with her peers. Carrying heavy bags like a backpack is not recommended; therefore, the patient should have two sets of schoolbooks (one at school and one at home).

Morbus Scheuermann—*Scheuermann Disease*

This disease usually occurs during the puberty growth spurt and is more common in boys than girls. The prevalence of Scheuermann disease in adolescents is about 5% Repetitive trauma during the growth period may be significant. The most probable cause of the disorder is aseptic bone necrosis, with a reduced blood supply to the growth zone. Necrosis is most pronounced in the front and causes the vertebral body to become wedge shaped (Figure 5.21). The changes are localized to the thoracic column in 70% of the patients.

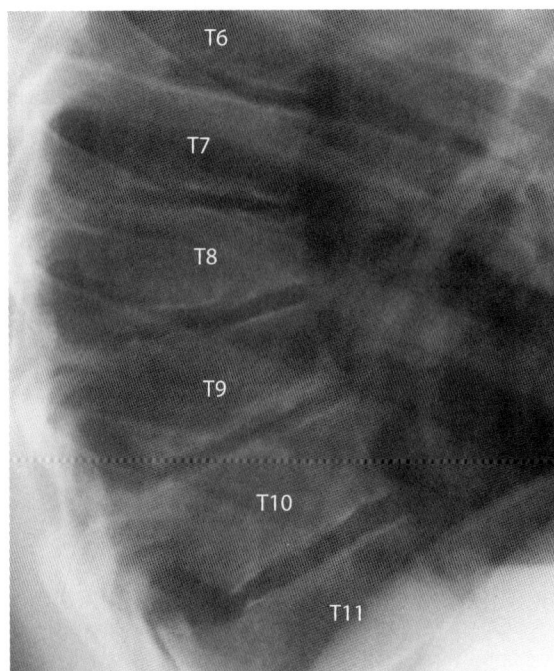

Figure 5.21 Morbus Scheuermann. Lateral X-ray shows an athlete with increased thoracic kyphosis, due to a wedge shape of the vertebral bodies of more than 5° in T7–T10. (Reproduced with permission from the Norwegian Sports Medicine Association.)

- Symptoms and signs: Increased kyphosis in the thoracic or thoracolumbar column. The normal curvature of the thoracic spine on the frontal plane (kyphosis) is 15°–30°. An increase greater than this is seen when there are congenital changes, fractures, growth disturbance (e.g., Scheuermann disease), and systemic diseases (e.g., Bekhterev disease). Sometimes it is difficult to distinguish between kyphosis and a normal relaxed posture. Most patients with moderate changes in the thoracic spine (which have been identified by X-ray) are pain free. Patients with Scheuermann disease in the thoracolumbar or the lumbar region usually have pain.
- Diagnosis: Scheuermann disease is defined by X-rays that show three or more vertebra with a 5° or more wedge shape. If the diagnosis is suspected during the growth period, the athlete should be referred for appropriate orthopedic care.
- Treatment: Physical treatment to strengthen the back and abdominal muscles is recommended. A brace can be used if the kyphosis is completely rigid. Surgery is rarely needed.

Morbus Bekhterev—*Bekhterev Disease*

Bekhterev disease occurs more often than Scheuermann disease and makes its first appearance earlier in men than in women. In Norway, the prevalence is about 1–2 per 1000 in the adult population, with 300–400 new cases annually. The condition is hereditary, and it is assumed that transmission is multifactorial.

- Symptoms and signs: Pain and stiffness gradually increase in the lumbar region. The pain is often localized to the entire spine and the iliosacral joints. Night pain and morning stiffness predominate. Symptoms often improve throughout the day and with physical activity.

- Diagnosis: A diagnosis is made if reduced range of motion in one or more sections of the back is present, as well as tenderness to palpation of the spinous processes and the iliosacral joints. Bekhterev disease affects the ischial tuberosity, the iliac crest, and the tendon insertions in the heel. It may make its first appearance with recurring eye inflammation (iridocyclitis), and it affects large joints (shoulders and hips). Chest excursion may be reduced early, but major limitations are usually present during the late stages. Thoracic kyphosis and the lack of lumbar lordosis (Figure 5.22) cause a characteristic posture and walk. A radiographic examination of the pelvis and vertebral column are diagnostic but rarely during the onset stage. Because Bekhterev disease is relatively rare, and only 1–2% of people who have a positive HLA-B27 test have the disease, a positive HLA-B27 test has no diagnostic value.

- Treatment: Patients who may have Bekhterev disease should be referred to a rheumatologist. Regular training is an important part of the treatment. NSAIDs are given during bad periods. Patients with severe pain should be evaluated by a rheumatologist for the use of medication. Surgical treatment may be indicated if the patient has major thoracic kyphosis that makes it impossible to maintain a normal visual angle.

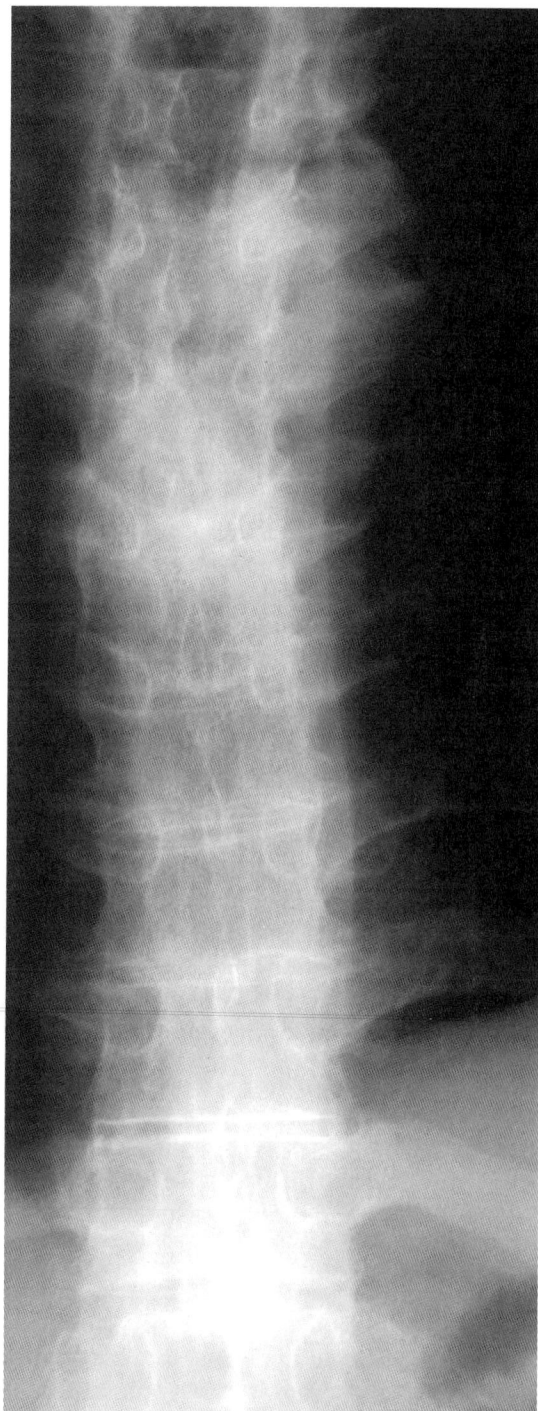

Figure 5.22 Morbus Bekhterev. The frontal X-ray view demonstrates significant sclerosis as an expression of ossification of the longitudinal ligaments. (Reproduced with permission from the Norwegian Sports Medicine Association.)

NECK AND BACK

Rehabilitation

Bjørn Fossan[1], Robert G. Watkins III[2], Robert G. Watkins IV[2], and Jens Ivar Brox[3]

[1]*Olympiatoppen, Oslo, Norway*
[2]*Marina Spine Center, Marina del Rey, California, CA, USA*
[3]*Oslo University Hospital, Rikshospitalet, Sognsveien, Oslo, Norway*

Table 5.10 lists the goals of rehabilitation.

Acute phase. Rehabilitation starts at the time of the acute injury and comprises the period of acute care, sport-specific training and return to competition. A thorough psychosocial evaluation to identify barriers to improvement is often helpful and it is recommended to include this early in the rehabilitation process. The treatment and information given to the patient depends on the diagnosis. The sports physician or physiotherapist should be aware that the information given about diagnosis and activity restriction in the acute phase will have an impact on the patient's understanding of the consequences of pain or injury. The acute phase may be dramatic and the evaluation should include a biomechanical and psychological evaluation in order to gain confidence and reduce fear. Imaging may be important in the acute or subacute phase, but the indication and interpretation should be evidence based. For example, abnormal findings may be normal according to age and not explain the pain and disability observed. The challenge is to promote confidence and understanding of the physical injury as well as the emotional reaction involved.

	Goals	Measures
Acute phase	Create calm and confidence, improve pain management, limit inflammation, invalidate red flags	Information, drug therapy, and PRICE (protection, rest, ice, compression, and elevation)
Rehabilitation phase	Create a rehabilitation plan	Create an overview of the diagnosis, prognostic factors, and sports activity, and create a plan in consultation with the athlete and trainer
	Restore normal function	Advice based on the anticipated natural course
	Maintain general strength and endurance	Individual, specific, and progressive exercise program
	Prevent recurrence	In case of chronic pain, chart yellow flags and counteract passive pain mastery
		Individually adjusted alternative training program
		Counteract the risk factors based on the sport-specific, individual, and general evaluation
Training phase	Lead the athlete back to sport activity	Exercise or training to meet sport-specific requirements
		Provide athletes with the information necessary to make independent evaluations of their career prospects

Table 5.10 Goals and measures for rehabilitation. (Reproduced with permission from the Norwegian Sports Medicine Association.)

In most cases, NSAIDs and paracetamol provide sufficient pain relief. It is often difficult to become completely pain free using relief from usual activities and drug therapy. It has not been documented that complete rest will shorten the acute phase. Therefore, the patient must be mobilized as quickly as possible. Short-term relief can be achieved by wearing a support belt. The exercise program should not be started during the acute phase.

Rehabilitation phase. In the natural course of acute neck and back injuries, the athlete should recover well in a short time. How long training and competition are interrupted will depend on the condition of the athlete and the requirements of the sport. Training to maintain general endurance and strength can often begin within a few days of injury. Function often improves significantly during the first week and makes treatment and rehabilitation unnecessary.

If the patient has recurring or persistent symptoms, a physician and/or a physical therapist must conduct a functional evaluation in consultation with the athlete or trainer to provide a basis for a rehabilitation plan. The functional evaluation should be done by a physical therapist or a physician who is very familiar with the sport to which the patient is returning. For example, because shoulder and hip movements are necessary in gymnastics, if movement is reduced, the athlete may increase lumbar lordosis to compensate and to satisfy the performance requirements. This may increase the load on the lumbar region. As this example demonstrates, treating the back alone is often an insufficient means of rehabilitating the patient so that she can return to sports. Simple methods, such as observation during various activities, testing muscle strength, and measuring the extent to which the joints are affected, provide a good basis for a goal-oriented rehabilitation process. If resources allow, video, ultrasound, and EMG can be used to evaluate movement and muscle use.

Rehabilitation Methods

It is essential that the sports physician and physiotherapist communicate and preferably include the athlete and the coach in this process. Disagreement upon the methods and strategies applied should be solved and not communicated to the patient. Realistic goals with the use of milestones to monitor the rehabilitation process are essential. Fear of pain, avoidant behavior, and depressive mood are commonly associated with persistent low back pain in athletes as well as in other patients. Evaluation of these aspects should be regarded equally important as imaging. Comprehensive multidisciplinary program that involve psychologist, physiotherapist, or manual therapist in addition to different medical specialists and intensive programs like functional restoration should be reserved for the most complicated cases.

When prescribing treatment for spine rehabilitation, the clinician must appreciate the important role of the entire cylinder of the trunk and its supporting muscles. The static ligamentous structures of the spine provide considerable resistance to injury, but this resistance in itself would be insufficient to produce proper strength without the additional support provided through the trunk musculature and lumbodorsal fascia. Muscle control of the lumbodorsal fascia allows a much higher resistance to bending and loading stresses. The lumbodorsal fascia and the muscles attaching to it must be considered of equal importance to the more specialized function of the intervertebral disk and facet joints.

NECK AND BACK

The trunk stabilization program may offer an early return to sports without the use of a lumbosacral brace. It comprises a combination of activities to bring the spine back to a position of balance and power in injured athletes. By training muscles of the trunk to work in coordination, the program produces biomechanically sound spinal function. Muscle function based on balance and coordination, not strength alone, is the result. Initially, the athlete is taught to maintain a safe, neutral, pain-free, and controlled position. He/she then moves through a series of exercises that combine balance and coordination. Gradually, the athlete, while maintaining good trunk control, is moved in incremental steps through increasingly advanced exercises. In each succeeding exercise, the patient gradually assumes more confidence and better coordination.

For the lower body, trunk control plays a vital role in the ability to rotate and transfer torque safely. Trunk strengthening exercises such as sit-ups and spine extensions produce strength. Flexibility produces a protective range of motion, but often the key is providing trunk strength and control at the proper moment during the athletic activity. For example, a baseball hitter goes from flexion through rotation to extension. You can have strong muscles but, if they do not fire in sequence, at the proper time, they will not protect the athlete from injury and certainly will not enhance performance. A key to producing a safe range of motion is to begin trunk control in the safe, neutral position, establish muscle control in that position and maintain it through the necessary range of motion to perform the athletic activity.

We recommend starting the identification of the neutral spine position with the dead-bug exercises. Dead-bug exercises are done supine with the knees flexed and feet on the floor. With the assistance of the trainer or therapist, the athlete pushes his lumbar spine toward the mat until he exerts a moderate amount of force on the examiner's hand. The next stage for torque transfer athletes is resistance to rotation, first supine, then sitting, then standing, in which the player maintains the neutral spine control position while resisting rotation of the upper body on the lower body. The player resists the rotational activity exerted by the therapist or trainer.

An additional benefit can be beach ball exercises. A ball with 4-ft diameter can be used to do partial sit-ups while maintaining control of the ball, and the trunk in neutral position, the sit ups and resistive sit-ups are done on the ball.

Functional strengthening is then performed according to the requirements of the specific sports. Extremity stretching exercises are an important part of any rehabilitation program. The more flexible the legs, arms, and upper body is, the more likely there will be a proportional decrease of motion stress on the injured lumbar spine.

Reduced range of motion may contribute to a change in loading of the other structures in the back. If the probable cause of reduced movement is muscular, stretching is indicated. If arthrogenic causes are suspected, joint mobilization and subsequent muscle stretching may be attempted (e.g., Figure 5.23). In both cases, activity with full range of motion and numerous repetitions are recommended (e.g., Figure 5.24).

The patient should be instructed to use the thigh muscles for heavy lifting. Therefore strengthening of the thigh muscles is an important part of rehabilitation of the spine.

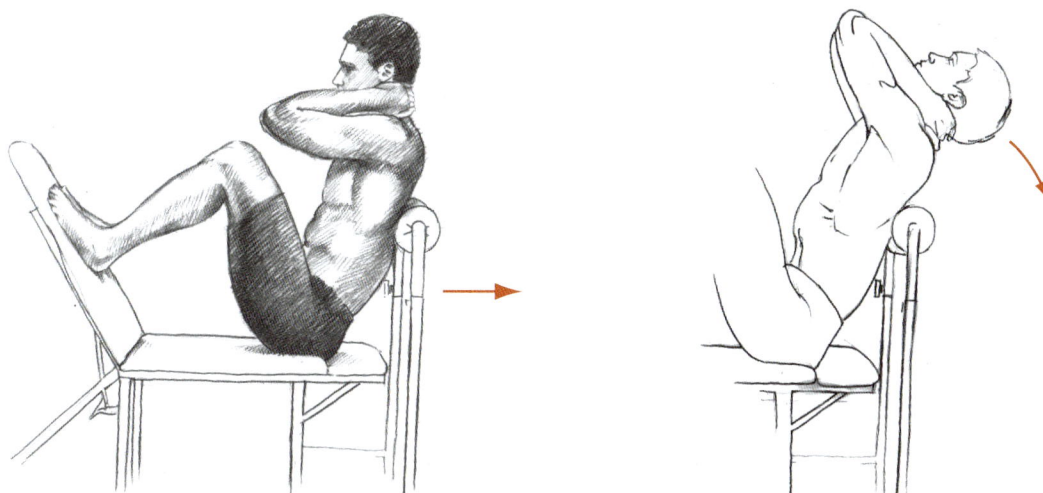

Figure 5.23 Mobilization/stretching the thoracic spine in extension

- Lock the lumbar region of your back by maximum flexion of your hips.
- Arch your thoracic spine backward over the pole in an extreme position.
- Do range of motion training and stretching.

(Reproduced with permission from the Norwegian Sports Medicine Association.)

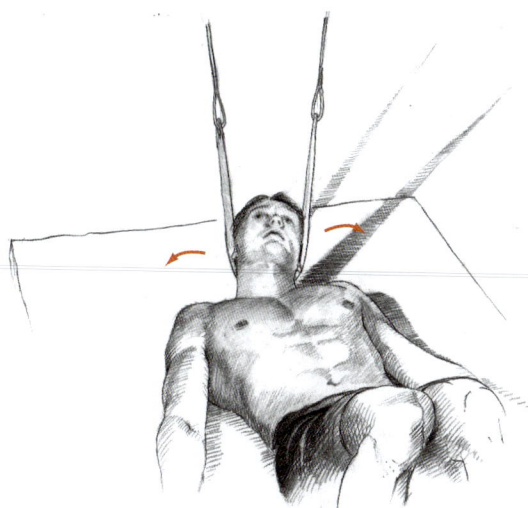

Figure 5.24 Active mobilization of the neck in lateral flexion

- Move your head gently between extreme positions in lateral flexion.
- Mobilize and stretch in the same manner in ventral flexion and extension (lying on your side) or in rotation.
- Do range of motion training.

(Reproduced with permission from the Norwegian Sports Medicine Association.)

On the other hand, the athlete should be informed that there is no reason to be too concerned about his back, by example by bending the knees in order to lift light objects. Positive information and advice may contribute to instilling confidence and gradually improving movement and muscular function.

As described previously, the deep musculature in the lumbar region and the neck are important for segmental stability and control. The deep-seated muscles (multifidus muscles) work together with the deep abdominal muscles (the diaphragm) and pelvic floor muscles as a functionally stabilizing unit. Recent studies suggest that activation and fatigability of the back musculature are different in people with healthy backs than in patients. Pain may have a reflex effect on muscle activity by

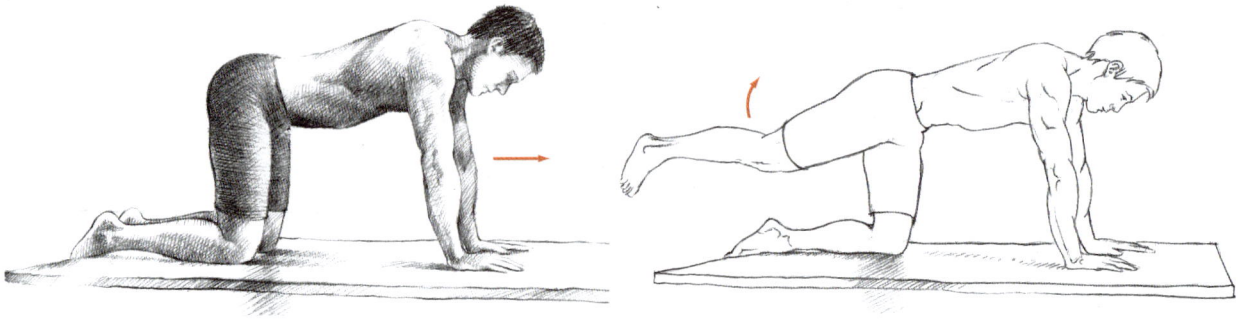

Figure 5.25 Deep trunk muscle exercises

- Position yourself on your hands and knees, slightly hollow backed.
- Pull in your abdomen without moving your lumbar region and without holding your breath.
- Alternately extend your right and left leg backward without moving your back.
- Release the tension in your abdomen between repetitions.
- Increase loading by placing your hands farther forward.

(Reproduced with permission from the Norwegian
Sports Medicine Association.)

inhibiting the deep stabilizing musculature while activating muscles like the ilio-psoas muscle and the erector muscle of the spine. Therefore, weakness of the deep musculature and increased activation of the superficial musculature can reinforce a dysfunctional pattern of movement. Back pain contributes to a changed activity pattern by affecting both the central and the peripheral mechanisms. Increasing awareness, practice, and automation of the deep musculature may begin at an early stage of the rehabilitation process. This type of training (e.g., Figure 5.25) has a documented effect on patients with spondylolisthesis and on the frequency of recurrence of subacute back pain. Its effectiveness has been studied over the last two decades, but there is a lack of uniformity about the definition of core stabilization and which exercises are most effective. Knowledge about dose-response, long-term effects, and patient selection, is limited. Current data do not support the prescription of lumbar stabilization exercises for all patients and the specific indication is a crucial area for further research. Core exercises may be important for prevention of back pain in certain sports, but core muscles are activated in a variety of movements, and the time that should be spend on specific exercises depends on several factors such as the time available, time of the year, previous back pain, and abdominal and back muscle strength.

Gradual repetition and integration into regular sport activity is necessary to automate the activation pattern. When great strength is required for stabilization, the superficial musculature will also contribute to stiffening the upper body and neck exercises. Therefore, training must be related to the requirements of the individual sport.

Sensory motor function training is an optimal form of stabilization training for athletes. For the lumbar spine, this should take place in a closed kinetic chain on a mobile surface. As shown in Figure 5.26, Sling Exercise Therapy is an ideal tool to exercise the neck and lumbar spine in a closed kinetic chain, and at the same time challenging neuromuscular control. At first, the training routine should take place while the athlete is sharp and in good form. It should be repeated as often as possible

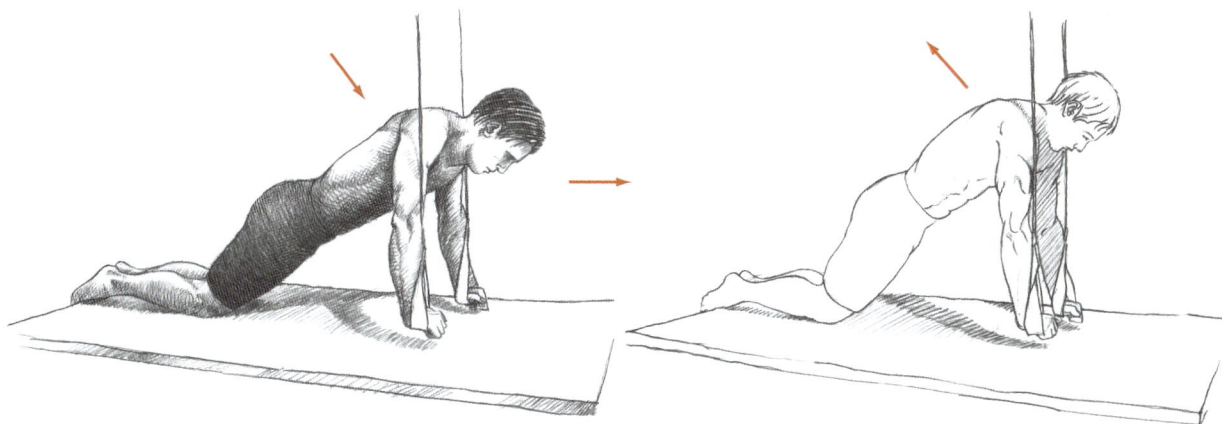

Figure 5.26 Functional stability training

• Allow your body to "fall through" your shoulders with your arms extended, and push up again.
• Increase loading by moving the contact point from your knees toward your toes.
• Avoid jerky movements of your neck and head.
(Reproduced with permission from the Norwegian Sports Medicine Association.)

and for a minimum of 10 minutes a day. As soon as the athlete masters this, strength and endurance training for the superficial musculature in an open and closed kinetic chain are integrated into the routine.

If the patient has chronic pain, in addition to medical diagnostics and the functional evaluation, it may be necessary to evaluate psychological factors to determine what needs to be emphasized during the rehabilitation process. Even for otherwise robust athletes, pain or fear of pain may be more significant than changes in the diagnostic images. In order to gain confidence it is essential to start rehabilitation at a very low level in patients with persistent pain.

When rehabilitation does not follow the anticipated course and there is no basis for surgery, the practitioner must change the rehabilitation plan. If it is impossible to begin active treatment, the so-called quota principle may be attempted. To apply this, the therapist chooses six to ten functional exercises. First, the patient does the exercises to exhaustion or until pain limits activity. The test is repeated in a day or two. The training dose should be set up to 50% of the average result of the two tests and is completed in a series three times a week. The dose is increased by one to five repetitions every other training day. The exercise regimen can be gradually adjusted according to normal physiological training principles. The key element of the quota principle is that activity is regulated by the test dose rather than by the pain limit. Rest follows training. In case of a relapse, the patient can return to the start dose but may increase the progression more rapidly if necessary.

For patients with chronic symptoms, aerobics or various group training is as effective as other exercise programs, and are more cost effective. Generally, long-term pain weakens cardiovascular function. Improving aerobic capacity may contribute to increasing the body's load tolerance.

Return to Sports

Most athletes will be able to return to their sport after an acute neck or back injury. The athlete needs to participate in normal training activity before participating in competition but does not need to be completely pain free. Nevertheless, the athlete should only stretch as far as he can, while still performing the movement in a technically correct manner. It may be appropriate to advise an individual athlete to switch to a different sport or to reduce his activity level. Young athletes are subject to injuries to the growth zones in the vertebrae, and these injuries may contribute to accelerated degeneration of the intervertebral disks. In addition to a diagnostic and a functional evaluation, young athletes with recurrent back pain should be evaluated for possible correction of risk factors before returning to normal training.

6 Chest and Abdomen

Thoracic Injuries

David Mulder[1], David McDonagh[2], and Mike Wilkinson[3]

[1]Montreal General Hospital, Montreal, QC, Canada
[2]St. Olavs Hospital, Trondheim, Norway
[3]Allan McGavin Sports Medicine Center, Vancouver, BC, Canada

Occurrence

Thoracic injuries have either an acute (traumatic) or insidious (chronic repetitive) etiology. The nature of the injury and thus its presentation is activity dependent. In sport, most traumatic thoracic injuries are blunt and occur in high-energy sports (such as equestrian sports, motorsports, ice hockey, football, alpine skiing), while in some sports there is intrinsic penetration danger (javelin, fencing, skiing). Repetitive strain injuries, particularly intercostal muscle strains, are the most common type of thoracic injury. They also account for the majority of time lost from practice or competition. These strains usually resolve rapidly but if they do not, your diagnosis may be incorrect—be aware of the possibility of costal stress fractures, particularly in sports such as rowing and golf (Table 6.1). Simple costal fractures are also seen in many sports; they are painful and usually keep athletes sidelined for many weeks, but are rarely associated with serious complications.

Serious chest injuries are extremely rare, but a sports physician must be able to correctly diagnose and manage these conditions in and around the field of play.

Diagnostic Thinking

Airway compromise may result from aspiration (chewing gum, teeth, blood, vomitus, etc.), a direct blow to the larynx or trachea, or from posterior sternoclavicular joint dislocations.

Most common	Less common	Must not be overlooked !
Simple rib fractures, p. 152	Pectoralis major rupture, p. 154	Intrathoracic injury
Rib stress fractures, p. 152	Sternoclavicular dislocation	Intra-abdominal solid organ injury
Costovetebral injuries, p. 153	Sternal & scapular fracture, p. 154	Female breast contusions, p. 157
	Pneumothorax, p. 155	
	Open pneumothorax, p. 156	
	Hemothorax, p. 157	
	Commotio cordis, p. 157	
	Major vascular injury	
	Lung contusion	

Table 6.1 Overview of differential diagnoses of thoracic injuries. (Reproduced with permission from the Norwegian Sports Medicine Association.)

The IOC Manual of Sports Injuries, First Edition. Edited by Roald Bahr.
©2012 International Olympic Committee. Published 2012 by John Wiley & Sons, Ltd.

The lung parenchyma may be damaged or compressed by a hemothorax, lung contusion, or pneumothorax. It is extremely difficult to make a precise diagnosis in the prehospital environment. Diagnosis and treatment go hand in hand. The main concern is to ensure that the airway is patent and that there is no pneumothorax, or worse, a tension pneumothorax. High-concentration supplemental oxygen and a strong suction system are essential. If there is a large pneumothorax or tension pneumothorax present, then the patient will remain in a critical condition until the pneumothorax is decompressed. Once adequate ventilation has been established, the athlete's clothing should be opened or removed so that a proper clinical examination of the chest, abdomen, back, and extremities can be performed. The next concern is that of major blood loss. Open wounds will be obvious, but intra-abdominal, pelvic, thoracic, or femoral artery bleeding less so. In the unlikely event of a life threatening thoracic injury, it is very often a complication of a bony skeleton injury (Figure 6.1) and in sport is almost always blunt. Establishment of a large bore intravenous portal is invaluable. The venue medical facility should have suitable emergency equipment available and be within easy access for the medical team.

The occult reality of the altered physiology of the elite athlete must always be considered with major thoracic trauma. Many clinical signs and symptoms may be masked by the adrenalin surge of professional competition. One must also consider the increased blood volume and stroke volume (50% above normal). Cardiac output may be six times normal and the resting heart rate may be below 50 beats per minute. Volume loss through sweating may be 5 kg or more. This altered physiology may lead to a sense of false security; the athlete may be far more ill than the vital signs would suggest. For a time, blood pressure may appear high or normal despite major hemorrhage.

Many less severe injuries are manifested by chest wall pain. These may include a simple undisplaced rib fracture or costochondral separation. A chest wall contusion may also result in local pain and swelling. Interscapular pain posteriorly may result from minor thoracic spine trauma such as a locked facet or compression fracture. Unexplained shortness of breath may be related to a small pneumothorax or an occult diaphragmatic injury. Assessing respiratory rate and measuring oxygen saturation are simple, valuable, and essential prehospital techniques, while a simple chest X-ray remains one of the most useful diagnostic aids after the clinical examination.

In athletes with less dramatic thoracic injury presentations, the history is of paramount importance to help make the diagnosis and direct any investigations or treatment. Intimate knowledge of the dynamics of the sport is an invaluable aid in this process. Athletes with chest wall conditions usually have pleuritic pain that is aggravated by deep inspiration, coughing, or sneezing and may be associated with dyspnea due to the pain restriction of deep inspiration.

Beware the athlete who presents with progressive dyspnea and pleuritic chest pain without any obvious precipitating event. A careful history will be needed to reveal forceful valsalva maneuvers during weight training, sprinting, or maximal effort intervals that would be a clear alert for a spontaneous pneumothorax.

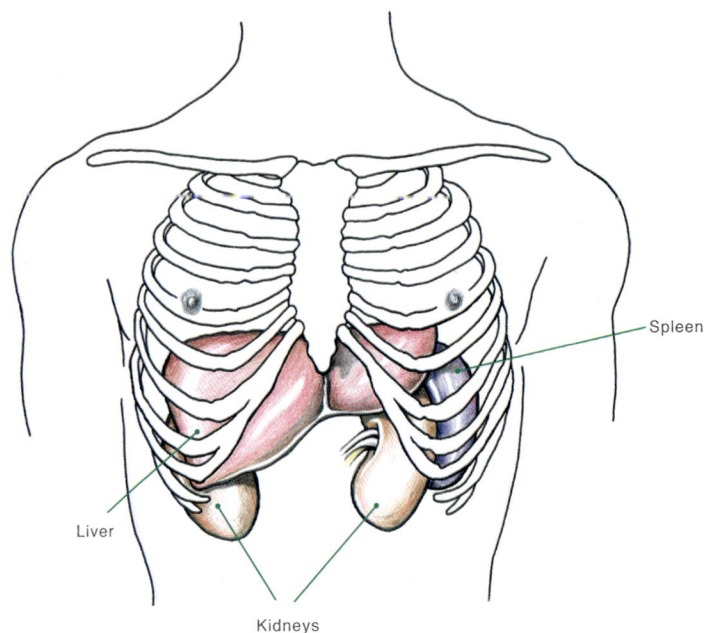

Figure 6.1 Relationship between thoracic cage and upper abdominal organs. (© Medical Illustrator Tommy Bolic, Sweden.)

Clinical Examination

Inspection. The primary survey with the player uncovered focuses on early identification of life threatening injuries. Of primary concern is the status of the airway as noted previously. If the athlete is able to talk, the airway is patent and the patient is conscious. A rasping voice, the choke sign, and/or swelling around the neck indicate an injury to the larynx or trachea in the neck. The larynx can be visibly displaced if fractured. Always inspect for dyspnea, cyanosis, and measure the respiratory rate. Rapid respirations with percussion hyperresonance may indicate the presence of a significant pneumothorax. Deviation of the trachea with distended neck veins suggests a tension pneumothorax with pericardial tamponade. Chest wall asymmetry or deformity may be a sign of multiple rib fractures, flail chest, a large pneumothorax, sternal fractures, or chest wall hematomas. Look for the paradoxical movement of a flail chest (the injured chest wall segment moving in with inspiration and out with expiration). An open pneumothorax is usually obvious though the presence of a skin flap should cause great concern due to the possibility of an underlying tension pneumothorax.

Palpation. Manual palpation of the chest wall can confirm the crepitus of subcutaneous emphysema (pneumothorax or larynx/pharynx fracture), the paradoxical chest wall movement of multiple rib (flail chest) fractures, the asymmetrical movement of the chest in the presence of a large pneumothorax, or sternal deformities associated with a fracture. Palpation of peripheral pulses can give useful information.

Percussion. Percussion of the chest wall may reveal hyperresonance with a large pneumothorax. Dullness to percussion at the lung bases may indicate a hemothorax. Percussion findings can be difficult to evaluate in the prehospital environment due to surrounding noise.

Auscultation. Auscultation of the chest may reveal absent breath sounds with a pneumothorax and/or hemothorax; the presence of muffled heart sounds may indicate cardiac tamponade although in the field-side situation these are often very difficult to assess. Regular repeated measurement of systemic blood pressure and assessment of peripheral pulses frequency and quality will help in assessing the circulation. Peripheral O_2 saturation measurement is also recommended.

Emergency Field-Side Treatment

If one identifies a life-threatening injury, then immediate treatment must be initiated before further clinical examination. The treating physician, paramedics, or helicopter medical staff should be able to accomplish the following procedures:

- Airway control
  - Mouth sweep
  - Oral airway, jaw thrust, chin lift
  - Suctioning of airway
  - Supplemental O_2
  - Helmet removal
  - Endotracheal intubation or cricothyroidotomy if airways are not patent
- Needle thoracentesis
  - Tube thoracostomy
- Ventilation
- Intravenous access
- Needle pericardiocentesis

The goal for venue medical staff intervention is to stabilize the patient before earliest possible safe transfer to an appropriate trauma care center. An emergency action plan should be developed before all major events and regular rehearsal is invaluable for all of the medical team.

Common Injuries

Simple Rib Fractures—*Costochondral Injury*

Simple rib fractures are among the most common thoracic injuries in high-energy contact sports. The costochondral and costosternal joints may also be affected, causing localized joint swelling or even subluxation.

- Symptoms and signs: Painful limitations of respiration along with local pain or crepitus are common findings in these conditions. In more subtle cases athletes may simply complain of pain when turning over in bed or on coughing/sneezing. There is usually localized pain with remote chest compression and chest expansion limitation due to pain. There may be a palpable step deformity of the involved joint or rib in severe cases. Commonly, when the sport involves significant repetitive collisions such as in ice hockey and rugby, there may be delayed presentation without recollection of a specific incident, as "bumps and bruises" are common post game.
- Diagnosis: Diagnosis is based on the mechanism of injury and the physical exam. The examination must exclude underlying lung injury and pleural injury. If only one rib fracture is suspected, and there is no suspicion of underlying thoracic injury, an X-ray is unnecessary. However, in the case of multiple rib fractures or if associated injuries to the chest are suspected, then an X-ray of the chest should be taken.
- Treatment by physician: A single fractured rib may be extremely painful but will heal by itself. It may take as long as 6 weeks before the patient can return to full activity. The only treatment required is rest and pain control. Intercostal anesthesia may provide some pain control in exceptional circumstances. Most cases are resolved in 3–4 weeks.
- Treatment by therapist: Treatment is directed by the pain level and should focus on trying to maintain normal chest function as much as possible. Avoid chest wall strapping due to the risk of atelectasis. Initial training will need to be altered with maintenance of aerobic fitness using, for example, a stationary bike and then graduated progression to sport-specific and resistance training.

Rib Stress Fractures

In a recent report from a major national rowing program approximately 32% of all lost training days in the 2 years prior to the summer Olympics were due to rib stress fractures. These fractures usually have a gradual (1–2 weeks) onset with no obvious precipitating event. Without rapid intervention they will result in up to 2 months of lost training and may even progress to a full displaced fracture, but when caught early and with appropriate training modification the athlete may be back to full training within 2 weeks. Despite numerous studies on forces, technique, and biomechanics no individual precipitating factors have been noted except for the volume of training and the introduction of the modern carbon shafted larger oars in the late 1980s and early 1990s.

- Symptoms and signs: In the initial phase the pain is relatively poorly localized and may mimic a simple intercostal strain or intercostal nerve irritation. Rib stress fracture pain tends not to resolve between sessions, depending on location will be aggravated at the "catch" (initial forceful part of each stroke) for the more common anterolateral fractures or at the "finish" (the end part of the drive phase of the stroke) for the less common posterior fractures. They are usually associated with classic pleuritic type pain and localized pain on remote rib compression. Costochondral strains and costochondritis are differentiated from rib stress fractures by the more acute onset and the very well localized pain at the associated costochondral joint. There may also be clinical evidence of associated subluxation of the joint.

- Diagnosis: In sports with repetitive chest wall forces (rotational, tractional, or compressive) such as rowing, canoe/kayak, tennis, golf, and throwing sports a high index of suspicion is required as stress fractures are often missed and treated as "chronic muscle strains." The gold standard for diagnosis is a bone scan though recent advances in MRI, ultrasound, and CT scan techniques have been made.
- Treatment by physician: Initial treatment is to control the local pain and to modify training. Bone healing may be promoted by using inhaled calcitonin and bone stimulators. Recent studies have shown a possible delay in bone healing with Nonsteroidal anti-inflammatory drug (NSAID) use, so these should be used with caution. In athletes with recurrent stress fractures other predisposing factors should be looked for, for example, osteopenia and the female athlete triad. Use of intravenous bisphosphonate treatment after recurrent fractures is still in the investigative phase and patients should be referred to an endocrinologist for a complete workup if this is considered.
- Treatment by therapist: Athletes should be withdrawn from the precipitating activity and may maintain fitness and pain avoidance through modified training such as the stationary bike. Once pain free, athletes may return to sport in a progressive nature. This time should also be used to address any biomechanical issues that have predisposed to the stress fracture.
- Prognosis: If diagnosed and treated early, athletes may return to sport in approximately 2 weeks but as noted previously, delayed diagnosis could result in a loss of 2–3 months training. In order to prevent recurrence it is essential to address the predisposing factors both in volume and biomechanics/equipment where present.

Costovertebral injuries—*Strains and subluxations*

These seemingly minor injuries can be very painful and debilitating to the athlete. They may occur after a single traumatic event, but are more commonly recurrent and associated with minor trauma, travel, or no obvious precipitant. They are sometimes a sequela to chest wall splinting due to a rib fracture/stress fracture or costochondral strain.

- Symptoms and signs: Athletes usually present with a constant sharp pain in the interscapular region with spasm of the rhomboids and local paravertebral muscles. In severe cases causing intercostal nerve impingement, there may be radiation of neural type pain along the dermatome. There is marked local tenderness in acute cases but may only be local muscle irritation in recurrent cases. Lateral flexion and thoracic rotation is limited locally with obvious limitation of movement at the affected level and associated decreased chest wall movement on inspiration.
- Diagnosis: This is a clinical diagnosis and investigations are usually not required. In atypical or resistant cases, imaging (X-ray) should be performed to rule out other occult causes such as minor vertebral fractures or other local pathology, for example, osteomyelitis.
- Treatment by physician: Initial treatment is aimed at pain control with ice, analgesics, local modalities, and taping and may require a local anesthetic injection or nerve block.

- Treatment by therapist: Manipulation by an experienced therapist will often have an immediate result with relief of the pain and spasm. Focus should then shift to correcting the underlying biomechanical predisposing factors when present.
- Prognosis: Once the joint is reduced and the pain sufficiently alleviated the athlete may return to sport but may require supportive taping in the initial phase. As these injuries are often recurrent the athlete should be put on a scapular stabilizing and postural exercise program with advice on prevention during travel.

Other Injuries

Pectoralis major rupture—*Chest Wall Muscle Injury*

Chest wall muscle injuries may occur. Total muscle ruptures are extremely rare but may occasionally be associated with weightlifting. Partial tears can sometimes occur in other sports such as American football, rugby, or ice hockey. Pectoralis major injury can be due to an avulsion near the musculotendinous junction with the humerus, although injures may also occur at the attachment to the sternum in weightlifting. Teres major and minor may be similarly injured.

- Symptoms and signs: The patient may hear or experience an acute "snap" and report pain, weakness, swelling, or muscular deformity.
- Diagnosis: Examination may reveal ecchymosis, a palpable defect, asymmetry of the axillary fold and weakness on resisted adduction, and internal rotation of the shoulder. MRI or ultrasound is invaluable in early diagnosis.
- Treatment by physician: The extent of muscle rupture and age of athlete will dictate surgical repair versus rest and immobilization. Patients should be referred to a specialist for evaluation.
- Treatment by therapist: Initial treatment will involve rest, ice, and anti-inflammatory agents. Resolution of local hematoma should be followed by passive shoulder range of motion programs and later focal muscle strengthening of the involved muscle groups (including the pectoralis minor, infraspinatus, and shoulder stabilizers) progressing to functional exercises and ultimately sport.
- Prognosis: Return to play after a major muscle injury is 6–12 weeks, longer if surgical repair is indicated.

Sternal & Scapular Fracture

The normal sternum/scapula requires high-energy blunt trauma to cause a fracture, so these fractures are often associated with cardiac, pulmonary or great vessel injuries. The patient may well be unconscious, but hemodynamically stable. The patient will need to be stabilized and evacuated urgently. Not all sternal fractures are associated with internal injury, but one needs to maintain a high index of suspicion. Sternal fracture combined with rib fractures may lead to a "flail chest" or a segment of chest wall that moves paradoxically with inspiration and expiration. This magnitude of blunt chest wall injury is best managed in the hospital setting as associated injuries will dictate management.

- Symptoms and signs: The patient may be unconscious. If conscious, there will be strong pain at rest and obviously with movement. There may be local deformity or crepitus. The patient's cardiovascular status must be regularly ascertained.
- Diagnosis: CT scanning or MRI reveals extent of bone injury and underlying cardiac or lung injury.

- Treatment by physician: In the prehospital environment the patient must be stabilized by ensuring airways patency, oxygenation, and ventilation. Pneumothorax must be diagnosed and decompressed. The patient must be transported to hospital in such a way as not to aggravate these fractures.

In-hospital observation must first exclude associated injury. Patients should be monitored with ECG for 24–48 hours. Epidural anesthesia has proven invaluable for pain control. Return to play ranges from 6 to 12 weeks.

Complicated Rib Fractures: Pneumothorax—*Air in the Chest Cavity*

A displaced rib fracture may penetrate intercostal vessels or the adjacent lung producing a pneumothorax (Figure 6.2) or a hemothorax. Air may leak under the skin causing subcutaneous emphysema or leak into the intrapleural space causing the lung to collapse. The amount of air leakage will decide the amount of lung collapse. A skin flap can act as a valve, allowing air to enter but not to exit the intrapleural space, thus causing pressure in this intrapleural space to constantly increase, forming a so-called tension pneumothorax. Total lung collapse, shift of the mediastinum to the opposite side of the injury and caval venous return interruption may occur. This is a potentially fatal condition and immediate decompression must be initiated before cardiorespiratory arrest occurs.

Remember, not all pneumothoraces are traumatic. A spontaneous pneumothorax may occur in the absence of trauma, usually in tall thin younger males. The clinical findings are usually not as pronounced as with traumatic injuries and they are usually treated conservatively.

- Symptoms and signs: Painful limitations of chest wall movement will worsen as the degree of lung collapse progresses. There may be palpable subcutaneous emphysema of the chest wall. Hemoptysis may also be noted. In events where there are multiple heats or a progression system of heats, semifinals, and finals over a short period close monitoring of any athlete with suspected rib fractures is mandatory as the pneumothorax onset may be delayed until further exertion occurs. Remember also that a pulmonary embolism can present with sudden-onset dyspnea, tachypnea, pleuritic chest pain, cough, and hemoptysis; pulmonary embolism is an alternative, though unlikely differential diagnosis in young female athletes on the contraceptive pill.
- Diagnosis: Percussion of the chest wall reveals a degree of hyperresonance whereas auscultation may reveal diminished breath sounds over the injury site or at the apex of the involved hemithorax. Deviation of the trachea away from the involved side and distention of neck veins are indicative of a tension pneumothorax. In a large pneumothorax, there may be reduced thoracic wall movement on the affected side. The patient will have an increased respiratory rate, reduced oxygen saturation levels, and even cyanosis. Chest X-ray confirms the diagnosis (Figure 6.2).
- Treatment by physician: Treatment consists of ensuring an open airway, supplemental O_2, thoracic decompression, pain control, treatment of other life-threatening injuries, and transport to hospital. On diagnosing a progressive and significant acute pneumothorax in the prehospital environment, a needle thoracentesis should be performed if the experience, equipment, and facilities are not available to perform a chest tube insertion. Insert one or several wide bore needles into the 3rd intercostal space in the anterior or midaxillary line and attached to a Heimlich valve. On arrival at hospital, a chest tube can be inserted and attached to underwater drainage with 20 cm of water suction to accomplish full decompression.

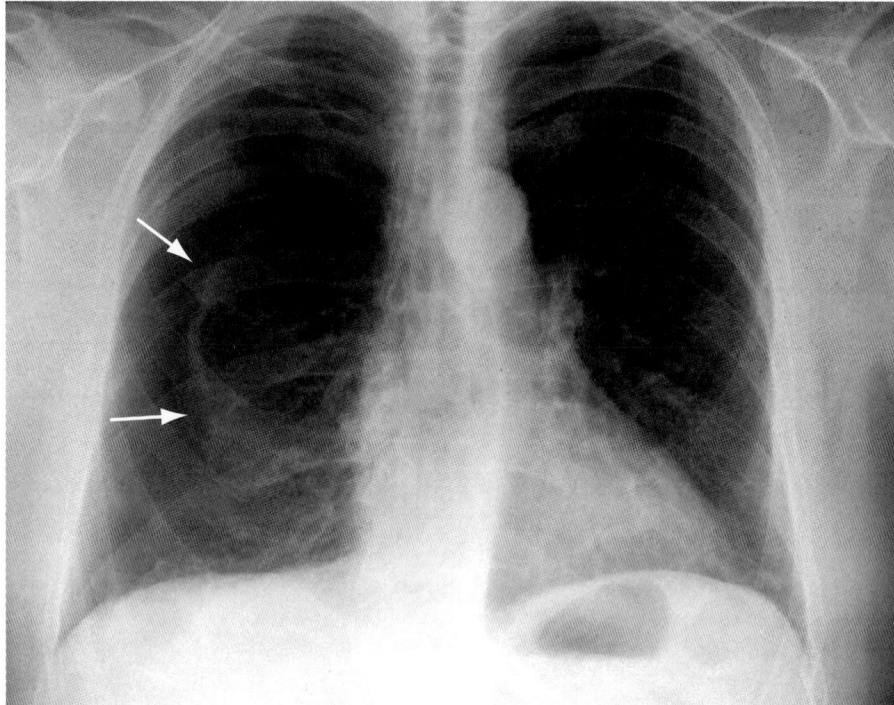

Figure 6.2 Pneumothorax after a rib fracture. The rib fracture is not visible on the X-ray, but the pleural edge is visible (marked by the arrows). (Reproduced with permission from the Norwegian Sports Medicine Association.)

• Prognosis: Resolution of the pneumothorax by chest tube alone will usually allow return to play in 3–4 weeks but in resistance sports may require up to 6 weeks. If a thoracotomy is required, return to play may be up to 3 months. Return to play requires a graduated progression as with all injuries; however, in this case breath holding and forced valsalva (e.g., in weight training) should be the final stage of progression with close monitoring for recurrence. If the sport involves significant ambient pressure changes such as skydiving or scuba diving/spear fishing then referral to a specialist in this field is essential due to the high risk of recurrence with potential catastrophic results.

Complicated Rib Fracture: Open Pneumothorax—*Open chest wound*

This rare injury occurs when the thorax has been penetrated by an object such as a javelin, ski pole, hockey stick, or venue protective devices. There is usually a visible defect in the chest wall related to the impaling weapon. As a general rule, the penetrating object should always be left in place and removed only in the operating room, due to the risk of intense bleeding on removal. A penetrating chest wound will probably cause both a pneumothorax and a hemothorax and may be associated with significant bleeding and hypotension. Injuries to other organs such as the heart, diaphragm, spleen, and liver may be also present and can be fatal. The event physician's major role is to (1) stabilize the impaled object; and (2) stabilize the patient (airways, oxygen, ventilate, cover the wound but do not create a tension pneumothorax, volume replacement) before rapid transportation to a trauma center for definitive imaging and operative intervention. A skin flap can act as a valve, allowing air to enter but not to exit the intrapleural space, thus causing pressure in this intrapleural space to constantly increase, creating the feared tension pneumothorax.

Complicated Rib Fractures: Hemothorax—*Blood in the chest cavity*

A rib fracture may also result in a hemothorax from associated lung parenchymal laceration or injury to the intercostal artery. This will produce dyspnea and dullness to percussion at the base of the involved hemithorax. Massive bleeding may be associated with systemic hypotension, unconsciousness, and coma. Prehospital treatment will be concentrated on maintaining patent airways, optimal oxygenation, and ventilation, while maintaining a minimum systolic blood pressure of 80 mm Hg. Hospital tube thoracostomy will be therapeutic, allow monitoring of continued bleeding and the need for surgical intervention. The patient with rib fractures involving the upper three ribs is at risk for neurovascular injury. Rib fractures from 9 to 12 may be associated with liver, spleen, renal, or diaphragmatic injury. Chest X-ray and CT scanning will guide therapy. Beware of the patient with hypotension after rib fractures!

Commotio Cordis—*Heart Contusion*

Commotio cordis is a rare, poorly understood, potentially life-threatening condition, which is seen in the young male athlete who receives a sudden blunt blow to the sternum or left chest wall resulting in ventricular fibrillation. The timing of the blow in relation to the T-wave is critical. Early defibrillation and resuscitation (within 1–3 minutes) improves an otherwise dismal survival rate. Some athletic venues have an automatic external defibrillator (AED) unit on site. It is imperative that all members of the medical team are trained in the recognition of this syndrome and the use of the local AED device.

Female Breast Contusion !

The female breast may be injured in contact sports such as martial arts, rugby, football, boxing, and ice hockey. A sports bra is protective, but contusion of mammary tissue may produce hematomas or fat necrosis. Conservative management is usually successful.

CHEST AND ABDOMEN

Abdominal Injuries

David McDonagh[1] and Mike Wilkinson[2]

[1]*St. Olavs Hospital, Trondheim, Norway*
[2]*Allan McGavin Sports Medicine Center, Vancouver, BC, Canada*

Occurrence

Acute traumatic injuries to the abdomen are usually of minor significance, though occasionally more serious, but rarely, life-threatening injuries can occur. The most frequent of these significant intra-abdominal organ injuries in sport are splenic, which can be seen in high-velocity sports such as skiing, snowboarding, equestrianism, American football, rugby, and mountain biking (Table 6.2). In society, in general, the most frequently traumatically injured abdominal organ is the liver. Blunt abdominal trauma in sport may cause renal injuries. Pancreatic trauma is rare, it is usually seen with injury to other organs. As injuries to these organs can be potentially fatal, it is important that sport physicians be able to recognize the early signs of sports-related intra- and extra-abdominal organ injury.

Diagnostic Thinking

While it is natural to assume that acute abdominal pain in an athlete is due to a sports-related injury, the pain may in fact be due to other abdominal conditions or due to referred pain from adjacent anatomical structures and may not be sports related at all. It is therefore essential to take a proper medical history, assess the athlete's hemodynamic stability, and perform a systematic quadrantic abdominal examination. Some patients with evolving major intra-abdominal injuries may be relatively asymptomatic initially and may manifest minimal physical signs. Though the event physician may seldom provide definitive treatment for many of these conditions, it is important to be familiar with current diagnostic and treatment modalities so that he or she can appropriately triage the patient. This information is also important in making return-to-play decisions.

Serious abdominal injuries are caused by blunt or penetrating trauma. The most common trauma mechanism in sport is when an athlete who is moving at speed,

Most common	Less common	Must not be overlooked ❗
Side stitches, p.161	Penetrating abdominal injury, p. 166	Any intra-abdominal organ injuries
Winding, p.161	Liver injuries, p. 167	Acute nontraumatic abdominal pain (multiple causes)
Abdominal wall contusion, p.162	Kidney injury, p. 167	
Rectus abdominis muscle tear, p.162	Gastrointestinal tract rupture, p. 168	
Other abdominal muscle tears, p. 163	Diaphragmatic rupture, p. 168	
Splenic injury, p. 164		

Table 6.2 Overview of differential diagnoses of abdominal injuries. (Reproduced with permission from the Norwegian Sports Medicine Association.)

has a sudden rapid deceleration due to being hit by another athlete or crashing into an object causing blunt trauma to the abdomen. This rapid deceleration can cause abdominal wall injury, intra-abdominal organ contusion or hemorrhage, and even organ shearing or laceration depending on the speed, angle of contact, and protective equipment. Approximately 5% of all mountain bike injuries are to the abdominal region, and more alarmingly, 26% of all cases with splenic injury required surgery. The greater the athlete's speed and weight, the greater the deceleration and the force translated. The organs most commonly involved are the spleen, liver, and small intestine. It is important to understand the actual accident mechanics or mechanism fully to help your diagnostic thinking and "alertness" for potentially severe occult injuries. One must be aware of these potential injuries particularly in high-velocity sports such as bicycling, alpine skiing, ski jumping, motor sports, and contact sports such as rugby, American football, soccer, boxing, and the martial arts.

Athletes who sustain a direct blow to the abdomen that results in injury to spleen, liver, or kidney may have immediate severe pain and can rapidly develop signs of shock and peritonism. Athletes who have sustained a direct blow causing slower bleeding may collapse later either on the field, at the sideline, or at home. At the time of hemodynamic compromise they will be pale, sweaty, may complain of thirst, and their pulse may be rapid and weak. If after blunt abdominal trauma an athlete complains of persistent or intense abdominal pain, they should be kept fasting and must avoid taking medications or fluids by mouth. If the athlete collapses or has clinical peritonism, then he or she should be placed in a recumbent position, with their legs elevated to assist venous return and standard Advanced Trauma Life Support protocols for stabilization should be initiated.

A major warning and red flag to any sports clinician—beware of the acute nontraumatic abdomen masquerading as an abdominal injury! On occasion an athlete will present with intense abdominal pain some hours after a sporting event in which the athlete may have had experienced a blow to the abdomen. The athlete is surprised by the intensity of the discomfort considering the force of the blow. This scenario can be quite dangerous as the patient may mislead the physician into believing that the insignificant trauma was in fact the cause of the patient's pain. The athlete may be presenting with an acute abdominal condition of nontraumatic origin. The commonest diagnosis of abdominal pain is still undifferentiated abdominal pain and 35–41% of emergency surgical admissions for abdominal pain receive this diagnosis, even after extensive tests and observation. Patients may also present with various forms of gastroenteritis, urinary tract, or gynecological infections. Acute appendicitis is always a potential diagnosis in the younger population and must always be considered. Amenorrheic athletes with abdominal pain may in fact be pregnant and presenting with an ectopic pregnancy! The list of possible causes is long and may require ongoing tests and monitoring to find the actual cause. We will not attempt to cover the full differential diagnosis for an acute abdomen here except to remind readers to be aware of this issue and to investigate and treat accordingly. Treatment varies depending on the cause and will range from simply putting an athlete under observation at a venue medical room, to full emergency stabilization and transportation to hospital.

Case History

Taking an adequate history is vital for evaluating any injury or condition, but this is particularly so in determining the cause of abdominal pain. It is important to emphasize that the physician should take a case history as he/she would otherwise do in the normal day-to-day nonsporting environment.

Start by enquiring about the onset of the pain. Was the pain possibly caused by trauma? Ask the athlete to describe the injury. Ask the athlete if they have had a similar injury previously and also ask if the pain experienced then was similar to that being currently experienced. Enquire about the onset of pain–was it of sudden or gradual onset. The athlete should precisely locate the pain and inform about pain radiation, if any. The character of the pain should be described; is it aching, dull, intense, burning, throbbing, knifelike, or colic-like pain? Pain intensity should also be enquired about; also how the pain has progressed, whether it is increasing or decreasing in intensity, if the pain is periodic or continuous. If the pain is of a more chronic nature then enquire about relieving or aggravating factors. Obviously, if appropriate, one must ask about bowel function, and other symptoms such as fever, anorexia, nausea, vomiting, dysuria, hematuria, hesitancy, melena, vaginal discharge, and dyspnea or chest pain. Is there a possibility of infection either from recent travel and food poisoning?

Taking a quick but precise previous medical history is vitally important, in particular to exclude infectious mononucleosis and other infections, coagulation disorders, and other conditions that may predispose athletes to intra-abdominal organ injury and hemorrhage. The importance of this part of the examination cannot be underestimated.

Finally, one should never forget to ask female athletes about their menstrual history. If they have a history of amenorrhea or irregular menses then pregnancy as a potential cause must be borne in mind.

Clinical Examination

Vital signs. One must always check the vital signs. Always evaluate pulse quality and frequency, measure the blood pressure, evaluate the quality and frequency of respiration, measure capillary oxygen saturation, measure the temperature if appropriate (e.g., in hypothermia). Rupture of the spleen, liver, and the extra-peritoneal kidneys can occur in various degrees but the presence of signs of shock or hemodynamic compromise such as low blood pressure, rapid pulse, increased respiratory rate, constriction of peripheral vessels combined with pain and guarding over the liver, spleen, or kidneys should give cause for alarm.

Inspection. Inspection includes a general inspection to see if the athlete is dyspneic, cyanotic, icteric, or pale and sweaty. Do not just inspect the suspected injured body part; a quick glance at other body parts may reveal surprising findings. When inspecting the abdomen, look for bruises or abrasions, lacerations, chest wall deformities and swellings, abdominal distension, and old scars. With major bleeding, abdominal distension may occur and this is obviously a critical situation requiring immediate intervention, stabilization, and patient evacuation. Regrettably, many intra-abdominal and pelvic hemorrhages are missed during the primary and secondary survey.

Palpation. Initiate palpation with light superficial examination before evaluating deeper structures. A quadrantic examination approach is usually recommended, in order to ascertain the presence of tenderness, rebound and contralateral tenderness, guarding, local rigidity, generalized rigidity, palpable masses, etc. The presence of a lower rib fracture should alert one to the possibility of underlying organ injury. The chest and pelvis must be palpated for tenderness or deformity. The spine and posterior thorax can be palpated after logrolling the patient before transport.

Percussion. Percussion may offer some important information in the prehospital environment, such as tympanic sounds with gastric distension or dull sounds with hemoperitoneum. Percussion tenderness may also be present.

Auscultation. Auscultation of the abdomen may reveal the presence or absence of either normal or tympanic bowel sounds.

Other examinations. The genitalia should be examined at some stage; similarly a rectal examination (for blood, masses, and tenderness) should be conducted in a secluded area and obviously not on the field of play. In emergency situations, it is not normal to perform these examinations in the prehospital environment. Hematuria may indicate injury to the kidney, bladder, or urethra.

Imaging. There is a recent trend to have ultrasound equipment at the stadium for major events to enable one to perform an immediate scan to help confirm the diagnosis. This however does not replace the need for a detailed history and examination with the appropriate monitoring.

Emergency Field-Side Treatment

Secure patent airways, ensure adequate oxygenation and ventilation, and evaluate the need for intubation. Blood volume should be restored by giving intravenous solutions such as Hartmann's solution, normal saline, or plasma expanders; however, rapid infusion is not advised as the sudden rise in blood pressure may disturb the natural wound hemostasis. A slow infusion is advised. If possible use wide bore intravenous catheters, two portals are better than one!

If the patient is becoming hemodynamically unstable, then rapid transportation to the nearest hospital is required. In flight treatment may also be necessary, so the athlete may need to be accompanied by a physician. Intravenous analgesia should be considered in conscious patients. Inhaled nitrous oxide should be avoided. The use of anti-shock trousers is usually contraindicated due to the risk of intra-abdominal bleeding. The old adage, *Never remove a foreign body,* still applies as removal almost always leads to increased bleeding (exceptions being penetrating injury to the cheeks). Penetrating foreign bodies should be left in place, but they must be immobilized to prevent further damage to internal organs (uncontrolled movement may cause a shearing effect) during transport. Open wounds should be covered with saline-dampened bandages.

Common Injuries

Side Stitches

Some athletes, particularly those who may be unconditioned or have recently eaten, may experience lateral abdominal pain while running, so-called side cramps or side stitches, or more precisely, exercise-related transient abdominal pain. The cause of this phenomenon is unknown and was previously assumed to be due to muscle cramping, though recent evidence seems to suggest that this is not the case. Diaphragmatic ischemia and/or rapid increase in venous flow to the liver have also been proposed as likely causes. Stitches can purportedly be prevented by proper warming up exercises but the response to this is variable at best. There is no treatment for the condition, other than verbal support, and the condition is usually resolves itself within a few minutes.

Winding

Winding is a relatively common injury in contact sports resulting from a blow to the solar plexus of the abdomen. The exact pathophysiological mechanism is unknown, however it is thought the external force seems to cause vagal stimulation and temporary diaphragmatic spasm. Typically, the winded athlete doubles up and has difficulty breathing. The situation resolves itself quickly without any residual symptoms. If symptoms persist, there may be internal injury requiring examination, observation, re-examination, and even hospital referral.

Abdominal Wall Contusion

Blows to the abdominal wall are not infrequent in sport and can be seen with "winding" or "solar plexus" punches. They may result in contusions in the abdominal wall muscles (usually the rectus abdominis muscle). Incidence varies from sport to sport; torso injuries are quite common in the English Premier League (soccer), 7% of all injuries. Contusions to the torso are also common in alpine skiing and snowboarding injuries. As with other contusions, early icing, NSAIDs treatment, and rest are the usual treatment modalities. Some athletes may need several days' rest, others several weeks. Other injuries, such as lateral and rotatory stretching injuries, sudden explosive weight lifting, and hyperextension of the spine can cause partial muscle tears and contusions.

Rectus Abdominis Muscle Tear—*Tearing the "Six-Pack"*

The rectus abdominis muscle originates in the xiphoid process and the cartilage of the 5th to the 7th ribs, and it inserts in the distal part of the pubic bone. Its main function is flexion of the lower trunk because it pulls the sternum toward the pubic bone, such as with a sit-up movement. The most common tear is proximally at the attachment to the anterior costal cartilages that results from sudden resisted anterior–posterior flexion such as in a rugby tackle, a linebacker in American football and a goalie in soccer, although a total tear is rare. When the resistance or tackle occurs in extension the tear will tend to be more distal (Figure 6.3) and may involve the attachment to the symphysis. Sports in which athletes are particularly vulnerable to this injury are tennis, weightlifting, rowing, and soccer (when training for shooting and heading the ball).

- **Symptoms and signs:** The athlete feels sudden intense pain corresponding to the area of the tear. Attempting to further load the muscle reproduces the pain.
- **Diagnosis:** During the acute stage, a tender defect in the muscle that corresponds to a tear may be palpated. The defect will gradually fill up with blood and edema, which turns into firmer scar tissue. Muscle fascia over the rectus abdominis is thick, so it rarely tears. Therefore, most injuries form intramuscular hematomas. The muscle can be tested by having the patient perform a head lift and a leg lift simultaneously from a prone position. The diagnosis can be confirmed with ultrasound imaging during contraction or MRI.
- **Treatment:** Treatment is essentially the same as for other muscle tears, with initial protection and

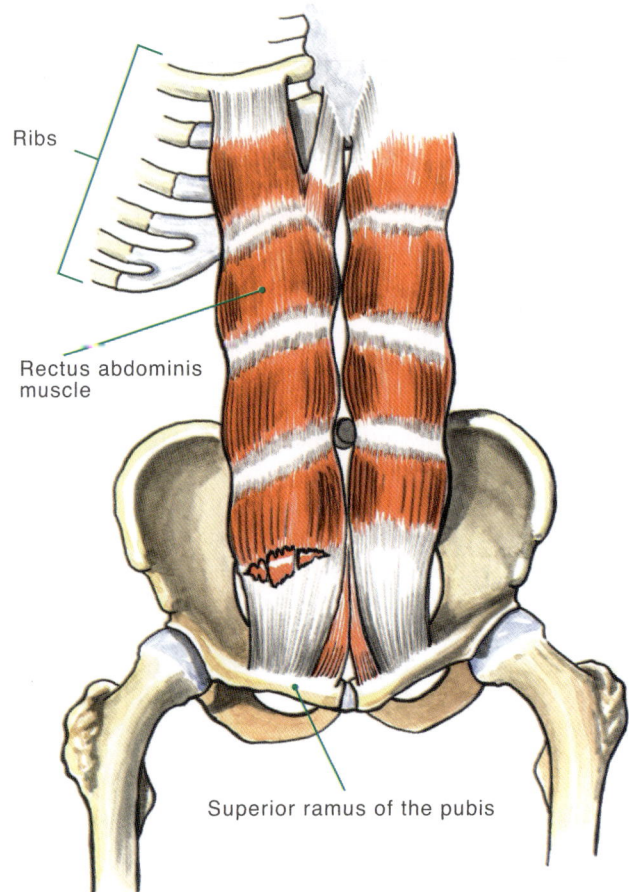

Figure 6.3 Partial tear distally in the right rectus abdominis muscle. (© Medical Illustrator Tommy Bolic, Sweden.)

Ribs

Rectus abdominis muscle

Superior ramus of the pubis

then early mobilization and rehabilitation as this helps in proper muscle healing. If symptoms are ignored and the athlete returns to sport activity too soon, tears in the distal muscle tendon junction may also develop into a chronic condition, which can be difficult to treat and may persist for a long period of time. This seems to be a particular concern for injuries to this muscle/tendon unit. Significant tears with a resultant defect, retraction, or post-traumatic herniation do poorly with conservative management with recurrent episodes of aggravation and weakness. In athletes these tears invariable require surgical repair by an experienced surgeon.

- Prognosis: Prognosis is good with early and proper rehabilitation. The athlete must not return to sport activity before he/she is pain free during sports-specific testing.
- Prevention: Prophylactic measures are regular strength training and stretching of the abdominal musculature. If there are recurring injuries, technique (e.g., for serving in tennis) should be evaluated and corrected.

Other Abdominal Muscle Tears

Most other acute abdominal wall strains are relatively minor, involving the external oblique and then the internal oblique muscles. Occasionally athletes will present with a more significant acute abdominal wall tear that results in either an avulsion of the attachment or a tear and resulting defect in the muscle close to the attachment. The wall component (or muscle) torn will depend on the mechanism and direction of force at the time of injury. Where the force is a combination of rotation and flexion the tear will occur in the transversus muscles (external more frequent than internal) and are more common proximally (usually in a more extended position) than distally or inferiorly (more flexed positions). These tears may occur in the same mechanism as the rectus tears above but more commonly where significant force or effort has been put into a flexion/rotation movement with added resistance, such as a hard tennis serve, spike in volleyball, golf swing, and the acrobatic sports such as gymnastics and freestyle skiing or a resisted slap shot in hockey.

- Symptoms and signs: Athletes present with an acute onset of localized pain, they often will recall the maneuver or incident and report a tearing sensation. In the acute on field assessment there is usually significant local tenderness and muscle spasm that will mask any abdominal wall defect. Later exam will reveal localized bruising, often a palpable wall defect or even hernia, weakness on opposed contraction with either an oblique or in-line sit up, and occasionally local muscle retraction. With minor tears, clinical findings are limited to local tenderness and local pain on resisted contraction without a palpable defect.
- Diagnosis: The diagnosis can be confirmed with ultrasound imaging during contraction or MRI.
- Treatment: Minor tears may be treated conservatively but the rehabilitation is often frustrating and slow. After control of the acute inflammatory response and early mobilization it is important to incorporate functional and sport-specific drills to the rehabilitation plan with a focus on not only strength but core abdominal function exercises and drills to minimize recurrence upon return to sport. As for rectus injuries, significant tears should be assessed by an experienced surgeon.
- Prognosis: Most athletes with an acute minor tear or strain will be able to return to sport within 1–3 weeks. Those with significant tears or those requiring surgery usually are able to return after 3–4 months, but may take up to 6 months for those with more complex proximal tears. All returning athletes will require continued maintenance treatment and functional strengthening to maintain function and prevent a recurrence.

CHEST AND ABDOMEN

Splenic Injury

Blunt trauma, often after a direct blow from a knee, shoulder, or kick to the upper left abdomen, may cause bruising, tearing, or even rupture of the spleen (Figure 6.4). The spleen has a rich blood supply, filtering 10–15% of the total body blood volume every minute, so trauma may cause varying degrees of bleeding within the encapsulated spleen. Splenic injury can be classified in several ways but for the event physician the most critical issue is to decide whether or not there is damage to the splenic blood vessels—in other words, is the athlete hemodynamically stable or not?

In milder injuries, there may be small capsular tears and small subcapsular hematomas, without any significant damage to the splenic parenchyma, where bleeding is limited and local. Larger contusions may occur, with bruising and bleeding, affecting larger areas of the spleen. Finally, lacerations can occur and if these involve the main splenic blood vessels (which they can do), there may be significant internal bleeding. The spleen filters 500–750 ml of blood per minute, so with such a high proportion of cardiac output, blood loss can be substantial and rapid. Should the spleen be damaged with penetrating injuries, great care must be taken in avoiding every type of infection. Reduced splenic function may lead to decreased white blood cell production and thereby reduce the body's ability to fight infection. Splenic trauma is more

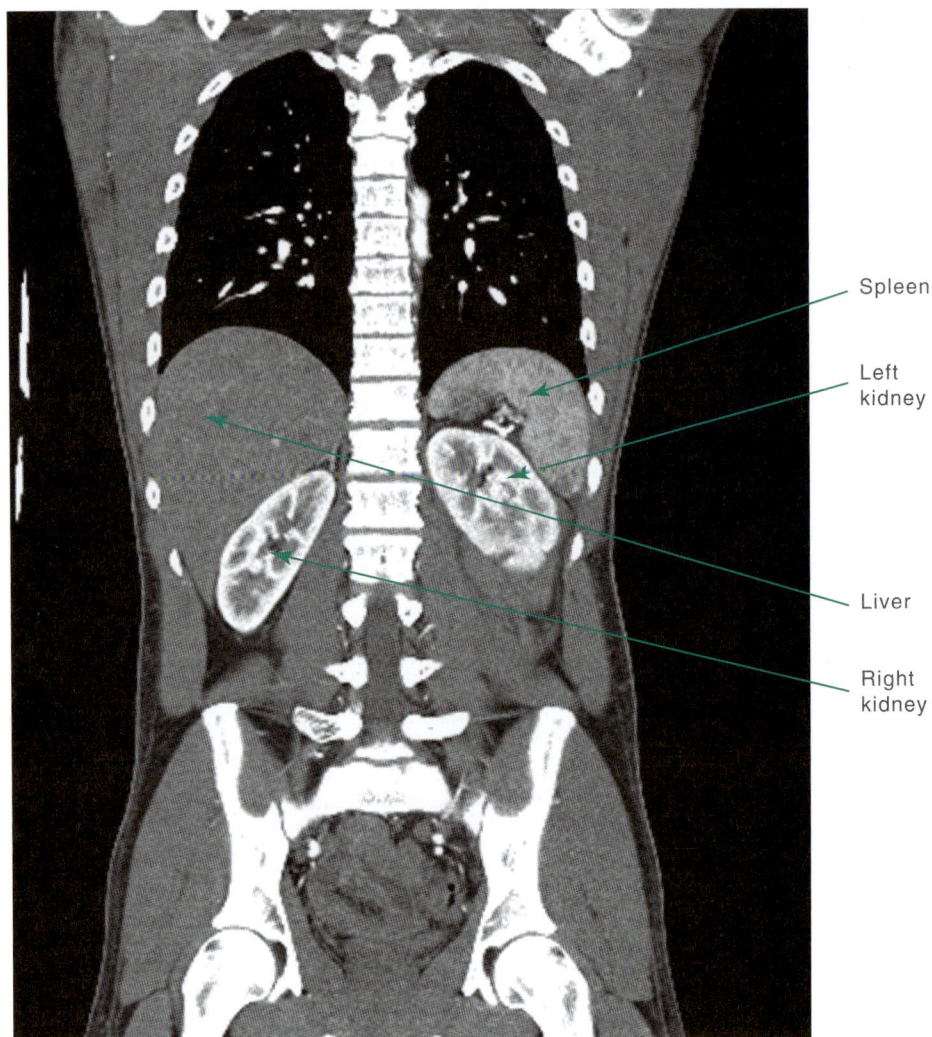

Figure 6.4 Coronal CT view showing small splenic contusion of the caudal splenic pole, without hemorrhage or sign of capsular or vessel injury, as well as laceration of the lower pole of the left kidney. (Reproduced with permission from the Norwegian Sports Medicine Association.)

common in children than in adults, probably due to the fact that they are more active than adults, but also because their abdominal organs are less protected by bone, muscle and fat. In young adults and adolescents, ruptured spleens are sometimes associated with splenomegaly caused by infections such as infectious mononucleosis, immune system disorders, malignancy and other splenic diseases. The diagnosis of splenomegaly and the ensuing decision on return to play is always a difficult one to be made by the sports physician. There are no hard and fast rules but in general the larger the spleen and the higher the level of physicality of the sport, the higher the risk for rupture and thus the greater the recommendation for withdrawal until the splenomegaly resolves. Atraumatic ruptures have been reported but are rare.

- Symptoms and signs: In the hemodynamically stable athlete there may be localized or generalized abdominal pain, tenderness, swelling, localized guarding. Surrounding ribs may be fractured. If the splenic blood vessels have been damaged then the patient may present with symptoms of shock or, more commonly in sport, gradual onset of shock symptoms and findings such as dizziness, vomiting, fainting, sweating, pale or clammy skin, rapid heartbeat, and weak pulse, falling blood pressure, dyspnea, increased respiratory rate and generalized deterioration of vital signs, and eventually loss of consciousness. As with any situation in collapse, always consider other causes of shock but with a history of sports trauma maintain a high index of suspicion for splenic injury.
- Diagnosis: A history of blunt trauma to the upper left abdomen, such as a knee or shoulder tackle in rugby or American football, or the butt of a stick in ice hockey, should raise concern. Always ask about previous or current Epstein Barr infections and other illnesses. Based on your clinical findings a decision must be made about the athlete's ability to immediately return to play or for the need for further evaluation in a hospital, where CT and/or ultrasound examinations and blood tests will usually confirm the extent of the injury.
- Field-side treatment: The main challenge for the event physician is to detect serious splenic lacerations, stabilize the patient as best one can and admit the patient urgently to hospital. With minor injuries, there is also concern regarding return to play issues, as undiagnosed capsular tears and contusions may worsen if re-exposed to trauma, especially if there is an underlying splenomegaly. These minor lesions must also be investigated. With severe splenic injury, treatment is simple but extremely demanding—ABC, stabilize as best you can, load, and go. Obviously ensure that airways are patent, give high-concentration O_2, at least 10 L/min, aiming to maintain O_2 saturation at a minimum of 94%, ventilate if necessary, insert a venous catheter, preferably two if you can, and administer fluid. Accompany the athlete to hospital if the medical staff in the ambulance does not have sufficient emergency training. If there are time or distance factors involved, order a helicopter. If there is a suspicion of minor splenic injury, the athlete should be withdrawn from sporting activity, stabilized, and transferred to hospital for a CT/ultrasound investigation. Ensure that airways are patent, give high-concentration O_2, insert a venous catheter, and administer intravenous fluid if in doubt. If you are unsure of the presence of splenic injury, and choose not to refer the athlete for further investigation, then it is important to regularly observe and re-evaluate the athlete's status for a period of time until you are confident they are stable and no longer at risk. Remember that athletes can appear to be in reasonably good form for some hours after injuring their spleen, before suddenly deteriorating. The athlete and coaching team should be informed of this possibility so that plans can be adapted, for example, with long air flights, return to remote locations.
- Prognosis: Athletes who have undergone a splenectomy should be able to initiate light physical training after 6 weeks, but should wait at least 3 months, preferably 6 months before participating in contact sports. Postsplenectomy athletes

will require a comprehensive vaccination program. For splenic lacerations without splenectomy the time to return is similar but they will require close monitoring. No athlete should return to play before normalization of splenic function and inflammation and infection parameters.

Other Injuries

Penetrating Abdominal Injury

Penetrating injuries occur when the abdominal region abruptly comes into contact with sharp objects. These objects can be part of the sporting apparel in fencing, hockey, or gymnastics but can also be any kind of stationery object—from picket fences, camera equipment, stanchions. With all penetrating abdominal injuries there is a risk of accompanying thoracic and diaphragmatic injury. These serious life-threatening injuries are rare in sport, though there have been several cases of judges, photographers, and even athletes, for example, Sadim Sdiri of France, being speared by javelins during athletic events.

- Symptoms and signs: The presence of a penetrating object must be noted and a presumption of internal organ injury must be made. There is always the possibility of a foreign body having entered the abdomen but this is unlikely in a sporting environment. The initial reaction is one of intense pain, which may be followed by vomiting, sweating with pale or clammy skin causing one to suspect the possibility of intra-abdominal bleeding. There may be increasing abdominal swelling. Guarding and pain may be present if the patient is conscious. There may be dull percussion sounds due to internal bleeding or tympanitic sounds with intestinal puncture. Auscultation of the abdomen may reveal the absence of normal bowel sounds. Obviously, one must evaluate the patient's respiratory function and hemodynamic status as internal organ damage will usually manifest as hemorrhage, leading to hypotension, tachycardia, increasing respiratory rate, decreased oxygen saturation and even shock. One must evaluate the neurological status if there is a possibility of spinal cord or major nerve injury.
- Diagnosis: Further diagnosis should be left until the patient arrives at the hospital. It is enough to know that there is potential internal organ injury and possibly respiratory dysfunction. Stabilization treatment is the main priority.
- Field-side treatment: All patients with penetrating wounds must be treated in the supine position, if possible. The impaling object must be stabilized to prevent further internal shearing. If the object falls out, then the wound must be covered with a sterile, saline bandage. If the wound is bleeding profusely, then pack the wound with sterile bandages but do not force bandages into body cavities. Count the number of bandages used. The patient needs high-concentration O_2 via a mask, assist ventilation if necessary, administer intravenous fluid via an intravenous portal, give analgesia if conscious, and transfer urgently to hospital. If the athlete is impaled upon a stationary object, such as a pole or picket fence, then it is better to try and cut the pole or fence part rather than withdrawing the foreign body. The fire brigade usually has the appropriate cutting equipment available, if needed. Maintaining adequate oxygenation, ventilation, and circulation is the main goal of treatment. Urgent referral to hospital by the most rapid means possible is recommended as rapid and sudden deterioration is not uncommon.
- Hospital treatment: A trauma team should be ready to meet the patient on arrival at hospital. The anesthesiologists will attempt to stabilize the patient while emergency CT and ultrasound examinations are being conducted. The abdominal surgeon will then make decisions regarding the probable need for investigative and corrective surgery.

Liver Injuries

Injuries to the liver, bile duct, and pancreas are once again rare in sport but if encountered may pose significant challenges to the sports physician in both terms of diagnosis and management. In the prehospital setting, these injuries require a high index of suspicion. It is essential to make a rapid diagnosis, initiate basic life support treatment, and to urgently refer the patient to hospital. Despite being relatively well protected, outside the sport setting the liver is the most frequently injured intra-abdominal organ. Liver injuries can be classified in many ways; anatomically, for example, the extent of vascular injury (subcapsular vessel injuries, transcapsular vessel injuries, and inflow/outflow vessel injuries); Organ Injury Scale, by CT classification. The most serious risk is that of hemorrhage. So defining the patient's hemodynamic status is, once again, the correct starting point. Is the athlete hemodynamically stable or unstable? The hemodynamically unstable patient requires urgent stabilization and evacuation.

- **Symptoms and signs:** Findings include local signs of injury, rib fracture, also pain and tenderness if the patient is conscious. If the patient has a normal and stable pulse and blood pressure but is dizzy, vomiting, feels faint or unwell, is sweating, or has pale or clammy skin, then there is a possibility of intra-abdominal bleeding. If significant injury is present, then the examiner will sooner or later find a rapid but weak pulse, falling blood pressure, dyspnea, and generalized deterioration of vital signs before eventual loss of consciousness. Always consider other causes of shock.
- **Field-side treatment:** The hemodynamically stable patient with a probable liver injury should be administered high-concentration O_2 via a mask after the airways have been made patent; the use of an oral airways is invaluable in the unconscious patient. Ventilation should be assisted if necessary, followed by the administration of intravenous fluid via an intravenous portal. Urgent transfer to hospital is essential. The patient with abdominal tenderness and any other symptom (dizzy, vomiting, fainting, malaise, sweating, or pale/clammy skin) should be withdrawn from the field of play and referred to hospital. The need for referral of a patient with abdominal tenderness but no other symptoms or signs (and who is of course hemodynamically stable) has to be made on an individual basis. But if the pain and tenderness are moderate and the case history does not suggest major impact trauma, then the patient can be observed and re-evaluated after 10–15 minutes. Once again, the importance of taking an accurate and detailed case history cannot be emphasized enough.

Kidney Injury

Due to their deep location, the kidneys are usually well protected by abdominal structures to the front and by the lower rib cage and back muscles to the side and back. Blunt trauma can however damage the kidneys (Figure 6.4) and injuries are seen in American Football, ice hockey, rugby, soccer, lacrosse, bicycle accidents and in equestrian sports. Some athletes have transplanted kidneys and these are often more caudally located than normal, and therefore at greater risk. Recurrent jarring such as with trail running or mountain biking may cause microscopic renal trauma presenting with hematuria that us usually self-limiting.

- **Symptoms and signs:** First look for abrasions or bruising over the loin or abdomen. There should also be pain and tenderness in the same area. There may be a loss of loin contour and look for the presence of a loin mass. Fractured ribs may also be found. Often, blood is found in the urine if there is renal damage; however, the absence of hematuria does not exclude kidney injury (as seen when there is disruption between the kidney and ureter). Bleeding can range from microscopic to macroscopic hematuria to profuse bleeding. The combination of macroscopic hematuria and relative hypotension is potentially serious and requires urgent referral to hospital even if the patient is hemodynamically stable. In milder cases a urine sample can be taken in the medical room. In severe cases the athlete may be unconscious with hypovolemic shock. Severe renal trauma is often accompanied by concomitant intra-abdominal organ trauma that should be looked for. It is impossible to correctly classify a damaged kidney in the prehospital environment.

- Field-side treatment: If you suspect renal trauma, then the patient should be stabilized and transferred to hospital for CT examination; ultrasound examination alone is not sufficient. Penetrating trauma is usually more serious. Stabilize the patient and the foreign body, following the basic life support procedures mentioned earlier and transfer the patient to hospital as soon as possible.
- Hospital treatment: Most blunt renal injuries are treated conservatively with strict bed rest until hematuria has resolved. Surgical repair is seldom needed after blunt sports trauma. Penetrating injuries or major blunt injuries often require surgical exploration, although accurate CT injury staging may allow conservative treatment if the patient is hemodynamically stable and has no other associated intra-abdominal injuries. Late complications of renal injury include hypertension, arteriovenous fistula formation, hydronephrosis, pseudocyst or calculi formation, chronic pyelonephritis, and reduced renal function among others.
- Prognosis: The athlete should be asymptomatic for several weeks and urine samples should test negative for blood on at least three separate occasions before being allowed to return to play. Light physical activity can be initiated once renal function and CT are normalized. Commencement of contact sports is controversial and many surgeons would recommend waiting a further 6 months before returning to play even with the addition of protective equipment.

Gastrointestinal Tract Rupture

In high-energy trauma injuries to the abdominal region, severe intra-abdominal lesions must always be suspected, though these injuries are unlikely in most sports. Asymptomatic patients must also be evaluated.

- Symptoms and signs: Rupture of the small intestine can give symptoms and findings similar to those of peritonitis. Rupture of the colon often causes pain and guarding initially. Precise field-side diagnosis is nigh impossible and patients should be transferred to hospital for further diagnostic investigation. Injuries of the pancreas are commonly associated and are often overlooked due to lack of clinical findings in the initial phase.
- Field-side treatment: Routine stabilization treatment is the goal; ensure that the patient's airways are patent, that high-concentration O_2 has been administered, that ventilation is satisfactory and that an intravenous infusion has been established. Analgesia should be administered if necessary. If there is a gastrointestinal rupture then the patient may deteriorate rapidly, so urgent transfer to hospital is advised. Due to the risk of occult injury, all high-energy abdominal injuries should be admitted to hospital for observation and/or advanced diagnostic imaging.

Diaphragmatic Rupture

Most diaphragmatic lacerations occur on the left hemidiaphragm and result from automobile accidents, but can potentially occur in high-velocity sports such as alpine skiing, luge, and skeleton. Respiration is restricted or absent. The stomach can herniate into the thorax and may undergo volvulus, causing the stomach to dilate, thus compressing the left lung. There is often a mediastinal shift to the right. Gastric distension can also result in perforation and should be prevented by inserting a nasogastric tube. Splenic and liver injury is also common with penetrating diaphragmatic injuries.

- Symptoms and signs: Clinical findings may reveal wound tenderness, impaired breathing, impaired respiratory sounds, loss of resonant percussion sounds over the lower lung region, as well as dyspnea, hypoxia, and abdominal pain. Bowel sounds may be found on lung auscultation. Diaphragmatic injury is often associated with other severe thoracic and abdominal injuries, so look for signs of other organ injury as detailed earlier.
- Field-side treatment: Secure airways, oxygenation, and ventilation. The patient may often require intubation before transportation. Hypovolemia must be corrected. Nasogastric tube insertion to prevent gastric distension is recommended though may be difficult to perform due to gastric displacement. Athletes may have severe pain that requires systemic analgesia. Rapid transportation is recommended—diaphragmatic injuries can be life threatening and will require surgical repair with a prolonged recovery.

7 Shoulder

Acute Shoulder Injuries

*Arne Kristian Aune[1], Ann Cools[2], Hilde Fredriksen[3], W. Ben Kibler[4],
Frank McCormick[5], Nicholas Mohtadi[6], Matthew T. Provencher[7],
and Marc R. Safran[8]*

[1]*Drammen Private Sykehus, Drammen, Norway*
[2]*Ghent University, Gent, Belgium*
[3]*Olympiatoppen, Oslo, Norway*
[4]*Lexington Clinic Orthopedics, Sports Medicine Center, Lexington, KY, USA*
[5]*Massachusetts General Hospital, Boston, MA, USA*
[6]*University of Calgary Sport Medicine Centre, Calgary, AB, Canada*
[7]*Naval Medical Center San Diego, San Diego, CA, USA*
[8]*Stanford University, Redwood City, CA, USA*

Occurrence

Acute shoulder injuries are common in athletes, especially in contact sports or those involving the risk of fall. The shoulder is the most commonly dislocated major joint in the body. Shoulder dislocations constitute 4% of all injuries in the 20- to 30-year-old age group, and most of these injuries occur during sport activity. Dislocations are three times more common among men than among women, and are predominantly anterior dislocations. In ice hockey, 20% of the injuries that occur are shoulder injuries, and of these injuries, 8% are dislocations. In skiing, 11% of all injuries are shoulder injuries: primarily dislocations, acromioclavicular (AC) joint injuries, and rotator cuff injuries. Twenty percent of all shoulder injuries are fractures, with fractures of the clavicle and of the greater tuberosity predominating among these injuries.

Differential Diagnoses

Shoulder diseases and injuries affect people in all age groups, and the age of the patient is crucial when making differential diagnoses (Table 7.1). In children, falls that result in direct trauma to the shoulder are the predominant cause of clavicular fractures. In young adults, especially athletes, AC injuries and dislocations are the most common type of shoulder injury. In middle-aged patients, painful subacromial conditions and rotator cuff tears and biceps tendonitis occur most often. In the elderly, particularly in women, osteoporotic fractures of the proximal humerus predominate. Osteoarthritis in the shoulder joint is relatively rare as a primary disease; usually, it occurs in secondary form after intra-articular injuries or chronic rotator cuff ruptures. This chapter describes the acute and chronic shoulder injuries that are most common in sport.

Most common	Less common	Must not be overlooked ❗
Clavicular fracture, p. 173	Rotator cuff rupture, p. 179	Posterior shoulder dislocation, p. 181
Acromioclaricular joint injury, p. 174	Fractures, p. 179	Plexus injuries, p. 181
Anterior shoulder dislocation, p. 176	Sternoclavicular joint dislocation, p. 180	Vascular injury

Table 7.1 Overview of differential diagnoses of acute shoulder injuries. (Reproduced with permission from the Norwegian Sports Medicine Association.)

The IOC Manual of Sports Injuries, First Edition. Edited by Roald Bahr.
©*2012 International Olympic Committee. Published 2012 by John Wiley & Sons, Ltd.*

Diagnostic Thinking

In the diagnosis of an acute shoulder injury, the key distinction is between a fracture and a soft-tissue injury (the ligaments and mucles). The injury mechanism and the clinical examination are the predominant determining factors. Vascular and nerve or plexus injuries must be excluded. The physician should make a tentative diagnosis, so that appropriate radiographs can be ordered. An acute shoulder injury should be evaluated at the primary-care level if radiography is available. Because it is easy to miss a shoulder dislocation, the practitioner must ensure that axillary or equivalent images are taken, in addition to frontal images. A key finding is the inability to externally rotate the arm. No other examinations are necessary during the acute phase. The need for referral depends on the expertise and experience available during the initial care and on access to radiography. The initial management is primarily oriented to achieving comfort once a fracture or dislocation has been ruled out.

Case History

It is important to determine the injury mechanism, the direction of the energy that caused the injury, and the amount of force involved. If a patient falls directly on her shoulder or on an outstretched arm, a fractured clavicle or a dislocated shoulder is most likely to result (Figures 7.1a and 7.1b). Direct trauma to the lateral side of the shoulder often causes an AC injury (Figures 7.2a and 7.2b). Powerful external rotation-abduction, such as that caused by overturning in motocross or falling in downhill skiing, increases the likelihood of neurovascular damage with an anterior

SHOULDER

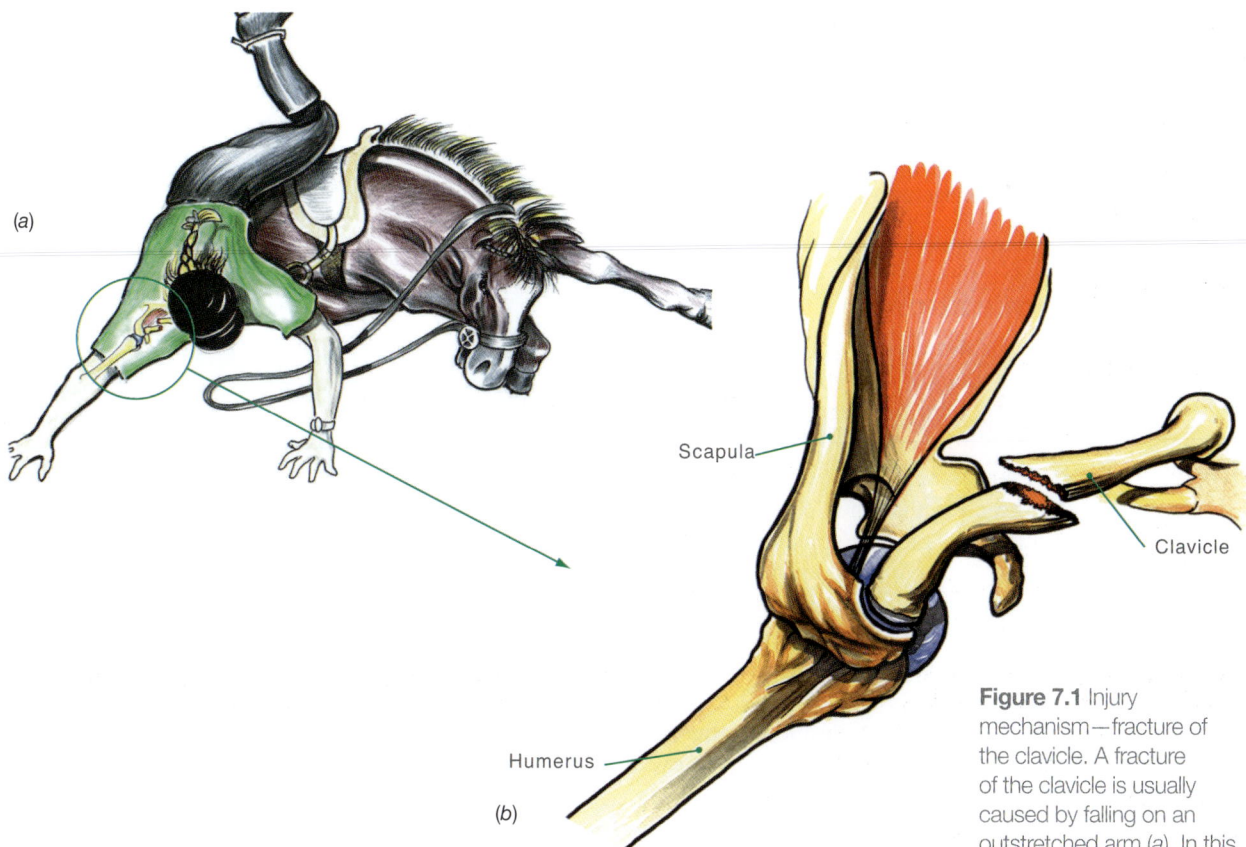

(a)

Scapula

Clavicle

Humerus

(b)

Figure 7.1 Injury mechanism—fracture of the clavicle. A fracture of the clavicle is usually caused by falling on an outstretched arm (a). In this example, the fall resulted in a medial fracture (b). (© Medical Illustrator Tommy Bolic, Sweden.)

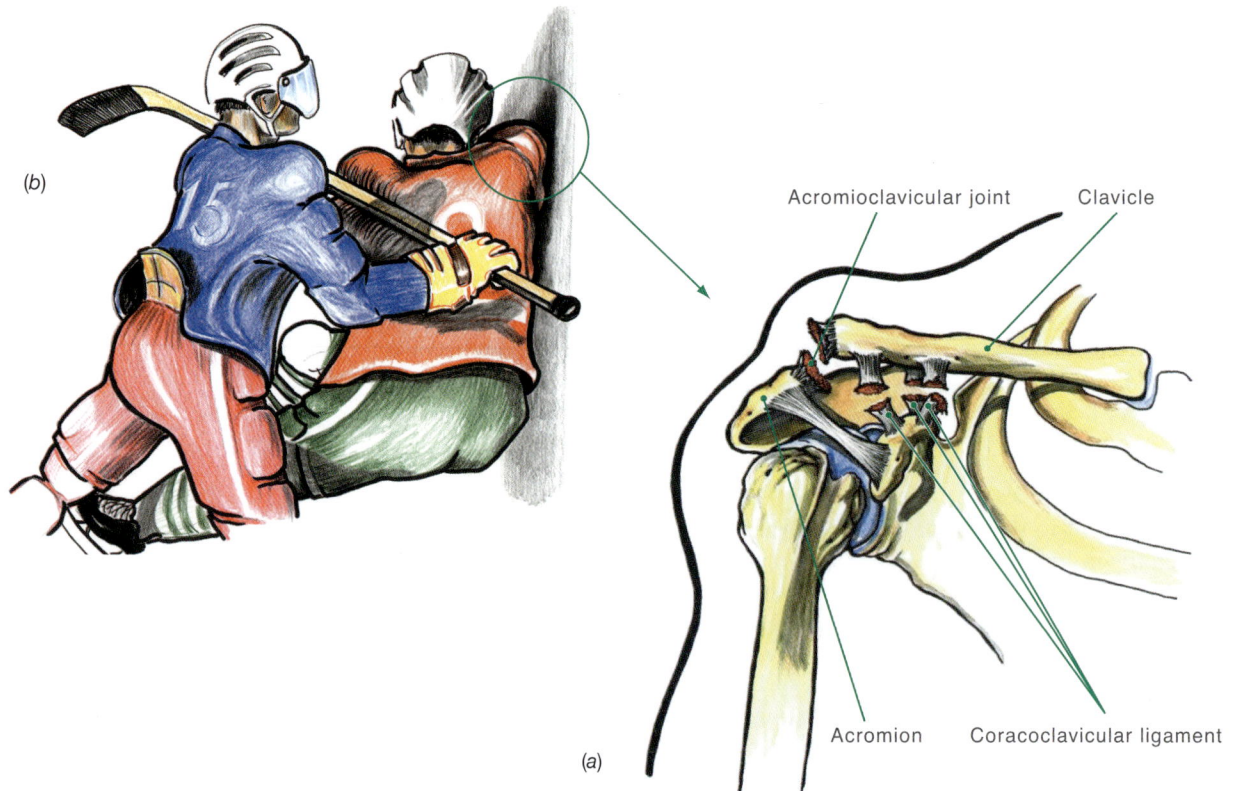

Acromioclavicular joint   Clavicle

Acromion   Coracoclavicular ligament

(a)

(b)

shoulder dislocation. It is important to ask the patient if he has suffered previous shoulder injuries or surgery or have had chronic shoulder problems. Middle-aged and older patients with degenerative changes in the rotator cuff commonly sustain rotator cuff ruptures.

Clinical Examination

Inspection. Changes in the contour of the shoulder under the deltoid and a fixed arm in slight external rotation and abduction are typical signs of an anterior dislocation. A dislocated AC joint or a fractured clavicle is easily detected by examining the patient. Hematoma and cranial dislocation of the lateral end of the clavicle are typical of AC joint injuries, but the patient may also have a lateral clavicular fracture. Hematoma above the clavicular metaphysis indicates a medial clavicular fracture. Swelling and subcutaneous bleeding must also be noted.

Palpation. The physician palpates all the important structures. He palpates the pulse distally and examines cutaneous sensibility, particularly laterally about the shoulder, to determine whether axillary nerve damage has occurred.

Functional tests. Range of motion should be checked. Generally, during the acute phase, it is neither possible nor necessary to perform functional tests, stability tests, or specific tests. However, these examinations are an extremely important tool in the evaluation of a chronic shoulder injury. Patients with acute rotator cuff injuries may have pseudoparalysis in connection with abduction and extension, and such a patient will shrug her shoulder (shrug sign). With dislocations, patients will often lose passive external rotation. This can be a sensitive tool identifying dislocation (especially posterior).

Figure 7.2 Injury mechanism—direct trauma to the shoulder. An acromioclavicular joint dislocation (a) is usually caused by direct trauma to the shoulder, such as being tackled into a sideboard (b). (© Medical Illustrator Tommy Bolic, Sweden.)

Supplemental Examinations

Radiographic examination. Radiographs should be taken of all acutely injured shoulders. Radiographs are ordered specifically on the basis of the clinical diagnosis. If a clavicular fracture is suspected, two radiographic views of the clavicle are taken using caudal and cranial angling. Both the sternoclavicular joint and the AC joint must be examined. If the patient is a child, it may be helpful to take the opposite side for comparison, so that it is possible to distinguish between fractures and a normal apophysis, if, for example, an acromial fracture is suspected. If the patient has an AC joint injury, images of the opposite side are taken for comparison. Images with cranial angling must be included. If the patient has a glenohumeral joint injury, such as a dislocation or suspected juxta-articular fracture, a trauma series is taken (i.e., frontal, axillary, and lateral radiographs). The axillary projection may be difficult to take if the patient has a great deal of pain and has difficulty with abduction. It is always possible to take a lateral projection. Axillary images can be facilitated by having the patient hold onto an IV pole with the arm only slightly abducted. Posterior dislocations are easily overlooked if no lateral or axillary views are taken. Radiographic verification must always be performed to check the position of the shoulder after a dislocation has been reduced, again using two opposite views.

Computer tomography (CT). CT scans may be useful to distinguish between juxta-articular fractures and fracture dislocations when determining whether surgery is necessary. However, CT is rarely advisable as an initial examination and is never indicated for care at the primary level.

Magnetic resonance imaging (MRI). MRI is seldom necessary for acute injuries but can be indicated in secondary-level care, to examine the patient for labral, plexus or rotator cuff pathology. Often in athletes, MRI imaging can be obtained promptly, but it is best done in consultation with the specialist to ensure the appropriate imaging sequences.

Angiography. If vascular damage is suspected, a vascular surgeon should be consulted to determine the appropriate imaging. MR angiograms, CT angiograms, and angiography are all considered options.

Common Injuries

Clavicular Fracture—*Collar Bone Fracture*

Clavicular fractures (Figures 7.3a and 7.3b) are extremely common in children and adolescents who fall on their shoulder or on an outstretched arm. The injury may also occur as a result of a direct blow to the clavicle. In lateral fractures, the trauma is usually directly above the outside of the shoulder, as happens with injuries to the AC joint, and clinically can look like an AC separation. The injuries are divided into medial and lateral fractures, depending on whether they are medial or lateral to the coracoclavicular ligaments. Another classification is based on dividing the clavicle in thirds.

- Symptoms and signs: Swelling and malalignment are easy to detect. If the patient has a lateral fracture, swelling, pain, and possibly malalignment are localized toward the AC joint.
- Diagnosis: Diagnosis is made on the basis of two X rays that must include the AC joint and the sternoclavicular joint.
- Treatment of medial (or mid-shaft) clavicular fractures: *Undisplaced fractures and fractures with minimal shortening (less than 1 cm)* are easy to treat, and they heal within a few weeks. A figure of eight bandage or collar'n cuff is used only for the purpose of pain relief, not to reduce the fracture. Movement exercise and the use of the

arm may begin as soon as the patient can tolerate it. Physical therapy is not necessary. Treatment may take place at the primary-care level. Surgery should be considered if there is significant shortening, displacement or angulation of the fragments, multiple fragments, open fractures, simultaneous fractures of the scapula (floating shoulder), and multiple trauma. Recent evidence has demonstrated that medial fractures with significant fracture fragment displacement respond better to surgical treatment, especially in active individuals or those involved with overhead activities. Thus, a low threshold should be had for referral to specialist or surgeons for athletes. In the interim, the fracture can be stabilized with a sling. In high-energy and comminuted fractures, the patient may have subclavicular vascular damage. A vascular surgeon may treat these types of injuries by means of simultaneous open reposition and fixation of the fracture using a plate osteosynthesis. Healing problems and pseudoarthrosis after fractures of the medial clavicle are rare and occur in fewer than 1% of patients. Shortening and deformity (bump above the healed fracture) may be cosmetically disfiguring but should not be treated surgically. There may be a great deal of callus reaction in children, but it will decrease with time. If a callus bump under the clavicle interferes with neurovascular structures, it should be removed.

Figure 7.3 Fracture of the clavicle. The radiographic views demonstrate a lateral clavicle fracture (a) and a medial clavicle fracture (b). (© Medical Illustrator Tommy Bolic, Sweden.)

- **Treatment of lateral clavicular fractures:** Stable fractures are treated conservatively at the primary-care level, in the same manner as medial fractures. If the fracture is displaced, surgery may be necessary because this type of fracture often causes healing problems and pseudoarthrosis. Therefore, lateral fractures with significant displacement should be referred to an orthopedic surgeon for evaluation.
- **Prognosis:** The prognosis is excellent, and returning to the original level of activity is common. However, lateral injuries may have sequelae with pain and reduced function over time. Some consider resection of the lateral end of the clavicle preventative for this problems. In these cases, the patient should be referred to an orthopedic surgeon for evaluation. Shoulder function is generally good after such an intervention.

Acromioclavicular Joint Injuries—*Injuries to the Joint between the Collar Bone and the Shoulder Blade*

The AC joint is often injured during sport activity, usually as a result of falling on the shoulder. If the trauma comes directly from outside the shoulder, the AC joint is compressed, and the articular surface and the intra-articular disk can be injured. If the energy comes at an angle from above, the shoulder, including the scapula, is pressed downward while the clavicle remains in place. This mechanism injures the coracoclavicular ligaments, increasing the degree of dislocation of the AC joint. AC joint injuries are graded according to the degree and direction of the malalignment (Figures 7.4a, 7.4b, 7.4c, and 7.4d).

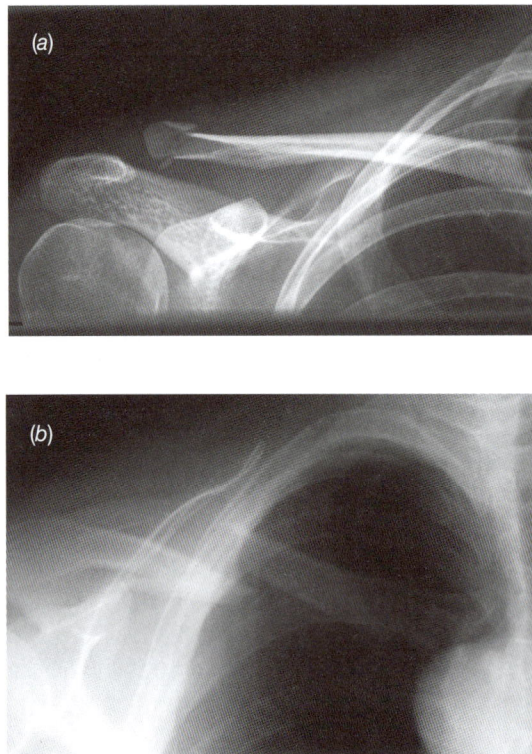

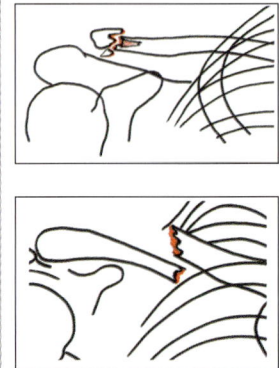

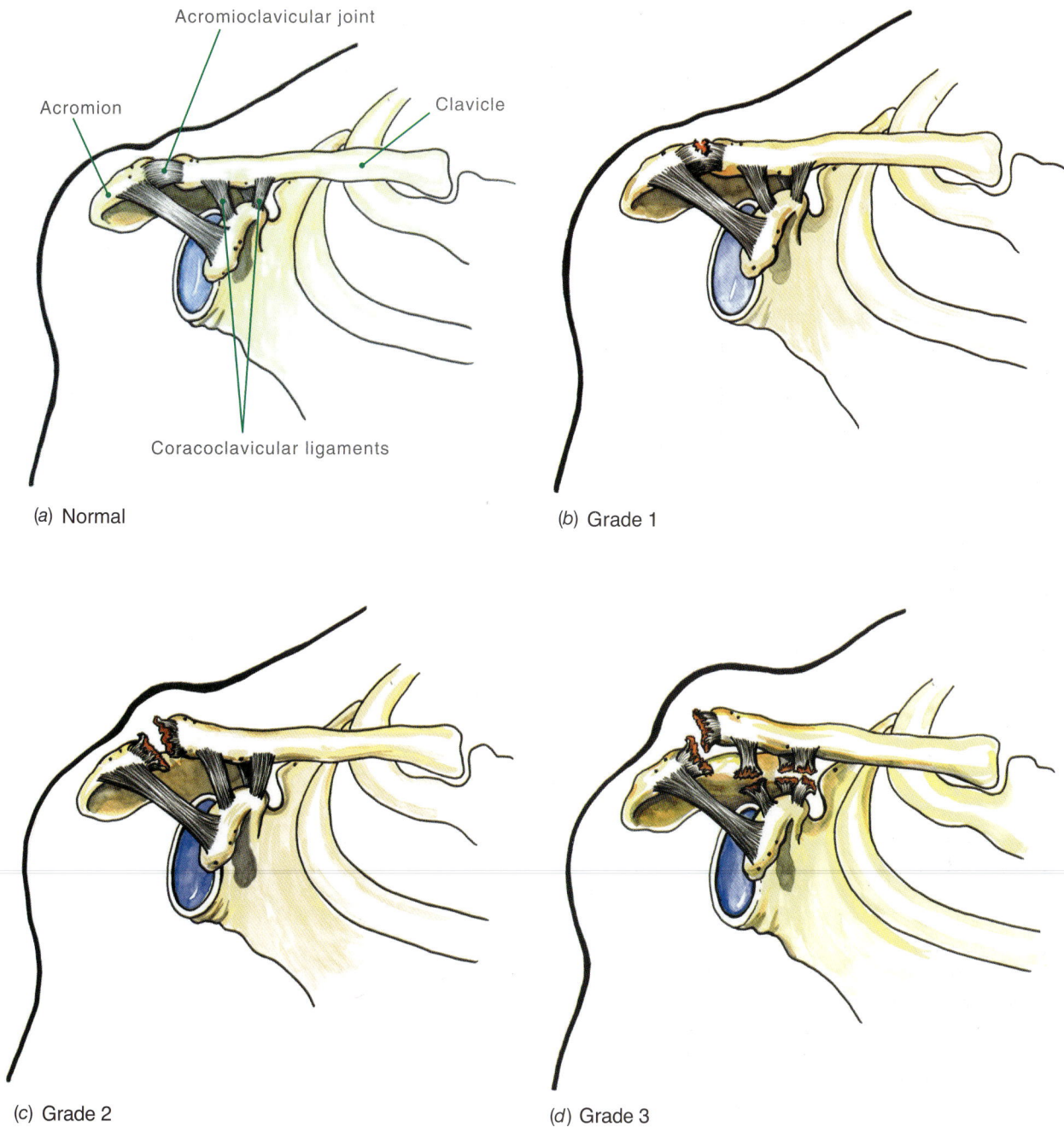

(a) Normal

(b) Grade 1

(c) Grade 2

(d) Grade 3

Figure 7.4 Grading AC joint injuries. (© Medical Illustrator Tommy Bolic, Sweden.)

Grade	Injury
1	Injury of the AC joint capsule without dislocation
2	Like 1, but with cranial subluxation or increased joint distance compared to the healthy side
3	Total dislocation where the AC joint capsule and the coracoclavicular ligaments are torn
4	Similar to 3, but with posterior dislocation where the clavicle penetrates the posterior trapezius muscle fascia
5	Like 3, but expressed cranial dislocation due to penetration through the trapezial fascia
6	Caudal dislocation—lateral clavicle is locked under the coracoid process

SHOULDER

- Diagnosis: The diagnosis is based on swelling and pain above the AC joint and possibly cranial, posterior, or caudal dislocation of the lateral clavicle in relation to the acromion. The injury is graded by a radiographic examination with and without loading, using the healthy side for comparison.
- Treatment: Grades 1–3 AC joint injuries can be treated conservatively at a primary-care level. The few patients who have late symptoms may be surgically treated at a later time. The natural course after a grade 1–3 AC joint injury is generally good. Most of the time, continuous malalignment and instability only cause cosmetic problems. If the injury is difficult to classify, or in a throwing athlete with a grade III sprain, the patient should be referred to an orthopedic surgeon for evaluation. Injuries with major dislocation (unstable grade 3 and grades 4–6) should be treated surgically. Otherwise, therapy consists of pain relief and short-term immobilization in a triangular bandage (or the like). Then, in accordance with the patient's level of tolerance, shoulder use is increased first to regain scapular retraction control, shoulder range of motion, then to regain strength. The patient returns to sport activity when the range of motion and strength are normalized and she can do sport-specific exercises without pain. Persistent pain and reduced function will make surgery necessary for some patients.
- Prognosis: The prognosis is good and return to the original activity level is common after conservative or surgical treatment.

Anterior Shoulder Dislocation—*Shoulder Out of Joint*

Most (95%) shoulder dislocations are anterior (Figures 7.5a, 7.5b, and 7.5c) and are frequently caused by sport-related shoulder trauma. The most common cause of anterior shoulder dislocation is a fall on an outstretched arm or strong external rotation of an abducted arm (such as when a team handball player is tackled while shooting the ball). Posterior dislocations are less common. The most common cause of posterior dislocation is positions of blocking or seizures.

- Symptoms and signs: When the shoulder (i.e., the humeral head) is dislocated anteriorly and out of the glenoid cavity on the shoulder blade, the patient holds her arm in a slightly externally rotated and abducted position without being able to move the shoulder or it is held in internal rotation. Frequently, there is a noticeable and palpable depression under the acromion due to the humeral head being out of the joint. The physician should examine innervation, especially cutaneous sensibility laterally on the shoulder (axillary nerve, called the deltoid patch). An injury of the brachial plexus caused by pressure from the humeral head may have serious consequences. The distal circulation should also be examined.
- Diagnosis: A radiographic examination (trauma series) is necessary to determine in which direction the humeral head is dislocated and to check for any simultaneous fractures. All three views are obtained. Axillary projections are strongly recommended. A simultaneous fracture of the greater tuberosity is involved in 5–13% of anterior shoulder dislocations. The incidence increases with age. Even if these fractures are displaced, they will usually be reduced exactly when the dislocation is reduced, though this must be confirmed with verification radiographs after reduction. If not, a surgical consultation should be made if the displacement is 5 mm or more. In the case of an anterior dislocation, the inferior glenohumeral ligament complex, including the labrum, is usually torn loose from the glenoid (Bankart injury). In 3–10% of these cases, the patient also sustains an intra-articular fracture avulsion from the anterior glenoid. This injury is usually minor and does not affect the initial treatment. Occasionally, the fracture involves a major portion of the glenoid, making surgical fixation to stabilize the shoulder necessary. Nearly all patients with a first-time dislocation sustain a compression fracture behind the humeral head when the head, in its dislocated position, is pressed posteriorly toward the glenoid

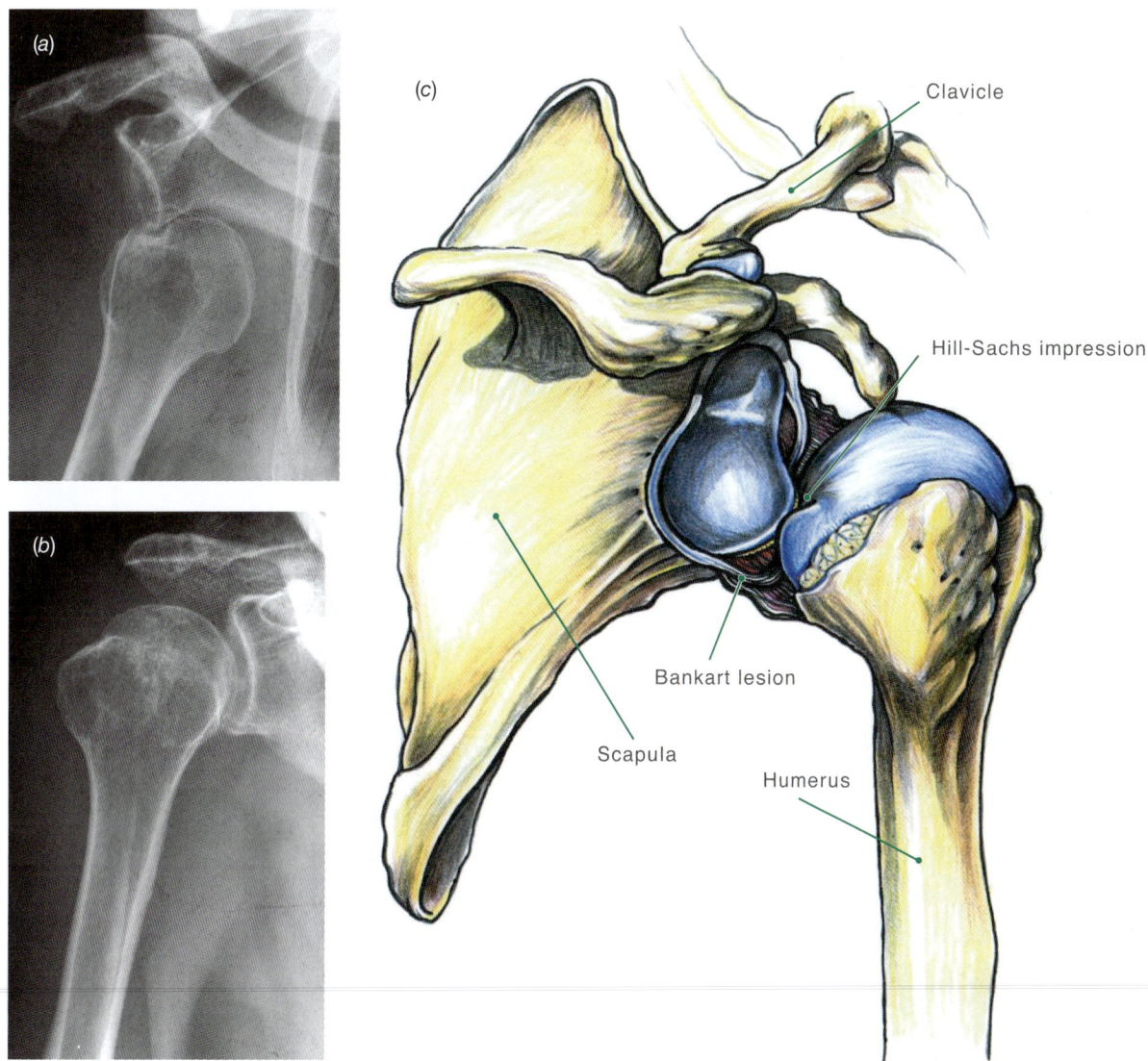

(a)

(b)

(c)

Clavicle

Hill-Sachs impression

Bankart lesion

Scapula

Humerus

SHOULDER

margin (Hill Sachs lesion). This may be a cartilaginous injury, which is not visible on radiographs or a skeletal impression. The injury does not affect the initial treatment. Posterior dislocation causes a reverse Hill Sachs impression fracture. Patients over the age of 40 will frequently have a rotator cuff tear. This should also be evaluated.

• Treatment: The level of treatment depends on the experience and competence of the caregiver, whether the patient has a primary dislocation or multiple recurrence, and on access to radiography. The physician must reduce the dislocation as soon as the diagnosis is made. Dislocations that remain untreated for a long time increase the risk of joint and neurovascular damage. Early reduction is easier because there is less muscle spasm. However, primary dislocations must be documented by radiography. In case of multiple recurrences, a radiographic examination is unnecessary. Before reduction, the patient may be given either 20 mL of 1% lidocaine intra-articularly via a direct lateral injection 1 cm below the acromion or intravenous sedation. Of the various methods of reduction, this author prefers the Stimson method (Figure 7.6). The patient is placed in a prone position with her arm hanging down from the side of the examination table. The arm is pulled downward in the longitudinal direction; the key is to get the patient to relax the musculature.

Figure 7.5 Anterior shoulder dislocation. The radiographic views demonstrate anterior-inferior dislocation of the humeral head with a Hill-Sachs impression (a) and reduction of the dislocation (b). The drawing (c) shows how the labrum–ligament complex is torn loose from the glenoid fossa by anterior dislocation in what is known as a Bankart lesion. (© Medical Illustrator Tommy Bolic, Sweden.)

177

The alternative is to tape a bucket to her wrist and increase traction by gradually filling the bucket with water. Reduction must be done slowly (it often takes 5–10 minutes before the shoulder is in place). In contrast to the "foot in the axilla" Hippocrates method, this method minimizes complications. It is also used for posterior dislocations. Another method of self-reduction, also complication free (Figures 7.7a and 7.7b), may be taught to patients who have a tendency for dislocation or for whom transport to the hospital will take time. In this method, after the shoulder is reduced, innervation and circulation are reexamined, and the reduction is confirmed by a radiograph. For pain relief (until the patient can comfortably move her shoulder) the shoulder is immobilized in an arm sling (or something like it) for as short a time as possible. The immobilization period is usually 3–4 days. There is some recent evidence that in patients who are strictly compliant to immobilization, the recurrence rate may be reduced by 35%. Increasing the period of immobilization beyond 3–4 weeks does not reduce the risk of recurrent dislocation.

Figure 7.6 Reduction of a dislocated shoulder—Stimson's method. Traction of the arm with the patient in a prone position on the bench. (© Medical Illustrator Tommy Dolic, Sweden.)

• Treatment by physical therapist: After a brief period of immobilization, exercises for scapular control range of motion, muscular balance, and strength begin.
• Return to sport: Before returning to sport, the patient must have achieved the same range of motion and strength in the injured shoulder as in the other shoulder, and the outcome of an apprehension test must be negative. Returning to sport too early involves a proven increased risk of recurrence. Therefore, a rehabilitation period of at least 3 months is recommended.
• Prognosis: Various studies report a high frequency of recurrence (46–95%) in young, active athletes. However, there is no routine indication for surgery after the first dislocation; otherwise, numerous athletes would have surgery unnecessarily. Surgical stabilization after a first dislocation is often considered in young patients who participate in throwing or contact sports and have dislocated their dominant shoulder because of the extremely high frequency of recurrence (up to 90%). Between 5% and 60% of patients with anterior shoulder dislocations sustain nerve damage. However, nerve damage is more common in older patients. Most nerve damage goes into spontaneous regression after 3–12 months. If axillary nerve function has not returned after 4 months, the patient is referred for nerve graft surgery evaluation. Rotator cuff ruptures occur in 40–90% of the middle-aged and elderly patients after the first dislocation. If this type of injury causes persistent pain and reduces strength, and if the athlete does not respond to exercise therapy, he should be referred for surgical evaluation. Recurrent dislocations have been linked to developing osteoarthritis over time.

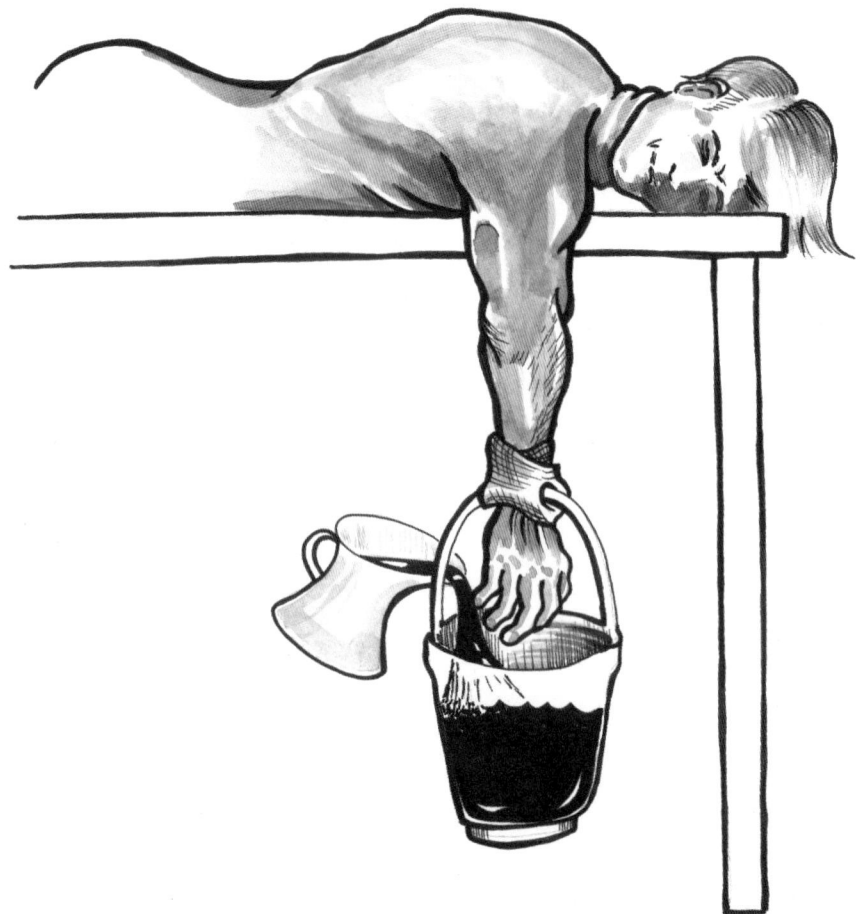

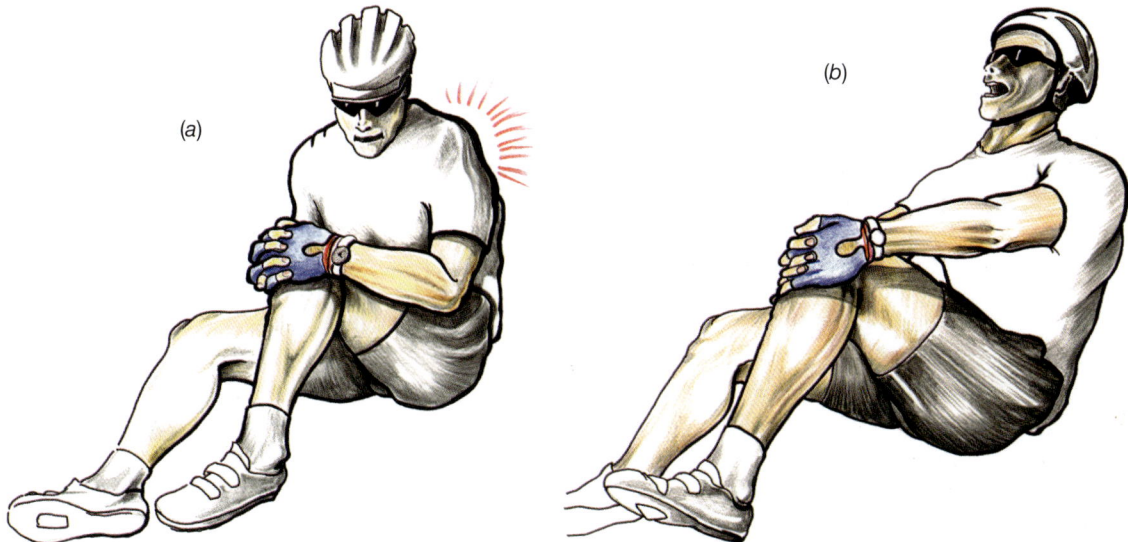

Figure 7.7 Reduction of a dislocated shoulder—self-reduction. The patient wraps his hands around his knee (a) and extends his hip while leaning backward (b). (© Medical Illustrator Tommy Bolic, Sweden.)

Other Injuries

Rotator Cuff Rupture

An acute rotator cuff rupture is rare among younger athletes, but a fall (e.g., while skiing) often causes a rupture in active older athletes with degenerative tendinous tissue. Rotator cuff ruptures are usually caused by a degenerative condition that is triggered by reduced circulation in the tendon because of age, tendinosis, and impingement. A fall may trigger a total rupture of the weakened tendinous tissue. Athletes in throwing sports may also sustain a partial rupture as a result of repeated eccentric loading of the tendinous tissue. Acute rotator cuff tears are very responsive to surgical repair. Thus, a history and physical exam suggestive of a tear warrant an expedient orthopedic surgeon evaluation. Evaluation and treatment of rotator cuff injuries is discussed in the section on chronic shoulder disorders.

Fractures

The most common juxta-articular fractures are avulsion of the greater tuberosity and intra-articular scapular fractures. These are discussed in connection with shoulder dislocation. A fracture of the greater tuberosity that is displaced more than 5 mm should be surgically reduced and fixed. Fractures without displacement are treated conservatively by short-term immobilization in an arm sling for pain relief, followed by range-of-motion exercises and strength training. If treated nonoperatively, weekly follow-up is necessary to assure the fracture does not displace during the healing process. The patient may be treated at the primary-care level. A proximal humeral fracture is a typical osteoporotic fracture in the elderly. In younger patients, fractures of the proximal humerus are less common. The rule is conservative treatment, as mentioned previously, but open reduction and fixation may be indicated for multiple fragment fractures and major dislocation. Therefore, this type of fracture should be referred to an orthopedic surgeon for evaluation. Fractures of the body of the scapula heal well. Treatment is conservative, with immobilization for pain relief, followed by range-of-motion exercises and strength training by a physical therapist at the primary-care level. Fractures that go into the scapular notch may lead to entrapment of the suprascapular nerve. In such cases, surgery may be necessary. Nerve lesions cause paresis in the supraspinatus muscle and/or the infraspinatus muscle, depending on the level of the injury. If this type of complication is suspected, the patient is referred for evaluation.

Sternoclavicular Joint Dislocation—*Collar Bone Dislocation (Injury to the Joint between the Collar Bone and the Breast Bone)*

Sternoclavicular joint dislocations (Figures 7.8a, 7.8b, and 7.8c) are rare. This joint is the only direct bony attachment of the shoulder to the axial skeleton. Its stability depends upon the costoclavicular, sternoclavicular and interclavicular ligaments as well as a sturdy joint capsule and intra-articular disc. The mechanism of injury is usually a blow to the shoulder from the front or behind leading to anterior or posterior instability. Posterior sternoclavicular dislocation may pose the threat of mediastinal vascular injury or airway compromise. Anterior instability is painful and disfiguring. There may be associated fractures of the clavicle. These injuries may be serious and difficult to treat if the clavicle dislocates posteriorly and threatens the large thoracic vessels behind it. Therefore, the patient should be evaluated and treated in the hospital.

- Symptoms and signs: Pain and deformity over the sternoclavicular joint are aggravated by any shoulder and anterior neck muscle movement. A posterior dislocation is characterized by a palpable or visible hollow and may be associated with difficult breathing or swallowing. This athlete is best transported to hospital for further imaging and treatment.
- Diagnosis: A radiographic examination may be completely negative, and CT scanning is essential in documenting associated injury.
- Treatment by physician: Anterior dislocations may remain untreated with satisfactory functional results. The prominence of the clavicle is only of cosmetic significance. It is not reduced because it rarely becomes stable. Children and adolescent patients often have a growth plate injury and no dislocation that will remodel. Posterior dislocation may threaten the structures in the mediastinum. Prominence of the sternoclavicular region is not necessarily always an anterior sternoclavicular injury—it may just be swelling from a posterior injury. Imaging with a CT scan will confirm the direction of injury. Treatment is reduction with preparedness for vascular surgery. These injuries are usually stable after reduction.
- Treatment by therapist: Shoulder sling and figure of eight bandage.
- Prognosis: Return to play usually requires 6–8 weeks if a closed reduction was possible. Open surgical reduction and repair will

Figure 7.8
Sternoclavicular joint dislocation. Normal anatomy (*a*), anterior dislocation (*b*), and posterior dislocation (*c*) are shown. Posterior dislocation may be life-threatening if it affects the large intrathoracic vessels. (© Medical Illustrator Tommy Bolic, Sweden.)

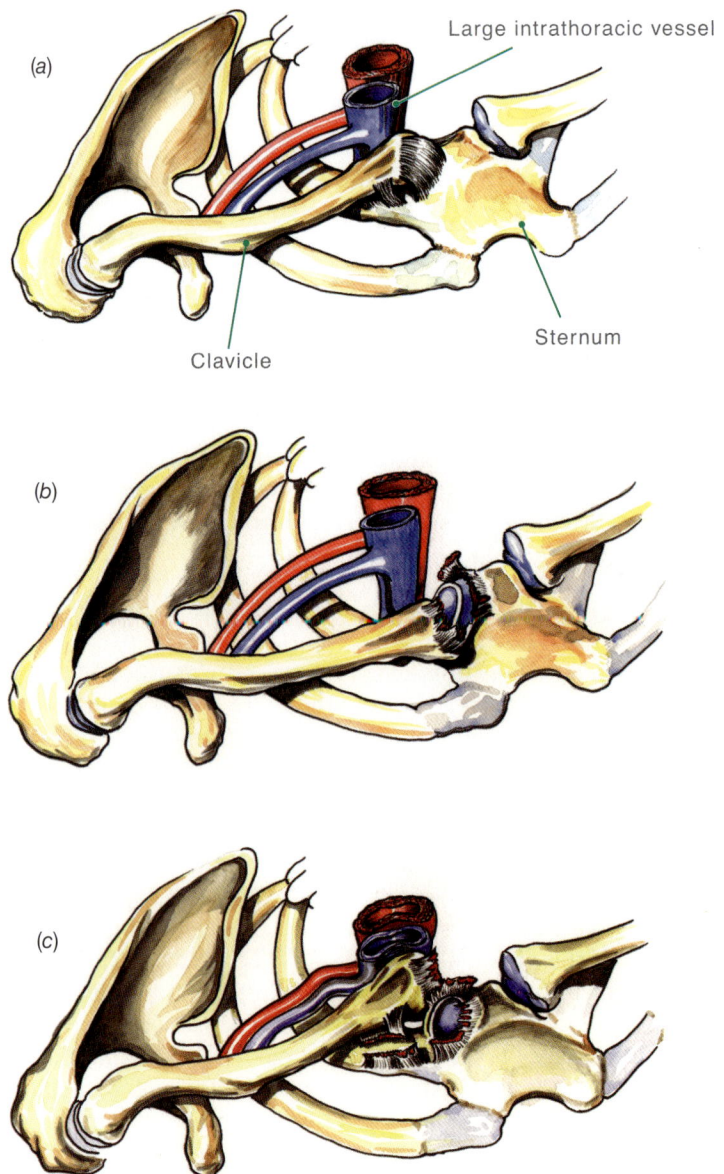

(a)

Large intrathoracic vessel

Clavicle

Sternum

(b)

(c)

require a minimum of 12 weeks but any return to play decision is also dependent on sternoclavicular joint stability, the absence of painful movement and the status of vascular repairs. Obviously, the physical nature of the sport will have to be taken into consideration.

Posterior Shoulder Dislocation—*Shoulder Out of Joint* !

Posterior shoulder dislocations represent less than 5% of all dislocations. The injury is often caused by a fall on an outstretched arm, an electrocution or by an epileptic seizure. Posterior dislocations may be overlooked, primarily because the radiographs are inadequate. A key physical exam finding is the loss of passive external rotation. Inspection from behind reveals an obvious change in the contour of the shoulder. The diagnosis is made using radiographic examinations with axillary and/or lateral images. The Stimson reduction method is used. The injury may be treated at the primary-care level in the same manner that anterior dislocations are treated–that is, depending on access to radiography and personnel with the proper expertise.

Plexus Injuries—*Nerve Root Injuries* !

Plexus injuries are divided into root avulsion injuries and more distal injuries. Root avulsion injuries cause the patient's arm and shoulder to become paralytic, and MRI or CT myelography typically show empty root cavities. This indicates a poor prognosis. The prognosis is better for more distal plexus injuries, and the injury should be observed for a while to see whether it spontaneously improves. However, after 3 months without improvement, surgery must be considered. Sural nerve graft surgery may improve elbow and hand function somewhat, but the effect on shoulder function is minimal. If a plexus injury is suspected, the patient should be referred to a neurologist or to a neurosurgeon or hand specialist.

SHOULDER

Chronic Shoulder Disorders

Arne Kristian Aune[1], Ann Cools[2], Hilde Fredriksen[3], W. Ben Kibler[4],
Frank McCormick[5], Nicholas Mohtadi[6], Matthew T. Provencher[7], and Marc R. Safran[8]

[1]*Drammen Private Sykehus, Drammen, Norway*
[2]*Ghent University, Gent, Belgium*
[3]*Olympiatoppen, Oslo, Norway*
[4]*Lexington Clinic Orthopedics, Sports Medicine Center, Lexington, KY, USA*
[5]*Massachusetts General Hospital, Boston, MA, USA*
[6]*University of Calgary Sport Medicine Centre, Calgary, AB, Canada*
[7]*Naval Medical Center San Diego, San Diego, CA, USA*
[8]*Stanford University, Redwood City, CA, USA*

Occurrence

Painful conditions in the shoulder caused by overuse, muscular imbalance, and instability are the predominant injuries in throwing sports and in sports such as swimming and tennis, with an incidence of between 17% and 26%. Overuse injuries to the shoulders of volleyball players and athletes in other throwing and racket sports are increasing, with a disproportionate share among female athletes. In fitness sports, shoulder overuse injuries are twice as common among older athletes as they are among younger athletes.

Differential Diagnoses

The injury spectrum (Table 7.2) depends on previous injuries and on the age and activity level of the athlete. Recurrent dislocations after a primary traumatic, anterior shoulder dislocation are common in younger athletes. But chronic shoulder pain is a problem in all age groups. In throwers, swimmers, and athletes who play racket sports or other athletes involved in activities that require extreme motion, shoulder pain is usually related to multidirectional laxity, muscular imbalance and the repetitive microtrauma of overhead sport. Subtle anterior instability can occur secondarily without overt subluxation or dislocation. In throwing athletes, and those involved in racquet sports, shoulder pain may be the result of muscular imbalance and stretching of the anterior joint capsule as a result of the unilateral activity and microtrauma. An alternative mechanism in these athletes is posterior capsular tightness that occurs as a result of chronic excessive overload from throwing. These results in posterior capsular contracture, leading to a glenohumeral internal rotation deficit (GIRD),

Most common	Less common	Must not be overlooked ❗
Posttraumatic shoulder instability, p. 192	Superior Labrum injury (SLAP lesion), p. 193	Radicular pain from the neck
Multidirectional laxity and anteroinferior instability, p. 194	Rotator cuff rupture, p. 199	Adhesive capsulitis, p. 204
Internal impingement, p. 196	Acromioclavicular joint osteoarthritis, p. 201	
Subacromial pain syndrome, p. 197	Entrapment of the suprascapular nerve, p. 202	
Recurrent posterior shoulder instability, p. 201		

Table 7.2 Overview of differential diagnoses of chronic shoulder disorders in athletes. (Reproduced with permission from the Norwegian Sports Medicine Association.)

producing altered humeral head motion with the throwing motion. Impingement and tendinosis of the rotator cuff and labral injuries in these athletes are usually secondary phenomena caused by instability and posterior capsular contracture.

Injuries to the glenoid labrum may cause pain and a feeling of instability. In middle-aged and elderly athletes, tendinosis, degenerative conditions, and rotator cuff tears are the primary causes of pain. Even if the natural course after AC joint dislocation is benign, pain in the joints and the development of osteoarthritis may occur as late sequelae. Weightlifters may have pain in the lateral clavicle caused by increased stress that may cause osteoarthritis and osteolysis in the lateral end of the clavicle. Entrapment of the suprascapular nerve is a rare differential diagnostic condition that may cause posterolateral shoulder pain and muscle atrophy, and is more commonly seen in athletes involved in volleyball and throwing sports.

Diagnostic Thinking

The main rule for most painful conditions in the shoulder, whether due to instability or tendinosis in the rotator cuff, is to treat them conservatively with a rehabilitation program. However, it is important to make the proper diagnosis including the anatomic injury and all alterations in muscle flexibility, strength, and strength balance so that the rehabilitation program can be adapted to the situation. For recurrent shoulder dislocation, treatment is often surgical. In this case, the goal of the evaluation is to determine what pathoanatomical changes have occurred to the joint so that appropriate surgical treatment may be planned.

One of the most frequent causes of chronic shoulder pain in the overhead athlete is "impingement." On the basis of the location of impingement, the symptoms are classified into subacromial versus internal impingement. Internal impingement comprises encroachment of the rotator cuff tendons between the humeral head and the glenoid rim in the late cocking position of throwing. Because of the specific position of this internal impingement, it is considered to be the primary cause of chronic shoulder pain in the overhead athlete.

Impingement can also be classified on the basis of the cause of the problem, dividing it into primary versus secondary impingement. In primary impingement, a structural narrowing of the subacromial space causes pain and dysfunction (see Subacromial pain syndrome on p. 197). In secondary impingement, there are no structural obstructions causing the encroachment, but rather functional problems, occurring only in specific positions, for instance the late cocking position of throwing or the tennis serve. Secondary impingement may occur in the subacromial space as well as internally in the glenohumeral joint, resulting from a variety of underlying conditions, for example, rotator cuff pathology, scapular dyskinesis, shoulder instability, biceps pathology, labrum lesions, and GIRD.

A thorough physical examination is the key for screening an athlete for impingement-related shoulder pain, prior to undertaking any imaging. The following algorithm (see Figure 7.9) offers a systematic approach to specific tests that can be used to elucidate impingement-related shoulder problems. Using a battery of specific shoulder tests (Jobe's empty can test, Hawkins, Neer, apprehension, relocation, release), the impingement symptoms may be classified into subacromial versus internal, and primary versus secondary. Subsequently, various tests can be used to clinically diagnose rotator cuff involvement (full can test), scapular dyskinesis (scapular assistance and retraction test), instability and underlying laxity (anterior, posterior and inferior laxity tests), biceps pathology and SLAP lesions (e.g., O'Brien test and Crank test), and GIRD (range of glenohumeral internal rotation).

SHOULDER

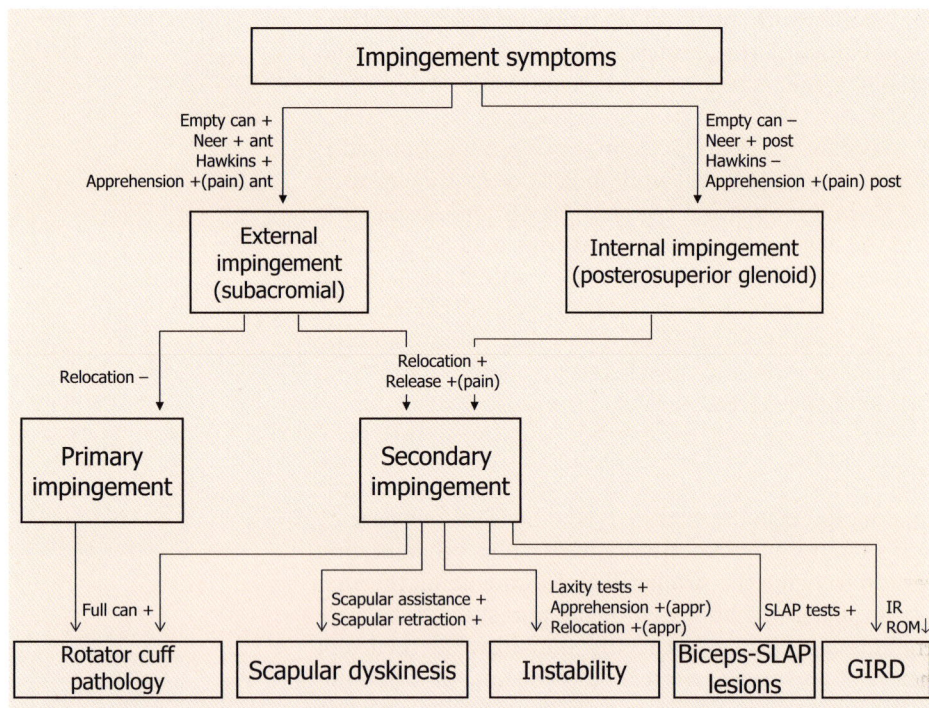

Figure 7.9 Algorithm for clinical reasoning in the examination of impingement-related shoulder pain in athletes. (Adapted with permission from Cools et al. Br J Sports Med 2008 (42): 628–635).

Case History

The case history is extremely important for chronic shoulder disorders. A good case history may contribute to narrowing down alternative diagnoses so that further evaluation, possibly with imaging diagnostics, becomes significantly easier.

First, it should be determined how the symptoms started. Did they result from a trauma? What type of activity was the patient engaged in when the symptoms first appeared? If the shoulder was dislocated previously, the problem is likely to be related to the previous instability. Did the patient hear or feel any click, sound, or crunching in his shoulder? If he did, the cause may be sequelae from a rotator cuff or a labral injury. Did the pain begin gradually, or did it arise suddenly? Is there a localization to the pain? This often helps to identify the injured area. Acute pain is typical of inflammatory conditions, whereas chronic pain is indicative of rotator cuff conditions or subtle instability. The practitioner should determine whether the athlete was able to continue his activity in whole or in part when the symptoms began.

The practitioner should record the medical history and symptoms and should indicate what therapy was attempted (e.g., physical therapy, drugs, surgery, or steroid injections). The patient should be asked specifically whether she had neck problems in the past.

The specific symptoms and the degree to which the symptoms affect sport activity, work, or daily life must be determined. Even if the shoulder has never been dislocated, the patient should be asked whether his shoulder feels unstable. If it was dislocated, he should be asked how many times, under what circumstances, and did he need to go to the hospital to have it reduced? If the patient has pain that may be caused by instability, the practitioner must determine whether the shoulder locks up and whether it clicks in certain positions. This points toward labrum pathology. In the case history, the patient should be asked about limited movement—for example, did he have trouble reaching behind his back or combing his hair?

Finally, the case history should be as specific as possible with respect to pain. Pain is often the main reason that the patient seeks help. The practitioner must distinguish between pain at rest or pain with activity. It is important to characterize the relationship of the activity to pain; specifically which activity and at what point during the activity particularly if it is an overhead sport. Expressed pain at rest with greatly limited movement indicates capsulitis (frozen shoulder or possibly arthritis. Patients with tendinosis or a rotator cuff rupture suffer from shoulder pain when lying on their arm, when lifting their arm, doing activities at or above shoulder level and even pain at night. Pain during activity in external rotation and abduction indicates anterior instability.

Clinical Examination

Inspection. It is very important to understand that asymmetry in the shoulder may be a direct result of changes that occur in the dominant shoulder in a sport such as tennis or in a baseball pitcher. This is a normal phenomenon. However, an abnormal position of the shoulder may indicate a change in the spinal column, a muscle injury, or neurological disease. Changes in position may also occur as a result of a painful condition that has lasted a long time. Muscular atrophy (e.g., of the supraspinatus and the infraspinatus muscles) may indicate a rotator cuff rupture or entrapment of the suprascapular nerve. Injury to the axillary nerve affects the deltoid muscle. There should be special attention to the resting posture of the scapula to evaluate dyskinesis. Observed prominence of the medial scapular border is a key diagnostic clue to abnormal scapular rhythm. This may indicate inflexibility or weakness in the supporting musculature, or joint internal derangement

Range of motion. When examining the active range of motion, the physician should note the scapulohumeral rhythm (i.e., the rotation of the scapula when the arm is abducted). He should stand behind the patient and compare the scapulohumeral rhythm to the other side. The active range of motion is not always the same as passive deflection. Disrupted scapulohumeral rhythm in the plane of the scapula indicates subacromial pain or weakness, or it may indicate changes in balance in the musculature, as happens when there is instability, labral injury or injury to the long thoracic nerve. The normal range of motion is flexion 180°, extension 30°, abduction 180°, adduction 30°, internal rotation in the neutral position 70°, and external rotation in the neutral position 60°. However, be aware of the asymmetrical increased external rotation and reduced internal rotation in the dominant shoulder of the overhead athlete when compared with the nondominant side. Although this is a normal phenomenon, it can become abnormal and should be addressed in circumstances where the shoulder becomes painful and the total combined internal and external rotation is limited. This condition is called GIRD. This is assessed by measuring glenohumeral internal rotation range of motion, preferable in the supine position with the shoulder abducted 90°, and the scapula stabilized against the table (Figure 7.10). Goniometric assessment as well as interpretation of the "end feel" is described as criteria for GIRD evaluation. A side-to-side difference of 20° is considered to be positive for GIRD.

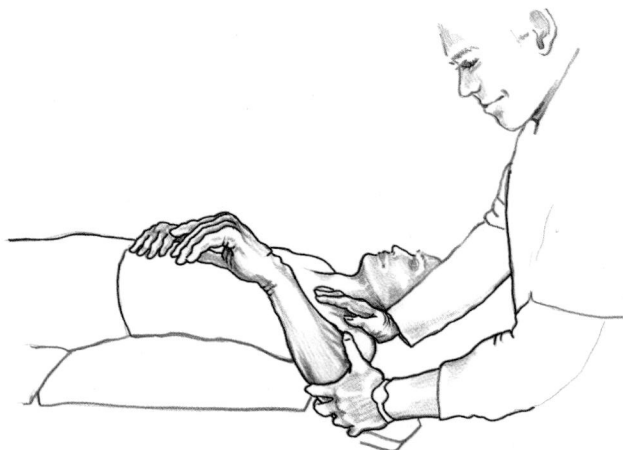

Figure 7.10 Assessment of glenohumeral internal rotation range of motion (GIRD). With manual fixation of the shoulder top, the arm is brought into maximal internal rotation in a 90° abducted position. Range of motion as well as decreased joint play or increased stiffness at end of range is assessed. (© Medical Illustrator Tommy Bolic, Sweden.)

Palpation. Several locations may be tender to palpation. Tenderness under the acromion corresponding to the greater tuberosity is a sign of rotator cuff or bursal pain, which may be rotator cuff degeneration or tendinosis with or without calcium deposits in the tendon insertion. Pain around the coracoid process is rare but may occur in the case of subscapular tendinosis or subcoracoid impingement, which frequently causes shoulder pain in swimmers, but if the pain is present along the pectoralis minor, it will indicate tightness in that muscle. Pain corresponding to the long biceps tendon is found when there is rotator cuff tendinosis or rupture and if the patient has impingement syndrome when the long biceps tendon is tender to palpation. Biceps tendon tenderness may also occur with primary biceps pathology or superior labrum (SLAP) lesions. However, if the patient has chronic rupture of the biceps tendon, the biceps sulcus is usually pain free. Pain above the AC joint and any thickening here is a sign of a degenerative condition in the joint–for example, as a result of previous trauma. Stability in the AC joint is examined by pressing the clavicle in the caudal direction, while the humerus is being pressed cranially or by eliciting pain at the joint as the arm is horizontally adducted. Pain at the AC joint when the arm is brought across the body is consistent with joint pathology, such as arthritis or distal clavicular osteolysis. Pain above the clavicle is rare but may occur if the patient has a late healing fracture or pseudoarthrosis. Tenderness to palpation above the sternoclavicular joint may be a sign of chronic instability. Sometimes the patient may spontaneously dislocate and reduce this joint. For various painful conditions, the muscle insertions around the shoulder should be palpated. However, some of these trigger points are uncharacteristic for diagnosing a possible injury, and they may be secondary to other pathology in the shoulder.

Neuromuscular function. A general neurological examination of the upper extremity should be performed, especially to look for accompanying injuries to the peripheral nerves, such as injuries to the suprascapular nerve and the axillary nerve (e.g., after shoulder dislocations). If the patient has injured the long thoracic nerve, the anterior serratus muscle becomes paralyzed. This causes what is known as winged scapula. This is determined by having the patient do push-ups against the wall, causing the prominence of the medial border of the scapula, which points out from the chest, to show clearly. The cervical spine should be examined for movement and root provocation, to determine whether the patient has any pain that radiates from his neck to his shoulder.

If the case history indicates recurrent dislocations or instability, the practitioner needs to examine shoulder stability by using specific tests.

Laxity Tests

Drawer test (anterior and posterior laxity test) (Figure 7.11). Normally, the humeral head can be translated anteriorly, posteriorly, and inferiorally. There is a great deal of variability in the magnitude of this translation in the athletic population. Therefore, it is necessary to compare the affected shoulder to the opposite side, to fully appreciate what is normal for each individual. If translation increases when the patient hangs his arm at his side, it is a sign of increased capsule laxity (Figure 7.7).

Sulcus sign (inferior laxity test) (Figure 7.12). Translation downward, or the so-called sulcus sign, is achieved by pulling the elbow distally, making a depression underneath the acromion, which indicates much laxity. This is particularly common in patients with multidirectional instability, where shoulder pain is caused by increased laxity.

Apprehension test (Figure 7.13). The test is done with the patient in a supine position or sitting with her arm at 90° abduction, 90° flexion in the elbow, and externally

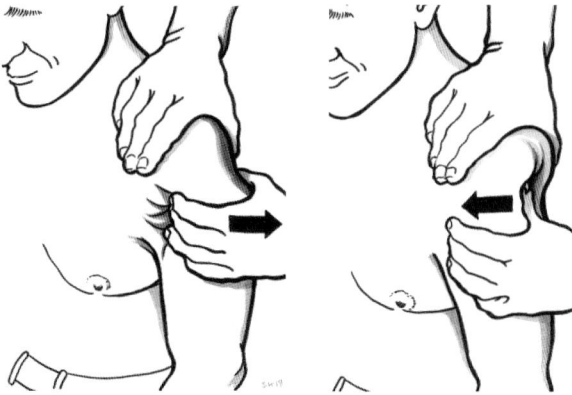

Figure 7.11 Drawer test (translation test). The patient's arm hangs by his side. One hand fixes the shoulder blade, while the other grasps the upper arm and pushes [it] backward and forward. (© Medical Illustrator Tommy Bolic, Sweden.)

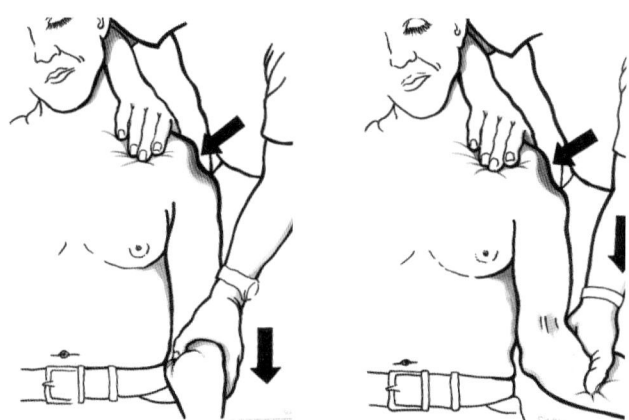

Figure 7.12 Sulcus sign. The patient's elbow, hanging by his side, is pulled in the distal direction. The test is positive when a depression is visible under the acromion. (© Medical Illustrator Tommy Bolic, Sweden.)

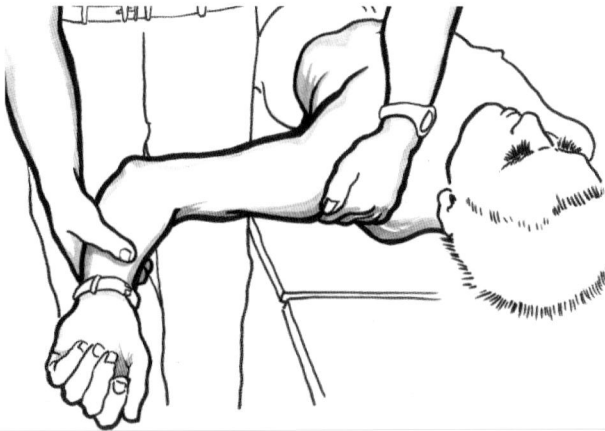

Figure 7.13 Apprehension test. With the shoulder in 90° abduction and 90° elbow flexion, external rotation is forced. The test for anterior instability is positive if the patient indicates discomfort, pain, or the fear that the shoulder is going out of joint. (© Medical Illustrator Tommy Bolic, Sweden.)

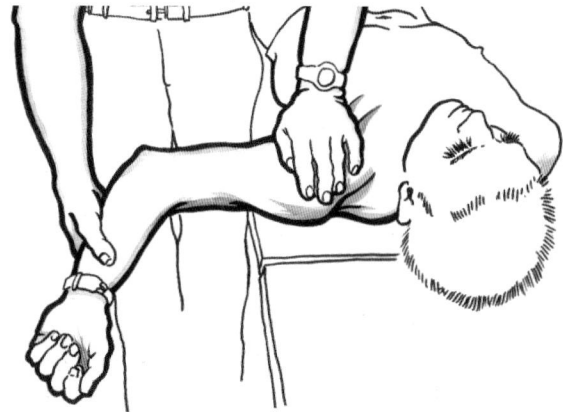

Figure 7.14 Relocation test. The examiner follows the same procedure as for the apprehension test but, in addition, applies support to the humerus from the front. If this brings pain relief in comparison with the apprehension test, the test is positive and indicates anterior instability. (© Medical Illustrator Tommy Bolic, Sweden.)

rotated. The examiner attempts to force external rotation further, and if the test is positive the patient will express discomfort, pain, and the fear that her shoulder will be anteriorly dislocated.

Relocation test (Figure 7.14). With the patient in the supine position, the examiner repeats the procedure for the apprehension test but applies even pressure on the upper humerus from the front so that the humeral head is held in place in the glenoid cavity. If this brings pain relief in comparison with a positive anterior apprehension test, the test is positive and a sign that the pain is caused by anterior instability.

Release test. The applied dorsal force on the humeral head during the relocation test is suddenly released. The test is positive if symptoms (pain, instability) reappear, and suggest the presence of secondary impingement and anterior instability.

Test for posterior instability. This test is conducted by having the patient sit or stand in a forward-leaning position, bending his arm to about 45° and internally rotating while the humeral head is pushed posteriorly along the axis from behind in the longitudinal direction of the humerus. The test is positive if there is posterior subluxation or dislocation of the humeral head.

General joint laxity. General joint laxity makes the connective tissue more flexible than normal. The patient should be examined for hyperextension of the knees and elbows of more than 10°, hyperextension of the fingers of more than 90°, dorsal extension in the ankle of more than 45°, and to find out if the thumb can be bent passively to the volar portion of the forearm. If the patient meets three of these five criteria, there is general joint laxity that makes the patient vulnerable to multidirectional shoulder instability.

Tests for Labrum Injury, Including SLAP (Superior Labrum) Lesion

O'Brien test. The O'Brien test (the active compression test) may be useful to test for a labrum injury or for AC joint pathology (Figures 7.15a and 7.15b). The test is conducted with the patient standing with his arm at 90° flexion, 10° to 15° adduction in relation to the sagittal plane, and with internal rotation, so that the thumb points downward. The examiner stands behind the patient and applies even pressure downward against resistance by the patient. The test is repeated with the patient in the same position but with the palm of the patient's hand up and fully externally rotated. The test is positive if the patient feels pain during the first part of the test and reduced or no pain during the second part. Pain or clicking in the shoulder joint indicates an injury to the labrum. Pain on top of the shoulder indicates damage to the AC joint. Results of this test must be taken with caution if there is concomitant rotator cuff involvement.

Crank test. Another test for a labrum injury is the crank test (Figures 7.16a and 7.16b). The patient lies supine with his arm abducted 160°, and the examiner stands behind the patient and applies compression and rotation internally and externally. The test is considered positive if the patient experiences pain or a clicking sensation.

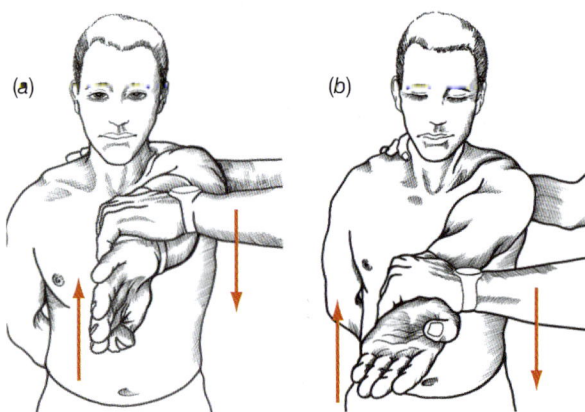

Figure 7.15 O'Brien active compression test. The examiner applies even pressure downward on a 90° flexed and 10° to 15° adducted and internally rotated arm (a). Pain in the shoulder joint and/or a click indicates a labrum injury. Pain over the acromioclavicular joint indicates pathology here. External rotation of the arm relieves the symptoms (b). (© Medical Illustrator Tommy Bolic, Sweden.)

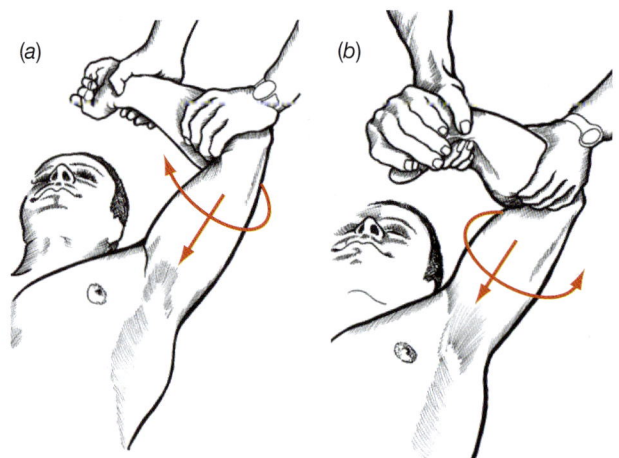

Figure 7.16 Crank test. With the arm abducted about 160°, compression is applied (a) and the humerus rotated (b). If the test is positive, the patient feels pain or a clicking sensation, indicating a labrum injury. (© Medical Illustrator Tommy Bolic, Sweden.)

(a)   (b)

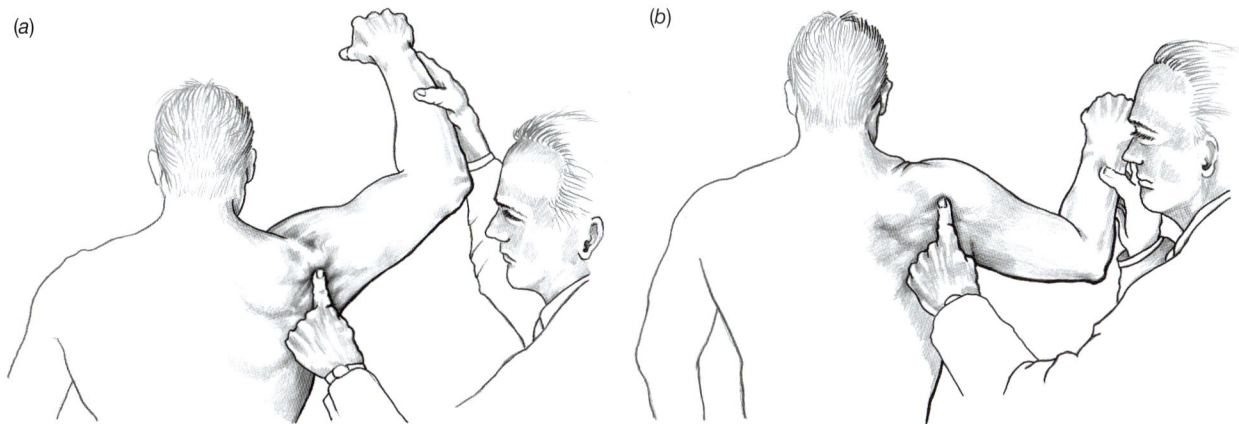

Figure 7.17 Dynamic labral shear (DLS) test. With the patient in a standing position, the involved arm is flexed 90° at the elbow, abducted in the scapular plane to above 120°, and externally rotated to tightness (a). It is then guided into maximal horizontal abduction. The examiner applies a shear load to the joint by maintaining external rotation and horizontal abduction and lowering the arm from 120° to 60° of abduction (b). A positive test is indicated by reproduction of the pain and/or a painful click or catch in the joint line along the posterior joint line between 120° and 90° of abduction. (© Medical Illustrator Tommy Bolic, Sweden.)

Dynamic labral shear (DLS) test. The test with the highest clinical utility for labrum injury is the DLS test (Figure 7.17). The arm is placed in 120° abduction, moved into horizontal abduction and external rotation, then brought inferiorly, shearing the arm along the posterior glenoid. A positive test is clicking and/or pain along the posterior joint that reproduces the symptoms.

Impingement Tests

Neer impingement test. If there is degeneration of the rotator cuff and entrapment under the acromion, specific examinations can be used to provoke pain. Pain that occurs when the arm is abducted, particularly between 70° and 130°, is defined as a positive painful arc. The examiner demonstrates the Neer impingement sign by stabilizing the acromion and pressing somewhat in the caudal direction, while passively forcing the arm into full flexion to 180°. The patient usually reacts with pain between 120° and 180°, as he does with a positive sign when the rotator cuff is trapped below the acromion.

Hawkins impingement test. This is somewhat simpler to test for than the Neer sign, particularly for patients with reduced range of motion (Figures 7.18a and 7.18b). The shoulder is forward flexed to 90° and internally rotated. If the patient reacts with pain, the sign is positive. To complete the impingement tests, the patient is given a subacromial injection of 5–10 mL of local anesthetic, and the examination is repeated. Pain relief is a positive test of impingement. A positive impingement test might help to distinguish between primary impingement and secondary impingement caused by instability.

Empty can and full can tests. In addition, the Jobe supraspinatus test, in which resistance is given against elevation in the scapular plane in internal

Figure 7.18 Impingement tests and injection technique. Hawkins impingement test is done with the upper arm at 90° flexion in the horizontal plane, with a flexed elbow, which is then internally rotated. If the test is positive, the patient has pain under the acromion (a). After a subacromial injection of local anesthetic (b), the test is repeated. If the injection brings pain relief, impingement is confirmed. (© Medical Illustrator Tommy Bolic, Sweden.)

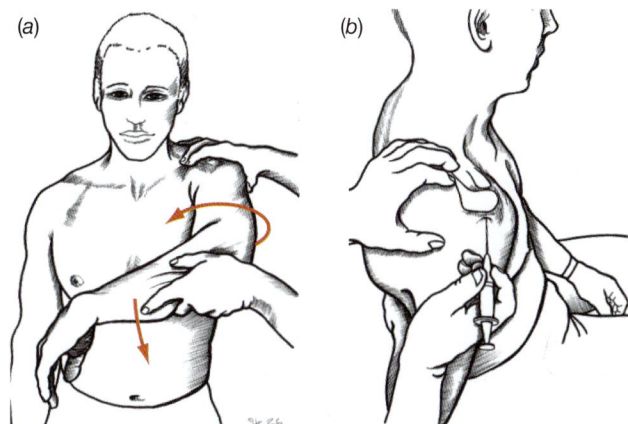

(a)   (b)

SHOULDER

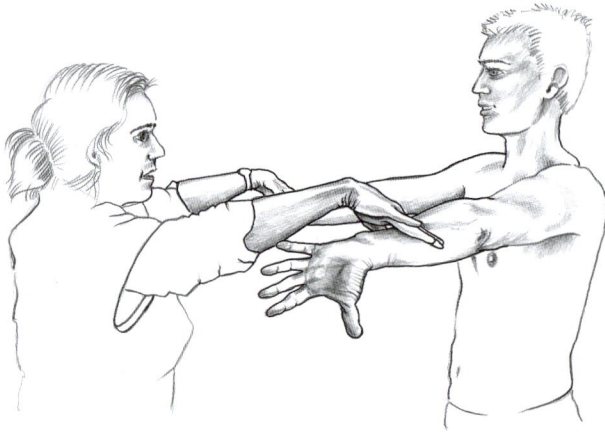

Figure 7.19 Empty can test (Jobe supraspinatus test). The shoulder is put into 90° abduction in the scapular plane and maximal internal rotation (thumbs down); resistance is given against further elevation. Pain and/or weakness confirm impingement and supraspinatus pathology. (© Medical Illustrator Tommy Bolic, Sweden.)

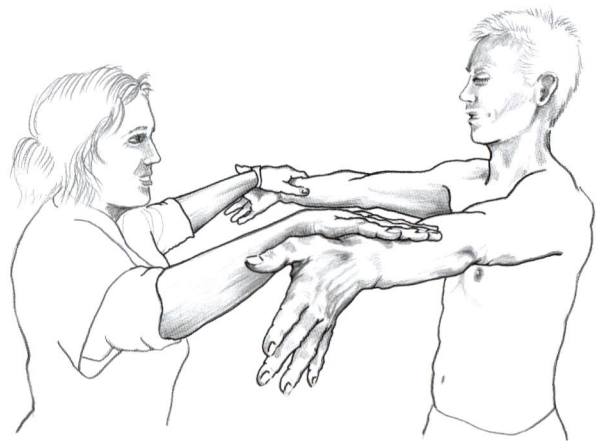

Figure 7.20 Full can test. The shoulder is put into 90° abduction in the scapular plane and external rotation (thumbs up); resistance is given against further elevation. Pain and/or weakness confirm supraspinatus pathology. (© Medical Illustrator Tommy Bolic, Sweden.)

rotation ("empty can" position, Figure 7.19), can provoke impingement-related shoulder pain, whereas the elevation in the scapular plane against resistance in external rotation ("full can" position, Figure 7.20), which requires high supraspinatus activity without excessive impingement of the tendon into the subacromial space, can provide information regarding supraspinatus integrity.

Testing of the AC joint (cross body test). The test (Figure 7.21) is conducted by having the patient raise his arm in the horizontal plane to 90° and compressing the upper arm axially toward the shoulder with maximum adduction of the arm at the same time. The test is positive if there is pain in the AC joint, which occurs if the patient has osteoarthritis, distal clavicular osteolysis or sequelae after an AC joint dislocation. To complete the test, inject a local anesthetic into the joint and repeat the test. The previously mentioned O'Brien test, in which pain is related to the AC joint, indicates joint pathology.

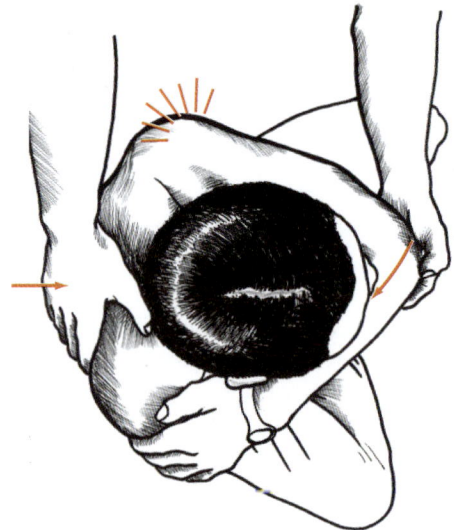

Scapular testing. Scapular involvement in impingement-related shoulder pain may be examined by the scapular assistance test (SAT) and the scapular retraction test (SRT). The SAT, in which scapular movement quality is examined, consists of manual assistance of correct scapular movement during elevation of the arm (Figure 7.22). Reduction of pain during this movement compared with nonassistance confirms scapular involvement in the shoulder complaints. In the SRT, in which scapular stability is examined, the empty-can test is performed while the examiner stabilizes the patient's scapula and shoulder in a position of retraction by placing the forearm along the medial border of the scapula (Figure 7.23). The test is positive for scapular involvement when the initial pain present in the empty can position disappears during the SRT.

Muscle strength. Reduced strength is usually related to pain, which indicates tendinosis or inflammation. Pain triggered by isometric tests for a specific muscle may be a sign of tendinosis. If strength is significantly reduced with a lesser element of pain, the patient may have a ruptured tendon. All muscles in the rotator cuff are tested. Maximum strength will only be generated off a stabilized, neutral scapula, so

Figure 7.21 Cross body test. The examiner applies compression on an arm that is adducted maximally in the horizontal plane. If the test triggers pain in the acromioclavicular joint, this indicates pathology in this joint. (© Medical Illustrator Tommy Bolic, Sweden.)

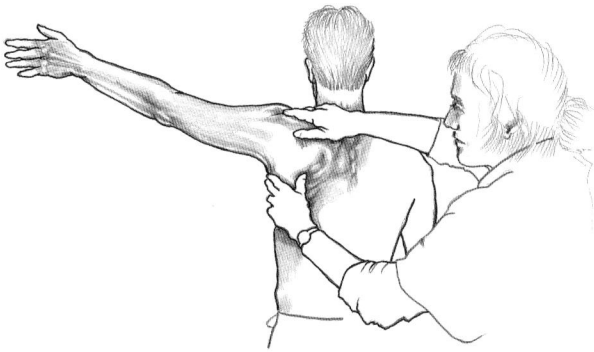

Figure 7.22 Scapular assistance test. The patient performs a painful movement (for instance abduction with painful arc) with manual assistance given by the examiner into correct scapular movement. The test is considered positive if complaints decrease with manual assistance, confirming scapular involvement in the impingement symptoms. (© Medical Illustrator Tommy Bolic, Sweden.)

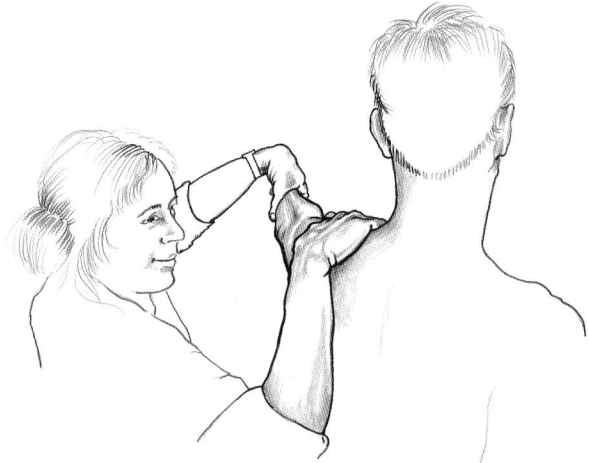

Figure 7.23 Scapular retraction test. The examiner performs a painful provocative test (for instance empty can) with manual correction of the scapular position against the thoracic wall. Increased strength or decreased pain during this test confirms scapular involvement in the impingement symptoms. (© Medical Illustrator Tommy Bolic, Sweden.)

all manual or measured strength testing should be performed off a stabilized scapula to estimate rotator cuff strength. The supraspinatus muscle is tested by having the patient abduct and internally ("empty can") or externally ("full can") rotate her arm on the plane of the scapula. The infraspinatus is tested by external rotation with the arm at the patient's side. The teres minor is tested by external rotation with the arm at 90° abduction. The subscapularis is tested by having the patient place her hand back on her lumbar spine and lifting her palm backward off the spine as well as with the belly press maneuver. The long biceps is tested by elbow flexion and supination.

Supplemental Examinations

Radiographic examinations. These examinations provide important information that is supplemental to the clinical examination. The routine radiographic examination always consists of two images, a frontal image and a lateral or axillary image. In addition, images of the AC joint can be taken, as can special images to look for shapes on the acromion (e.g., if the patient has subacromial pain).

MRI. Magnetic resonance arthrography is the best supplemental examination to the usual radiographic images for diagnosing shoulder diseases. However, the indication for an MRI should be limited, because the examination is expensive. MRI is not indicated for manifest instability in the shoulder, except in patients older than 40 years, more than half of whom also have a cuff rupture. If the patient has an unclear painful condition where instability is suspected, an MRI is indicated. MRI is not indicated for subacromial pain syndrome but is useful as a preoperative examination if it is suspected that the patient has a rotator cuff rupture that requires treatment.

CT. A CT scan with double contrast (in the form of contrast medium and air) is a good test for a Bankart lesions and additional osseous injuries after dislocation. Because this information is seldom of any practical value to treatment (as a supplement to information obtained about clinical symptoms and from radiographic images), CT scans are not routinely performed during the evaluation of an unstable shoulder or other chronic painful conditions in the shoulder. The CT scan can be a helpful tool for surgical planning.

SHOULDER

Ultrasound. Ultrasound is a good screening method for rotator cuff disease, but a skilled operator must administer the examination.

Common Injuries

Post-traumatic Shoulder Instability—*Instability after a Previous Injury*

After the first dislocation, it is quite usual for the shoulders of active young athletes to be repeatedly dislocated as a result of trauma or when the shoulder is in external rotation and abduction. The frequency of dislocations varies from a few times a year to several times a day. More than 80% of the patients have a Bankart injury (tearing of the joint labrum and the glenohumeral ligaments from the anterior lower portion of the glenoid cavity). This causes the labrum and the ligament to lose their stabilizing functions, and the head may glide out of the socket. In addition to a Bankart injury, stretching of the capsule and ligament is probably of greater significance to repeat dislocations than previously believed. Indications of instability may vary; some patients feel only uncertainty or pain when the arm is in an externally rotated position.

- Diagnosis: The diagnosis is based on the information in the case history (i.e., recurrent anterior shoulder dislocation or pain). Examination findings are increased anterior translation, a positive apprehension test, and a positive relocation test. Generally, no sulcus sign is present. If pain is the only symptom, the diagnosis may be somewhat more difficult to make. However, in these cases the apprehension and relocation tests are usually also positive. Frontal and axillary radiographs should be taken. The best way to demonstrate an osseous Bankart injury or Hill Sachs lesion is by means of an axillary radiograph or a CT scan. A finding of a supplemental osseous injury it is a bad prognostic sign and generally points toward surgery. It also shows the direction of the dislocation and may be of significance for the choice of surgical method. MRI is seldom necessary in evaluating recurrent shoulder dislocations.
- Treatment: Recurrent shoulder dislocation is not a benign condition. The greater the number of dislocations, the greater the risk of joint damage, more capsular injury, and osseous lesions. Surgical treatment should be considered if there have been more than three dislocations and the patient exhibits functional limitations and apprehension (guarding with motion). Primary caregivers do not need to refer the patient for surgery until the patient is unable to tolerate the subjective difficulty caused by the shoulder instability. Surgery to repair the Bankart injury consists of repairing the labrum ligament complex back to the glenoid rim (Bankart operation). It is usually also necessary to tighten up the joint capsule and the glenohumeral ligaments. For younger patients with associated osseous lesions more extensive surgical repair and reconstruction may be necessary using bone block transfer to the anterior-inferior glenoid.
- Treatment by physical therapist: The initial phase of rehabilitation after surgery should protect the repaired structures until sufficient healing has taken effect. This usually occurs within 6 weeks, and external rotation and abduction should be restricted to what was determined to be safe at the time of the surgery. Subsequently, the patient retrains range of motion, muscular balance, neuromuscular control, and strength, in addition to doing sport-specific exercises. The patient may return to full activity after 3–6 months, depending on the type of activity and sport. Every attempt should be made to restore normal strength and proprioceptive control before returning the athlete to sport.
- Prognosis: A surgical repair is usually successful when the patho-anatomical lesions are addressed. There is debate with respect to how the surgery should be performed but most of the evidence would favor an open repair compared with an arthroscopic repair for recurrent dislocators, particularly in the younger athlete

involved in contact sport. The prognosis for recurrence is poorer in younger patients (<25 years old) with bony pathology. There is a current trend to be more aggressive surgically in these patients.

Superior Labrum Injury (SLAP Lesion)—*Injury to the Meniscus of the Shoulder Joint*

In addition to Bankart injuries, trauma often results in other injuries to the glenoid labrum. If the patient falls on an outstretched arm or is involved in repetitive overhead throwing motions subject the labrum-biceps tendon complex may be torn from the upper portion of the glenoid cavity, which is known as a superior labral anterior to posterior (SLAP) lesion (Figure 7.24).

- Symptoms and Signs: Patients with a superior labrum (SLAP) lesion often have pain in the upper or posterior part of the shoulder, especially when they externally rotate or abduct their shoulder. They may also have a feeling of instability, sliding, or clicking in the joint.
- Diagnosis: Diagnosis is based on the case history and on a positive O'Brien test, a positive crank test and the DLS test. The patient often has clinical signs of anterior instability. However, the diagnosis may be difficult to make and sometimes it cannot be verified in patients with chronic painful shoulder conditions after trauma until arthroscopy is performed. Magnetic resonance arthrography may be used.
- Treatment: Patients who are suspected of having this condition having failed rehabilitation should be referred for arthroscopy of the shoulder and possible repair of the lesion.
- Treatment by physical therapist: Rehabilitation follows the same principle as that given after surgery on a Bankart injury, but it is also necessary to restrict eccentric loading of the long biceps tendon for 6–8 weeks after the operation.
- Prognosis: In most cases, the prognosis is satisfactory. If the mechanism of injury is due to repetitive microtrauma in the overhead athlete, care must be taken to maximize the rehabilitation, correct any imbalances and address technique in order to be ultimately successful.

SHOULDER

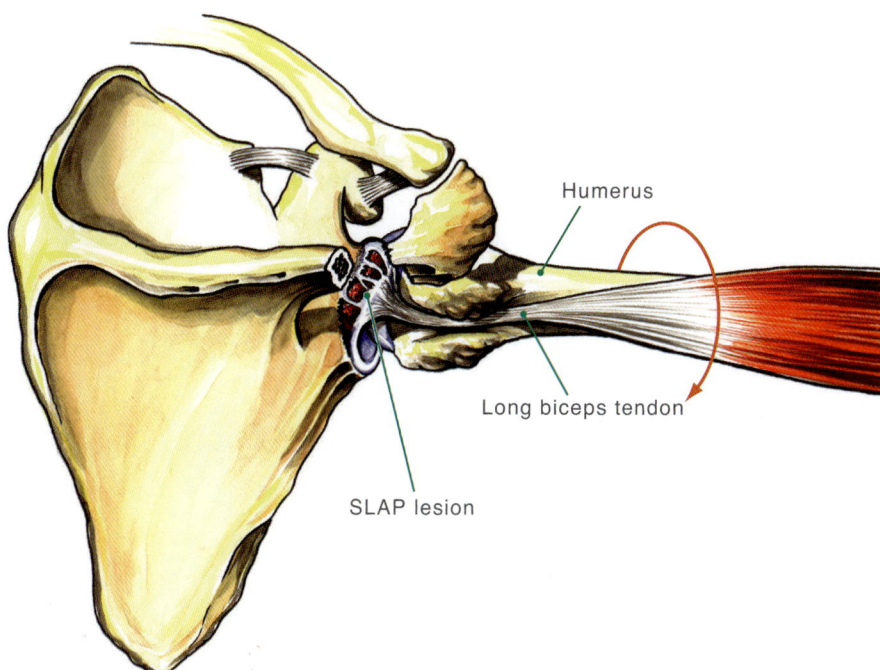

Humerus

Long biceps tendon

SLAP lesion

Figure 7.24 SLAP lesion. Tearing of the labrum-biceps tendon complex from the upper portion of the glenoid cavity. (© Medical Illustrator Tommy Bolic, Sweden.)

Multidirectional Laxity and Anteroinferior Instability—*Unstable Joint*

This condition never results from a single injury but is caused by a longer process in which repeated minor injuries stretch out the joint capsule and the ligaments. Congenital, general joint laxity is also a predisposing factor. This is common in younger athletes, especially girls, but symptoms first appear after a great deal of loading or repeated trauma—for example, if an athlete trains more for throwing or swimming than her tissue can tolerate. Throwers often have increased external rotation and reduced internal rotation, which also predisposes them to stress on the anterior and lower capsule and ligaments. Therefore, the condition occurs most often in sports that require particularly large movements of the shoulder joint, such as throwing motions and swimming strokes. When loading exceeds the ability to tolerate it, the capsule and ligaments are gradually stretched out (Figures 7.25a, 7.25b, and 7.25c). Initially, dynamic stabilizers can compensate through increased muscle activity, but continued activity results in rotator cuff fatigue, making it impossible to stabilize the humeral head in the glenoid cavity. The situation generally worsens because the scapulothoracic muscles cannot stabilize the scapula in an optimal position with respect to the humerus. The pectoralis minor and latissimus dorsi are hyperactive, and the serratus anterior and lower trapezius are inhibited.

This may result in rotator cuff injury. Direct contact may be made between the rotator cuff, the acromion, and the coracoacromial ligament at the end of a throwing motion, which may cause inflammation in the subacromial space and damage to the bursal side of the rotator cuff. This condition is called secondary impingement. At the extreme cocking phase of the throwing motion, when the arm is abducted and externally rotated, the head slides forward because the capsule is slack, and contact might occur between the articular side of the supraspinatus and the upper posterior portion of the glenoid. Over time, this may result in a superior labrum injury and so-called internal impingement of the supraspinatus tendon (Figure 7.25).

• Symptoms and signs: *Anteroinferior* instability in active young patients with secondary rotator cuff injuries is often the most difficult problem to diagnose. The shoulder has usually never been dislocated before, and the symptom is most often pain. Therefore, this condition may be thought to be simply subacromial pain and it is easy to treat incorrectly. An accurate case history is important. The clinical examination usually produces a positive translation test both anteriorly and posteriorly. A positive sulcus sign is often present, and the apprehension and relocation tests are positive. Signs of tendinosis and impingement of the rotator cuff, with positive isometric tests and impingement tests, are often present. These may be distinguishable from primary subacromial impingement because patients have a positive relocation sign (unlike in patients with subacromial impingement), and they generally affect young patients. Scapular dyskinesis is a frequent exam finding.
• Diagnosis: Diagnosis is made on the basis of the clinical examination. A normal radiographic examination is included so that skeletal injuries can be excluded. Magnetic resonance arthrography may demonstrate increased joint volume, and secondary impingement may cause an increased signal, which corresponds to the posterior portion of the glenoidal labrum and the supraspinatus tendon at the same time. However, laxity testing comparing both shoulders under general anesthesia and confirmation of the pathology at arthroscopy is the best method of making the proper diagnosis.
• Treatment by physical therapist: The main therapy for multidirectional laxity and secondary rotator cuff pain is a long-term, goal-oriented rehabilitation program. The patient should be removed from the activity or sport that caused the condition and should be allowed relative rest. Good communication is necessary between the

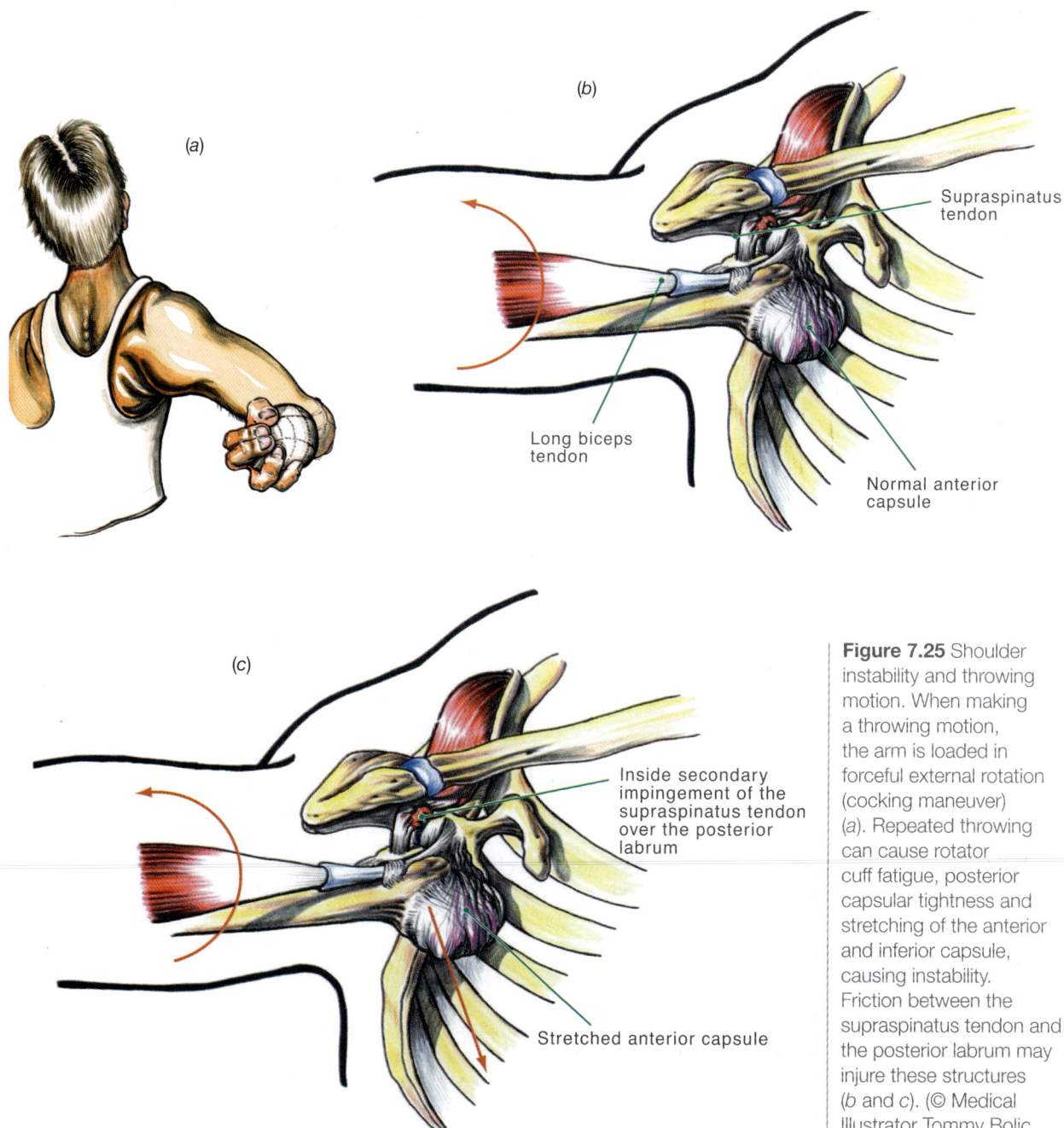

Figure 7.25 Shoulder instability and throwing motion. When making a throwing motion, the arm is loaded in forceful external rotation (cocking maneuver) (*a*). Repeated throwing can cause rotator cuff fatigue, posterior capsular tightness and stretching of the anterior and inferior capsule, causing instability. Friction between the supraspinatus tendon and the posterior labrum may injure these structures (*b* and *c*). (© Medical Illustrator Tommy Bolic, Sweden.)

caregiver, the athlete, and the trainer or coach, because a standardized rehabilitation may take 3–6 months before the patient may return to sport training. Therefore, everyone involved in the rehabilitation process (including the athlete and the physical therapist), needs to be highly motivated. Treatment should be coordinated with a physical therapist who specializes in providing this treatment. The rehabilitation program is based on stretching the tight posterior structures, strengthening the rotator cuff and scapular stabilizing musculature and in particular improving the neuromuscular control of the shoulder complex. This specific therapy should be combined with addressing any sport specific technical concerns in order to prevent further problems. Once the specific deficits have been corrected progressive training for throwing or other sport-specific training may begin.

- Treatment by physician: If symptoms are still present despite a well-coordinated rehabilitation program, surgery may be indicated. If surgery is required, it will be necessary to tighten up the joint capsule. Rehabilitation follows the same guidelines as described for the primary conservative treatment. Throwers should not throw at full speed for a prolonged period of time, up to 1 year after the operation.
- Prognosis: The prognosis is worse for this type of instability than after operations in which there is posttraumatic instability, and only 50% of the throwers return to their original activity.

Internal Impingement

This condition results from repeated overuse in an overhead athlete, such as a baseball player, tennis player, or volleyball player. After contact with the ball, or release of the ball in the throwing athlete, the phase that follows, where the remaining energy is released, results in large forces on the shoulder to resist distraction and slow the arm down. This may result in degeneration of the posterior rotator cuff and capsule. To excel in these sports, the athlete must stretch out the anterior soft tissues to help gain external rotation, as this improves their ability to perform overhead sports. Oftentimes, there is a concomitant decrease in internal rotation. The tendon changes that occur may worsen the internal rotation of the shoulder. When this happens the normal mechanics of the shoulder are altered. When the athlete moves in to the throwing position (abduction/external rotation), the humeral head shifts posterosuperiorly. This may result in a SLAP lesion, through a peel back mechanism. Also, the posterosuperior rotator cuff may impinge against the posterosuperior glenoid, resulting in rotator cuff and labral injury.

- Symptoms and signs: With internal impingment, there is a loss of more than 25° of internal rotation of the affected shoulder as compared with the unaffected shoulder, with the arm in 90° of abduction. The shoulder has usually never been dislocated before, and the symptom is most often pain. Therefore, this condition may be thought to be simply subacromial pain and it is easy to treat incorrectly. The clinical examination may produce a positive anterior translation test. Signs of tendinosis and impingement of the rotator cuff, with positive isometric tests and impingement tests, are often present. These are distinguished from primary subacromial impingement because they have a positive relocation sign (unlike in patients with subacromial impingement), and they generally affect young patients. There may be a positive O'Brien's test as well.
- Diagnosis: Diagnosis is made on the basis of the clinical examination. A normal radiographic examination is included so that skeletal injuries can be excluded. MRI may demonstrate bone cysts in the posterosuperior humeral head, thickening of the posterior band of the inferior glenohumeral ligament, posterosuperior labral injury, and tendinosis and/or partial tearing of the posterosuperior rotator cuff.
- Treatment by physical therapist: The main therapy for internal impingement and GIRD is a long-term, goal-oriented rehabilitation program. The patient should be removed from the activity or sport that caused the condition and should be allowed to rest. Good communication is necessary between the caregiver, the athlete, and the trainer or coach, because a standardized rehabilitation program takes a minimum of 20 weeks before the patient may return to sport training. Therefore, everyone involved in the rehabilitation process (including the athlete and the physical therapist), needs to be highly motivated. Treatment should be centered on a physical therapist who specializes in providing this treatment. The rehabilitation program is based on stretching the posterior structures, on strength training of the rotator cuff and musculature stabilizing the scapula, and on improving the neuromuscular control of the shoulder complex. Once the GIRD is corrected, and there

is pain free strength and rotator cuff testing, progressive training for throwing or other sport-specific training may begin.

• Treatment by physician: If symptoms are still present despite a well-coordinated rehabilitation program, surgery may be indicated. If surgery is required, it will be necessary to cut the posterior capsular ligaments and repair the superior labrum lesion, if necessary. Rehabilitation follows the same guidelines as described for the primary conservative treatment. Throwers must not throw at full speed until 6 months after the operation.

• Prognosis: The prognosis is guarded with any high-level throwing athlete undergoing surgery for their shoulder.

Subacromial Pain Syndrome—*Impingement Syndrome*

In the subacromial pain syndrome, the pain is related to the rotator cuff muscles, including the long biceps tendon, the supraspinatus tendon, and the infraspinatus tendon with the subacromial bursa (Figures 7.26a, 7.26b, and 7.26c). In the classic description of primary subacromial impingement, these soft-tissue structures become painful—either as a result of degeneration or inflammation—and increase the amount of occupied area in the subacromial space. Impingement of these structures underneath the acromion and the coracoacromial ligament with the shoulder in the abducted position will occur. With time and repeated injury the supraspinatus tendon suffers damage, particularly in the patient over the age of 30 years. The diagnosis may be difficult to make in younger athletes because the symptoms and signs may be identical but the process of impingement is a secondary one as described earlier. Subacromial pain syndrome weakens the function of the rotator cuff (which is to stabilize the head in the glenoid fossa). This causes the deltoid muscle to pull the humerus even further in the cranial direction, worsening subacromial impingement syndrome. It also reduces function, limits movement even further, and changes the scapulohumeral rhythm. When this happens, the acromion fails to move posteriorly and superiorly with arm motion, increasing the impingement position. Another etiology is scapular dyskinesis. If the scapula does not move with normal range and rhythm, then the acromion cannot rotate out of the way of the proximal humerus, and impingement may occur. The course of the pathology starts with tendinosis and may reach the final stage when the rotator cuff degenerates and eventually may result in partial and full thickness rotator cuff tears. The classic description of primary subacromial pain syndrome/impingement is described in stages. Stage 1 is acute inflammation, with swelling and edema in the rotator cuff. Stage 2 is scar formation and a chronic irreversible change in the rotator cuff. Stage 3 is the final stage, with increasing degeneration and rupture. However, whether inflammation is actually involved in the initial stage, is poorly documented.

• Symptoms and signs: The patient is usually older than 40 years of age. However, if the patient is an 18-year-old swimmer or athletic thrower with subacromial pain syndrome, this syndrome is often secondary to labral injury, posterior shoulder tightness, scapular dyskinesis, or multidirectional instability with secondary impingement. The onset of symptoms is often related to minor or to repeated trauma, to a long career in sport, or to a job that may cause overuse of the shoulder. Pain is often unspecific at first but is later localized anterior and lateral to the acromion and the AC joint. Pain at night is typical for this condition, and the patient often has difficulty lying on the affected shoulder. It is painful to carry, and especially to lift, objects with the elbow extended above shoulder level. The typical painful arc is between about 70° and 130° of abduction where the affected subacromial soft-tissue structures are trapped between the acromion and the humeral head. Both active and passive shoulder movements are often reduced because of pain and decreased strength. The movement rhythm in the glenohumeral joint is generally

SHOULDER

(a)

Supraspinatus

Acromion

Deltoid

(b)

Infraspinatus

Coracoacromial ligament

Supraspinatus

Long biceps tendon

Greater tubercle

(c)

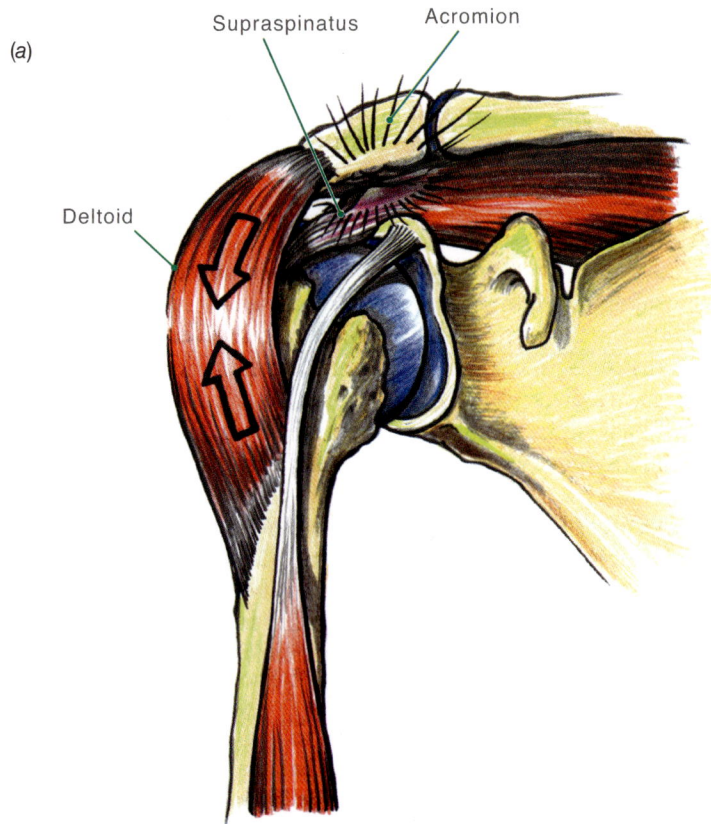

Figure 7.26 Subacromial impingement of the rotator cuff. Impingement weakens the depressive function of the supraspinatus and the infraspinatus on the humeral head. The deltoid pulls the head up toward the acromion and makes subacromial impingement (a) worse. When the arm is at the patient's side, the insertion of the supraspinatus and infraspinatus tendons to the greater tuberrosity is lateral to the acromion (b). When the arm is abducted, the tendons will come into contact with the anterior underside of the acromion and the coracoacromial ligament and impingement occurs (c). (© Medical Illustrator Tommy Bolic, Sweden.)

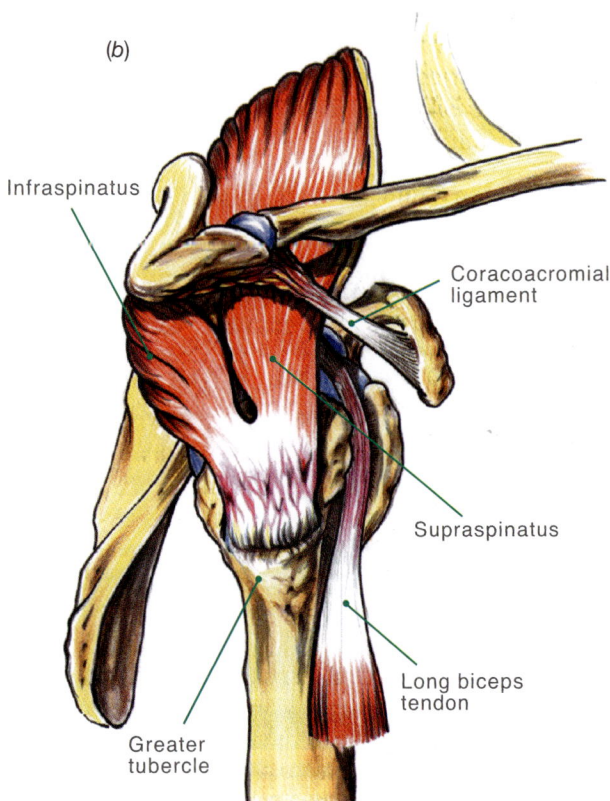

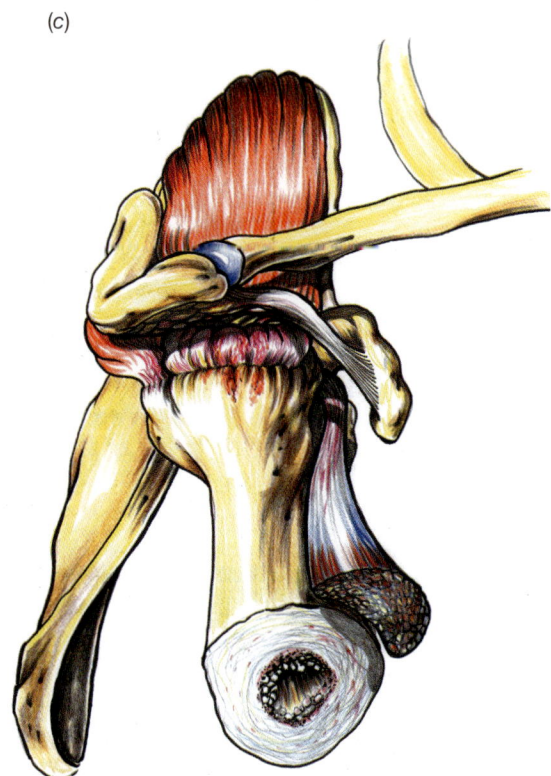

compromised. In addition to that, there is often contracture of the posterior joint capsule. The patient also experiences somewhat reduced strength during flexion, abduction, and external rotation of the arm. Assessment of scapulohumeral rhythm is also important, by observing the patient from behind while they forward elevate their arm repeatedly.

- Diagnosis: The diagnosis is made after a general clinical examination of the shoulder, including an examination of stability. Weakness in the supraspinatus muscle may be present, particularly if the patient has a chronic painful condition. Palpation findings may be uncharacteristic, but generally palpation tenderness is present above the supraspinatus tendon's insertion to the greater tuberosity underneath the anterolateral corner of the acromion. The range of motion is generally limited, especially abduction, internal rotation, and flexion. The scapulohumeral rhythm is also changed. Evaluation for scapular dyskinesis should be done. Symptoms can be relieved by manual repositioning of the scapula in retraction. Muscle strength is generally reduced, especially when the supraspinatus is tested. Pain during isometric testing is suggestive for tendinosis particularly with positive Neer and Hawkins signs. To confirm the diagnosis, the impingement tests can be repeated after the patient is given a subacromial injection of local anesthesia. This will usually bring pain relief. Sometimes the patient has long-term problems with osteophytes under the acromion, which is ossification of the coracoacromial ligament insertion. Although uncommon, calcium deposition may occur on the tendon insertion. The osteophytes and calcium deposits are visible as a shadow on the radiographs. A special radiograph, known as a supraspinatus outlet view, may help determine the shape of the acromion. In type 1 the acromion is very flat, allowing for satisfactory subacromial space. Type 2 with a curved shape or type 3 with a hooked shape tends to reduce the amount of subacromial space. Types 2 and 3 acromions are more common in patients with rotator cuff disease. Diagnostic ultrasound in experienced hands is very helpful in determining whether the rotator cuff is torn. More detailed evaluation with magnetic resonance arthrography may be required to determine the size and location of rotator cuff damage and at the same time address associated pathology.

- Treatment: Treatment is mainly conservative, with a program that aims to improve the function of the rotator cuff and the musculature that stabilizes the scapula. Nonsteroidal anti-inflammatory drugs (NSAIDs) may be used to ease rehabilitation. Subacromial injection of cortisone is controversial. Repeated injections cause the risk of degenerative rotator cuff ruptures. If conservative treatment does not produce a satisfactory result within 3–6 months, the patient is referred to a specialist for surgical evaluation. Surgery for primary impingement was commonly performed in the past but should be restricted to patients who have failed nonsurgical management, have the specific anatomical findings of a narrowed subacromial space and bursal sided rotator cuff pathology. In these patients, the subacromial bursa is debrided and the impinging structures are resected. Subsequent treatment follows the same principles as primary conservative treatment, with retraining for range of motion and muscular control. The rehabilitation period is between 6 and 12 weeks, depending on the type of work or activity the patient is going to return to.

- Prognosis: The results are good in about 80% of the patients, but it is not possible to predict whether the patient will return to work or sport activity that requires the use of the shoulder, particularly if the patient is in stage 3.

Rotator Cuff Rupture — *Injury of the Rotator Cuff*

An injury to the supraspinatus tendon (Figures 7.27a and 7.27b) is a common cause of subacromial pain and limited shoulder function in middle-aged athletes and patients who do jobs that require the use of the shoulder. There is relatively poor blood

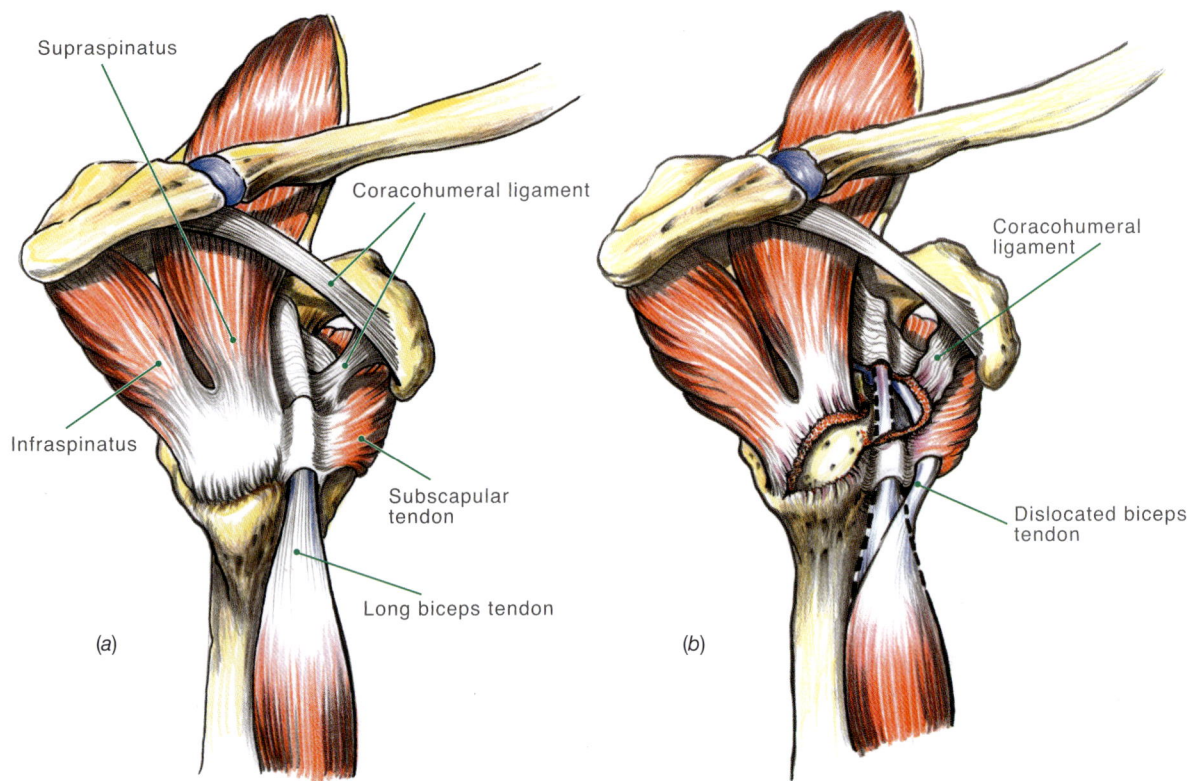

Supraspinatus

Coracohumeral ligament

Coracohumeral ligament

Infraspinatus

Subscapular tendon

Dislocated biceps tendon

Long biceps tendon

(a)

(b)

circulation in the supraspinatus tendon, and repeated trauma with micoruptures and degeneration may lead to a full thickness rupture. This usually begins anteriorly in the supraspinatus tendon in the area where the biceps tendon penetrates the sulcus and may gradually spread backward and down into the infraspinatus tendon. If the rupture is massive, the biceps tendon will also be affected, either ruptured or dislocated out of the sulcus, particularly when the upper portion of the subscapularis tendon is involved. Athletes in throwing sports may also sustain partial supraspinatus tendon ruptures as a result of great eccentric loading of the tendon during the throwing motion. These ruptures are usually located on the underside of the tendon close to the shoulder joint.

- Symptoms and Signs: The typical patient is older than 40 years and has a case history that includes repeated trauma or loading. Often the patient states that he has had several episodes of acute shoulder inflammation and possibly local injections of corticosteroids. Clinical examination findings are often the same as the findings in patients with subacromial pain syndrome, often with impingement. The strength of muscles of the rotator cuff may be reduced, depending on the size of the tear. An ultrasound examination may be useful if it is performed by an experienced examiner. The patient should be given a dynamic examination; then both partial and total ruptures may be found. Radiographic examinations are done in the same manner as they are for subacromial impingement. Leakage through the rotator cuff into the subacromial space may be visible on a CT arthrography scan. An MRI examination is sensitive to both partial and total rotator cuff ruptures. The disadvantage is the high cost, though it does not require injection of contrast to identify the tear.
- Treatment: The primary treatment of a chronic rotator cuff rupture is conservative and follows the same guidelines as treatment for subacromial pain syndrome. Treatment is given at the primary-care level. Since the outcomes for return to sports in athletes is better when surgery is performed for smaller tears as compared with larger tears, there

Figure 7.27 Rotator cuff rupture. Normal anatomy of the rotator cuff, seen from the side, is shown (a). A rotator cuff rupture usually begins anteriorly in the supraspinatus tendon and may expand posteriorly into the infraspinatus tendon. If the rupture goes anteriorly through the biceps tendon sheath, the coracohumeral ligament, and down into the subscapularis tendon, dislocation of the biceps tendon often follows (b). (© Medical Illustrator Tommy Bolic, Sweden.)

is a tendency to be more aggressive about surgically repairing rotator cuff tears in athletes of any size or chronicity. For long-term symptoms that do not respond to exercise therapy, the patient is referred for evaluation to consider surgery. Surgical treatment is repair of the rotator cuff and sometimes subacomial decompression. Surgery is more often indicated in acute or acute on chronic cases in young and active individuals.

• Prognosis: A rotator cuff rupture does not mean the end of the athlete's sport career. Most athletes who have a rotator cuff problem have a minor partial rupture. The outcome of conservative or of surgical treatment is usually good in these patients. Total ruptures are degenerative disorders that occur in the elderly and rarely in connection with sport activity. When there is a full thickness rotator cuff tear in the overhead athletes, the results are less predictable. In other words, there is a relatively high failure rate. The return to sports in these patients is better when the tear is smaller, as compared with larger tears that undergo repair. For the nonathlete with a degenerative tear, and for those not wishing to return to overhead sports, the functional outcome of a rotator cuff repair is generally satisfactory. However, the results depend on how large the injury is, how many tendons are torn, and how far the degeneration of tendons and muscles have progressed. Patients often have to change their activity or their job.

Other Conditions

Recurrent Posterior Shoulder Instability — *Shoulder Out of Joint*

Recurrent, posterior shoulder dislocation or subluxation is a less common sport injury. The patients present in a variety of different ways. Some present after an acute traumatic episode of dislocation or subluxation. These patients typically have a posterior labral tear (i.e., so-called reverse Bankart lesion) and although the prognosis is not as bad as the similar anterior traumatic instability surgery may be required. They have signs of instability as their arm is in front of them, such as in blocking, pushing or lifting weights (bench-press). In this scenario arthroscopic repairs are advocated and the prognosis is usually good. More often athletic patients present with pain or loss of function and associated clinical signs of posterior instability. In these scenarios, there is a history of repetitive microtrauma. An example would be the lead shoulder in the golfer. The condition generally causes moderate discomfort and sometimes a feeling of instability. Treatment is conservative at first, with training for muscular balance, and is administered as primary-level care. If the patient has persistent, major pain, surgery may be indicated. However, the frequency of recurrence and the risk of complications are higher than they are after surgery for anterior dislocation.

Acromioclavicular Joint Osteoarthritis — *Arthritis in the Joint between the Collar Bone and the Shoulder Blade*

Even if the natural course after an AC joint injury is good, sometimes athletes present chronically with pain in the joint due to instability or degenerative changes in the intra-articular disk. This can subsequently lead to distal clavicular osteolysis and in some patients post-traumatic osteoarthritis (Figures 7.28a and 7.28b). It should be pointed out that distal clavicular osteolysis can also occur without a preceding acute traumatic event. This is common in athletes who train with weightlifting, particularly bench pressing.

• Symptoms and Signs: The case history is generally related to a previous AC joint injury or to long-term weight bearing, as in the case of weightlifters. Patients usually localize their pain and tenderness directly to the joint.

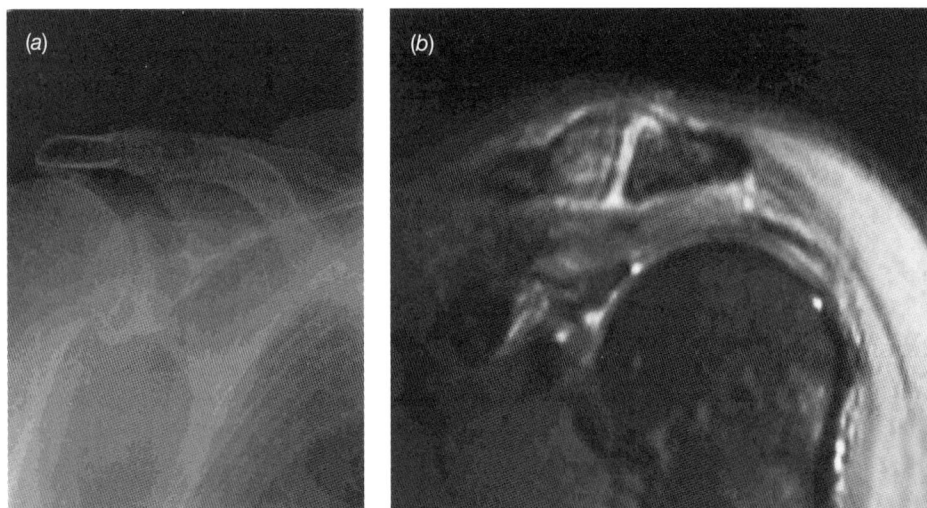

Figure 7.28
Acromioclavicular joint arthritis. The radiographic view shows a narrow and uneven joint space and often subchondral sclerosis (a). MRI demonstrates reactive changes in the soft tissue and signal changes in the distal clavicle (b). (Reproduced with permission from the Norwegian Sports Medicine Association.)

• Diagnosis: The diagnosis is based on palpation tenderness directly over the joint, positive provocation tests and pain relief when local anesthesia is injected. In addition, there may be instability similar to that which occurred after a previous dislocation. The diagnosis is confirmed by plain radiographs of the AC joint, which may demonstrate instability or the development of osteoarthritis.
• Treatment: Initial treatment is conservative. The patient is cared for at the primary-care level with activity modification, nonsteroidal anti-inflammatory medications and cortisone injections into the joint for pain relief. If this does not succeed, the patient is referred for possible surgery.

Entrapment of the Suprascapular Nerve

The suprascapular nerve begins at the upper portion of the brachial plexus and passes through the scapular notch and the spinoglenoid notch (Figure 7.29). The nerve may be compressed in this passage, because of traction of the nerve from repeated activity with the arm above shoulder level, especially in volleyball players but also in throwers, tennis players, and swimmers. Another cause of entrapment is compression from a ganglion cyst, which may develop in connection with a superior labrum lesion.

• Symptoms and signs: The clinical symptoms are atrophy (Figures 7.30a and 7.30b) and reduced strength in the infraspinatus muscle (shoulder external rotation) and possibly in the supraspinatus muscle (abduction strength in the scapular plane, in addition to pain posteriorly in the shoulder.
• Diagnosis: If the nerve is entrapped at the scapular notch in front of the origin of the motor branch to the supraspinatus, testing of both the supraspinatus muscle and the infraspinatus muscle will reveal atrophy and weakness, and forced external rotation and abduction may cause pain. If the infraspinatus is affected in isolation, the nerve is affected more distally in the spinoglenoid notch. EMG may be used to confirm the diagnosis. An MRI should be performed to exclude a ganglion cyst.
• Treatment: If the patient has a ganglion cyst, decompression of the cyst is indicated and surgical treatment of the associated superior labrum lesion if present. Otherwise, treatment is conservative with an interruption in, or modification of, activity and a rehabilitation program for the rotator cuff. This includes stretching the posterior shoulder and rotator cuff strengthening. However, if the onset of symptoms is not known then MRI and EMG analysis should be performed in order to help

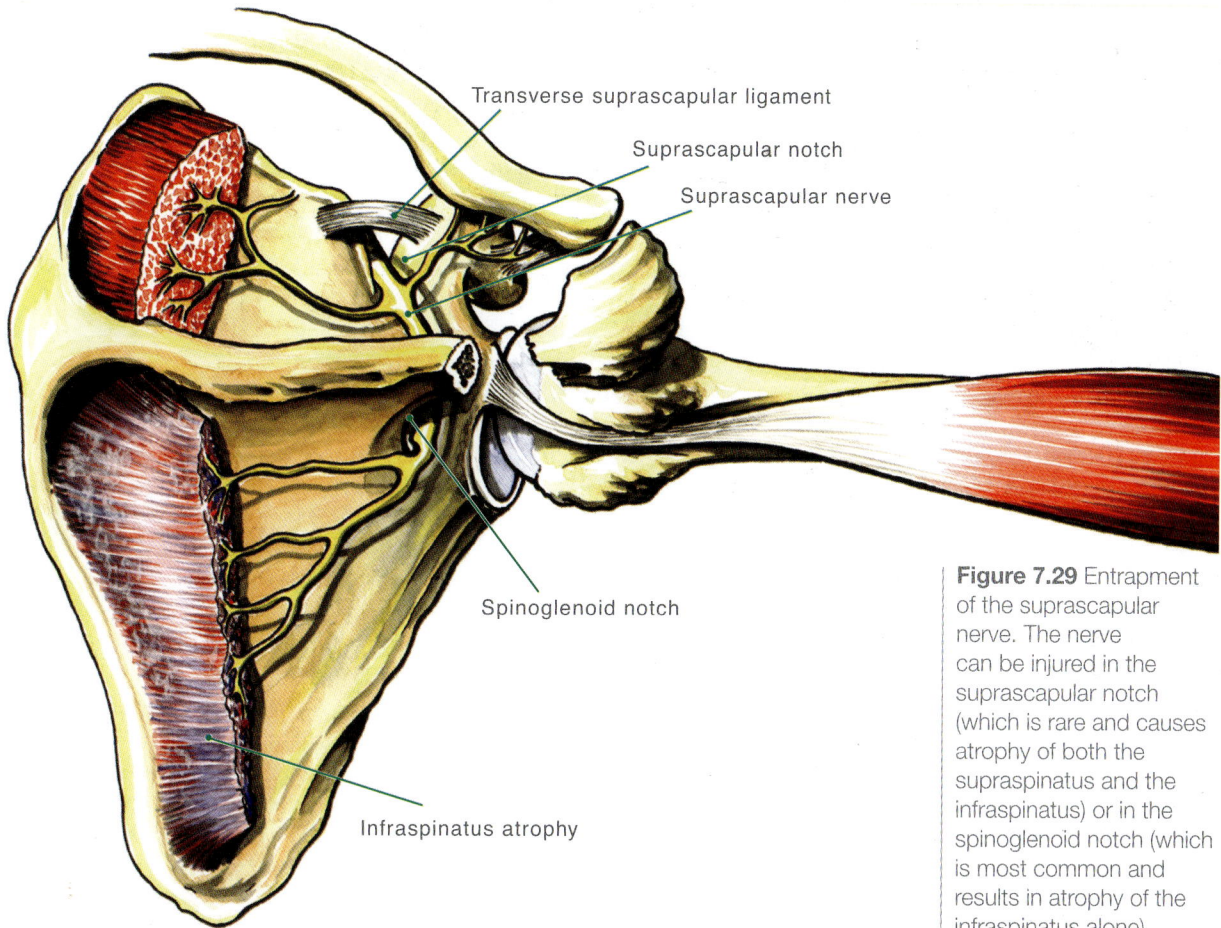

Transverse suprascapular ligament

Suprascapular notch

Suprascapular nerve

Spinoglenoid notch

Infraspinatus atrophy

Figure 7.29 Entrapment of the suprascapular nerve. The nerve can be injured in the suprascapular notch (which is rare and causes atrophy of both the supraspinatus and the infraspinatus) or in the spinoglenoid notch (which is most common and results in atrophy of the infraspinatus alone). (© Medical Illustrator Tommy Bolic, Sweden.)

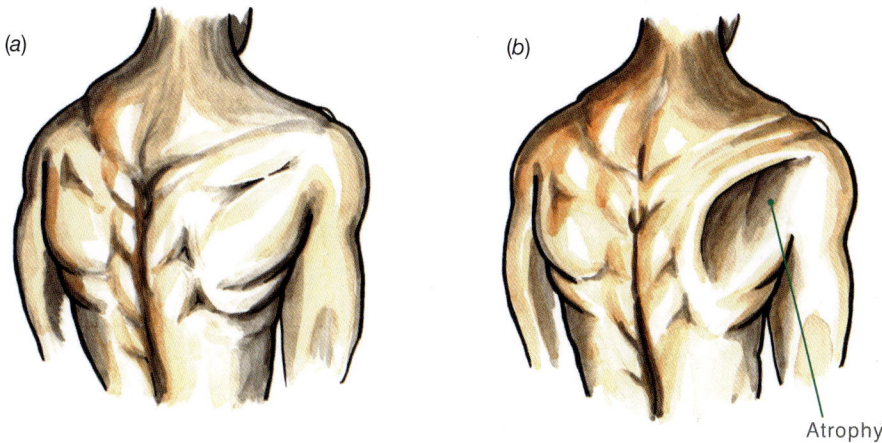

(a)

(b)

Atrophy

Figure 7.30 Infraspinatus atrophy. Normal muscle volume (a); atrophy of the infraspinatus (b). (© Medical Illustrator Tommy Bolic, Sweden.)

determine the prognosis for nerve recovery. If satisfactory function has not been achieved after 3–6 months, surgery should be considered. Surgical release of the nerve often relieves pain and sometimes hypotrophy as well. Surgery will have absolutely no benefit in resolving muscle atrophy if not performed in a timely fashion, that is, before extensive fatty atrophy of the infraspinatus as demonstrated on MRI.

Adhesive Capsulitis—*Frozen Shoulder* !

Adhesive capsulitis, or frozen shoulder, is a relatively rare condition in athletes. The joint capsule becomes inflamed, resulting in intra-articular adhesion and stiffness in the joint capsule, causing typical joint contracture. The cause is unknown. The condition is described as painful, restricted shoulder movement.

- Symptoms and signs: The patient has significant pain, and movement has practically stopped. Movement generally follows a capsular pattern where abduction takes place almost exclusively between the scapula and the chest wall. External rotation has usually stopped completely. The course can be divided into three stages, each of which lasts up to half a year. The first stage is the stiffening stage, during which there is pain and restricted movement. In the second stage the condition is stationary, and in the third stage the pain ceases and the shoulder "thaws out." These three stages often last from 1 to 2 years in total.
- Diagnosis: Typical clinical examination findings are limited movement and the capsular movement pattern. It is necessary to distinguish between this condition and a rotator cuff rupture with a secondary stiff shoulder or limited motion due to pain. Measuring external rotation with the arms at the sides may be a clue, as this motion should not be limited by pain. Supplemental radiographic and MRI examinations are of limited value, but magnetic resonance arthrography may demonstrate reduced capsule volume or a rotator cuff rupture.
- Treatment: The natural course of the condition is benign. In the first stage, intra-articular steroid injections can be used following a careful stretching program. Surgery is seldom indicated, but cases with severe stiffness in stage 2 can be treated with manipulation under anesthesia or arthroscopic capsular release.

Rehabilitation of Shoulder Injuries

Ann Cools[1] and Hilde Fredriksen[2]

[1]*Ghent University, Gent, Belgium*
[2]*Olympiatoppen, Oslo, Norway*

Goals and Principles

Table 7.3 lists the goals of shoulder injury rehabilitation.

Each acute injury causes dysfunction, especially in the shoulder, where an injury easily causes changes in the scapulohumeral rhythm. To prevent this from changing the athlete's movement pattern (which in turn could predispose the athlete to new injuries), the athlete must have an individually adapted training program to normalize function again.

Important Factors in Shoulder Injury Rehabilitation

Rotator cuff training. The rotator cuff balances the humeral head in the glenoid fossa, so that the joint rotates on physiological axes. For example, the subscapularis muscle and the pectoralis muscle are both internal rotators in the shoulder. If their insertions and action angles on the humerus were examined, it would be obvious that in their function as internal rotators have very different functions in the glenohumeral joint (Figure 7.31).

Whereas the subscapularis muscle contributes to centering the humeral head in the glenoid fossa, activation of the pectoralis major muscle causes anterior translation

	Goals	Measures
Phase 1	Reduce swelling	PRICE principle
Phase 2	Reduce pain	Possibly short-term immobilization
	Improve the movement pattern in the shoulder girdle as a whole:	Exercise within the limits of pain, with emphasis on scapulohumeral rhythm, range-of-motion training, and sensory motor training
	• Strengthen the rotator cuff	
	• Stabilize the scapula	
Phase 3	Restore the normal movement pattern in the shoulder girdle as a whole:	Functional exercises
	• Strengthen the rotator cuff	Sport-specific training
	• Stabilize the scapula	Recover completely before engaging in maximum activity
	• Improve range of motion	
	• As a minimum, reach the same sensorymotor function, strength, and range of motion as before the injury	
	Reduce the risk of reinjury	

Table 7.3 Goals and measures for rehabilitation of shoulder injuries. (Reproduced with permission from the Norwegian Sports Medicine Association.)

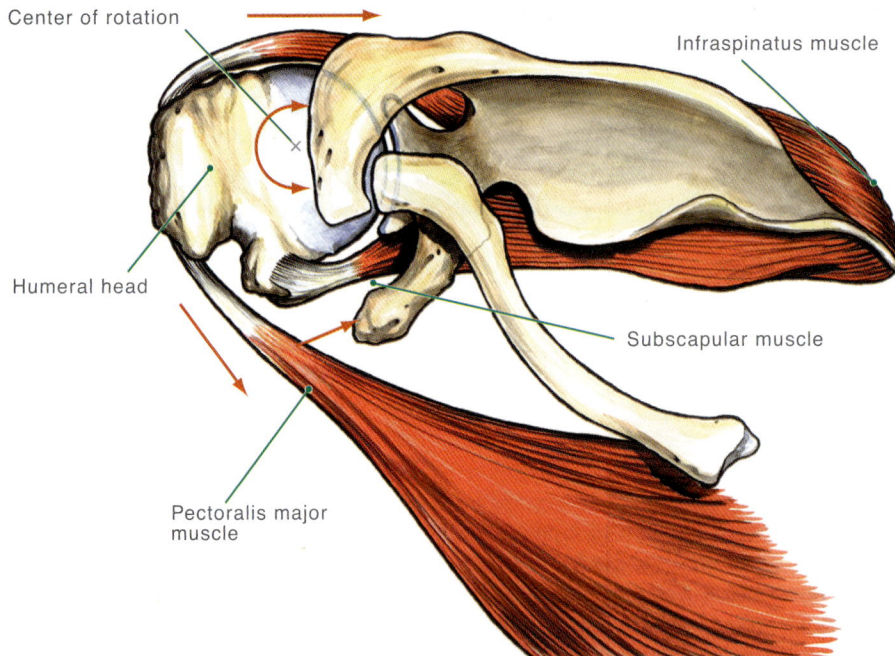

Center of rotation

Infraspinatus muscle

Humeral head

Subscapular muscle

Pectoralis major muscle

Figure 7.31 Role of internal rotation. The pectoralis major muscle has an anterior force component that contributes to anterior translation of the humeral head. (© Medical Illustrator Tommy Bolic, Sweden.)

of the humeral head. Like the subscapularis muscle, the posterior muscles of the rotator cuff also play an important role in centering and stabilizing the humeral head in the glenoid fossa, while larger muscles, such as the pectoralis major, the deltoid, and the latissimus dorsi, may develop into major destabilizing elements in the shoulder. Hence, the role of the rotator cuff as juxta-articular, stabilizing musculature is extremely important to shoulder balance. However, the external rotators are both stabilizers and main external rotators, and as a consequence, they also need exercises for strength and endurance. Early in the rehabilitation period it may be necessary to exercise the rotator cuff in isolation, while supporting the arm, to isolate movement as much as possible (e.g., Figure 7.32). However, as soon as possible, the rotator cuff should be exercised in larger movements that also require the ability to

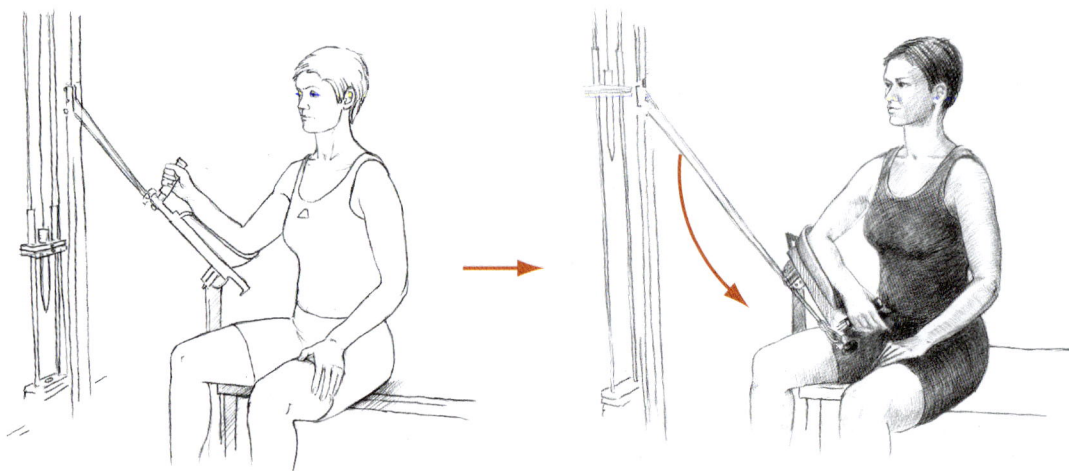

Figure 7.32 Sitting shoulder rotation (with support).

- Internal rotation: Attach rope at the hand (as shown in the figure).
- External rotation: Attach rope at the elbow.
- In the final position the rope needs to be almost parallel to the forearm.
- Progression: Increase degree of abduction (in the plane of the scapula) in the shoulder joint.

(Reproduced with permission from the Norwegian Sports Medicine Association.)

stabilize the scapula (e.g., Figure 7.33). When throwers are at the end of rehabilitation, eccentric training of the posterior portion of the rotator cuff is important. The quality of the manner in which the exercises are done is crucial because it controls the progression of rehabilitation.

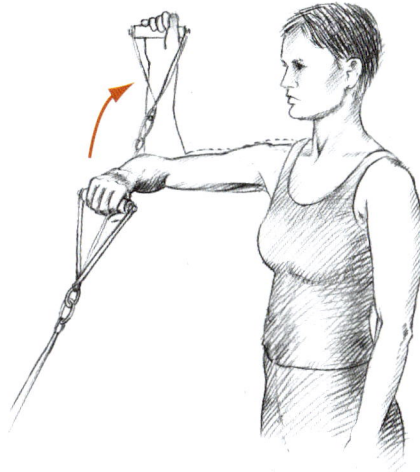

Figure 7.33 Standing shoulder rotation (without support).

• This exercise requires a great ability to stabilize the scapula.
• External rotation: Stand facing the pulley apparatus (as in the figure).
• Internal rotation: Stand with your back to the pulley apparatus.
• In the final position, the rope must be almost parallel to your forearm.
• Progression: Increase degree of abduction (in the plane of the scapula) in the shoulder joint.
(Reproduced with permission from the Norwegian Sports Medicine Association.)

Restoring normal coordinated scapular movement. It is of limited help to center the humeral head in the glenoid fossa if the ability to stabilize the scapula is compromised. Good scapular control is necessary to provide a stable base for arm movement, both by holding the glenoid fossa in a position that provides the greatest possible congruence with the humeral head and by ensuring proper positioning of the scapula. The ability to stabilize the scapula is often reduced after injury because of pain-based inhibition of the anterior serratus muscle and the trapezius muscle. The initial goal is to develop good coordination between movements of the humerus and scapula, and to reduce flexibility deficits, causing abnormal scapular position. Figure 7.34 summarizes a clinical algorithm for the treatment of scapular dyskinesis.

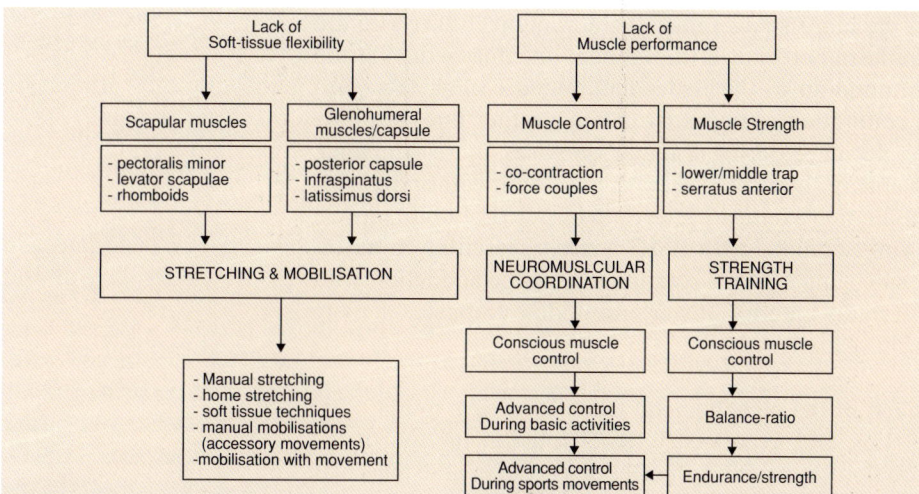

Figure 7.34 Treatment algorithm for scapular dysfunction. (Reproduced with permission from Ellenbecker & Cools. Br J Sports Med 2010 (44): 319–327).

The upper part summarizes possible causes for scapular dyskinesis, in the lower part therapeutic strategies are suggested. A patient presenting with scapular dyskinesis may have flexibility problems or muscle performance problems, or both. In case of flexibility problems these may involve the scapular muscles, in particular the pectoralis minor and the levator scapulae, or at glenohumeral level, in particular stiffness and tightness of the posterior shoulder structures (the capsule as well as the external rotator muscles). Both of these flexibility deficits may lead to scapular malpositioning, especially anterior tilting and downward rotation.

Muscle performance problems may be divided into neuromuscular deficits (a lack of co-contraction and force couple activity) or strength deficits. In the latter case, the serratus anterior, lower and middle trapezius in particular have been found to be weak, whereas the upper trapezius often shows hyperactivity.

Each side of the algorithm needs a specific approach regarding rehabilitation. Flexibility deficits need to be addressed by stretching and mobilization techniques, whereas muscle recruitment normalization is the main goal for the patient who has muscle performance problems. Of course, if both flexibility deficits and muscle dysfunction are responsible for the scapular dyskinesis, both problems should be addressed. However, to obtain proper muscle control and motor learning in a corrected scapular position, flexibility deficits should be addressed first, before starting the muscular rehabilitation program.

The pectoralis minor, levator scapulae and posterior shoulder muscles very often induce scapular dyskinesis because of tightness and hyperactivity. Stretching should be performed of all these structures; however, taking into account that often a position might compromise shoulder stability and cause symptoms. For instance, the open door stretch for the pectoralis minor, in which the patient passively brings his shoulder into 90° abduction and external rotation, increases the stress on the anterior capsule, and should be avoided. Direct stretches on the coracoids pushing the scapula into posterior tilting might increase the length of the pectoralis minor without putting the shoulder at risk for pain and instability symptoms. With respect to muscle performance enhancement and neuromuscular training, exercises on unstable surfaces like slings, wobbleboards and Swiss balls are ideal tools to exercise the shoulder in a closed kinetic chain, and at the same time provide a significant challenge on proprioception and neuromuscular control. At the beginning of the rehabilitation process, it may be helpful to do exercises in the plane of the scapula—that is, with the humerus in abduction at about 30° flexion anteriorly. In this plane, conditions are good for stabilizing the humeral head in the glenoid fossa. At more than 90° abduction, there will be more space under the acromion if exercises are done in the plane of the scapula rather than at full abduction, thus reducing the possibility of impingement. In addition to the issues mentioned earlier, the clinician should also focus on (a) restoration of muscular balance rather than absolute muscle strength, (b) increasing demands during scapular exercises, increasing load, functional demands, and challenging shoulder positions, and (c) integrating the kinetic chain into shoulder rehabilitation exercises. Exercises for restoration of muscle balance have been described and examined with EMG analysis, resulting in movements (for instance push-ups, side lying external rotation and prone abduction with external rotation) increasing serratus anterior, lower and middle trapezius activity with inhibition of upper trapezius activity.

Sufficient internal rotation motion of the glenohumeral joint. Throwing sports often involve increased external rotation and decreased internal rotation motion of the shoulder. Reduced internal rotation is caused by posterior capsular and muscular contracture and may increase anterior translation of the humeral head and contribute to anterior instability. In addition to stretching of the posterior shoulder capsule, by performing the sleeper's stretch or the cross body stretch, soft tissue techniques on the posterior rotator cuff and hold-relax stretches for that muscle group may increase range of motion into internal rotation and decrease anterior tilting of the scapula.

Sufficient range of motion of the spine. Increased thoracic kyphosis and reduced extension reduce arm movement as a whole and worsen the working conditions for the scapular musculature, thus increasing the risk of poor glenohumeral joint function. In that case, the physical therapist should perform both mobilization and exercise therapy.

Integrating the kinetic chain. The term kinetic chain refers to the sequential activation of muscles and movement of bones and joints (body segments) to achieve the motions, positions and velocities required for a special movement. Proper sequencing results in efficient force and motion production. Weakness of the contralateral hip abductors and trunk muscles are often seen in throwers with shoulder dysfunction, and should be addressed. Integrating the kinetic chain in shoulder rehabilitation can be initiated early in the rehabilitation, by doing weight shifting, combined with trunk flexion/extension and rotation and scapular protraction and retraction. Progression can be adding movements of the arm and subsequently resistance.

Pain and quality of function are used to guide the progression of the rehabilitation.

During the last stage of rehabilitation, increasing demands can be implemented using more challenging shoulder positions (throwing position), highlighting the stretch shortening cycle through plyometric exercises, and involving diagonal patterns into open chain exercises (e.g., Figure 7.35). There should also be more emphasis on

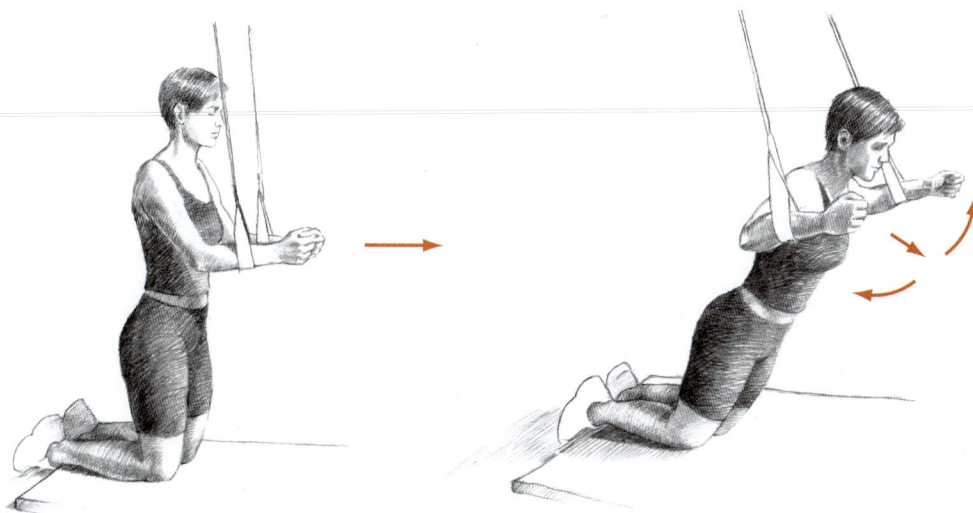

Figure 7.35 Horizontal abduction and adduction in slings.
- Kneel, with the body leaning forward over the elbows bent at 90°.
- Tense your abdominal and back muscles, gently extend your arms out to the sides and lean your body forward. Focus on control in the extreme position; hold. Pull your body back again by pressing your arms together.
- Progression: Gradually extend your arms farther out to the sides.
- Position yourself farther back from the plumb line of the rope.
- Keep less distance between the sling and the floor.
- Increase the speed of movement.
(Reproduced with permission from the Norwegian Sports Medicine Association.)

sport-specific training. Collaboration with coaches, particularly during this phase is important, to make sure the training is adjusted to the demands of the sport and managed with respect to what the shoulder can tolerate.

Return to Sport

It is advisable to compare the strength, sensory motor function, and flexibility of the injured side with the healthy side before the player is considered to be fully rehabilitated. Athletes in throwing sports need to realize that the throwing arm normally has increased external rotation and reduced internal rotation and is stronger than the arm on the other side. In throwing sports, the athlete must have completed a throwing training program (throwing and catching) with increasing intensity and must have trained at maximum intensity before being allowed to compete. Athletes in team sports also should train in practice games before being allowed to compete. Specific functional tests must be adjusted according to the requirements of the individual sport.

Preventing Reinjury

It is possible to reduce the risk of reinjury by means of optimal rehabilitation, paying attention to the factors mentioned previously. This involves the healing of all structures and ensuring that the patient has normal scapulohumeral rhythm and sensory motor function, as well as strength and range of motion. Elimination of GIRDs (side to side difference of less than 25°, with similar total rotational arc of motion between the dominant and nondominant shoulders) is an important step in prevention of shoulder reinjury. Further, having appropriate core strength is important to maintain efficiency of the kinetic chain, and thus in reducing stresses to the shoulder. Posttraumatic and multidirectional instability are the greatest challenges in sport-related shoulder injuries. Athletes often have very strong muscles designed for power and speed, including the pectoralis major muscle and the latissimus dorsi muscle. Therefore, the physician must make sure that the rotator cuff and scapular muscles function correspondingly well. This will ensure that the instantaneous axis of rotation of the glenohumeral joint is kept within physiological ranges through the ranges of motion. It is important to establish a coordinated movement pattern throughout the whole range of motion, with the shoulder as an integrated part of the whole kinetic chain.

8 Elbow and Forearm

Acute Injuries of the Elbow and Forearm

Mark R. Hutchinson[1], James R. Andrews[2], Babette M. Pluim[3], Kevin E. Wilk[4], and Stein Tyrdal[5]

[1]*University of Illinois at Chicago, Chicago, IL, USA*
[2]*Andrews Sports Medicine and Orthopaedic Center, Birmingham, AL, USA*
[3]*Royal Netherlands Lawn Tennis Association, Amersfoort, The Netherlands*
[4]*Champion Sports Medicine, Birmingham, AL, USA*
[5]*Oslo University Hospital, Oslo, Norway*

Occurrence

The elbow and forearm are essential anatomic structures in virtually all sports that require throwing, lifting, pushing, pulling, or catching. The elbow's flexion and extension with associated forearm pronation and supination places the hand in a position to grip a handle, hold a ball, or simply place the upper extremity in a position to assist balance. It is, therefore, not a surprise to realize that acute and chronic injuries of the forearm and elbow can severely affect an athlete's performance in most sports. The following sections are dedicated to acute and chronic injuries of the elbow and forearm.

By definition, an acute injury is one that occurs over a short period of time. Most athletes can define the moment that the pain began or when they felt a pop, instability, or weakness. While minor acute injuries of the elbow and forearm are common in contact and collision sports, significant and catastrophic injuries are, fortunately, uncommon. The incidence of elbow injuries in sports depends on the specific demands and risks of the sport. Skeletal maturity is also a key factor related to acute injuries. In children, the weakest link to injury about the elbow is the growth plate in comparison to adults where the weakest link is the ligamentous structures.

Most common	Less common	Must not be overlooked	!
Sprains and strains, p. 218	Medial collateral ligament rupture, p. 219	Apophyseal avulsion	
	Elbow dislocations, p. 221	Olecranon fracture, p. 227	
	Distal biceps tendon rupture, p. 223	Monteggia, essex-Lopresti and Galeazzi fractures, p. 230	
	Triceps tendon rupture, p. 224	Acute vascular and nerve injury, p. 231	
	Acute olecranon bursitis, p. 225	Lateral ligament injury	
	Supracondylar and intra-articular fractures of the humerus, p. 226		
	Radial head or neck fractures, p. 228		
	Fractures of the forearm, p. 229		

Table 8.1 Overview of the differential diagnoses for acute elbow and forearm injuries. (Reproduced with permission from the Norwegian Sports Medicine Association.)

The IOC Manual of Sports Injuries, First Edition. Edited by Roald Bahr.
©2012 *International Olympic Committee. Published 2012 by John Wiley & Sons, Ltd.*

In children, the elbow joint is the joint that is most frequently dislocated. Among adults, the elbow is the second most commonly dislocated joint (after the shoulder).

Differential Diagnoses

Table 8.1 provides an overview of the most common differential diagnoses of acute elbow injuries. When creating a differential diagnosis of acute elbow and forearm injuries, the clinician should consider both structural anatomy and specific anatomic region. The key structural components include bone, cartilage, ligament, muscle, tendon, nerve, and artery. Bone fails via fracture. Acute fractures about the elbow include supracondylar, intra-articular, radial head and neck, olecranon, and avulsions of tendon insertions. In children, fractures usually involve the growth plate that is their structural weak link. In adults ligament injures are more common than fractures. The ultimate ligament injury is a joint dislocation in which the articular surfaces are no longer aligned. This can only occur with complete injury of the ligaments and capsule about the elbow. In every case of a fracture or dislocation, the clinician should be keenly aware of the potential associated injury to the brachial artery or nerve structures that cross the elbow joint. Intra-articular fractures should always raise concern of traumatic injury to the articular cartilage, which in turn increases the risk of future arthritis.

On the lateral aspect of the elbow, the clinician should consider lateral condyle fractures, avulsions of the extensor mechanism, radial head fractures, radial head dislocations, acute posterior lateral rotatory instability, and direct contusions to the lateral epicondyle or extensor muscle mass. On the medial aspect of the elbow, athletes can have an avulsion of the medial epicondyle, medial condyle fractures, medial collateral ligament tear (acute associated with dislocation or chronic associated with overuse), contusion of the flexor muscle mass, or contusion of the ulnar nerve. Posteriorly, olecranon fractures can occur with direct impact but may be associated by a prodrome of pain and a stress fracture. Direct impact can also lead to acute olecranon bursitis or bleeding into the bursa. Triceps tendon ruptures more often have a chronic prodrome or a history of steroid use but always have an acute catastrophic failure. Anteriorly, coronoid fractures are commonly associated with elbow dislocations and may predispose to recurrent disability. Rupture of the distal biceps tendon usually occur acutely with eccentric loading but may also have a chronic predisposition.

The forearm lies immediately distal to the elbow and is intimately related to the function of elbow pronation and supination. Acute injuries of the forearm range from simple contusion, to muscle tendon ruptures, compartment syndrome, and fractures. Forearm fractures can involve isolated injuries to the radius, ulna or both. However, the astute clinician must also recognize the common association of an isolated forearm fracture with joint instability proximally or distally. A Monteggia fracture is a fracture of the ulna with a proximal radio-ulnar instability, a Galleazi fracture is a fracture of the radius with distal radio-ulnar instability, and an Essex–Lopresti fracture is a radial head fracture with distal radio-ulnar instability. Each of these MUST be recognized due to the high risk of dysfunction if left untreated.

Diagnostic Thinking

Most elbow injuries can be treated at the primary-care level. The practitioner rarely has a problem distinguishing between contusions, muscle strains, and sprains (such as partial ligament ruptures) in comparison to complete dislocations or major fractures. The challenge is to determine which injuries may cause problems later on, and which should be referred to an orthopedic surgeon without delay. It is important to be completely knowledgeable of the broad differential of acute elbow and forearm injuries because overlooked injuries or inappropriately treated and rehabilitated injuries can lead to permanent disability. A complete neurovascular evaluation including a careful assessment of distal pulses should be performed on every patient to avoid missing the diagnosis of an arterial injury, compartment syndrome, or nerve injury. An acute hemarthrosis should raise suspicion of a more severe intra-articular or supracondylar injury. Therefore, patients with limited range of motion, focal bone pain, acute hemarthrosis, or gross instability must be x-rayed. If an intra-articular fracture, joint instability, displaced fracture, or neurovascular injury is identified or strongly considered, referral is indicated.

When potential catastrophic injuries can be ruled out of the differential diagnoses by imaging and clinical examination, a conservative course of treatment can be initiated. Advanced studies can be obtained with a high degree of suspicion, but most minor injuries will resolve with observation and simple conservative treatment of rest, ice, compression, and elevation. Since the elbow tends to get stiff, early mobilization is also important to optimal outcomes. The practitioner must avoid unnecessary and long-term immobilization. The elbow joint of an adult cannot be immobilized for longer than 3 weeks without a significant risk of permanently reduced range of motion. If the patient continues to improve then no additional studies are necessary. However, if complaints persist, more advanced evaluation including stress radiographs, MRI scan, MR arthrography, or bone scans can be considered.

Case History

One of the most common injury mechanisms in sport is an indirect trauma to the elbow caused by a fall on an outstretched arm. With the fall, the elbow is in near full extension with simultaneous valgus stress and supination of the forearm (Figure 8.1).

Most often this type of trauma causes only a sprain. If greater force is involved, total ligament ruptures with dislocation also occur, sometimes combined with fractures. In the case of dislocations, the lateral ligament complex is almost always torn first, and the medial collateral ligament may remain intact. Compression will cause most dislocations to be posterior. Compression may cause accompanying fractures in the lateral column (the capitellum and the radial head) and in the coronoid process. When falling on an outstretched arm, the athlete often lands on the wrist first with forces being transferred up the entire upper extremity. Therefore, the physician should also check for associated injuries at the wrist, through the entire length of both bones of the forearm, and in the shoulder area.

Another common acute injury mechanism in sport is direct trauma. Athletes may be hit directly on the elbow by a ball, puck, or

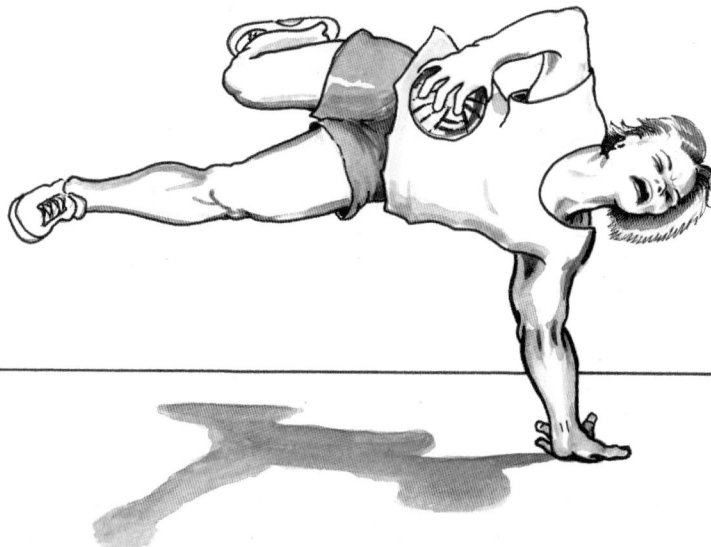

Figure 8.1 Injury mechanism. Falling on a nearly outstretched arm is the most common cause of elbow dislocations. (© Medical Illustrator Tommy Bolic, Sweden.)

bat or they may land directly onto their elbow during a fall. Direct impact onto a muscle belly can lead to a deep bruise or hematoma. Direct impact onto the posterior aspect of the elbow can cause bleeding into the olecranon bursa, an olecranon fracture, an intra-articular fracture, or supracondylar fractures.

Muscle tendon injuries can be chronic or acute. The ultimate failure or rupture is invariably an acute event that can occur with pushing or pulling. Distal biceps tendon ruptures are more common when the muscle is firing eccentrically. Both triceps tendon and biceps tendon injuries are usually accompanied by some preinjury risk factors including an old injury, preexistent tendinopathy, or a history of anabolic steroid use.

Clinical Examination

When faced with an acute injury, the practitioner must determine whether the patient has a severe injury–that is, a dislocation or fracture. Hemarthrosis and limited range of motion (ROM) are signs of severe intra-articular injuries that necessitate radiographic examinations. The clinician should always make an assessment of neurovascular function by checking pulses and nerve function. If the joint or bones require manipulation or reduction, neurovascular evaluation should always be performed both pre- and post-reduction. When elbow fractures and dislocations occur or both bone forearm fractures occur, consideration of an acute compartment syndrome should always be included in the examination and ruled out.

Inspection. Dislocated elbows, major elbow fractures and both bone forearm fractures will cause diffuse swelling, malalignment, deformity, significant pain, with limited function including reduced active and passive ROM of the elbow and forearm. Direct inspection and comparison with the opposite side may reveal obvious differences. There is usually a 15°–20° valgus carrying angle of the elbow. If this is not present, then a fracture or dislocation is likely present.

Palpation. For acute injuries palpation is usually painful, which may make it more challenging to perform an adequate examination. Effort should be made to palpate bony landmarks and bony alignment. Sharp edges or deformity may indicate fracture of dislocation. Direct palpation should include: (1) the medial epicondyle, (2) the distal humeral physis in children, (3) the lateral epicondyle, (4) the radial head, (5) the olecranon, (6) the sublime tubercle (insertion of the medial collateral ligament onto the ulna), (7) the mobile wad (flexor muscle mass), (8) the extensor muscle group, (9) the triceps insertion onto the olecranon, and (10) the biceps tendon. Intra-articular effusion or hemarthrosis may be detected by palpating the "soft spot," which is located in the middle of the lateral triangle (the three corners of this triangle are the lateral epicondyle, the anterior margin of the radial head, and the tip of the olecranon) (Figure 8.2). Demonstrating fluctuation in the "soft spot" means that there is intra-articular fluid. The biceps should be able to be "hooked" with one finger reaching from lateral to medial in the cubital tunnel. If you cannot hook the biceps tendon, it likely represents a distal rupture (Figure 8.3).

Neuromuscular function. One of the most important portions of the examination regarding acute

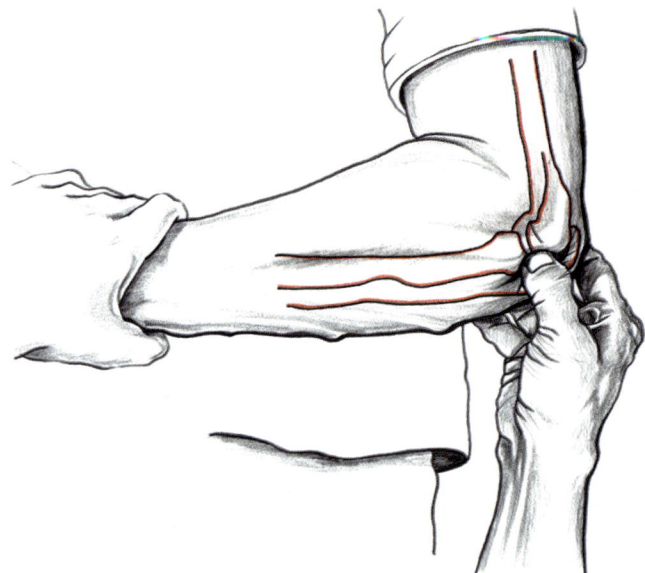

Figure 8.2 Palpation of the elbow to detect intra-articular fluid in the elbow. Fluctuation in the soft spot is a definite sign of joint effusion. The easiest way to find this point is to allow the thumb to slide anteriorly from the tip of the ulna along the lateral edge of the ulna. (© Medical Illustrator Tommy Bolic, Sweden.)

elbow and forearm injuries is an evaluation of neuromotor function. Admittedly motor examination can be difficult or limited due to associated patient guarding. Nonetheless, it is imperative to demonstrate that the major nerves that cross the elbow are still functioning. Sensation should be assessed on the palmar radial aspect of the hand (median nerve), the palmar ulnar aspect of the hand (ulnar nerve) and the dorsal aspect of the hand (radial nerve). Distal motor function can be assessed by extending the wrist, fingers, and thumb (radial nerve), thumb opposition (making the OK sign is median nerve) and abduction and adduction of the fingers (crossing fingers is ulnar nerve). Complete nerve function is examined as described in Chapter 9 (see Figure 9.3, p. 260). Ideally a complete motor evaluation about the elbow should also assess resisted elbow extension (triceps), resisted elbow flexion (brachialis and biceps), resisted elbow supination (biceps and supinator), resisted elbow pronation (pronator teres), wrist extension, and wrist flexion.

Circulation. The physician must also evaluate circulation; especially when fractures and dislocations have occurred. It is easiest to palpate the pulse by palpating the radial artery or the ulnar artery, just proximal to the wrist. Because of pain and swelling, it can be far more difficult to palpate the brachial artery in the elbow region. The capillary refill and hand warmth may also be used to evaluate circulation to the hand. With more severe injuries, the examiner should also make an assessment for compartment syndrome. Bleeding or swelling into the volar or dorsal compartments can build up so much pressure that circulation is compromised. Classically the patient will have pain beyond a level that would be expected by the injury, tight and tense compartments, pain with direct palpation of the compartments, pain with passive motion of the muscles in the compartments, and paresthesias of associated sensory nerves. Late and ominous findings of compartment syndrome include paralysis or pulselessness. Intra-compartmental pressure elevation can be measured to confirm elevated pressures. If present, surgical fascial release must be performed emergently to save the muscles and hand.

Movement. The normal ROM in the elbow joint is from full extension (0°) to 140°–150° flexion, 75° pronation, and 85° supination. The best way to evaluate the ROM is by comparing it with the opposite side and by using a goniometer. If the ROM is reduced with a hard "end point," it indicates that there is probably a mechanical block. If the "end point" is soft or absent, then pseudo-locking may be occurring in which the joint ROM is being limited by pain and not by a structural block. When evaluating pronation and supination the elbow should be flexed and held at the side in an effort to isolate the motion away from associated shoulder rotation. If an elbow dislocation occurred, a careful ROM should be performed after reduction to document a safe ROM that might be used during post-reduction rehabilitation.

Stability tests. In full extension, the most important stabilizing structures of the elbow are the bony articulation. When the elbow is flexed, the collateral ligaments play a more important role. Varus and valgus stability are examined starting at 20°–30°

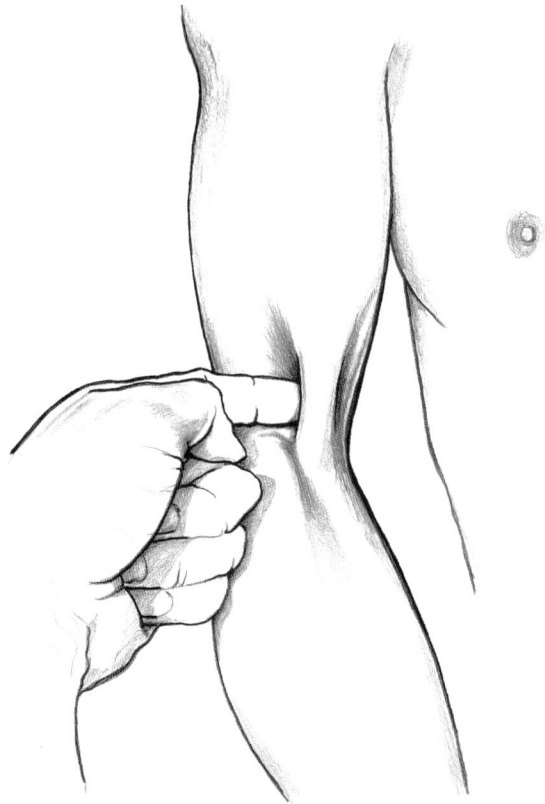

Figure 8.3 Biceps hook test. The examiner draws his hooked finger across the antecubital fossa from lateral to medial while the athlete attempts to flex his biceps muscle. If the biceps is intact, the examiner will hook the biceps tendon. If the biceps is torn, the examiner will be unable to hook the tendon. (© Medical Illustrator Tommy Bolic, Sweden.)

ELBOW AND FOREARM

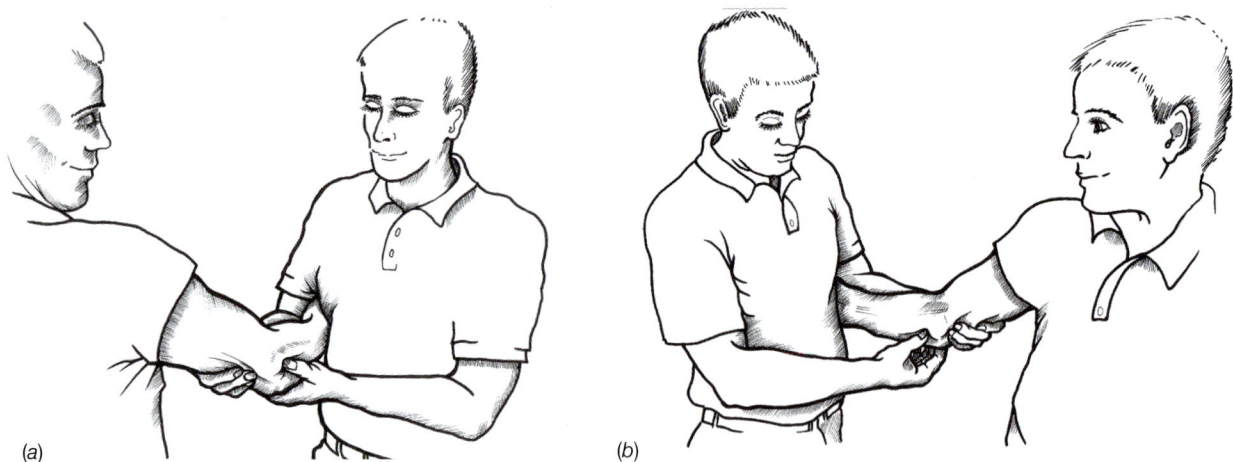

Figure 8.4 Moving valgus stress test (*a*) and milking maneuver (*b*). (© Medical Illustrator Tommy Bolic, Sweden.)

flexion of the elbow (Figure 8.4a and b). If the elbow can be hyperextended, lateral elbow instability may also be tested on an extended elbow. The examiner should apply stress by locking the patient's forearm between the examiner's upper arm and thorax. Then the examiner should place the tip of the thumb into the joint space medially or laterally, and apply valgus and varus stress, respectively. The test is positive if there is a palpable, and possibly a visible, opening of the joint with or without discomfort or pain.

The moving valgus stress test (Figure 8.5a) starts with the arm in full flexion. The examiner applies a constant valgus torque and then quickly extends the elbow. The test is positive when the patient reproduction of his painful symptoms with an apprehension-like response between 120° of flexion and 70° of extension.

In the milking maneuver (Figures 8.5b and 8.6), the athlete's elbow is flexed to about 90° or the same angle at which they throw. The examiner exerts a valgus

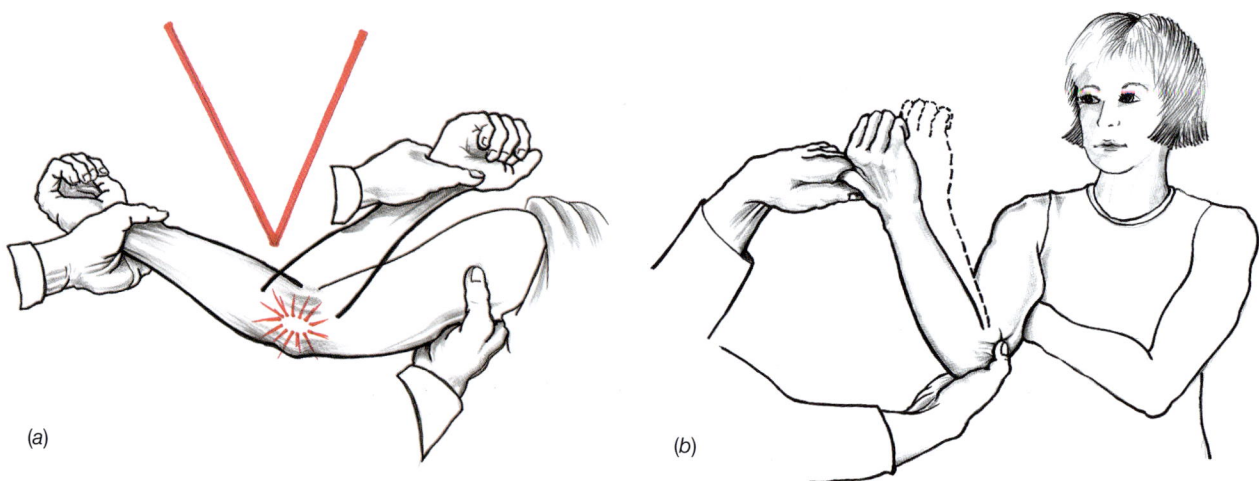

Figure 8.5 Technique for examining varus/valgus instability: With the elbow in 20°–30° flexion, the examiner checks for varus (*a*) and valgus (*b*) instability by grasping the patient's right upper arm with his left hand. The examiner places the tip of his right thumb on the joint line laterally (*a*) or medially (*b*) and applies valgus and varus stress, respectively. The patient's forearm is locked between the examiner's own forearm and thorax. The test is positive if a palpable (possibly visible) joint opening is found. (© Medical Illustrator Tommy Bolic, Sweden.)

torque by holding the patient's thumb and pulling creating a valgus stress force across the elbow. Pain that reproduces complaints is considered a positive finding. During the acute phase, it may be difficult to assess stability because of acute pain. Formal ligamentous testing may need to be delayed until after there is confirmation of no associated fracture and the soft tissues are allowed to settle down or under anesthesia.

The posterolateral instability (pivot shift) test is used to assess insufficiency of the lateral collateral ligament (Figure 8.7). This test is performed by flexing the elbow to 90° with the patient supine and his arm over his head. The forearm is fully supinated and slowly extended while applying valgus stress with supination movements and axial compression. The test is positive if a posterior prominence appears during extension (the dislocated radiohumeral joint) or when the patient experiences pain or apprehension. Valgus and supination creates a force that subluxates the lateral aspect of the elbow and radial head in extension that is reduced with a clunk with flexion.

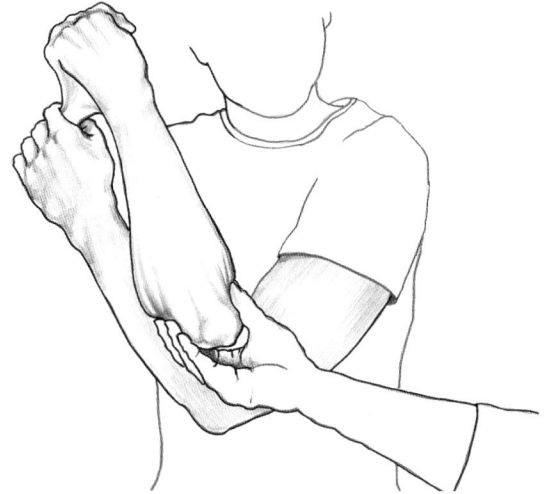

Figure 8.6 Milking maneuver is performed with the elbow flexed about 90°, then the examiner pulls on the patient's thumb causing a valgus stress at the elbow. Pain over the medial collateral ligament is considered positive. The moving valgus stress test is a dynamic variation of the milking maneuver in which the elbow is ranged from 30°–120°while simultaneously applying valgus stress. (© Medical Illustrator Tommy Bolic, Sweden.)

Supplemental Examinations

Radiographic examinations. Making the decision of when to obtain additional imaging is based on both the clinical suspicion of more severe injury and the potential risk that a significant injury is missed. Patients with a joint effusion, hemarthrosis, gross deformity, pain over a bony prominence, locked or reduced ROM after an acute injury, or crepitus with limited ROM should always be examined using anterior/posterior and lateral radiographs. Classically for any injury involving the forearm the joints above and below the site of injury should be included in the evaluation. For elbow injuries, the physician must make sure that the forearm and the wrist are clinically examined to assess whether they should be included in the diagnostic imaging. For skeletally immature athletes, a comparison view of the opposite side should always be obtained. Comparison views may also be helpful in adult patients when the diagnosis is less clear.

When to order additional studies. Occasionally, the initial radiographs are normal, but the patient's complaints persist or the clinician remains suspicious of a more severe injury. In this case additional studies should be obtained to rule out unrecognized problems.

- Oblique views will increase the accuracy of demonstrating minor accompanying fractures and can be helpful if the regular frontal and lateral views are difficult to interpret. Pronation and supination views will provide new aspects of the radial head and neck. Stress views may reveal joint instability or physeal injuries in children.
- Ultrasound can be a valued adjunct when evaluating muscle tendon injuries and can confirm the continuity of the triceps tendon, the extensor tendons or the biceps tendons. Bone scans are rarely used in the acute phase since it takes several days for them to become positive; nonetheless, they may assist in making the diagnosis of stress injuries of the bone such as an olecranon stress fracture. CT scans may be obtained by orthopaedic surgeons for preoperative planning of complex bone fractures but it is rarely necessary for the primary-care physician to order these.

• The clinical indication for when to obtain an acute MRI scan is open to debate. In many countries, MRI imaging is prohibitively expensive and not readily available. Most of the diagnoses should be able to be made by a complete history and physical exam and basic radiographs. With that understood, the MRI is a wonderful diagnostic tool that can identify the presence of loose bodies, provide a more defined prognosis of stress injuries than a bone scan, make the determination between partial and complete ligament and tendon injuries, and guide surgical intervention by better defining all injured structures with an acute injury. Care must be taken not to over interpret those findings. For example, the MRI scan of an athlete with an elbow dislocation will reveal diffuse edema and injury of the capsule, ligaments, muscles and even bone edema; nonetheless, most will have an excellent outcome with a conservative treatment plan.

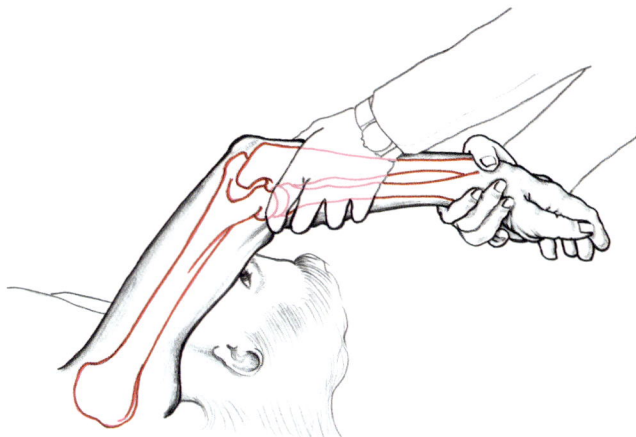

Figure 8.7 Pivot shift test. This exam is best performed with the patient supine and the arm extended above the head. The examiner stands above the athlete's head and ranges the elbow from extension to flexion with the forearm maximally supinated and a simultaneous valgus load. If the examiner feels a clunk as the radial head reduces from a posterior subluxated position, then the patient has posterolateral rotatory instability. (© Medical Illustrator Tommy Bolic, Sweden.)

Specific Diagnoses—Common Injuries

Sprains and Strains—*Partial Ligament and Partial Muscle—Tendon Injuries*

By far the most common injuries about the elbow are simple ligament sprains and muscle strains. Most athletes do not seek medical assistance because the subjective symptoms are moderate and temporary. The swelling and pain that accompanies such injuries usually subside after a few days. The basic approach to treatment is rest, ice, compression, and elevation. An astute clinician should always rule out associated intra-articular fractures and avulsions in adults as well as physeal injuries in children.

• Symptoms and signs: Pain, tenderness, swelling, and limited range of motion.
• Diagnosis: Sprains and strains should be focally tender over the appropriate anatomy. Partial ligament sprains will hurt when the ligament is tested in tension. Partial muscle strains will hurt with resisted motor function of the specific muscle tendon unit. If there is joint effusion or reduced range of motion, the patient *must* be referred for a radiographic examination. If the physician does not find objective signs of skeletal or ligament injury during the clinical examination, but the patient indicates that she is in a great deal of pain, she *should* be given a radiographic examination. If pain and swelling do not improve within a week, the patient *must* be referred for a radiographic examination and possibly for supplemental examinations. The clinical examination may demonstrate swelling and limited range of motion, but a sprain will often be an exclusion diagnosis after supplemental examination(s) have excluded fractures or dislocations.
• Treatment by physician: Rest, ice, compression, and elevation (RICE) treatment during the acute phase is customary. The use of nonsteroidal anti-inflammatory drugs (NSAIDs) is debatable since the early phase of healing depends on the inflammatory response. Nonetheless, they are still commonly used. Acetaminophen or paracetamol can be used as an alternative to manage pain. Immobilization is not mandatory but may be necessary for a few days for symptomatic pain relief. Be careful not to immobilize the elbow for extended periods due the high risk of residual stiffness. Sprains are treated using active ROM exercises within the limits of pain, muscle strength training, and protection against new trauma until activity is pain free.

- Treatment by therapist: The patient should be instructed to do self exercises that are within the limits of pain. All types of passive stretching should be avoided. The guiding fundamental in rehabilitation is to first regain motion, then strength, and then functional skills (see Rehabilitation of Elbow Injuries). The elbow has a propensity to getting stiff so early ROM is usually emphasized. When full, pain-free ROM (or a ROM acceptable for the athlete) is achieved, strength training may begin.
- Prognosis: Most athletes with mild injuries return to full training in less than 3 weeks. Complete ligament ruptures and tendon tears are described below and can take significantly longer or require surgical reconstruction. Premature return while the athlete is still painful or the collagen has not completely healed increases the risk of recurrence or more severe injury progression.

Other Injuries

Medial Collateral Ligament Rupture—*Injury to the Medial Ligament*

The medial collateral ligament rupture (Figure 8.8) is at risk of failure due to valgus load, which exceeds the functional strength of the native ligament. This can be secondary to a fall leading to either a valgus load or a hyperextension injury that loads the ligament. In overhead throwing sports (such as javelin, baseball, handball) repetitive valgus loading during the cocking phase of throwing can lead to chronic changes within the ligament that in turn weakens the structure. Ultimately a load, which in a healthy ligament would not cause ligament rupture, can be strong enough to cause failure in the weakened ligament. A number of other factors have also been correlated to the risk acute medial collateral ligament failure in throwing athletes including athlete fatigue, poor kinetic chain coordination, and poor throwing technique. Complete rupture of the medial collateral ligament is commonly associated with elbow dislocations.

- Symptoms and signs: The most common symptom is medial elbow pain usually exacerbated by throwing or valgus load. The key clinical findings are tenderness to palpation just distal to the medial epicondyle and pain with valgus stress. If a total rupture has occurred, acute pain will be accompanied by swelling, ecchymosis, and a feeling of instability. Complete rupture of the MCL can lead to a traction injury

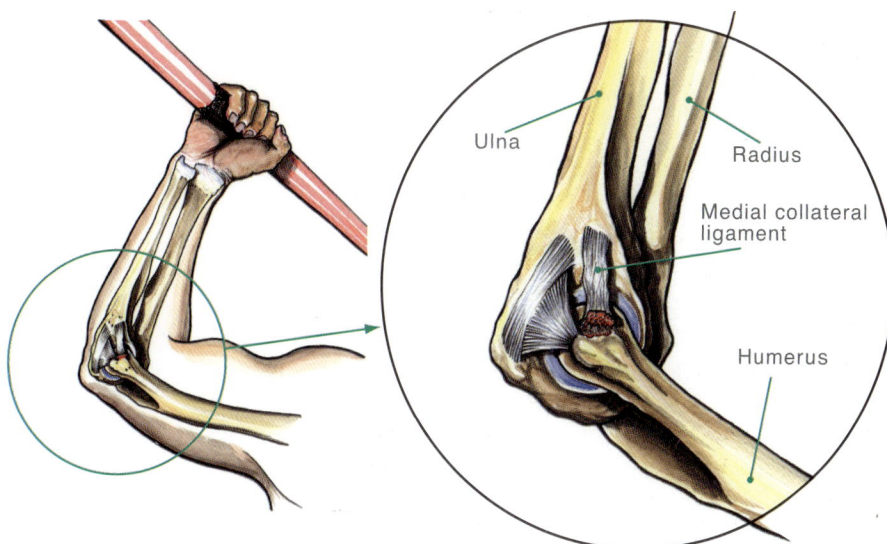

Ulna

Radius

Medial collateral ligament

Humerus

Figure 8.8 Medial ligament injury. Javelin throwing is a classic injury mechanism for tearing the medial collateral ligament in the elbow. Tearing usually occurs at the insertion to the humerus with repeated valgus stress and rotation. (© Medical Illustrator Tommy Bolic, Sweden.)

of the ulnar nerve at the cubital tunnel with associated clinical findings of tingling in the two ulnar fingers or weakness of the intrinsic muscles of the hand.

- Diagnosis: The physical finding noted in the preceding text should make the clinician suspicious of the diagnosis but it must be acknowledged that feeling instability is difficult in isolated ligament ruptures even in the most experienced hands. Valgus stress radiographs may reveal asymmetric joint space widening when compared to the contralateral elbow. The best two tests to confirm dysfunction of the MCL are the milking maneuver and the moving valgus sheer test. The most conclusive diagnosis is generally made with magnetic resonance arthrography. Examination with standard elbow views should always be performed to exclude associated fractures.
- Treatment: Initial treatment of isolated medial ligament injuries is the classic RICE (rest, ice, compression, and elevation). Partial injuries may heal with a period of rest followed by gradual return using a gradually progressive throwing protocol. Approximately 50% of those will fail if the patient returns to high level throwing demands. Surgical reconstruction of the ligament may be necessary for complex injuries and gross instability. Isolated MCL injuries in elite throwers will require reconstruction if the athlete wishes to return to their previous sport. Gymnasts may also require reconstruction due to their repetitive upper extremity weight-bearing demands. For most patients and athletes with little to no throwing demand, surgery reconstruction is rarely required.
- Prognosis: Prognosis for MCL injuries depend on whether the injury is partial or complete and, more importantly, on the specific sports demand. Many athletes with less throwing and upper extremity weight-bearing demand can do very well without surgical intervention. With modern reconstruction techniques, return to play can be expected in 75% of patients but it may take 1–2 years to return to their full preinjury performance.

Lateral Ligament Injury !

Injuries to the lateral collateral ligament are less common than the medial collateral ligament. Injuries to the ligament structures on the lateral/outside part of the elbow are usually the result of a fall on an outstretched arm or forced hyperextension of the elbow usually with the forearm supinated. Ligament sprains are classified according to how great the instability is (Figure 8.9a–d). In I and II grade injuries, most are minor partial ruptures without significant instability, and most will be diagnosed as a sprain without recognition of the ligament injury. In grade III injuries, there is also a risk of simultaneous medial ligament injury, instability of the radial head or complete joint dislocation. Partial ruptures are probably the cause of many painful conditions on the lateral side after minor trauma, such as a hyperextension injury. True lateral instability may be secondary to an isolated ligament injury or be a chronic complication of a dislocated elbow.

- Symptoms and signs: Athletes will generally complain of a sensation of lateral elbow instability or popping that is effected by forearm position. Extension and supination will lead to posterolateral rotatory instability while flexion and pronation leads to reduction.
- Diagnosis: The key clinical finding is posterolateral rotatory instability (Figure 8.7). On plain radiographs, the examiner needs to make sure that there is not an associated fracture of the capitellum, radial head or radial neck fracture. Varus stress radiographs may reveal lateral joint line gapping.
- Treatment and Prognosis: For mild injuries of the lateral complex of the elbow, the treatment is conservative with use of a sling and guarded ROM to allow the partially injured ligament to heal. After 4–6 weeks when the patient has achieved a pain-free full range of motion, the athlete can usually gradually return to full

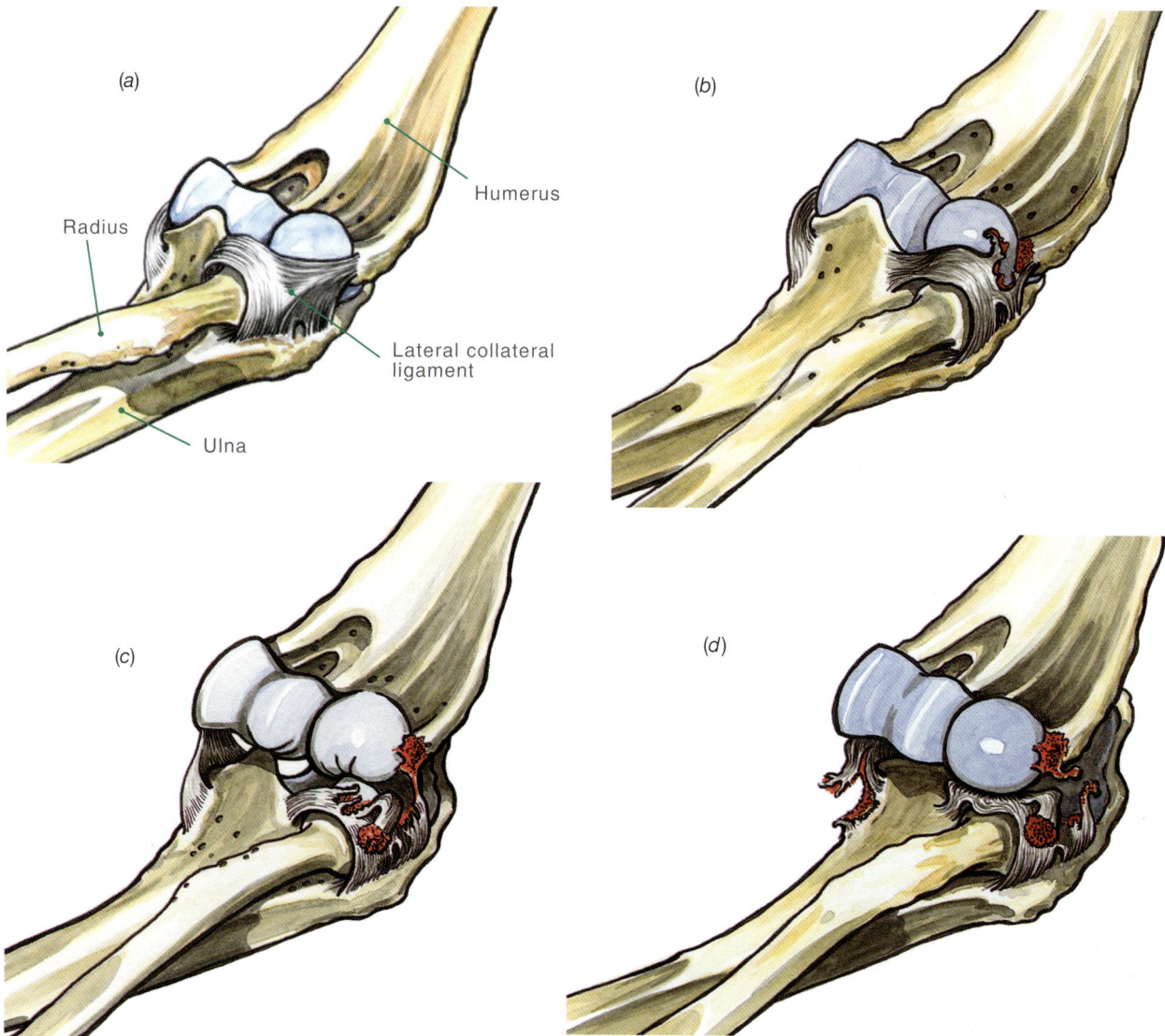

Figure 8.9 Spectrum of instability. Lateral ligament complex injuries are classified according to the degree of instability: Grade I (*a*): distortion, partial ruptures without instability; Grade II (*b*): posterolateral rotation instability—that is, subluxation of the head of the radius with supination, axial compression, and valgus stress; Grade III: dislocated elbow. In Grade IIIa (*c*), the humerus "rests" on the top of the coronoid process; in Grade IIIb (*d*), the entire elbow is dislocated. (© Medical Illustrator Tommy Bolic, Sweden.)

activities with no long-term deficits. For complete injuries especially those in which the diagnosis has been delayed and recurrent stability is present, surgical reconstruction may be required to stabilize the elbow.

Elbow Dislocations

Dislocations are by definition the most severe of ligament injuries in which not only is the ligament completely torn but the ligament has completely failed in its primary function of keeping the joint stable. Elbow dislocations are always associated with ligament ruptures of the medial and/or lateral collateral ligaments as well as the capsule of the elbow joint. Careful evaluation of radiographs must always be performed because elbow dislocations are frequently accompanied by fractures, including fractures of the radial head (5–10%), avulsion injuries involving one of the condyles (medial or lateral, about 12%), and fractures of the coronoid process (10%). Intra-articular fractures will predispose the athlete to arthritis and must be anatomically reduced. Elbow dislocations with associated fractures are at increased risk of recurrent dislocations when compared to purely ligamentous dislocations. Injuries of the chondral surface are commonly associated with elbow dislocations and may be missed on standard radiographic evaluation since there is no bone attached to the cartilaginous fragment.

- Symptoms and signs: Elbow dislocations generally present with gross deformity. They are rarely open but are commonly associated with decreased sensation in the radial, ulnar or median nerve distribution. These neuropraxias are usually transient and related to stretching of the nerve at the time of injury but permanent nerve injury can occur. It is essential that the clinician carefully evaluate distal neurovascular function before and after a reduction is performed.
- Diagnosis: The diagnosis is made clinically due to the gross deformity, but standard anterior/posterior and lateral radiographics may not only reveal the joint dislocation but also associated fractures. Frequently, these prereduction radiographs are difficult to read due to the overlapping shadows of mal-aligned bones. Immediate post-reduction radiographs are essential to confirm anatomic reduction as well as the presence or absence of associated fractures. The joint space should be symmetric throughout. A widened joint space post reduction may indicate and interposed cartilage fragment or soft tissue. The radial head should point to the center of the capitellum on all views if the radiohumeral joint is anatomically reduced.
- Treatment by physician: Reduction of an elbow dislocation should be performed by a knowledgeable and experienced clinician. Due to three bones involved in the articulation, the elbow is not the easiest of joint dislocations to reduce and, therefore, sideline attempts by an inexperienced clinician should be avoided. In most cases when distal neurovascular function is intact, the elbow can be splinted where it lies and transported to the nearest emergency room. If transport is unavailable, distal vascular function is poor, and the clinician is confident, a single attempt on the sideline can be performed with in line traction. Some doctors like to push the olecranon into place and some prefer to pull it in to a reduced position. Either is acceptable. Dislocated elbows that cannot be reduced require surgery. Associated fractures that remain displaced after reduction also require surgical intervention.

  After reduction, stability should be tested to assess the safe and acceptable ROM that can be performed in early rehabilitation. The elbow is immobilized in accordance with Table 8.2. Early movement prevents post-traumatic stiffness. Adults can tolerate a maximum of 3 weeks of immobilization; children can achieve full mobility even after 6 weeks of immobilization. Retraining should be pain free; otherwise, minor bleeding, which leads to capsule shrinkage and reduced range of motion, may ensue. If full ROM has not been achieved in 6–8 weeks, more aggressive therapy should be started (see Section Post-traumatic Stiffness).
- Treatment by therapist: The patient should be instructed in exercises he can do alone that are within the limits of pain. It is very important to communicate with the physician regarding the safe ROM that should be allowed immediately after reduction. All types of passive stretching must be avoided. When full ROM (or ROM acceptable to the athlete) is achieved, strength training may begin.
- Prognosis: Up to 50% of all dislocations (with and without fractures) will have late symptoms, such as reduced ROM and strength, pain, or instability. The symptoms are related to the extent of the primary injury, or accompanying injuries. It is possible to tolerate a slight limitation of extension in most sports. In general, the prognosis is good for posterior dislocations that have no

Stability after reduction	Treatment	Duration
Stable in all directions	Immediate active exercises	
Stable with pronation	Orthosis that prevents supination but allows flexion and extension	3 weeks maximum
Unstable with pronation	Orthosis (or possibly a cast) that prevents extension in the direction of instability	3 weeks maximum

Table 8.2 Guidelines for immobilization of dislocated elbows. (Reproduced with permission from the Norwegian Sports Medicine Association.)

accompanying fractures and that have been immobilized for only 2–3 weeks. Due to the potential association of a medial collateral ligament injury with the elbow dislocation, throwing athletes may have a more guarded prognosis after elbow dislocation.

Distal Biceps Tendon Rupture—*Injury to the Tendon of the Biceps Muscle*

Ruptures of the distal biceps tendon (Figure 8.10) are rare, accounting for only 3–10% of the biceps tendon ruptures and less than 1% of injuries about the elbow. Nonetheless, it is an important injury not to miss since delayed repair can be more difficult. Indeed if left untreated, patients will have a loss of both elbow flexion and forearm supination power and strength. Distal biceps tendon ruptures primarily affect men compared to women, and in 80% of cases, it is localized to the dominant arm. The injury appears suddenly when the elbow is forcefully extended and supinated from a 90° flexed position while the elbow's flexors and supinators work eccentrically. Previous tendinopathy secondary to overuse predisposes the tendon to rupture, as does a history of anabolic steroid use. Body builders are most susceptible to this injury.

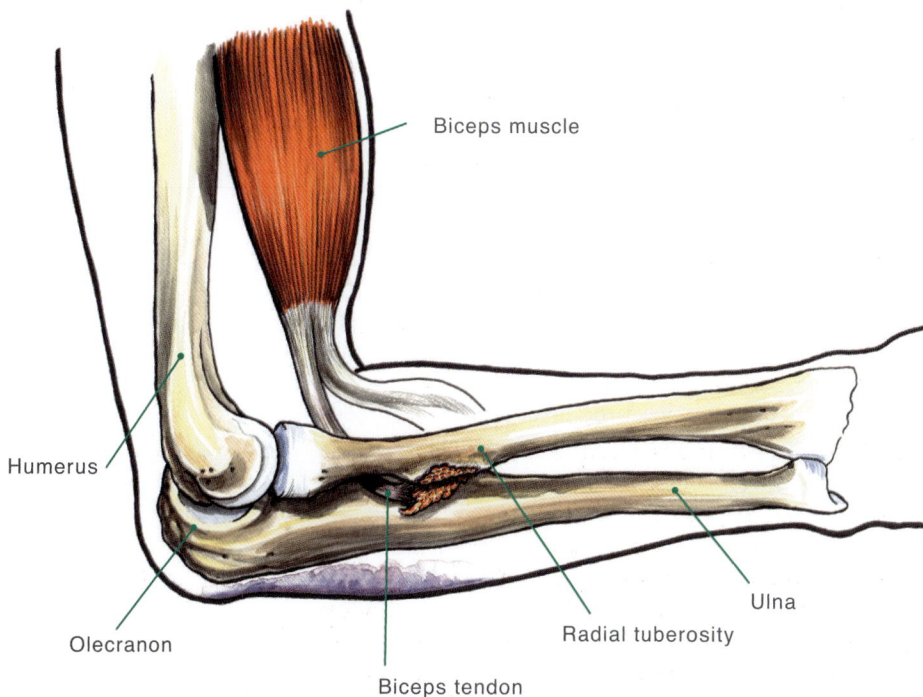

Figure 8.10 Distal biceps tendon rupture, a rare injury, occurs in the radial tuberosity. It is palpated laterally while the forearm is pronated. (© Medical Illustrator Tommy Bolic, Sweden.)

- Symptoms and signs: The most common presentation of an acute biceps rupture is a sudden, sharp pain in the antecubital fossa of the elbow, followed by discomfort in the forearm or the lower portion of the upper arm. The intense pain subsides within a few hours, while aching pain continues for weeks with cramping of the biceps muscle belly. Clinically, the patient will have pain and weakness with resisted elbow flexion and forearm supination. Ecchymosis is frequently present on the volar aspect of the elbow and into the forearm. A defect can be palpated in the distal biceps tendon, when the muscle is contracted. A proximal "Pop-eye" sign can be visualized as the biceps muscle retracts proximally when compared to the contralateral biceps. The hook test (see Figure 8.3) is a great clinical test to confirm the absence or continuity of the distal biceps.
- Diagnosis: The diagnosis is based on the symptoms and the clinical examination as noted in the preceding text.
- Treatment by physician: Early surgical repair (in 1–2 weeks) is recommended for people with high activity levels who require full function of the arm. Conservative treatment will provide satisfactory function for only 50% of patients. In sedentary, low demand patients, the outcomes of non-surgical treatment may be acceptable. For the athletic population, repair is strongly recommended. The exact surgical approach (single incision or double incision) is dependent on surgeon preference and each approach is subject to unique risks and benefits. Partial ruptures may heal without surgery but should be followed carefully since the remaining bundle may become painful and ultimately fail.
- Treatment by therapist: Partial injuries to the distal biceps must be treated with a period of protected against resisted exercises to avoid progressing to a complete injury. Post-surgical rehabilitation is dependent on the strength of the construct. Most patients should avoid resisted exercises for 6–8 weeks but motion is encourage early in recover to avoid elbow stiffness.
- Prognosis: Long-term prognosis for surgical repair of complete injuries is excellent. Specific surgical approaches carry unique risks of nerve injury or heterotopic ossification with associated stiffness. Partial injuries have a guarded prognosis, as many will develop chronic pain complaints with resisted elbow flexion. Non-surgical treatment of complete injuries will lead to moderate loss of elbow flexion strength but significant loss of supination strength.

Triceps Tendon Rupture—*Injury of the Tendon of the Triceps Muscle*

A rupture of the triceps tendon (Figure 8.11) is even uncommon than a biceps rupture; but without proper diagnosis and adequate treatment, elbow dysfunction may become significant. The injury affects women almost as often as men (2–3). The injury mechanism is usually a fall on an outstretched arm (sudden eccentric loading of the elbow) or direct trauma. Previous tendinopathy predisposes it to rupture. Body builders are most vulnerable to this injury. Anabolic steroid abuse significantly increases the risk of triceps tendon ruptures.

- Symptoms and signs: The athlete complains of pain at the insertion of the triceps onto the olecranon. If extensor function is lost, a total rupture has occurred. The most common findings are ecchymosis and swelling. A defect may be palpated just proximal to the olecranon.
- Diagnosis: The diagnosis of a triceps rupture is based on symptoms and clinical findings. Advanced imaging is rarely required but standard radiographs may reveal an avulsion of the bony attachment, which may alter treatment options or techniques. The practitioner should distinguish clinically between partial ruptures and total ruptures. A variation of the Thompson test (commonly used to

diagnosis Achilles tendon ruptures) can also be used for triceps tendon ruptures. While supporting the arm and bending the elbow to 90°, the triceps muscle can be squeezed mimicking a triceps contraction. If the elbow extends, then the triceps tendon is intact. If no movement occurs, then a complete rupture has occurred. In challenging cases in which the diagnosis is less clear, either MRI or ultrasound may be used to confirm the diagnosis.

- Treatment by physician: Complete ruptures require surgical repair. Partial ruptures may be treated conservatively with active exercises that are within the limits of pain.
- Treatment by therapist: Rehabilitation of partial injuries of the triceps should first be treated by regaining full motion followed by a gradual progression of resistance training and strength. Premature return to play may predispose the athlete to either chronic tendinopathic complaints or a completion of the triceps rupture. If the athlete has no pain, ROM and resistance can be advanced ad lib. Functional training and challenges should be observed before release to return to play. Post-surgical rehabilitation is guided by the quality of the repair at the time of surgery. It is important for the therapist to communicate with the surgeon regarding the pace at which rehabilitation can occur postoperatively.

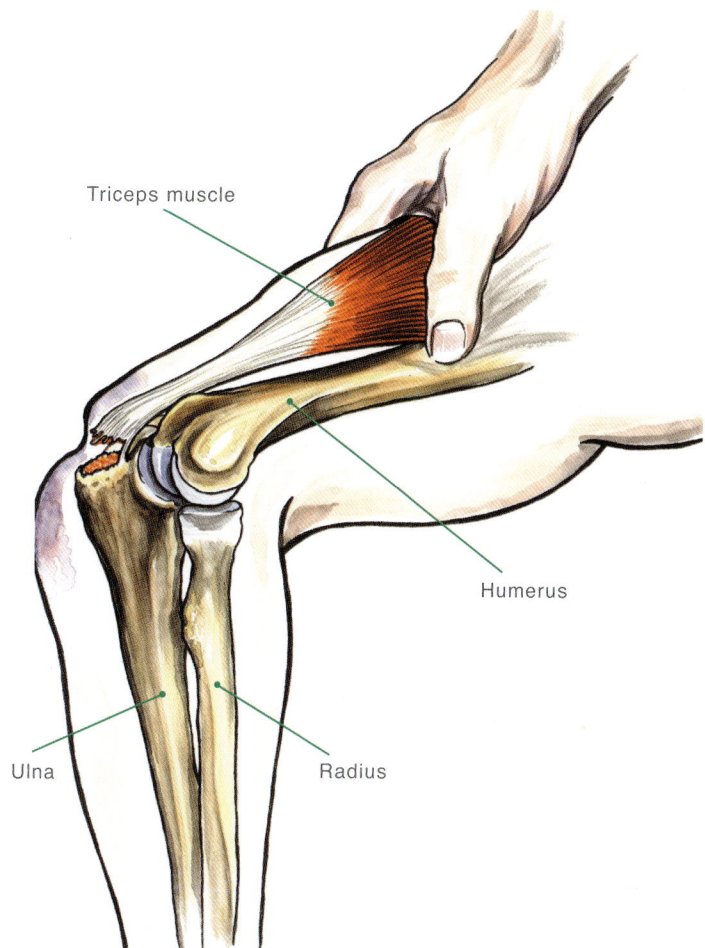

Triceps muscle

Humerus

Ulna

Radius

Figure 8.11 Triceps tendon rupture. The Thompson test is shown. By supporting the arm and flexing the elbow 90°, it is possible to quickly squeeze the triceps muscle to cause a reflex contraction. A lack of extension indicates a total rupture. (© Medical Illustrator Tommy Bolic, Sweden.)

Acute Olecranon Bursitis—*Bursa Inflammation at the Tip of the Elbow*

The olecranon bursa serves as a protective pad over the posterior aspect of the elbow. The elbow has several small bursae but the large olecranon bursa is by far the most common injured or inflamed. The olecranon bursa is subject to direct trauma due to a fall when the athlete lands on their flexed elbow or collides with retaining walls in such sports as ice hockey or handball. Acute injuries may be accompanied by intra-bursal bleeding and a hematoma. If synovial irritation continues, the condition may become chronic. The olecranon bursa lies beneath the skin with very little protective fat tissue making it subject to becoming infected with minor scrapes or abrasions.

- Symptoms and signs: Acute olecranon bursitis usually presents after an appropriate history with exquisite tenderness superficial to the olecranon. The bursa is usually fluid filled and baggy. Intra-bursal bleeding is usually accompanied by echymotic changes and discoloration. Septic bursitis usually presents with redness, tenderness, local warmth, and fever. The practitioner must be aware that these symptoms can develop very quickly.
- Diagnosis: The diagnosis is usually based on the case history and the demonstration of a fluid filled boggy bursa. Fever and local warmth should alert the examiner to the potential of an infection. If the diagnosis is unclear, aspiration is recommended.

The aspirate will be clear or mixed with blood if the patient has sterile bursitis, whereas pus may be aspirated if the patient has septic bursitis.

- Treatment by physician: For non-septic, acute olecranon bursitis, treatment is generally conservative with ice, non-steroidal medications, compression dressings, and elbow pads to prevent recurrence. Aspiration is reserved for those suspicious of sepsis for fear of seeding a simple hematoma or bursitis. If the bursa is tense, blood may be aspirated during the acute stage but it is imperative that each aspiration is performed with sterile technique. If the patient has septic bursitis, the bursa must be incised and drained. In recurrent cases, more formal excision may be required.

Supracondylar and Intra-articular Fractures of the Humerus

In children, supracondylar (Figure 8.12), bicondylar, transcondylar, and intercondylar fractures of the distal humerus total 50–60% of all fractures about the elbow. The injury occurs more commonly in boys than girls and is like related to increased participation in collision sports or other at-risk behaviors. The most common mechanism is a fall on an outstretched hand. These fractures have a high risk of persistent deformity and neurovascular injury. They require anatomic reduction and careful assessment of neurovascular function both pre- and post-reduction.

Complex supracondular fractures may extend into the joint increasing the instability and leading to a risk of arthritis in the future. Isolated intra-articular fractures such as fractures of the capitellum or isolated condyle fractures may be subtler than supracondylar fractures and require careful examination of the radiographs. The general presentation is similar.

- Symptoms and signs: For significant injuries, gross malalignment of the elbow is obvious; however, the clinician should carefully look for subtle findings of non-displaced injuries. Signs of non-displaced injuries include swelling and focal tenderness proximal to the joint line. The athlete will be resistant to flex and extend the joint. It is imperative that the clinician assesses nerve and circulation function since the neurovascular structures lie very close to the site of injury. If there is gross displacement with fracture edges threatening to pierce or if pulses are absent, the clinician may attempt a reduction even before radiographic studies can be obtained.
- Diagnosis: The diagnosis is made by standard AP and lateral radiographs of the elbow. Extra oblique views may be helpful if the standard views are difficult to interpret. When a fracture line is not obvious careful inspection for the anterior and posterior fat pads may signal a non-displaced supracondylar fracture. For children, it is strongly recommended that comparative views of the opposite elbow be obtained. This is particularly helpful when assessing growth plate injuries. Once again, the physician should always check skin color, capillary filling distally, distal pulses, and distal nerve function.
- Treatment principles: The main goal of treatment is prevention of displacement in non-displaced fractures and restoration to normal alignment for those that are displaced. When non-displaced fractures are present with intact neurovascular function, the patient can be treated with cast immobilization for a short period of

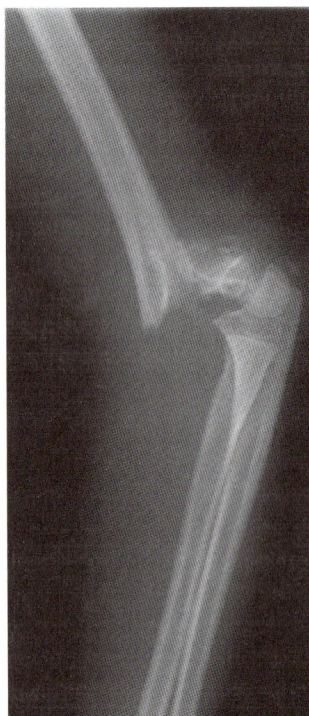

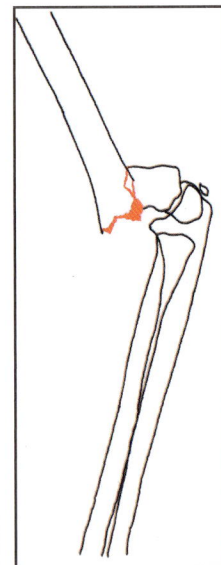

Figure 8.12
Supracondylar fracture of the humerus with significant malalignment, usually caused by hyperextension of the arm when blocking a fall. (© Medical Illustrator Tommy Bolic, Sweden.)

time. Beware extended immobilization can lead to permanent loss of motion. For displaced fractures, reduction under anesthesia in the operating room is required. In children percutaneous pinning is frequently added to maintain reduction and allow earlier motion. In adults, formal open reduction and internal fixation is usually performed. If an athlete is hurt on the playing field, emergency transport is not readily available, and pulses are absent; alignment can be improved by applying longitudinal traction followed by splinting, before the patient is transported to the hospital. Definitive stabilization will be performed in the operating room.

Olecranon Fracture !

Because of its superficial location, the olecranon is vulnerable to injury from direct trauma, such as falling on the elbow. In sports, stress fractures can occur in the olecranon secondary to repetitive throwing and lifting. Olecranon fractures are divided into three types, according to the Mayo classification (Figure 8.13). Type I fractures are nondisplaced, with no or minimal crushing. Type II fractures are stable with displacement, with or without crushing. Type III fractures (the least common) are unstable, with or without crushing, and may have accompanying fractures in the radial head. If this is the case, it can be difficult to distinguish between a type III olecranon fracture and a Monteggia fracture.

- **Symptoms and signs:** If no dislocation has occurred, swelling is usually moderate. If a dislocation has occurred, more swelling is usually present because of bleeding from the fracture and the displaced olecranon fragment. Elbow extension is reduced. Maximum tenderness is experienced at the level of the fracture. Because the olecranon is superficial, a defect can often be palpated.
- **Diagnosis:** The diagnosis is made clinically, but a standard X-ray series of the elbow is required to assess the extent of injury as well as look for associated injuries. If there is any pain of the forearm or wrist, radiographs should include the entire forearm and wrist.
- **Treatment by physician:** The goals of treatment are to (1) reconstruct the articular surface, (2) maintain muscle strength, (3) re-establish joint stability, (4) avoid joint stiffness, and (5) avoid complications. To achieve these goals, most olecranon fractures must be surgically treated at a hospital. The exceptions are simple,

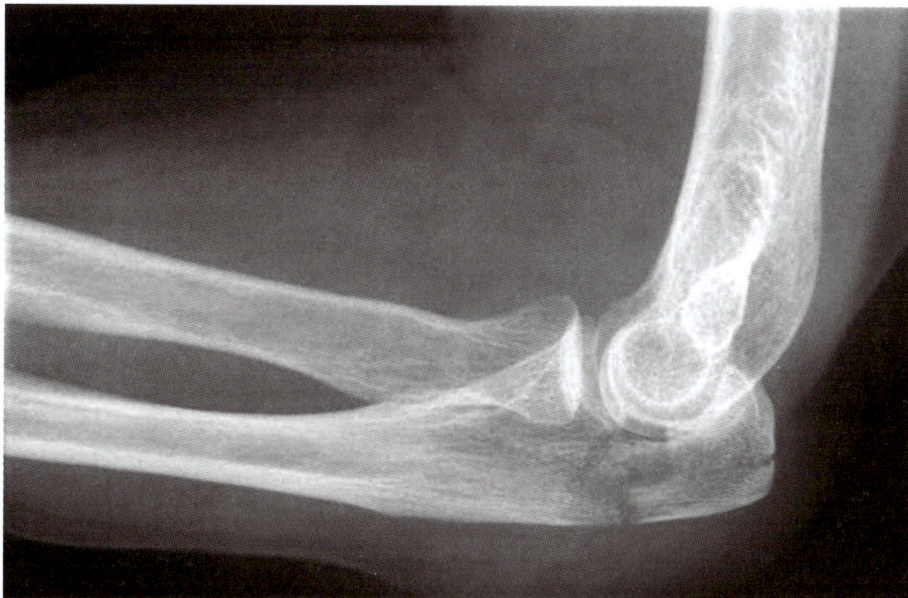

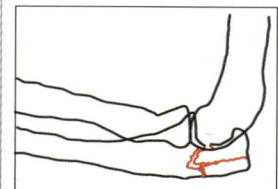

Figure 8.13 Olecranon fracture, usually caused by falling on the tip of the elbow and often requiring surgery. (© Medical Illustrator Tommy Bolic, Sweden.)

ELBOW AND FOREARM

227

non-displaced, and stable fractures (type I), which can be immobilized for 2–3 weeks. Repeat radiographs should be taken after about 1 week to make sure that the fracture does not become displaced.

- Treatment by therapist: It is important that the physical therapist communicate with the physician before aggressively regaining motion. In non-displaced, stable fractures, gentle motion can begin after 2–3 weeks of immobilization. Initially the exercise program emphasizes instruction in selfexercises within the limits of pain. After the fracture is healed, exercises to improve the ROM are emphasized. Strength training begins after satisfactory ROM is achieved.
- Prognosis: Overall the prognosis is good; however, any intra-articular irregularity can lead to arthritic changes. If open reduction and internal fixation was required, painful retained hardware is common due to the subcutaneous location of the olecranon. In those cases, a second surgery may be required to remove the hardware. Other potential complications include ulnar neuropathy, elbow instability, or fracture nonunion with pseudoarthrosis.

Radial head and neck fractures

Fractures of the radial head and neck may occur in isolation, with elbow dislocations, or with complex forearm fractures. It is important for the clinician to carefully evaluate the athlete for all possible associated injuries. Isolated cases usually occur secondary to a fall on an outstretched hand. When associated with injuries of the medial collateral ligament, the elbow tends to be unstable.

- Symptoms and signs: Athletes will present with pain over the lateral aspect of the proximal forearm exacerbated with pronation and supination. The radial head is a subcutaneous structure and can easily be palpated. Focal pain should raise suspicion of a radial head or neck fracture. Valgus stress of the elbow will also exacerbate lateral joint line pain.
- Diagnosis: Anterior/posterior and lateral radiographs of the elbow will commonly be diagnostic. Subtle fractures may require additional oblique views to visualize the fracture. If the athlete has any pain of the forearm or wrist, complete imaging of the forearm and wrist should be obtained to rule out associated injuries.
- Treatment by physician: Treatment options depend on the size, location, angulation and displacement of the fracture as well as the presence or absence of associated injuries. Intra-articular radial head fractures involving more than 1/3 of the head, that have more than 3 mm displacement and are more than 30° angulated require surgical fixation. Comminuted fractures or those associated with medial elbow instability or midshaft ulna fractures may require radial head replacement.

Physeal and apophyseal fractures—*Little Leaguer's Elbow*

When a child falls on an outstretched arm, he may sustain an avulsion fracture of the ligaments or tendon insertion of the elbow flexors or extensors (Figure 8.14). Children may also sustain partial avulsion with growth zone of the medial epicondyle from intensive periods of repeated throwing (little leaguer's elbow). Approximately 12% of all growth zone injuries occur in the elbow. Avulsion injuries of the medial epicondyle related to throwing are more common in boys than girls.

- Symptoms and signs: In throwing athletes, an acute pop may be perceived during a single hard toss. Subsequent attempts at throwing exacerbate the pain. If the mechanism is a fall on an outstretched hand, the athlete will have an acute onset of pain over the medial or lateral epicondyle immediately after the fall. Pain with resisted wrist flexion for injuries of the medial epicondyle or pain with resisted wrist extension for injuries of the lateral epicondyle is common. The primary finding is distinct tenderness of the epicondyle.

- Diagnosis: Anterior/posterior and lateral radiographs are the key to diagnosis. It is strongly recommended that for all children comparative radiographs are obtained with the contralateral elbow to better assess what may be subtle displaced growth plate injuries compared to a normal growth plate.
- Treatment by physician: For minimally displaced injuries, the athlete should stop loading the epicondyle; that is, throwers should stop throwing and gymnasts should cease weight-bearing activities. Early elbow ROM is allowed within the limits of pain. Resistive exercises should be withheld for at least 6–8 weeks. If the fragment is displaced by more than 2 mm or is rotated, surgery may be recommended especially in throwing athletes.
- Prognosis: Prognosis is good. Even when the fracture heals with a fibrous union, patients are able to function with little disability or pain. Growth disturbances are rare, because the epicondyles do not affect longitudinal growth nor do they articulate with the elbow joint.

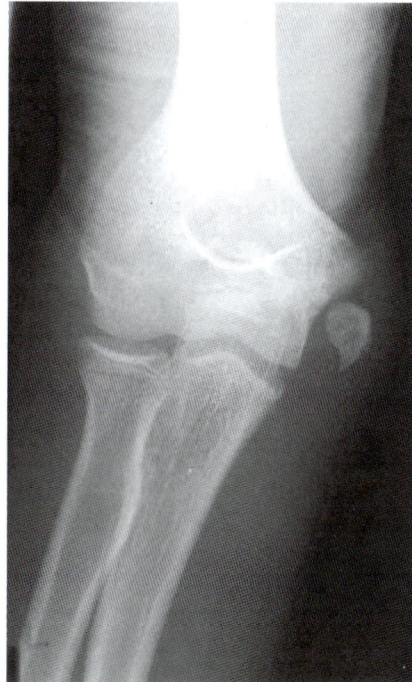

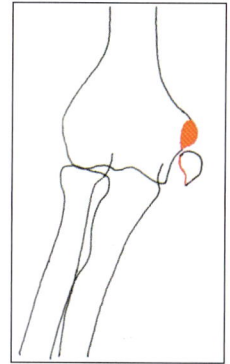

Figure 8.14 Apophysis fractures. When a child falls on an outstretched arm, an avulsion fracture may occur through the growth zone. (© Medical Illustrator Tommy Bolic, Sweden.)

Fractures of the Forearm

Forearm fractures involve shaft fractures of either the radius, ulnar or both. (Figure 8.15a–c). In adults these tend to be unstable and require open reduction and internal fixation. Children frequently sustain these injuries as the result of a fall. Direct trauma (blows and kicks) may also result in fractures in one or both forearm bones. Isolated non-displaced fractures of the ulna may be caused by direct impact (night stick fracture) and maybe treated with casting although athletes will return to play earlier with surgical fixation. A fracture of the proximal aspect of the ulnar with associated radial head instability is called a Monteggia fracture. These are unstable and require surgical fixation.

- Symptoms and signs: Symptoms and signs are moderate swelling, obvious malalignment, total dysfunction, and significant pain. If circulation or the skin is threatened, the fracture should be reduced and stabilized immediately before the patient is sent to the hospital.
- Diagnosis: The diagnosis is based on the apparent malalignment. Anterior/posterior and lateral radiographs are necessary to confirm the diagnosis and to demonstrate associated injuries. A general rule is to always obtain radiographs of the joint above and below the fracture to assure that those joints are not hiding associated injuries. The practitioner must check skin color, distal capillary filling, the pulse in the radial artery, as well as distal skin sensation.
- Treatment by physician: The patient is referred to the hospital immediately to be evaluated for probable open reduction and internal fixation. Some fractures in

ELBOW AND FOREARM

229

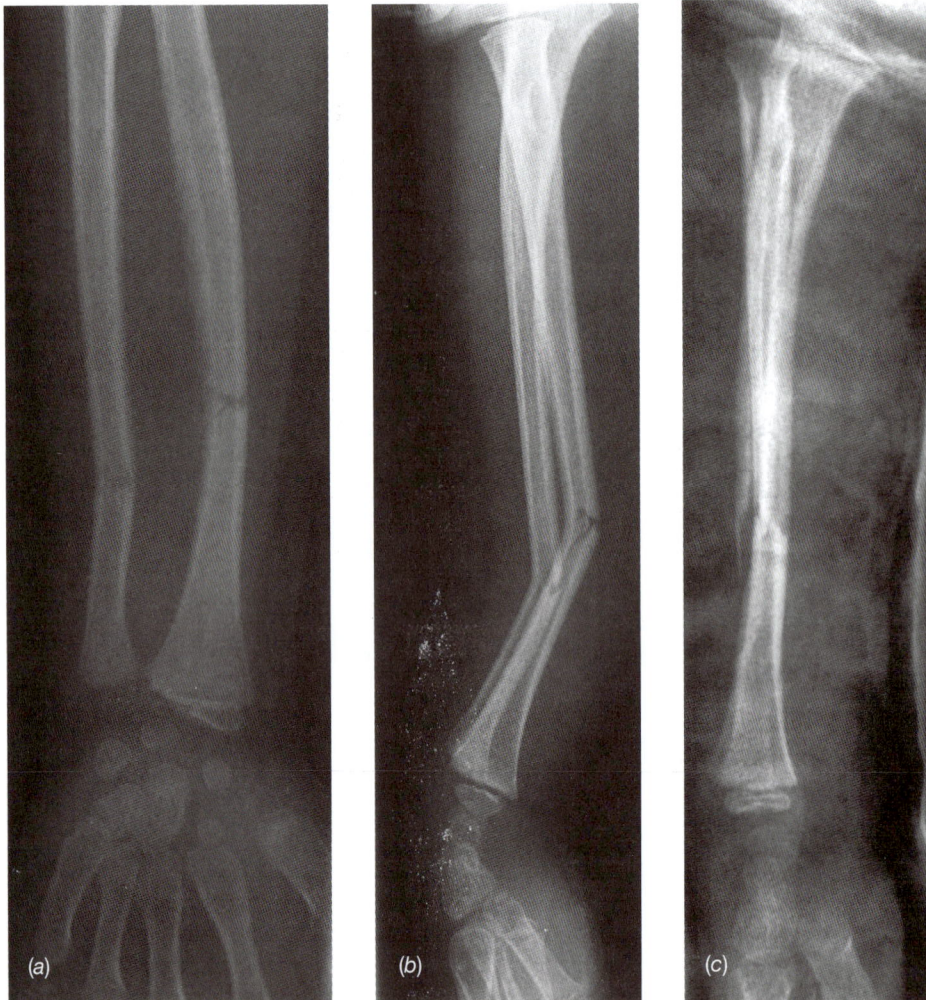

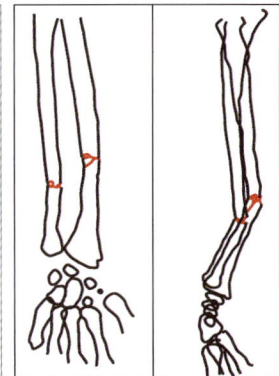

Figure 8.15 Forearm fractures are usually caused by a child falling on an outstretched hand. The anterior/posterior view shows the fracture lines of both the radius and the ulna, but with what appears to be acceptable alignment (a). The lateral view reveals malalignment (b). After reduction, the lateral plane shows good alignment (c) (NOTE: An anterior posterior view must also be taken routinely after reduction to assure anatomic reduction in all planes). (© Medical Illustrator Tommy Bolic, Sweden.)

children can be treated with closed reduction and casting but most in adults are treated with open reduction and internal fixation.

Monteggia, Essex–Lopresti and Galeazzi Fractures !

The cause of Monteggia fractures is disputed, but they are probably the result of direct trauma or a fall. The injury consists of an ulnar fracture in the proximal third, with simultaneous dislocation of the proximal radius (Figure 8.16). The injury is uncommon (7% of ulnar fractures and 0.7% of elbow injuries), but it may cause significant sequelae and can easily be overlooked. This can happen if radiographic studies of the wrist or forearm alone are taken without complete visualization of the elbow or if the position of the radial head is misinterpreted. The practitioner must also be aware of the possibility of an Essex–Lopresti fracture (which is a fracture in the radial head, with simultaneous dislocation of the distal radioulnar joint) and of a Galeazzi fracture (which is a fracture in the shaft of the radius, with simultaneous dislocation of the distal radioulnar joint). A Galeazzi fracture is caused by a fall on an outstretched arm. Because the symptoms at the wrist dominate, it is easy to forget that the elbow joint needs to be examined clinically and if necessary by radiography. Each of these forearm fracture variations are unstable, commonly missed, and lead to significant dysfunction if left untreated.

- Symptoms and signs: Symptoms and signs are severe pain localized to the forearm, significantly reduced function, swelling, discoloration, and malalignment. The clinician should carefully palpate for associated pain in either the wrist or elbow for every forearm fracture encountered. In addition the practitioner should be aware of associated injuries of neurovascular structures such as injuries to the deep branch of the radial nerve, which can be tested by assessing extension strength of the wrist. A complete neurovascular evaluation should be done before and after any attempted reduction.

Figure 8.16 Monteggia fracture. Fracture in the proximal ulna with simultaneous dislocation of the radial head. This injury may result from a fall or direct trauma. (© Medical Illustrator Tommy Bolic, Sweden.)

- Diagnosis: Diagnosis is made by radiographic examinations of the forearm on long film including the elbow joint in two planes and the wrist joint in two planes. The general rule is to always obtain radiographic images of the joint above and below a fracture. The practitioner should be aware that if a line is drawn through the shaft of the radius, it should always meet the middle of the capitulum humeri in all planes. If this is not the case, the radial head is fully or partially dislocated.
- Treatment by physician: The patient with this type of injury must be referred to an orthopedic surgeon. The fracture must be reduced and the position monitored. If reduction of the radial head is insufficient, open reduction and possibly fixation using a plate on the ulna and suturing of the ligament complex is necessary.
- Treatment by physical therapist: Treatment by a physical therapist is the same as for dislocations.

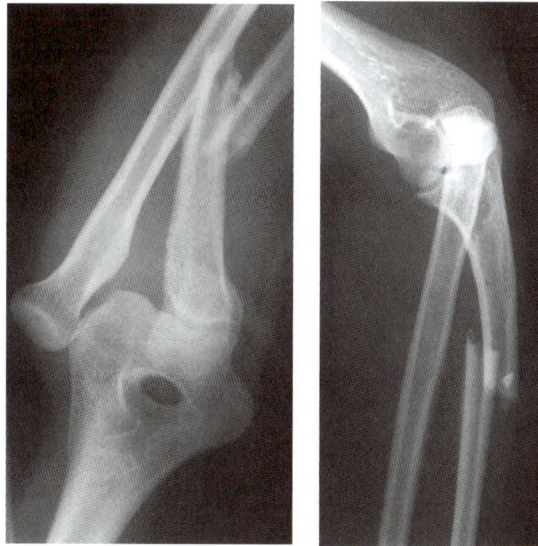

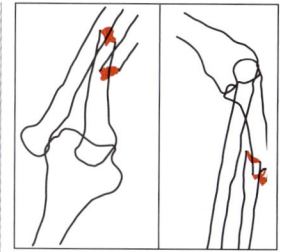

Acute Vascular and Nerve Injury !

Acute vascular and nerve injuries are severe injuries that occur primarily in combination with major upper arm, elbow, and forearm injuries. Minor trauma may also cause these types of injuries. Therefore, it is a good habit to always screen for these injuries whenever the elbow is examined. This is always necessary before and after repositioning of fractures or dislocations.

Acute vascular injury involves torn vessels with a dramatic progression of symptoms, or as thrombosis, such as in the subclavian artery with a more chronic course. Complete injuries are surgical emergencies that if left untreated can lead to limb loss, compartment syndrome or permanent dysfunction.

Acute compartment syndrome can be caused by crush injuries, fractures, or direct trauma that leads to increased pressures in a restricted fascial compartment. The pressure can be so great that it cuts of circulation and leads to muscle and nerve ischemia. If unrecognized and left untreated, permanent dysfunction or limb loss can occur.

ELBOW AND FOREARM

231

- Symptoms and signs: An acute arterial injury may be partial or complete. Pulses may be diminished or absent. Ischemic pain in the muscle is exacerbated by passive stretching. The skin may be pale and cool with poor capillary refill. The distribution of sensory or motor loss will point to specific nerve involvement. Classic presentation of a compartment syndrome involves severe ischemic pain which is described as pain out of proportion of what would normally be expected of a similar trauma, palpably tense compartment, pain to deep palpation of the compartment, pain with passive motion of the muscle compartment, and pallor. In the late phases paralysis and pulselessness may also be present but these are ominous signs.
- Diagnosis: The diagnosis of an acute arterial injury is based on a case history and a weak or absent pulse. Compartment syndrome occurs as discussed in the preceding text and can be confirmed with intra-compartmental pressure measurements.
- Pressures within 20 mm of diastolic pressure are considered positive. If the diagnosis is obvious, immediate surgical decompression should be performed.
- Treatment by physician: Patients with suspected vascular or nerve injury should be referred to a specialist for immediate evaluation and surgical repair of vascular injury or fascial release of compartment syndrome.

Overuse Injuries of the Elbow and Forearm

Babette M. Pluim[1], Mark R. Hutchinson[2], James R. Andrews[3], Kevin E. Wilk[4], and Stein Tyrdal[5]

[1]*Royal Netherlands Lawn Tennis Association, Amersfoort, The Netherlands*
[2]*University of Illinois at Chicago, Chicago, IL, USA*
[3]*Andrews Sports Medicine and Orthopaedic Center, Birmingham, AL, USA*
[4]*Champion Sports Medicine, Birmingham, AL, USA*
[5]*Oslo University Hospital, Oslo, Norway*

Occurrence

In contrast to the acute injuries, a chronic injury (generally) develops slowly and is intermittent but persistent. Chronic injuries result from repetitive overuse of a joint or muscle group and result from repeated microtrauma and stress. In sports, this is usually caused by activities that involve throwing, hitting with a racket or bat, or put strong pressure on the elbow joint, such as gymnastics. Athletes commonly complain of a gradual onset of pain with exercise and find it hard to identify exactly when it started. Typically, the symptoms become more frequent and severe and eventually inhibit the ability of the athlete to train or compete at their chosen sport.

Acute elbow injuries constitute only a small portion (3–6%) of the total number of injuries in sport; however, in throwing and racket sports and sports with weight-bearing through the upper limbs, overuse injuries in the elbow area are much more common. In a prospective cohort study of 298 junior baseball pitchers (9–14 years) over two seasons, the frequency of elbow pain was 26%. Their risk of sustaining a serious throwing injury within 10 years was 5%. The repetitive stress of high valgus and extension loads on the elbow during throwing may cause structural changes and result in minor or major elbow injury. These injuries have a tendency to become chronic. In athletes that have elbow complaints for longer than 2 months, the distinction between acute injuries and overuse injuries may have less clinical importance since the treatment protocols will be similar. Nonetheless, careful analysis of the mechanism of injury and pathophysiology is important to target rehabilitation and avoid recurrence of problems.

Most common	Less common	Must not be overlooked ❗
Lateral epicondylopathy (Tennis elbow), p. 237	Triceps tendinopathy, p. 240	Ulnar stress fracture, p. 240
Medial epicondylopathy (Golfer's elbow), p. 239	Chronic olecranon bursitis, p. 242	Olecranon stress fracture
Valgus extension overload/posterior medial impingement, p. 241	Ulnar nerve entrapment/neuropathy, p. 243	Radial nerve entrapment, p. 243
Post-traumatic stiffness, p. 247	Partial or chronic medial collateral instability	Median nerve entrapment, p. 244
	Hyaline cartilage problems, p. 245	Chronic compartment syndrome, p. 244
	Panner's disease, p. 246	
	Osteochondritis dissecans, p. 246	

Table 8.3 Overview of the differential diagnoses of overuse elbow injuries. (Reproduced with permission from the Norwegian Sports Medicine Association.)

Differential Diagnoses

Table 8.3 provides an overview of the differential diagnoses. The practitioner should be aware that the athlete might have symptoms from several parts of the elbow at the same time. Patients with symptoms from multiple tendon insertions are more difficult to treat. In young, active patients, symptoms from several joints may be a sign of systemic disease, such as rheumatoid arthritis. Symptoms of hemophilia and tumors may be seen for the first time in connection with (minor) trauma. Children may sustain apophyseal fractures. Loose bodies with or without cartilage injuries occur alone or in combination with ligament injuries or fractures.

The most common chronic elbow injuries involve the extensor tendons (lateral) and flexor tendons (medial) origins and are commonly known as tennis elbow and golfer's elbow, respectively. Overuse of the cartilage leading to osteochondritis of the capitellum, overuse of the bone leading to stress fractures, and chronic irritation of nerve tissue (entrapment syndrome) are less common but potentially disabling for athletes In the skeletally immature, overuse can lead to growth plate injuries or chronic traction of the medial epicondyle apophysis (little leaguer's elbow). Many activities may cause muscle soreness that usually resolves. When muscle pain recurs with continued use, the clinician should consider exertional compartment syndrome within the differential diagnosis. Elbow pain, stiffness, and dysfunction may also occur secondary to old injuries with untreated residual pathologies such as loose bodies or chronic degenerative changes such as spurring or intra-articular degeneration, which can lead to chronic swelling, stiffness, and pain.

Diagnostic Thinking

The goal of the examination is to make the most precise diagnosis possible that can, in turn, guide a targeted and effective treatment plan. The examination should be conducted the same way every time, according to a standardized procedure, to avoid overlooking key symptoms and signs. It is especially important for chronic injuries for the clinician to evaluate the entire kinetic chain (core strength and balance, scapular function, and shoulder function) for potential contribution to the chronic resistant elbow complaints. In athletes with chronic elbow injuries, careful attention should be made regarding old injuries, the mechanism of the initial injury, and the baseline status of the athlete prior to any recent flair of complaints. The degree of impairment in function and the athlete's level of ambition are decisive for the amount of diagnostic work that is initiated. With greater disability and persistent pain, a more thorough work-up is necessary. While tumors and pathologic processes are rare, they should be considered within the differential when elbow complaints are unrelenting despite an appropriate time frame of treatment.

Case History

The case history must be as short, clear, and concise as possible, but several factors need to be evaluated. Localization of the symptoms usually provides a good basis for evaluating which structure(s) are affected. The activity patterns and activity types that provoke symptoms should be mapped carefully. This is especially true for chronic injuries. Establishing the pattern of training or overuse is important in preventing recurrence. In throwers, the case history should include the number of tosses per event as well as the frequency of competition or events. Prior injuries of the elbow or of any site along the kinetic chain (knee, hip, core, scapular, and shoulder) are important to document to be able to optimize treatment and recovery.

Sport	Most common injury
Golf	Flexor tendinopathy
Handball (goalies)	Partial or complete medial collateral ligament injury due to valgus hyperexten-sion, valgus extension overload
Baseball	
Tennis	Extensor carpi radialis brevis tendinopathy
Javelin	Medial collateral ligament (MCL) ruptures
Gymnastics	Anterior capsular injury due to hyperextension, MCL injuries
Water skiing	Valgus injuries, chondromalacia
Weightlifting	Medial collateral ligament rupture, ulnar neuritis, biceps and triceps tendinopathy or ruptures from overuse
Volleyball	Partial medial collateral ligament injury and posterior impingement due to hyper-extension

Table 8.4 Connection between various sports and typical injuries. (Reproduced with permission from the Norwegian Sports Medicine Association.)

The typical injury panorama varies by sport (Table 8.4). The case history should, therefore, include documenting the specific sport, the athlete's position and role in the sport, and the loading pattern including throwing style. Knowledge of the various sports and the associated loads makes it easier to determine which structures will be involved. For example, many people think of the elbow joint as strictly a hinge joint allowing only flexion and extension. Elbow dynamics and the forces across the elbow during athletic participation is, however, much more complex. During an overhead throwing motion, the elbow proceeds from flexion and extension, is subjected to valgus loads during cocking and varus loads during follow-through, and rotates from neutral pronation and supination to a more pronated position. Chronic overuse can lead to failure of muscle-tendon units or stabilizing ligaments through-out this range of motion.

The activity that provokes the symptoms is often the one that causes them—for example, repetitive valgus loads lead to ten-sion of the medial elbow structures such as in baseball or javelin throwing; repetitive extensor loading such as in the back hand in tennis leads to tendinopathy of the extensor tendons (Figure 8.17). Each overuse injury has its distinct pattern, and it is easier to make the diagnosis if the patient's case history is precise.

Clinical Examination

Most structures in the elbow are superficial and easy to pal-pate. This is especially true for common chronic pathologies including medial and lateral tendinopathy, biceps and tri-ceps tendinopathy, stress fractures, and medial apophysitis. Good knowledge of anatomy is crucial to a meaningful clini-cal examination. It is recommended that the examination be performed in the same manner every time, so that necessary examinations are not overlooked or omitted. The general ex-amination technique for the elbow region is described under acute elbow injuries and includes motor testing and ligament stability testing. For chronic elbow injuries, in particular, at-tention should target sensations of crepitus or locking that may represent degenerative changes and loose bodies. Re-sisted motor function is essential to assess for tendinopathies. Several specific tests are used to come up with a more specific

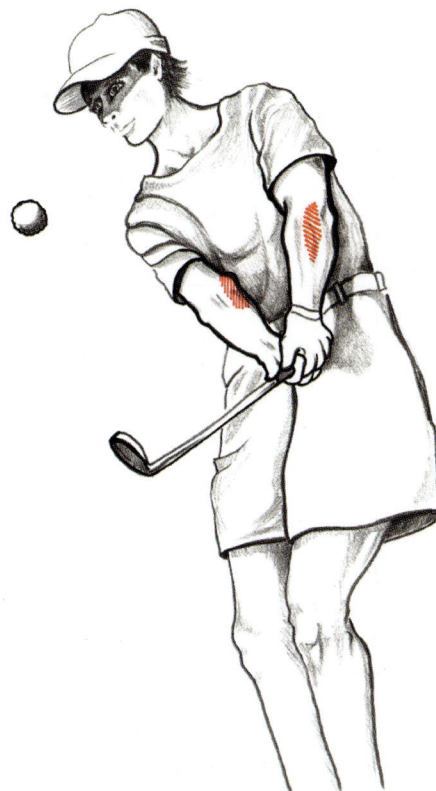

Figure 8.17 Injury mechanism in golf—medial and lateral epicondylopathy. Lateral epicondylopathy or extensor carpi radialis brevis tendinopathy can occur in the golfer's left arm, which leads the motion, whereas medial epicondylopathy could occur in the right arm, which is the trailing arm in a right-handed golfer. (© Medical Illustrator Tommy Bolic, Sweden.)

diagnosis. For chronic injuries, it is important to complete an analysis of the entire kinetic chain looking for any contributing cause to the elbow pathology.

Range of motion. One of the most common findings in patients with chronic elbow problems is a loss of motion particularly that of loss of extension. ROM is best documented by use of a goniometer, which improves reproducibility of the measure as well as provides the best assessment regarding response to treatments attempting to regain full motion.

Varus and valgus instability tests. Varus and valgus stability tests are described in the section on acute elbow injuries (see Figure 8.5a and b). In chronic cases, the same testing is performed but the findings may be more subtle. Gross instability is rarely present. Valgus stress testing, moving valgus sheer test, and milking maneuver, more commonly reproduce pain but not gross instability in chronic cases. Formal stress images documenting side-to-side differences of greater than 2 mm or MRI arthrograms that reveal leaking along the ligament and confirm chronic instability.

Valgus extension overload test. This test is used to demonstrate posteromedial osteophytes along the medial margin of the olecranon (Figure 8.18). This is seen as sequelae after years of intensive throwing, and has been described in baseball pitchers and tennis players. The test is started at full extension, placing the fingertip on the posteromedial edge of the olecranon and applying valgus stress. The test is positive if it causes tenderness and palpable posteromedial crepitation.

Radiohumeral chondromalacia. Degenerative changes in the radiohumeral joint may be demonstrated by starting at full extension (Figure 8.19). Palpate the radial head and apply steady pressure in supination and pronation. The test is positive if there is palpable crepitation, locking, and pain.

Supplemental Examinations

Radiographic imaging. A standard elbow series should be taken for all athletes with chronic elbow pain. Anterior/posterior and lateral views are standard; however, oblique radiographs will increase the probability of demonstrating accompanying joint space irregularities, degenerative spurring, calcifications, or loose bodies. A reversed axial projection allows better visualization of the posterior elbow, olecranon and trochlea. Stress radiography, as noted previously, may be helpful in identifying or quantifying instability patterns.

Fluoroscopy. Fluoroscopic imaging is helpful for acute injuries and to assist in assessing dynamic stress testing; however, standard imaging is preferred in chronic cases of elbow pathologies as the images are more distinct than fluoroscopic images.

Ultrasound. Ultrasound has become increasingly popular as a diagnostic tool for musculoskeletal injuries in both the radiology suite and the clinician's office. Joints, tendons, and muscles can be evaluated dynamically and it is quite simple to compare to contralateral side. In chronic cases about the elbow, ultrasound is most commonly used to evaluate the extent of medial or lateral tendinopathy. Another key benefit is to assist in the accuracy of therapeutic injections.

Magnetic resonance imaging (MRI). MRI is very useful for the evaluation of soft tissue lesions and can be used to assess the integrity of capsular and ligamentous structures around the elbow. If intra-articular lesions are suspected, MRI is preferred over ultrasound. MR arthrography may be useful if a total ligament

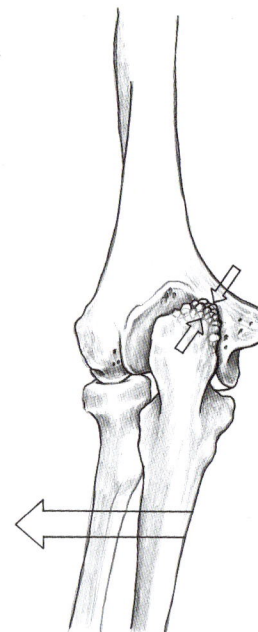

Figure 8.18 Valgus extension overload of the elbow occurs with repetitive valgus loading of the elbow as it approaches full extension. Lateral compression can lead to osteochondritis dissecans. Medial tension can lead to MCL laxity that in turn leads to posterior impingement of the lateral edge of the olecranon in the olecranon fossa. (© Medical Illustrator Tommy Bolic, Sweden.)

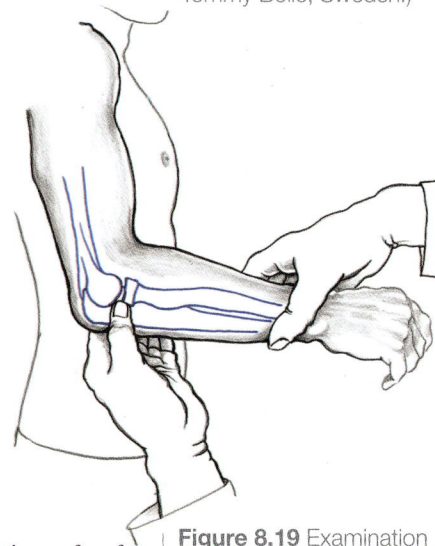

Figure 8.19 Examination of radiohumeral chondromalacia. (© Medical Illustrator Tommy Bolic, Sweden.)

rupture without dislocation is suspected. Leakage of contrast from the joint is considered an indication of a rupture. The indications are acute ruptures without dislocation or preoperative evaluation of chronic ligament injuries.

Computer tomography (CT). CT is useful for the assessment of osteochondritis dissecans, stress fractures, loose bodies, chondral, and bony lesions and the medial collateral ligament. Multidetector computer tomography (MDTC) is very efficient to detect small intra-articular loose bodies, soft tissue calcifications and avulsion fractures. CT arthrography will increase the sensitivity for the detection of loose bodies and can identify defects in the inner layer (undersurface) of the MCL.

Specific Diagnoses—Common Injuries

Tendinopathy of the Extensor Carpi Radialis Brevis (Lateral epicondylopathy)— *Tennis Elbow*

Repetitive and long-term loading (flexion/extension and pronation/supination of the wrist) creates the risk of hyaline degeneration of the origin of the extensor tendons (Figure 8.20). The histological changes are characteristic of tendinosis, and inflammatory cells are not found. Currently the names epicondylopathy or tendinopathy of the extensor carpi radialis brevis, which are more neutral with respect to cause, are preferred. The extensor carpi radialis longus and extensor carpi ulnaris are less commonly affected by the overuse tendinopathy. The incidence in general practice is 4 to 7 per 1000 patients a year, and the prevalence in the general population ranges from 1–3%, with a peak between the ages of 35 and 54. Tennis elbow is clearly more common in the mature club player than skeletally immature player. In tennis, the pathomechanics have been associated with hitting a one-handed backhand; hitting the ball late with the wrist flexed, wet tennis balls, rigid racquets and more tightly strung racquets. Players who use a two-handed backhand are less commonly affected. The prevalence increases with age and career duration. Women and men are equally affected. Athletes in other sports may also develop lateral epicondylopathy, including golfers, throwers, swimmers, fencers, and baseball players (Figure 8.21). It is likely related to the repetitive wrist extension demands in those sports. Lateral pain is five to ten times as common as medial pain.

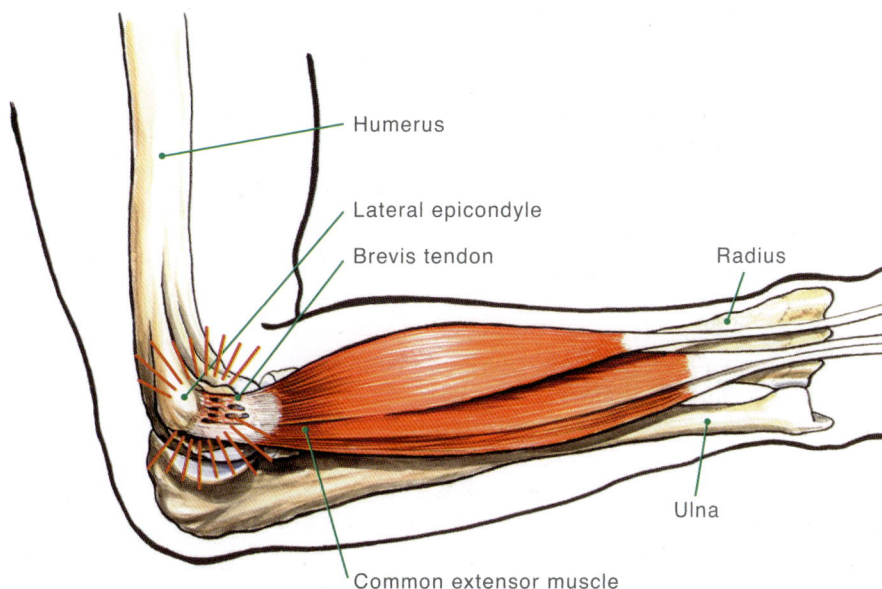

Figure 8.20 Extensor carpi radialis brevis (ECRB) tendinopathy, usually caused by repetitive and long-term loading. The extensor tendon insertions undergo hyaline degeneration that may become visible macroscopically. (© Medical Illustrator Tommy Bolic, Sweden.)

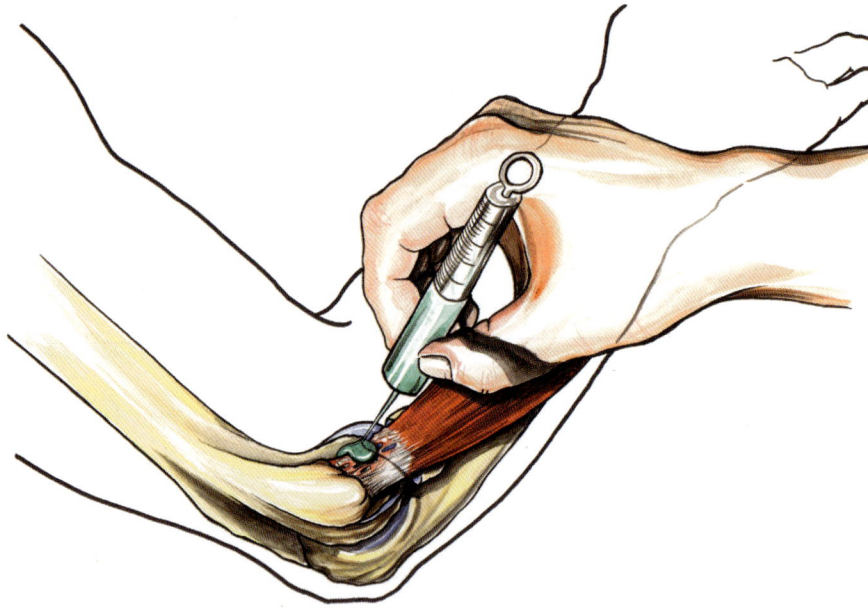

Figure 8.21 Injection technique for lateral epicondylopathy: local anesthetic is injected below the extensor longus tendon and above the extensor brevis tendon. The fluid is injected without resistance. (© Medical Illustrator Tommy Bolic, Sweden.)

- **Symptoms and signs:** The symptoms are pain on the lateral side of the elbow and weakness when using the extensor muscles of the forearm. The pain may radiate down the forearm to the fingers or into the upper arm. The onset of pain may be acute or more gradual. Simple daily activities such as turning a doorknob, shaking hands or holding a cup may be extremely painful.

- **Diagnosis:** The diagnosis is made clinically with a typical history, palpation of tenderness near the origin of the wrist extensors, and pain with resisted wrist extension. Testing of the extensor carpi radialis longus is performed with the elbow flexed to 30° and resistance given to the second metacarpal bone. The extensor carpi radialis brevis is tested with the elbow fully extended and resistance given to the third metacarpal bone. In addition, the extensor carpi ulnaris can be differentiated by resisting ulnar deviation. Sonographic examination can provide information about the severity of the diseases and may show a focal hypoechoic area, calcifications, or a discrete tear.

- **Treatment by physician:** The condition is usually self-limiting, and most patients (90%) recover within1 year. There is no single intervention that has been proven to be most efficient. Treatment begins with rest from offending activities and cold therapy (ice). Initial pain management may be supplemented with paracetamol or NSAIDs. The concept of the use of anti-inflammatory medications and corticosteroids has been debated secondary to the absence of inflammatory cells within the pathologic tissue. Nonetheless, peripheral tissues may have some associated inflammation and anti-inflammatory use has the potential of reducing pain and allowing the patient to successfully perform an eccentric training program. Counterforce bracing (tennis elbow strap), extensor stretches, and deep friction massage have been successful in some cases. Evidence to support alternative treatments of tendinopathy including extracorporeal shockwave therapy (ESWT), autologous blood injections or injections with platelet-enriched plasma have been inconclusive. In resistant cases, surgery may be indicated. Outcome studies have revealed positive outcomes when ECRB debridement is performed percutaneously, arthroscopically, or open.

- **Treatment by therapist:** Programs of eccentric strength training exercises and stretching have shown promising results. The patient should be instructed in active exercises (that are within the limits of pain), stretching, and strength training. Playing technique should be reviewed, and a fitted orthosis (possibly tape) should be applied. The benefits of electrotherapy, ultrasound, and laser therapy are poorly documented. The use of an extension brace may be attempted for pain relief.

• Prognosis: ECRB tendinopathy (lateral epicondylopathy) is frequently self-limited with most patients (90%) responding to conservative treatment and recovering within1 year. Athletes with an acute onset, a specific triggering cause, and rapid onset of therapy have the best prognosis. In resistant cases, surgery can be effective in 80–90% of patients.

Medial Epicondylopathy—*Golfer's Elbow*

Medial epicondylopathy is a disorder that is characterized by pain localized to the origin of the wrist's flexor musculature insertion onto the medial epicondyle of the humerus (Figure 8.22). It has been associated with golfer's who take a large divot or who have repetitive forearm pronation during the golf swing. It has also been correlated with climbers secondary to the repetitive flexor load associated with climbing. In tennis pain occurs with service and when hitting a forehand. Medial epicondylopathy occurs less commonly than lateral epicondylopathy. Histologically, it is the same condition as tennis elbow—that is, hyaline degeneration and tendinopathy within the tendinous tissue. Both golfers and tennis players (forehand and service) may get both conditions simultaneously.

• Symptoms and signs: Pain is present with palpation just distal to the medial epicondyle and with resisted flexion and pronation of the wrist. The clinician should always also assess the ulnar nerve secondary to its anatomic proximity in the cubital tunnel.

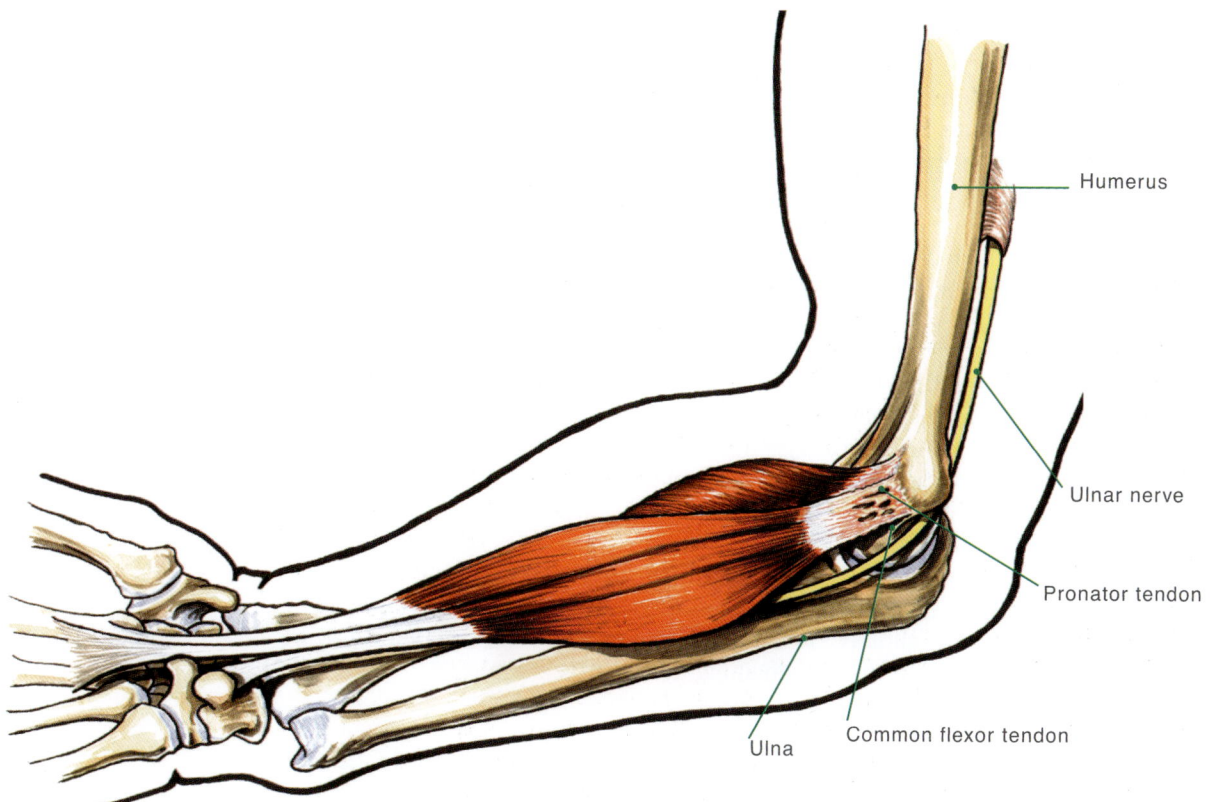

Figure 8.22 Medial epicondylopathy, usually caused by repetitive and long-term loading. The flexors and/or pronator tendon undergo hyaline degeneration that may be visible macroscopically. (© Medical Illustrator Tommy Bolic, Sweden.)

Humerus

Ulnar nerve

Pronator tendon

Common flexor tendon

Ulna

- Diagnosis: The diagnosis is made with a typical case history, palpation of tenderness at the medial epicondyle, and pain provocation when the wrist is flexed against resistance. Manual resistance of wrist flexion should be performed as well as pronation to determine whether a pronator strain has occurred. Insufficiency of the medial collateral ligament should be ruled out. Sonographic examination maybe used to confirm the diagnosis, although it may be negative in early stages or in mild cases.
- Treatment by physician: The physician should advise the patient to change his activity pattern and may recommend the player to have his playing technique and equipment reviewed. In acute cases, paracetamol and NSAIDs (preferably topical) may provide temporary, symptomatic relief. Similar to the treatment of lateral epicondylopathy, corticosteroid injections are no longer recommended. Indeed, they should always be avoided about the medial epicondyle secondary to the risk of weakening the medial collateral ligament.
- Treatment by therapist: The patient should be instructed in active exercises (that are within the limits of pain), stretching, and strength training. Playing technique should be reviewed, and a fitted orthosis (or tape) should be applied. The benefit of electrotherapy, ultrasound, or laser therapy for medial epicondylopathy is inconclusive.
- Prognosis: The prognosis for medial epicondylopathy is good when identified early and rest, ice, and physical therapy are instituted. Surgical debridement is less commonly performed compared to lateral tennis elbow surgery either because the incidence of medial symptoms is less or because conservative treatment is more effective. Patients with associated ulnar symptoms have a less favorable outcome.

Other Injuries

Ulnar Stress Fracture—*Stress Fracture in the Forearm Bone*

Stress fractures in the elbow region are rare. The practitioner should distinguish between stress fractures that are caused by repetitive stress (e.g., in javelin throwers and baseball pitchers) and separation of the growth zones around ossification centers due to trauma, such as from one particular throw. Stress fractures occur mainly in the ulnar shaft or in the olecranon. They may affect all parts of the olecranon but are usually localized to the middle portion where there is a natural lack of cartilage thickness. Although displacement of stress fractures can occur, this is rarely the case.

- Symptoms and signs: Athletes present with focal tenderness over the olecranon or directly over the bone the forearm for distal or midshaft ulnar stress fractures. Pain may be exacerbated by loading across the stress fracture as with throwing, lifting weights, or the weight-bearing demands of gymnastics.
- Diagnosis: Radiographs should be obtained but may be negative. Definitive diagnosis is confirmed with bone scan or MRI.
- Treatment by physician: Distal and midshaft ulnar stress fractures are treated conservatively. Stress fractures of the olecranon often require surgery to allow early ROM and avoid elbow stiffness. An avulsion of the tip of the olecranon can be excised with primary repair of the remaining triceps attachment.

Triceps Tendinopathy—*Posterior Tennis Elbow*

Triceps tendinopathy is a relatively uncommon problem of the posterior aspect of the elbow related to repetitive overuse and chronic intra-substance breakdown or

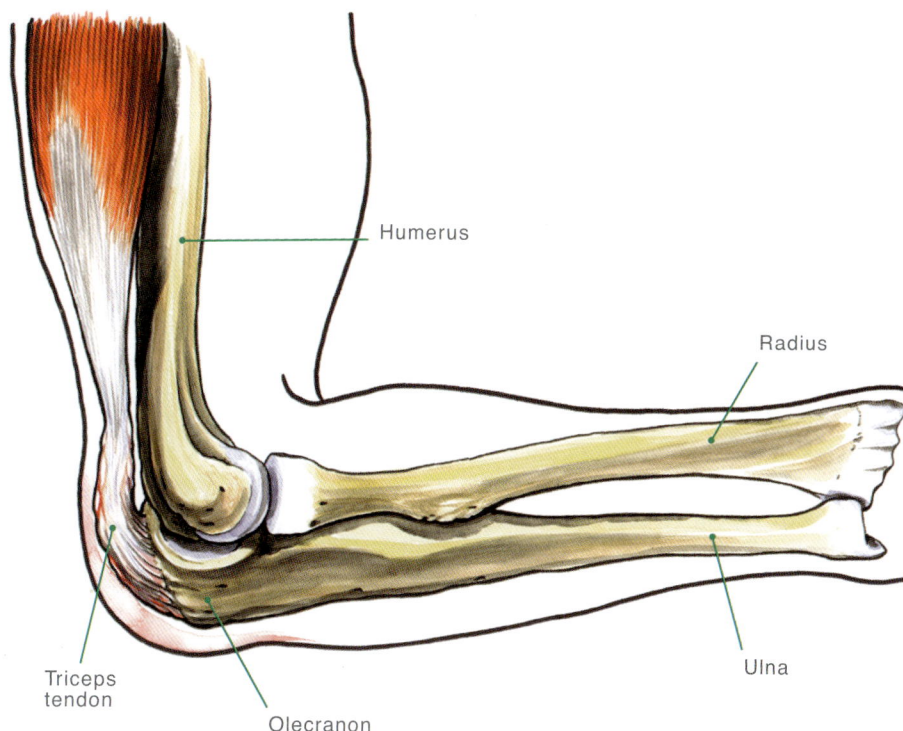

Figure 8.23 Triceps tendinopathy. The tendon becomes swollen and tender at the insertion to the olecranon. (© Medical Illustrator Tommy Bolic, Sweden.)

tendinosis in the triceps insertion onto the olecranon (Figure 8.23). It has been seen in throwers, tennis players, weight lifters, and gymnasts.

- Symptoms and signs: There is pain on active elbow extension and pain with palpation of the triceps insertion at the tip of the olecranon.
- Diagnosis: The diagnosis is usually made by typical case history and by demonstrating pain during active extension against resistance.
- Treatment by physician: Initial treatment includes rest and ice followed by modified training when the athlete returns to play. Paracetamol and NSAIDs may provide pain relief in acute cases. Any corticosteroid injections directly into a tendon or ligament are discouraged for fear of weakening collagen and leading to complete rupture. Eccentric training for tendinopathy in other locations has evidence based support and therefore should also be attempted for the triceps.
- Treatment by therapist: The patient should be instructed in active exercises (that are within the limits of pain), stretching, and strength training. Eccentric rehabilitation programs are preferred. The benefits of electrotherapy, ultrasound, extracorporal shock wave therapy, laser therapy and injection of platelet rich plasma are controversial and not clearly supported by evidenced based medicine.

Valgus extension overload/Posterior medial impingement

Both repetitive hyperextension trauma and a singular acute trauma can lead to posterior medial elbow impingement. It is commonly seen in football linemen, gymnasts, rodeo riders, weight lifters, fast-pitch softball pitchers, and shot putters.

- Symptoms and signs: Athletes typically present with pain along the posteromedial aspect of the elbow that is exacerbated with forced extension and valgus stress, In sports, the pain usually occurs during throwing or serving. There may be locking or loss of extension caused by loose bodies, bone spurs or soft tissue impingement.

- Diagnosis: The clinical test for valgus extension overload involves the clinician grasping the elbow in a flexed position. As the clinician forces the elbow into extension, a valgus stress is simultaneously applied to the elbow. The clinician palpates the posteromedial joint for tenderness and/or crepitation. Pain over the posteromedial olecranon process signifies a positive test result in true posterior impingement; there is no instability, whereas in postero–medial impingement there is. Imaging will show posterior osteophytes.
- Treatment: Conservative treatment consists of activity modification with relative rest and anti-inflammatory medication. A tape or extension brace can be used to limit maximal extension. Surgery may be necessary to remove loose bodies, deepen the fossa olecrani or even remove the tip of the olecranon. This can be done open or arthroscopically.

Chronic Olecranon Bursitis—*Student's Elbow or Miner's Elbow*

Chronic olecranon bursitis occurs with repetitive direct trauma to the olecranon that can occur in such sports as weight lifting, ice hockey or soccer goalies (Figure 8.24). There may be an acute event that did not resolve or it may simply have a gradual onset of repetitive overuse. It is often possible to palpate moveable fragments in the bursa. They usually represent synovial tissue or scar tissue.

- Symptoms and signs: Athletes present with tenderness, swelling or a soft tissue mass on the posterior aspect of the elbow. If the swelling is red and warm or the patient has associated fever, chills, or adenopathy, consideration of an infected bursa must be entertained.
- Diagnosis: Diagnosis is usually made on the basis of case history and by palpation of the enlarged olecranon bursa.
- Treatment by physician: Elbow pads are the usual first line of treatment. Occasionally, fluid can be aspirated, and cortisone injected. A compression bandage should then be applied to avoid recurrence of the swelling. Aspiration and injection may need to be repeated 2–3 times to achieve resolution. If the problem persists, surgical excision of the olecranon bursa may be indicated.

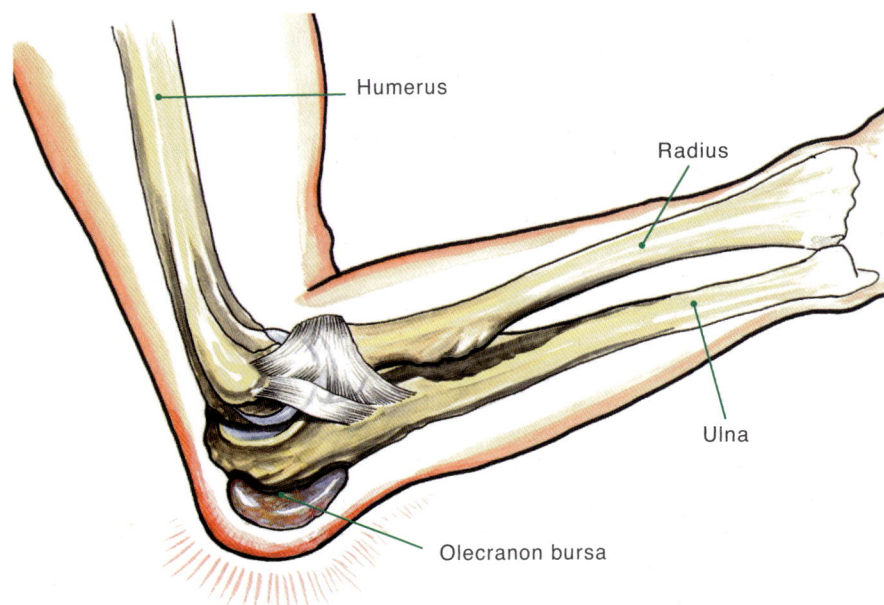

Figure 8.24 Olecranon bursitis, usually caused by a friction injury of the bursa, which swells up and becomes painful. (© Medical Illustrator Tommy Bolic, Sweden.)

Ulnar Nerve Entrapment/Neuropathy

After carpal tunnel syndrome, ulnar neuritis in the elbow (cubital tunnel syndrome) is the most common nerve entrapment syndrome. Pathoanatomic contributions include: (1) compression of the nerve due to external pressure or secondary to scar tissue from a previous-traumatic injury; (2) friction in the muscular tunnel distal to the medial epicondyle; (3) subluxation of the ulnar nerve; or (4) medial collateral ligament instability. Cubital tunnel syndrome is seen most often in tennis players, baseball players with medial collateral ligament instability, and in 60% of the patients who have had surgery for medial epicondylopathy.

• Symptoms and signs: Athletes present with paresthesia in the little finger and on the ulnar side of the ring finger. Symptoms are usually worse with elbow flexion. There is rarely pain in the hand, but achy pain radiate up the forearm up to the elbow. Tinel's sign is usually positive as the examiner taps over the ulnar nerve at Guyon's canal or over the cubital tunnel. In chronic cases, atrophy of the interossei muscles and weakened thumb-index finger pinch may be seen (Froment sign).

• Diagnosis: Diagnosis is made on the basis of classic history and by clinical evaluation. Loss of skin sensation is easiest to determine on the two outermost joints of the little finger. Strength of the ulnar hand and forearm muscles should also be assessed. The most important muscles to assess are the first dorsal interosseous, the abductor digiti minimi, the flexor digitorum profundus of the fourth and fifth digits and the flexor carpi ulnaris. Electromyography can help to localize the site of the compression and secure the diagnosis. Ultrasound imaging can show a change in diameter of the nerve and be used to support the clinical and electrophysiological diagnosis. Additional work up may be needed to rule out systemic causes of the peripheral neuropathy, such as diabetes or thyroid problems, depending on the clinical situation.

• Treatment by physician: Conservative treatment is indicated for patients with intermittent symptoms that occur with repeated elbow flexion and extension. In these cases, the activity pattern should be changed to avoid provoking symptoms. The athlete should avoid leaning on the elbows, using an armrest, and crossing the elbows. A night splint that prevents flexing of the elbow more than 30° may be of benefit. Surgery may be performed if conservative measures fail or if there is a progression of symptoms including motor weakness or atrophy. Surgical options include simple decompression and ulnar nerve transposition. Comparative studies have shown both to be equally effective. Transposition is required if ulnar nerve subluxation is also present.

Radial Nerve Entrapment !

Entrapment of the motor (deep) branch of the radial nerve, the posterior interosseous nerve, may cause symptoms that resemble lateral epicondylopathy or tennis elbow. The condition is described under several different names: atypical epicondylitis, interosseous posterior syndrome, and supinator syndrome. Nerve compression may be secondary to a tumor or ganglion, synovitis, or compression by the arcade of Frohse. Up to 5% of patients diagnosed with tennis elbow actually have a radial nerve entrapment.

• Symptoms and signs: Athletes with radial nerve entrapment have: (1) lateral, aching pain, often at night, which radiates down into the forearm and up into the upper arm and (2) weakness in the extensor muscles. The pain tends to be focused more distal and within the muscle mass compared to the more proximal classic tendinopathy of the extensor carpi radialis brevis.

- Diagnosis: Clinical presentation may be difficult to distinguish from tennis elbow. Three findings indicate entrapment of the radial nerve: (1) maximum tenderness deep in the extensor musculature 2 cm distal and 2 cm medial to the lateral epicondyle, (2) increased pain with active supination against resistance, and (3) pain provoked by extending the middle finger against resistance while the elbow and wrist are held in extension. Muscle weakness can be verified using electromyography. Ultrasound imaging can be used to localize the area of entrapment and to determine if there are any mass lesions compressing the nerve.
- Treatment: Alternative training may be attempted with a gradual resumption of sport activity. If this does not provide relief from symptoms or if the weakness progresses, surgery is usually indicated. The difficulty lies in securing a definite diagnosis.

Median Nerve Entrapment—*Entrapment of the Median Nerve in the Elbow Region* !

The median nerve can be compressed proximally at the elbow and distally in the carpal tunnel. Clinical syndromes at the proximal elbow are the anterior interosseous nerve syndrome and the pronator teres syndrome. These three conditions cause distinct symptoms. Distal entrapment in the carpal tunnel, carpal tunnel syndrome, is discussed in the chapter on wrist and hand injuries.

- Symptoms and signs: Symptoms of median nerve entrapment syndrome at the elbow are often vague and consist of discomfort and weakness. Patients with anterior interosseous nerve primarily complain of weakness in pinch. This is caused by weakness of the flexor pollicis longus muscle and the radial part of the flexor digitorum profundus muscle. Patients with pronator teres syndrome offer complaints of pain and paresthesias in the first three fingers and radial aspect of the ring finger. Symptoms may be exacerbated by activity and more specifically to repeated resisted pronation. Reduced skin sensation is a late sign.
- Diagnosis: Tinel's sign is usually positive with percussion over the course of the nerve proximally in the forearm. For anterior interosseous nerve syndrome, pain can sometimes be provoked by flexion of the middle finger against resistance (the elbow is held at 90°). In pronator syndrome, pronation of the forearm against resistance and flexion and supination of the elbow against resistance (weight lifting) may provoke the symptoms. Ultrasound imaging and electromyography can be used to support the diagnosis.
- Treatment by physician: The physician can recommend a period of alternative training. Surgery can also be considered if this does not provide relief from symptoms.
- Prognosis: The outcome of surgery is usually good with full return to athletic activity in about 6 weeks.

Chronic compartment syndrome !

Chronic compartment syndrome in the forearm is a condition that can be seen in sports characterized by prolonged static muscle contractions, including motor cycle riders in road racing or motocross, gymnasts and mountain climbers. The condition can be difficult to distinguish from entrapment of the radial or median nerve. If the athlete tries to continue despite and through the pain, it is possible that exertional related compartment syndrome can convert to an acute compartment syndrome that requires urgent surgical release.

- Symptoms and signs: Athletes present with gradually increasing cramp-like pain with prolonged static arm use, reduced strength, and paresthesia in the forearm and all fingers. Muscle compartments may be tense to palpation. In cases of chronic exertional compartment syndrome, symptoms are relieved a few minutes after cessation of activity. If resolution does not occur then emergent fascial release may be necessary to address an acute compartment syndrome.

- Diagnosis: The diagnosis is based upon the history and palpation of tight forearm muscles. While the exact pathophysiology is not known, the most common presentation is of increased intra-compartmental pressures confirmed by pre- and post-exertional compartment pressure measures. Baseline pressures and normal pressures are usually below 20 mmHg. Exertional measures that are above 25 mmHg or elevate 10 mmHg more than baseline are considered positive.
- Treatment: Surgical fasciotomy is warranted if the symptoms are so severe that the athlete cannot continue to perform. Associated injuries including direct muscle trauma or stress fractures should be ruled out and treated prior to considering surgical release.
- Prognosis: Good after surgery. Athletes can usually return to sport 2–4 weeks after fasciotomy. Nerve release usually requires another two weeks of recovery.

Hyaline Cartilage Problems

Injuries and problems of the hyaline cartilage covering the articular surface of the elbow joint may result from long-term overuse, a genetic predisposition, or previous-traumatic injury to the joint itself (Figure 8.25a–c). Ultimately, the cartilage loss can lead to pain, stiffness, locking, and permanent disability. Posteromedial osteophytes along the medial margin of the olecranon may develop as sequelae of years of intensive throwing. Degenerative changes in the radiohumeral joint are seen in throwers in a variety of sports (e.g., baseball, javelin, tennis, etc) and after hyperextension trauma (e.g., handball goalies). Loose bodies may develop from previous intra-articular fractures, posterior olecranon osteophytes and impingement or from osteochondritis dissecans.

- Symptoms and signs: Symptoms of cartilage injury include pain, swelling, grinding sensations or crepitus, as well as catching or locking. Initially the pain may be mild and associated with the unique demands of the sport. Over time, the pain may progress and may linger after play. Ultimately, loss of motion and pain can lead to disability and inability to play.
- Diagnosis: If a patient has an appropriate history and physical findings, radiographic studies should be obtained and carefully reviewed. In younger patients comparative radiographs of the contralateral elbow may be helpful. Careful inspection may reveal osteophytes, joint space narrowing, subchondral sclerosis, radiolucencies,

Figure 8.25 Cartilage injury in a boxer's elbow. A loose body is located in the posterior and lateral portion of the humerus (a). It is attached by scar tissue (b) and is arthroscopically removed using grasping forceps (c). (Reproduced with permission from the Norwegian Sports Medicine Association.)

ELBOW AND FOREARM

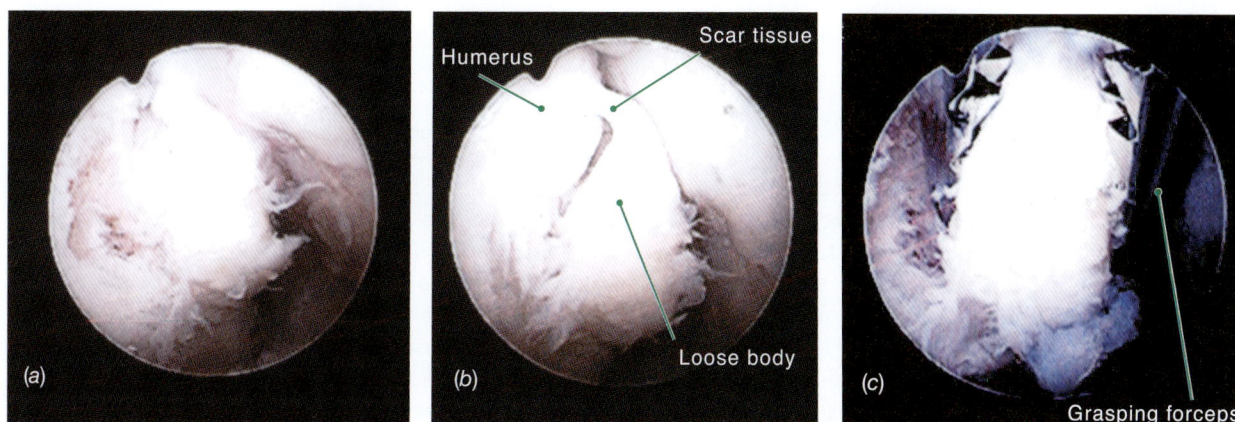

or loose bodies. MRI arthrography is more sensitive but ultimately the extent of cartilage injury can only be made via direct inspection with arthroscopy.

• Treatment by physician: Initial treatment is focused on optimizing motion and pain control. Paracetamol and NSAIDs may provide pain relief when the condition is acute. Intra-articular corticosteroid injections may be attempted for synovitis, but the long-term effect is controversial. A history of mechanical locking usually indicates an intra-articular loose body that can be surgically removed (by arthroscopy or arthrotomy). With focal full thickness cartilage lesions, cartilage restoration procedures have been attempted with guarded prognosis regarding return to play.

• Treatment by physical therapist: The main goal of rehabilitation is to optimize range of motion.

• Prognosis: The prognosis is dependent on the extent of cartilage damage as well as the loading, throwing, upper extremity weight-bearing demand of the athlete. Simple loose bodies are easily removed with arthroscopy and generally have a good prognosis. More extensive cartilage damage implies a poor prognosis with increased risk of developing progressive arthritis, stiffness, swelling and pain. Athletes with high loading and throwing demands and larger lesions may have to give up their sport.

Panner's Disease

Panner's disease is an osteochondrosis of the developing humeral capitellum and usually affects the dominant elbow of 5–10-year-old children. The blood supply to the growth plate of the capitellum is temporarily disrupted, resulting in cell death (avascular necrosis) and flattening of the capitellum. This is followed by rebuilding and remodeling in the course of 1–2 years.

• Symptoms and signs: Symptoms are pain on the outer side of the elbow that worsens with activity and eases during rest. The elbow may feel stiff and the child may be unable to completely straighten the elbow. Pronation and supination may be limited. Although the symptoms gradually go away in the course of 1–2 years as the bone matures, it may leave the child with some limitation of elbow extension.

• Diagnosis: X-rays are required to confirm the diagnosis and may show flattening of the humeral capitellum and an irregular and fragmented growth plate. MRI may show a diffuse capitellar signal. After healing, the capitellum will have resumed its normal shape and X-rays will have normalized.

• Treatment: Panner's disease is usually self-limiting and activity modification is commonly all that is required. In severe cases a cast or splint is prescribed for 3–4 weeks in order to allow the arm to rest completely and control pain. Long-term prognosis in most patients is excellent, although a long time is required for healing and some extension limitation may remain.

Osteochondritis Dissecans

Osteochondritis dissecans (OCD) of the elbow is a disorder in which the subchondral bone of the capitellum is compromised potentially leading to a loose or unstable osteochondral fragment. OCD occurs after the capitellum has ossified. This is an older age group than those seen with Panner's disease with an age range of 10–15 years old. Pathophysiology is felt to be the result of repetitive axial loading, repeated valgus stress, and a tenuous blood supply that in turn leads to avascular necrosis, subchondral fracture, and fragmentation. The humeral capitellum is affected most often, although lesions have also been found in the radial head, trochlea and olecranon. It occurs most commonly in throwing sports, gymnastics, racquet sports, and weight lifting. OCD occurs more frequently in males than females with a male incidence of 4 per 1000.

- **Symptoms and signs:** Common presenting symptoms are pain, catching and locking, and, in advanced cases, there may be crepitations. In the beginning, the pain may only be a slight discomfort during sports, which disappears at rest. Over time, the pain worsens, is dull, is difficult to localize and may linger after play. There may be stiffness of the elbow, with limited extension. The joint may be warm and swollen. In about 20% of the cases, the onset is acute; in the remainder of the cases, the symptoms develop gradually.

- **Diagnosis:** A history with intermittent locking of the elbow joint is common. Clinical examination may reveal local tenderness over the lateral elbow, swelling and joint effusion, loss of extension with the classic catching and locking of the elbow. The valgus extension overload test and the test for radiohumeral chondromalacia are usually positive. Anterior/posterior, lateral and oblique radiographic views should be taken and assessed for lesions in the capitellum and loose bodies. Documenting the state of the growth plate maturation as well as fragmentation of the medial epicondyle is also important. Radiographs may reveal no abnormalities in the early stages, but later they may show a sclerotic rim of subchondral bone, irregular ossification, and/or a bony defect adjacent to the articular surface. Only 30% of loose bodies can be seen on plain radiographs. In late stages, lateral radiographs may show flattening of the capitellum. MRI is used for early detection of OCD and for determining the size and extent of the lesion. MR arthrography is useful for detecting loose bodies. CT scanning can detect changes in body anatomy.

- **Treatment by physician:** In the acute phase, activity modification, rest, cooling with ice and pain killers will provide pain relief. An elbow sling can temporarily be used. Further treatment depends on the characteristics of the lesion. Rest is appropriate for patients with stable lesions, an open capitellar growth plate, localized flattening of the subchondral bone and good elbow function. Patients with a fragmented lesion, a closed growth plate, or more than 20° loss of elbow function do not respond well to conservative treatment and may benefit from surgery. Surgery may consist of arthroscopic debridement and fragment removal, subchondral bone drilling, fragment fixation, or osteochondral autograft transplantation.

- **Treatment by therapist:** The patient should be instructed in active exercises that do not provoke pain. Post-operative rehabilitation will be discussed in more detail in the rehabilitation section.

- **Prognosis:** The prognosis varies based on the extent of lesion and the age of patient. Younger patients have a better prognosis while extensive lesions with larger loose fragments have a less favorable prognosis. The athlete's sports demand may also play a role in prognosis with throwers and particularly gymnasts having a poorer prognosis.

Post-traumatic Stiffness

Reduced ROM in the elbow joint is common after elbow injury and may lead to chronic disability. For activities of daily life a ROM from 30° extension to 130° flexion and a combined pronation and supination of 90° is sufficient. Certain sports like gymnastics may require full extension to optimally perform while other athletes in less motion dominant sports may be able to continue their career with some reduction of end range of motion. The elbow is particularly vulnerable to post-traumatic stiffness, because of the unique tendency of the joint capsule to shrink, the short distance between the capsule and the muscle, and the great risk of comminuted fractures. The degree of stiffness is usually related to the extent of the trauma and how well the congruence of the articular surface can be recreated.

• Symptoms and Signs: The main sign is stiffness in the elbow. Pain may suggest intra-articular injury, such as osteoarthritis.
• Diagnosis: Diagnosis is made clinically. Standard radiographs of the elbow joint in two planes are necessary to demonstrate any osseous joint injury or bony block. A goniometer is used to measure the total arc of motion. Use of the goniometer is especially helpful when monitoring patient's response to treatment.
• Treatment by physician: The key to avoidance of post-traumatic stiffness is early ROM as soon as ligament, muscle tendon, and osseous stability allows. The physician should avoid immobilizing the elbow for longer than 4–6 weeks unless absolutely necessary. If results are unsatisfactory, surgery may be indicated. If surgery is required, it is usually necessary to release the adhesions by cutting the capsule anteriorly and/or posteriorly.
• Treatment by physical therapist: The physical therapist should give the patient instruction for selfexercises and should check to make sure that the exercises are done correctly, without provoking pain. Qualified therapists may attempt mobilization.

Rehabilitation of Elbow Injuries

Kevin E. Wilk[1], Leonard C. Macrina[2], James R. Andrews[3], Mark R. Hutchinson[4], Babette M. Pluim[5], and Stein Tyrdal[5]

[1]*Royal Netherlands Lawn Tennis Association, Amersfoort, The Netherlands*
[2]*Champion Sports Medicine, Birmingham, AL, USA*
[3]*Andrews Sports Medicine and Orthopaedic Center, Birmingham, AL, USA*
[4]*University of Illinois at Chicago, Chicago, IL, USA*
[5]*Royal Netherlands Lawn Tennis Association, Amersfoort, The Netherlands*
[6]*Oslo University Hospital, Oslo, Norway*

Introduction

Participation in sport can lead to numerous acute and chronic injuries to the elbow as has been presented in the first two sections of this chapter. Rehabilitation after these injuries is often challenging because of the unique anatomy and the significant stress applied to this complex during sport-specific movements. The ultimate goal of any rehabilitation program is to gradually restore function and return the athlete to symptom-free competition as quickly and safely as possible. Functionally, the elbow plays an integral role in the interplay between the shoulder, wrist/forearm, and hand. Successful rehabilitation of the elbow joint must address this kinetic linking to compliment the usefulness of the elbow in sport. Rehabilitation requires a thorough knowledge of the anatomy, biomechanics, and pathomechanics of athletic participation. Each patient should be progressed individually, driven by the patients symptoms and the clinicians continuous assessment during the rehabilitation process. A team approach including family, physician, therapist, athletic trainer, coach, and biomechanist should be instilled to enhance compliance and promote proper

	Goals	Measures
Acute phase	1 Minimize the effects of immobilization	1 ROM within 75% contralateral extremity
	2 Re-establish non painful range of motion	2 Diminishing pain scale
	3 Decrease pain and inflammation	3 Progressing from isometric to isotonic activities
	4 Prevent muscular atrophy	
	5 Do not overstress healing tissues	
Intermediate phase	1 Enhance elbow and upper extremity mobility and function	1 Full Range of motion
	2 Improve strength and endurance	2 Minimal pain or tenderness
	3 Re-establish neuromuscular control and dynamic stability	3 Good manual muscle test (at least 4/5)
Advanced Rehab Phase	1 Progression of activities prepare the athlete for sports	1 No pain or tenderness
	2 Progress strength, power, endurance and neuro-muscular control	2 Full, pain-free range of motion
	3 Sports specific functional drills in preparation for return to sport	3 At least 70% strength compared to contralateral extremity per isokinetic test or handheld dynamometry

Table 8.5 Acute elbow injury rehabilitation goals and measures. (Reproduced with permission from the Norwegian Sports Medicine Association.)

education and management related to the rehabilitation process. Continuous feed-back/communication is a necessary step in the promotion of a successful outcome regarding elbow injury. In this chapter an overview of several non-operative and post-operative rehabilitation programs will be discussed for specific sport injuries, which use a multiphased, progressive rehabilitation approach based on current scientific research and clinical experience to ensure a safe and timely return to sport.

Goals and Principles

Rehabilitation after elbow injury or elbow surgery follows a sequential and progressive multiphased approach. The ultimate goal of elbow rehabilitation is to return the athlete to his or her previous functional level as quickly and safely as possible. Several key principles must be addressed when the athlete's elbow is rehabilitated: (1) the effects of immobilization must be minimized, (2) healing tissue must not be overstressed, (3) the patient must fulfill certain criteria to advance through each phase of the rehabilitation, (4) the program must be based on current scientific and clinical research, (5) the process must be adaptable to each patient and his or her specific goals, and (6) the rehabilitation program must be a team effort between the physician, physical therapist, athletic trainer, and patient. Communication between each team member is essential for a successful outcome. The following section will provide an overview of the rehabilitation process after elbow injury and surgery. Discussion of rehabilitation protocols for specific pathologies will follow this general overview. In Table 8.5, the rehabilitation goals and criteria for entering each phase of rehabilitation are summarized.

Phase I: Acute Phase

The first phase of elbow rehabilitation is the immediate motion phase. The goals of this phase are to minimize the effects of immobilization, re-establish non-painful ROM, decrease pain and inflammation, and retard muscular atrophy. The rehabilitation specialist must not overstress healing tissues during this phase.

Early ROM activities are performed to prevent loss of motion and joint contractures, nourish the articular cartilage and assist in the synthesis, alignment, and organization of collagen tissue. ROM activities are performed for all planes of elbow and wrist motions to prevent the formation of scar tissue and adhesions. ROM activities can be performed passively using only the examiners assistance to gain motion or dynamically as the athlete uses their own motor power to gain motion (examples are shown in Figures 8.26 and 8.27).

Re-establishing full elbow extension is the primary goal of early ROM activities. These interventions are designed to minimize the occurrence of elbow flexion contractures. The elbow is predisposed to flexion contractures because of the intimate congruency of the joint articulations, the tightness of the joint capsule, and the tendency of the anterior capsule to develop adhesions after injury. More specific stretching techniques that target either loss of flexion or extension may be of particular benefit (examples are shown in Figures 8.28 and 8.29). The brachialis muscle also attaches to the capsule and crosses the elbow joint before becoming a tendinous structure. Injury to the elbow may cause excessive scar tissue formation of the brachialis muscle as well as functional splinting of the elbow.

Gentle joint mobilizations may be performed during this early phase of rehabilitation as tolerated. These mobilization techniques are used to neuromodulate pain by stimulating Type I and Type II articular receptors. Posterior glides with oscillations are performed in the midrange of elbow motion to assist in regaining full extension.

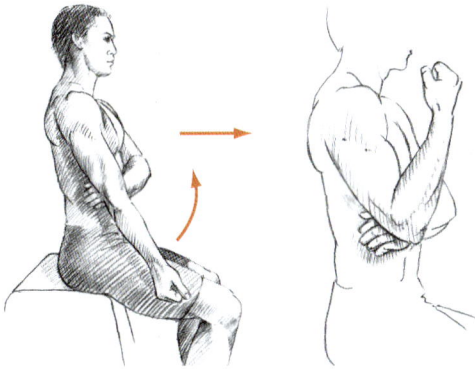

Figure 8.26 Dynamic elbow flexion

- Starting position: Allow the elbow to fall into full extension. Gravity will assist and elbow extensors can be fired to maximally extend the elbow. Next, the athlete should actively, with contraction of the biceps and elbow flexors, maximally bend/flex the elbow. Maximum flexion can be assisted by using the opposite hand.
- Practice resistance with tension band or dumbbells.
(Reproduced with permission from the Norwegian Sports Medicine Association.)

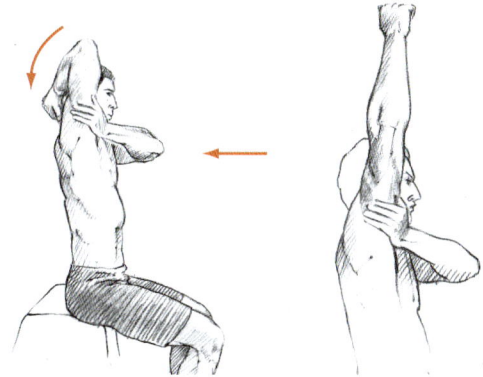

Figure 8.27 Dynamic elbow extension

- Starting position: Begin with the humerus elevated 180° with the elbow pointing to the ceiling and the elbow bent in maximum flexion. From this position the athlete can extend the elbow using triceps contraction until reaching full extension.
- Practice resistance with tension band or dumbbells.
(Reproduced with permission from the Norwegian Sports Medicine Association.)

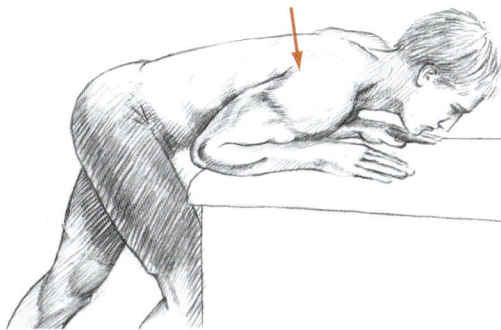

Figure 8.28 Targeted stretching to increase elbow joint flexion

- Starting position: Begin by facing a table or counter top and place the athlete's forearms flat on the surface. As the athlete leans forward and lowers his chest to the table, he can stretch elbow extensors and gain improved ROM in flexion.
(Reproduced with permission from the Norwegian Sports Medicine Association.)

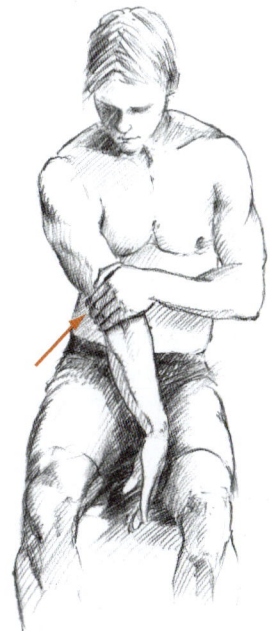

Figure 8.29 Targeted stretching to gain elbow extension

- Starting position: The athlete is asked to extend the arm as much as possible and place their back of their hand on the inner surface of their contralateral thigh. With the hand locked into place, they can reach across with their opposite hand and gently pull and stretch the elbow into fuller extension.
(Reproduced with permission from the Norwegian Sports Medicine Association.)

Aggressive mobilization techniques are not used until the later stages of rehabilitation when pain has subsided. If the patient continues to have difficulty achieving full extension using ROM and mobilization techniques, a low-load, long-duration (LLLD) stretch may be performed to produce a creep of the collagen tissue, which will result in tissue elongation. This intervention is extremely beneficial in regaining full elbow extension. The athlete lies supine with a towel roll placed under the brachium to act as a cushion and fulcrum. Light resistance exercise tubing is applied to the wrist of the patient and secured to the table or a dumbbell on the ground (Figure 8.30). The patient is instructed to relax as much as possible during the duration of the treatment, which should be performed for 10–15 min at a time and 3–4 times per day. The amount of resistance applied should be of low magnitude to enable the athlete to tolerate the stretch for the entire duration without pain or muscle spasm.

The aggressiveness of stretching and mobilization techniques is dictated by the healing constraints of the involved tissues as well as the amount of motion and end-feel of the joint complex. If the patient exhibits a decrease in motion and hard end-feel without pain, aggressive stretching and mobilization techniques may be used. Conversely, a patient exhibiting pain before resistance or an empty end-feel progression should be slow with gentle stretching.

Cryotherapy and high-voltage pulsed stimulation may be performed as required to assist in reducing pain and inflammation. Once the acute inflammatory phase has passed, moist heat, warm whirlpool, and/or ultrasound may be used at the onset of treatment to prepare the tissue for stretching and improve the extensibility of the capsule and musculotendinous structures.

The early phases of rehabilitation must also focus on retarding muscular atrophy. Subpainful and submaximal isometrics are performed initially for the elbow flexors and extensors, and for the wrist flexor, extensor, pronator, and supinator muscle groups. Isometrics should be performed at multiple angles for 2–3 sets of 10 repetitions, holding each contraction for 6–8 s. Shoulder isometrics may also be performed during this phase with caution against internal and external rotation exercises if painful. Alternating rhythmic stabilization drills for shoulder flexion/extension/horizontal abduction/adduction and shoulder internal/external rotation are performed to begin re-establishing proprioception and neuromuscular control of the upper extremity.

Phase II: Intermediate Phase

Phase II, the intermediate phase, is initiated when the patient exhibits full ROM, minimal pain and tenderness, and a good (4 over 5) manual muscle test of the elbow flexor and extensor musculature. The emphasis in this phase includes enhancing elbow and upper extremity mobility, improving muscular strength and endurance, and re-establishing neuromuscular control of the elbow complex.

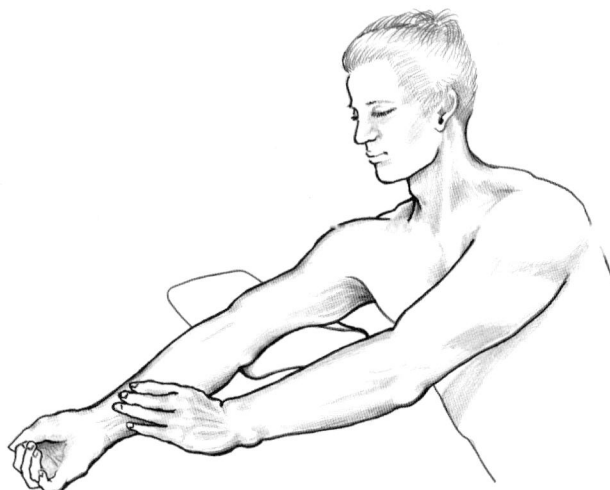

Figure 8.30 A low-load, long-duration (LLLD) stretch may be performed to produce a creep of the collagen tissue. (Reproduced with permission from the Norwegian Sports Medicine Association.)

Stretching exercises are continued to maintain full elbow flexion and extension. Mobilization techniques may be progressed to more aggressive grade III techniques as needed to apply a stretch to the capsular tissue in end range. Flexibility activities are progressed during this phase to focus on wrist flexion, extension, pronation, and supination excursion. Shoulder flexibility is also maintained in athletes with emphasis on flexion, external and internal rotation, and horizontal adduction.

Strengthening exercises are advanced during this phase to include isotonic movements. Emphasis is placed on elbow flexion and extension, wrist flexion and extension, and forearm pronation and supination. The weight of the arm is initially used before progressing to a 1-pound dumbbell. Resistance is then advanced in a controlled progressive resistance fashion by 0.5 kg per week to gradually stress the involved tissues. The shoulder and scapular muscles are also included in a progressive resistance program during the later stages of this phase. The Thrower's Ten program is an example of a program that emphasizes strengthening the shoulder external rotators and scapular muscles. Shoulder internal and external rotation are performed with exercise tubing at 0° of abduction; standing scaption with external rotation (full can), standing abduction, prone horizontal abduction, and prone rowing are all included in this phase. The overall goal is to restore neuromuscular control and strength of the surrounding musculature.

Muscular endurance activities are also incorporated during this phase of the rehabilitation program. High repetition, low resistance dumbbell exercises, and the upper body ergometer may be used to accomplish these goals.

Neuromuscular control exercises are initiated in this phase to enhance the ability of the muscle to control the elbow joint during athletic activities. These exercises include proprioceptive neuromuscular facilitation exercises with rhythmic stabilizations and slow reversal manual resistance elbow/wrist flexion drills.

Phase III: Advanced Rehabilitation Phase

The third phase involves a progression of activities to prepare the athlete for sport participation. The goals of this phase are to gradually increase strength, power, endurance, and neuromuscular control to prepare the athlete for a gradual return to sport. Specific criteria that must be met before the athlete enters this phase include full non-painful ROM, no pain or tenderness, and strength that is 70% of the contralateral extremity.

Advanced strengthening activities during this phase include aggressive strengthening exercises emphasizing high-speed and eccentric contractions as well as plyometric activities. Strengthening exercises are progressed to include the Advanced Thrower's Ten Exercise Program. These exercises were designed based on numerous electromyographic studies to strengthen all of the shoulder, scapular, elbow, and wrist muscles that are used during upper extremity athletic activities. Internal and external rotation exercises with exercise tubing are progressed to a functional position of 90° of shoulder abduction with 90° of elbow flexion. Exercises should be performed at both slow and fast speeds. Scapulothoracic exercises are progressed to include prone horizontal abduction at 100° and full external rotation as well as prone rows into external rotation.

Elbow flexion exercises are advanced to emphasize eccentric control of elbow extension. The biceps muscle is an important stabilizer during the follow-through phase of overhead throwing to eccentrically control the deceleration of the elbow, preventing pathologic abutting of the olecranon within the fossa. Elbow flexion can be performed with elastic tubing to emphasize slow and fast speed concentric and eccentric contractions. Aggressive strengthening exercises with weight machines are also incorporated during this phase. These most commonly begin with bench press,

ELBOW AND FOREARM

seated rowing, and front latissimus dorsi pull-downs. Neuromuscular control exercises are progressed to include side-lying external rotation with manual resistance. Concentric and eccentric external rotation is performed against the clinician's resistance with the addition of rhythmic stabilizations. This manual resistance exercise may be progressed to standing external rotation with exercise tubing at 0° and finally at 90° of shoulder abduction. Plyometric drills are an extremely beneficial form of exercise for training the upper extremity musculature. The physiologic principles of plyometric exercise use an eccentric prestretch of the muscle tissue, thereby stimulating the muscle spindle to produce a more forceful concentric contraction. Plyometric exercises are performed using a weighted medicine ball during the later stages of this phase to train the upper extremity musculature to develop and withstand high levels of stress. Plyometric exercises are initially performed with two hands performing a chest pass, side-to-side throw, and overhead soccer throw. These may be progressed to include one-hand activities such as 90/90 throws, external and internal rotation throws at 0° of abduction, and wall dribbles. Specific plyometric drills for the forearm musculature include wrist flexion flips and extension grips.

Return to Activity Phase

The final phase of elbow rehabilitation, the return to activity phase, allows the athlete to progressively return to full competition using an interval sport program. Sport-specific functional drills are performed to prepare the athlete for the stresses involved with each particular sport.

Before an athlete is allowed to begin the return to activity phase of rehabilitation, he or she must exhibit full ROM, no pain or tenderness on clinical examination, a satisfactory isokinetic test, and a satisfactory clinical examination. Isokinetic testing is commonly used to determine the readiness of the athlete to begin an interval sport program. Athletes are routinely tested in elbow flexion/extension, shoulder internal/external rotation, and shoulder abduction/adduction at 180° and 300° per second.

Upon achieving the criteria that have been outlined, a formal interval sport program should be initiated. The athlete may perform the program three times per week with a day off in between each step. If the athlete experiences symptoms at a particular step within the program, he or she is instructed to regress to the prior step until symptoms subside. Typically, the athlete should warm-up, stretch, and perform one set of their exercise program before throwing, followed by two additional sets of exercises after throwing. This provides an adequate warm-up but also ensures maintenance of necessary ROM and flexibility of the elbow joint.

9 Wrist, Hand, and Fingers

Hand and Wrist Injuries

Jan-Ragnar Haugstvedt[1], Vaughan Bowen[2], and Loris Pegoli[3]

[1]*Østfold Hospital Trust, Moss, Norway*
[2]*University of Calgary, Calgary, AB, Canada*
[3]*University of Milan, Milano, Italy*

Occurrence

Hand injuries represent 20–25% of all injuries that are treated at emergency clinics. The injury panorama ranges from "innocent" sprains to complicated fracture dislocations. An injury causing stiffness of the wrist and eventually a fusion as a result of a missed diagnosis and treatment, results in a higher medical disability as compared to loss of the anterior cruciate ligament in the knee. Therefore, the physician must strive for good and accurate diagnostics and treatment of hand injuries.

Differential Diagnoses

Table 9.1 provides an overview of current diagnoses of hand and wrist injuries. The most common is a sprained wrist. The athlete falls and puts her hands out for protection resulting in twisting, stretching, or hyperextension. This may cause pressure, contusion, and partial overstretching of the skin, the musculature, and/or the capsule apparatus.

Major forces may cause ligament or skeletal injury. A partial rupture of a ligament causes pain, swelling, and discoloration of the skin, but no signs of instability or fracture. A fracture is more common in elderly people than in youths, the quality of the bone being better in younger people. Depending on the force at the time of the injury, a fracture in the distal forearm or a ligament injury within the carpus with or without a fracture in the carpal bones may be the result. The practitioner must

Most common	Less common	Must not be overlooked ❗
Wrist sprain, p. 262	Distal radius fracture, p. 263	Scaphoid fracture, p. 266
	Wrist fracture	Dislocations in the wrist
	Carpal bone fracture, p. 267	
	Ligament injury in the wrist, p. 268	
	Injury of the distal radioulnar joint	
	Carpal dislocation, p. 270	
	Distal radioulnar joint injury, p. 271	
	Triangular fibrocartilage complex rupture, p. 272	
	Tendon injury, p. 273	
	Nerve entrapment, p. 274	

Table 9.1 Overview of diagnoses of injuries of the hand and wrist. (Reproduced with permission from the Norwegian Sports Medicine Association.)

The IOC Manual of Sports Injuries, First Edition. Edited by Roald Bahr.
©2012 *International Olympic Committee. Published 2012 by John Wiley & Sons, Ltd.*

examine for a scaphoid fracture that may not always be possible to diagnose at the first examination. However, if overlooked and untreated, these fractures may cause changes in the wrist and carpus that might require future surgery.

People in all age groups may sustain a distal radioulnar joint (DRUJ) and/or triangular fibrocartilage complex (TFCC) injury, and a wrist fracture at the same time. These injuries are often overlooked as an arthroscopic examination, considered the gold standard for diagnosing intra-articular injuries of the radiocarpal joint, is rarely performed in acute injuries. Studies have shown that more than 50–70% of patients with a distal radius fracture simultaneously sustain a TFCC injury or an intracarpal ligament lesion. If a patient is suffering from wrist pain after healing of a fracture of the distal radius, these structures are generally the ones that are affected.

Tendon injuries at the wrist level without a simultaneous open wound are very rare. Occasionally, the patient's extensor pollicis longus (EPL), the long extensor tendon of the thumb, spontaneously ruptures.

Diagnostic Thinking

Some injuries in the hand and wrist present with obvious abnormalities such as: laceration, bruising and swelling, skeletal deformity, and postural abnormalities. These features usually make the problem easy to localize and evaluate. Other injuries, particularly those involving the wrist, may have very subtle features making them difficult to diagnose.

Upon initial inspection of the hand and the wrist, the physician should look for a deformity. If this is found, it may indicate a fracture or a dislocation. A classic "dinner fork" or "bayonet" deformity on the distal forearm is typical of a distal radius fracture. Swelling or discoloration should be looked for, indicating bleeding from a fracture hematoma or a ligament rupture. If there is deformity and/or swelling, the patient should be referred for a radiographic examination. The same is true if signs of instability are found during a clinical examination.

Generally, however, deformity, major swelling, or definite signs of instability are uncommon—quite unlike tenderness from direct palpation. Tenderness to palpation is suggestive of a sprain (an injury of the soft tissue and the capsule apparatus). A sprain is an exclusion diagnosis used when the patient indicates mild discomfort and pain and when no evidence of instability or skeletal damage is found during an objective examination including radiography.

If a patient returns several days or a week after an injury complaining of pain and discomfort, a referral for radiographic and clinical examination by specialists should be performed.

After falling on his hand with great force, the patient may suffer from major swelling over the wrist, pain caused by attempts at hand motion, and tenderness on palpation with or without simultaneously passive motion of the wrist. These symptoms and findings make it necessary to examine the patient for a ligament injury in the wrist or a carpal bone fracture. It is not possible to distinguish between a fracture and a ligament injury by means of a clinical examination, and the patient may often have a combination of the two. The patient must be referred for a radiographic examination in which additional views (other than standard posteroanterior (PA) and lateral views) may be ordered. The area of maximum tenderness should be described to guide the radiologist in focusing on the area that needs to be examined. If the patient is suspected of having, or is found to have, a carpal bone fracture or a ligament injury in the wrist, then the injury was likely caused by great force, and the patient should be referred to a specialist for further diagnostics and treatment.

In the case of an open wound, particularly one caused by a sharp object, the possibility of a tendon and/or nerve injury should always be considered. Each individual tendon should be examined separately. An injury of the median nerve will cause reduced sensation in the thumb, index finger, middle finger, and the radial half of the ring finger. The athlete will typically soon notice this and seek medical advice. However, an ulnar nerve injury at the wrist level might be overlooked. This will cause a significant reduction in the function of the intrinsic muscles of the hand, with muscle atrophy as the result. Therefore, an accurate examination of sensory function and muscular activity in any case of a possible nerve disturbance should be performed. The nerve injury can be diagnosed by *clinical examination,* and reduced nerve function should not be "observed." If reduced function in one or more tendons is found by clinical examination, or the patient indicates reduced sensation in all or part of her hand, she *must* immediately be referred to a hand surgeon for further treatment.

When a patient presents with an unusual injury with unexpected severity of symptoms, the "medical problem" may be a way of explaining poor performance. Some patients present with what they perceive to be an injury, but in reality the problem is related to some other cause.

Case History

The mechanism of injury—such as a fall on an extended (Figure 9.1) or flexed hand while the hand is kept in a pronated or supinated position; a direct blow; or twisting of the wrist, with a strong extension or flexion motion in the wrist—may reveal something about the type of injury that was sustained. Other indicators are a deformity, a crunchy sound, or major swelling that occurred at the time of the injury. Have discoloration or reduced tendon or nerve function occurred after the injury?

Injuries may result from single or repetitive events. In acute injuries, details of the mechanism of injury may suggest which anatomical structures have been damaged. A fall on the outstretched hand produces forced hyperextension of the wrist, whereas other types of injury may be associated with excessive flexion, ulnar or radial deviation, or rotation, all mechanisms of possible fractures, ligament injuries, or dislocations in the hand and wrist.

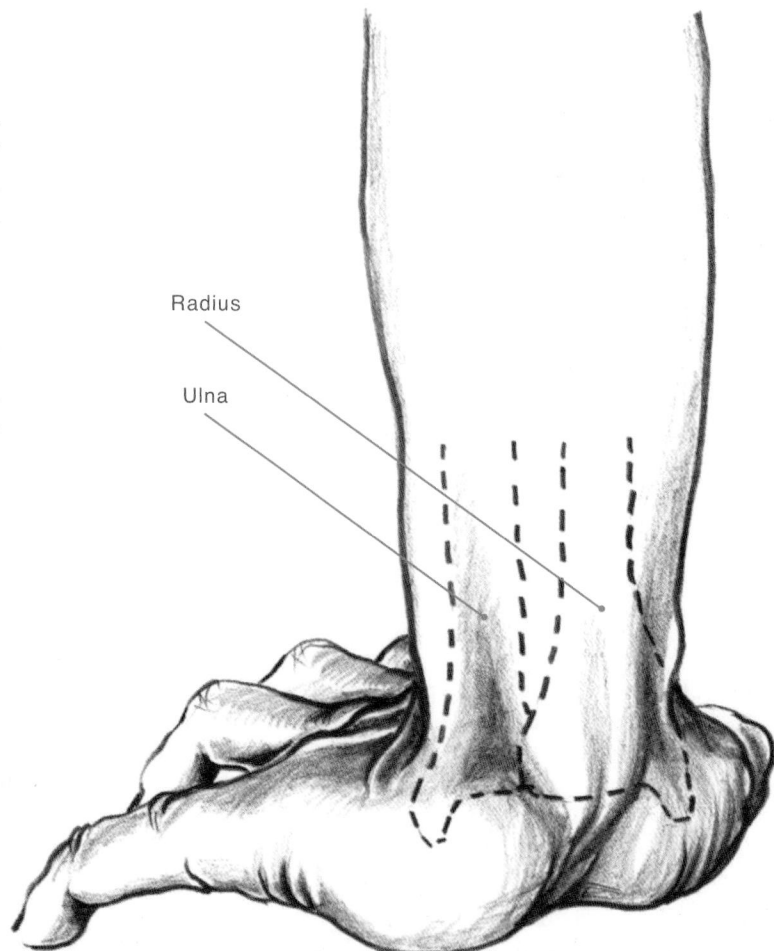

Figure 9.1 Typical mechanism for wrist injury: falling on an extended hand can cause a distal radius fracture, a fracture in the carpus, or a ligament injury in the wrist. (© Medical Illustrator Tommy Bolic, Sweden.)

Radius

Ulna

A fall on an outstretched hand may cause a fracture through the distal radius. The type of injury caused by a fall depends on (1) the position of the hand at the time of the fall, (2) the direction and intensity of the force that occurs during the fall, and (3) the age of the person falling (related to bone quality). In addition to a fracture, the athlete may also sustain ligament injury that causes instability in the wrist and/ or in the DRUJ.

A fracture of the scaphoid is the most common type of fracture in the carpal bones. As in the case of a fracture of the distal radius, the mechanism of injury is a fall on an extended hand. A scaphoid fracture is more common in young, active men. Children and the elderly may, however, sustain them as well. A scaphoid fracture may be associated with other injuries in the wrist. An isolated fracture of other carpal bones is rare. A dorsal avulsion fracture or a transverse fracture may be seen in the triquetrum. The hook of the hamate (projecting into the palm of the hand) may be injured playing golf or as a result of a strong blow to a racket or club that a player is holding in his hand. A direct blow to the ulnar side of the hand may also cause a fracture of the pisiform bone.

Several ligaments stabilize the various carpal bones to each other and to the radius and the ulna. Depending on the mechanism, direction, and force of the injury, various parts of the ligaments may be torn. Falling on a hyperextended, ulnar-deviated, and slightly pronated hand may cause a significant ligament injury in the wrist. The ligament injury may occur alone or in combination with a fracture or dislocation of one or more carpal bones. The scapholunate (SL) ligament may rupture, there may be a fracture of the scaphoid, a rupture of the lunotriquetral (LT) ligament, a fracture of the triquetrum, a dislocation of the lunate, or a combination of these. Other ligaments may also be injured, but they are rarely diagnosed and treated as isolated injuries.

The TFCC is one of the most important structures in the wrist, consisting of a meniscus-like structure, the articular disk, and the palmar and dorsal radioulnar ligaments. The TFCC may be injured, frequently seen when there is a combination of rotation and hyperextension of the wrist, or in combination with a fracture of the distal radius.

Clinical Examination

The chief aim of clinical examination should be to find the exact location of the problem. In the hand, look for abnormalities in size, shape, and posture. In open wounds pay close attention to functional loss and postural abnormalities distal to the injury. When examining the painful wrist, imagine the skeleton as a pile of stacked boxes covered by soft-tissue layers like an onion. Answer the question, "In which container and in which layer does the problem lie?"

Inspection. Start by looking. Note any alteration in contour, either in the soft tissues or bony skeleton. Is the color and texture of the skin altered in any way? Are there any surface imperfections such as scars or draining sinuses? A classic "dinner fork" or "bayonet" deformity on the distal forearm is typical of a distal radius fracture. Swelling or discoloration should be looked for, indicating bleeding from a fracture hematoma or a ligament rupture.

Palpation. Next, gently palpate (Figure 9.2). Are the texture and contour of the soft tissues and the skeleton normal? Is there tenderness on superficial or deep palpation? Is the temperature elevated? Be systematic; start at the radial styloid and work

(a)

(b)

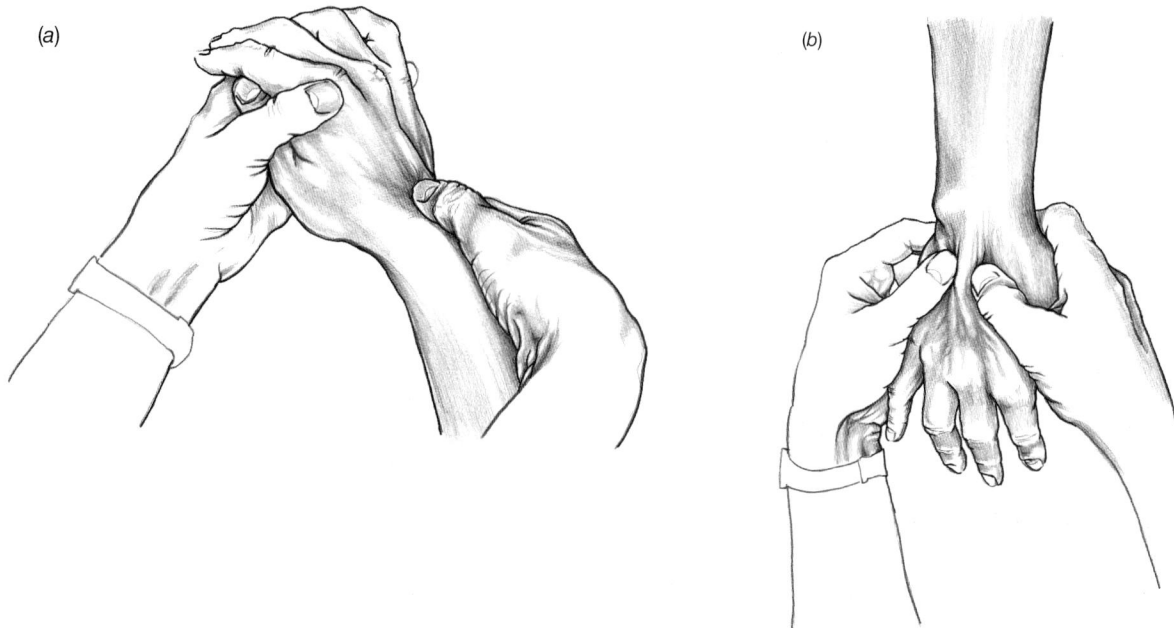

your way over the dorsum to the ulna styloid. Next, turn the hand over and palpate across the palmar surface. Knowledge of anatomy is essential; with practice it is possible to identify almost every important structure.

Next, proceed to the examination of specific areas. In the wrist, test the DRUJ for stability. Then check the extensor carpi ulnaris (ECU) tendon for instability (seen in tennis players). Palpate for tenderness and clicks around the TFCC, a positive fovea sign (TFCC injuries) and feel for tenderness on the proximal articular surface of the triquetrum (ulna carpal impingement). Flex the wrist and see if pisotriquetral glide is associated with pain, instability, or crepitus (arthritis or intra-articular fractures). Press on the hook of hamate, which will be tender in acute fractures and nonunions (a problem seen in batting injuries). Check the body of hamate and the body of capitate for tenderness. Palpate for tenderness in the anatomical snuffbox—at the scaphoid waist (scaphoid nonunion), proximally toward the SL joint (static and dynamic dissociations), and distally toward the scaphotrapezoidtrapezium (STT) joint (arthritis). Move the thumb basal (carpometacarpal, CMC) joint, examining it for pain, crepitus, arthritis, fractures, and instability. In the hand, check each digit in turn and examine each anatomical structure: bone, joint, tendon, pulley, nerve, vessel, and skin.

Range of motion and strength. Range of motion and strength should then be checked in all directions and the results should be compared to the noninjured side. Wrist extension is normally about 70°, flexion is about 80°, and pronation and supination are both close to 90°. Normally, the wrist can be deviated radially to approximately 20°; ulnar deviation is approximately 30°.

Special tests. There are more specific tests for tenosynovitis, possible dislocations, and instabilities, these tests require regular training to perform and could be difficult to interpret. There are also tests to investigate nerve problems (compression and local injury). These tests should be reserved for a specialist to perform and interpret.

Grip strength. Testing grip strength is a useful diagnostic tool. This is best done objectively using a dynamometer. Several readings should be taken from both the symptomatic and normal sides. Results not only tell us about grip strength but can also be used as a measure of consistency, an important parameter if there is concern about secondary gain.

Figure 9.2 The entire wrist, the dorsal and volar side, should be systematically examined such as here for (a) scapholunate (SL) and (b) lunotriquetral (LT) ligament injuries. (© Medical Illustrator Tommy Bolic, Sweden.)

Neurovascular status. Nerve injury in the hand or at the wrist level reduces sensation in all or part of the hand. In addition, there may be a loss of motor (muscle or tendon) function. By touching a finger with a cotton ball, a paper clip, or some similar object, or by testing for two-point discrimination, it is possible to examine for sensation. This is typically tested for on the palmar side (flexor side) of the hand. The *median nerve* innervates the entire thumb, the index finger, the middle finger, and the radial side of the ring finger. The motor branch of the median nerve (at the wrist level) may be injured after it branches off the trunk of the median nerve, resulting in lost opposition of the thumb (i.e., the thumb cannot be flexed and rotated into the hand so that the pulp of the thumb comes into contact with, and in the same plane as, the pulp of the little finger) (Figures 9.3a–9.3d).

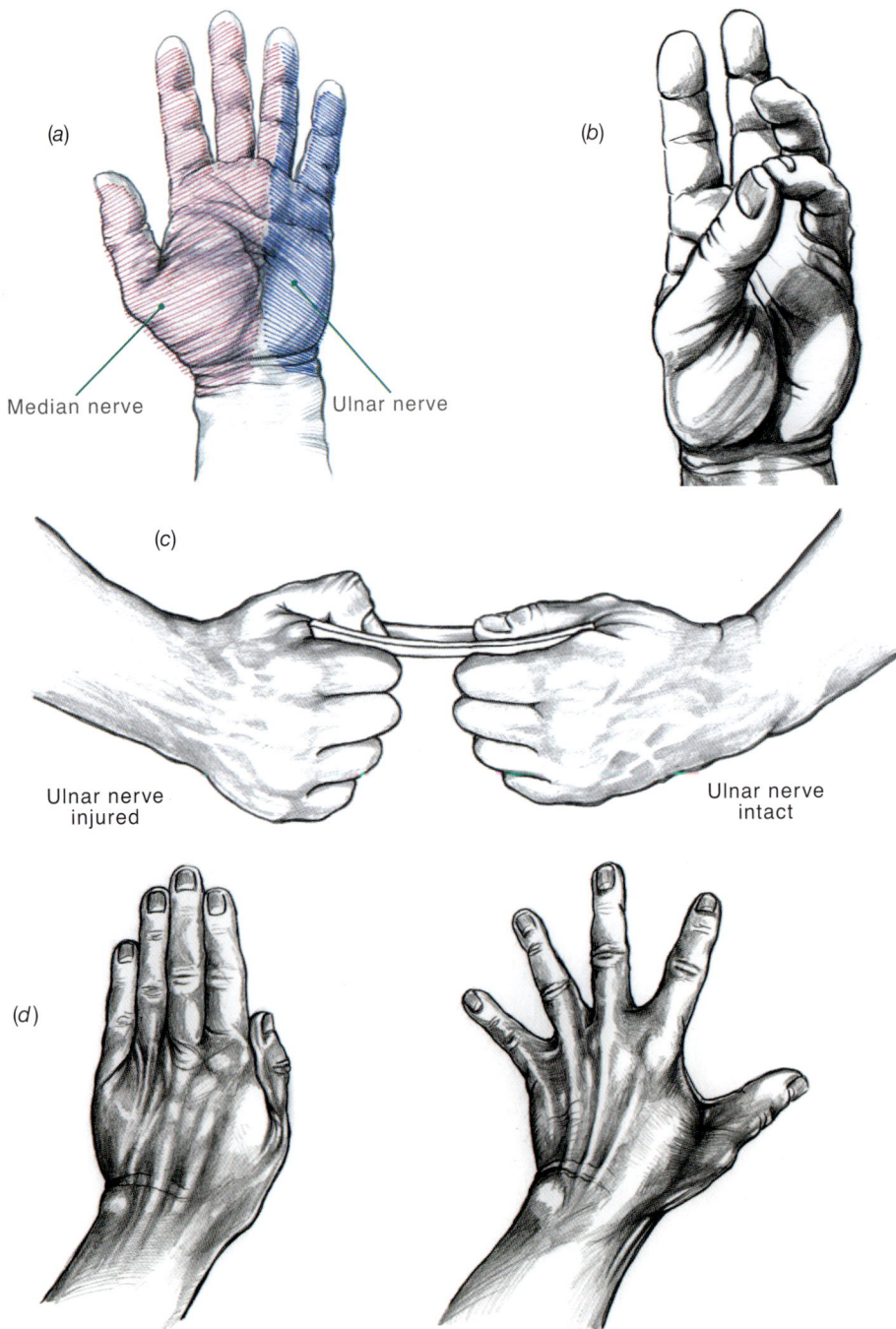

(a)

Median nerve   Ulnar nerve

(b)

(c)

Ulnar nerve injured   Ulnar nerve intact

(d)

Figure 9.3 Median and ulnar nerves—innervation areas and functional tests. The median nerve innervates the thumb, the index finger, the middle finger, and the radial side of the ring finger (red) on the palm of the hand, whereas the ulnar nerve innervates the ulnar side of the ring finger and the little finger (blue) (a). If the median nerve is intact, the thumb can be rotated and flexed toward the pulp of the little finger (function of the opponens pollicis muscle) (b). If the ulnar nerve is intact, it can activate the adductor pollicis longus muscle, so that it is possible to hold a piece of paper between an extended thumb and the index finger. If the ulnar nerve is injured, the paper can be held using the flexor muscles of the thumb (which are innervated by the median nerve) (c). An intact ulnar nerve allows normal abduction and adduction of the fingers (d). (© Medical Illustrator Tommy Bolic, Sweden.)

If there is an injury to the *ulnar nerve* at the wrist level, the patient may lose sensation in the little finger and in the ulnar side of the ring finger. In addition, there may be a loss of function of the intrinsic muscles of the hand. The ability of the patient to adduct and to abduct her fingers, as well as to extend her proximal interphalangeal (PIP) joints (function of the intrinsic muscles) (Figure 9.3) will be reduced. In addition, there is reduced strength in the adductor pollicis longus muscle, leading to loss of the ability to hold a piece of paper between the thumb and index finger when the thumb is extended and pressed against the index finger's metacarpophalangeal (MCP) joint.

Tendon function. A tendon rupture at the wrist level without a simultaneous open wound is rare. However, after a radius fracture, the tendon of the EPL may rupture at Lister's tubercle (a bony prominence on the dorsal side of radius proximal to the wrist). To test for EPL muscle function, the patient is asked to place the palm of his hand on a surface and then lift his thumb from the surface. This is not possible if the tendon is torn (see Figure 9.14).

Additional Examinations

Plain radiographs. A radiographic examination is necessary if the patient has pain, swelling, and tenderness in the wrist after being injured, and especially if a patient returns several days or a week after an injury complaining of pain and discomfort. A wrist fracture is usually visible on "standard" radiographs (PA and lateral views should always be taken as a minimum). On the lateral view, the articular surface of the distal radius normally shows a 10°–12° of palmar tilt. In the PA view, the length of the ulna and the radius should be the same. The radioulnar inclination (examined on an PA view, reflecting the angle between a line running through the distal radial and ulnar corner of the radius and another line perpendicular to the longitudinal axis of the radius) should be about 22°. In some cases it is useful to obtain comparative images of the other side. Beware, however, of the patient who is very sore or apprehensive because he/she may not position the wrist correctly for these views to become positive.

Specialized plain radiographs. These are used to examine particular areas not well seen on regular films. Focused PA and lateral views are obtained for injuries to digits. There are also specialized views for the scaphoid and the pisotriquetral joint. A carpal tunnel view may show the hook of hamate, and a clenched fist view and/or motion study series may show intercarpal instability.

If injuries of the wrist are suspected, at least four different radiographic views of the carpus should be performed. These include:

- A PA view: This is obtained when the styloid process of the ulna and the styloid process of the radius are as far apart as possible.
- A true lateral view: When the palmar edge of the pisiform is between the palmar edge of the capitate and the scaphoid, the view is within about 10° of a true lateral view.
- A PA view with the hand in a clenched fist and at maximum ulnar deviation: This allows the scaphoid to extend, producing a good image of the bone and making a possible dissociation between the scaphoid and the lunate more easy to see.
- An oblique view with the hand in 45° of pronation.

Other imaging methods:

- CT scans are used when detailed information is needed on a part of the skeleton and is the best technique for finding fractures in the distal carpal row. The DRUJ

can also be demonstrated using this technique that also can be used for three-dimensional images for planning management of comminuted fractures or complicated malunions.
- Tc99 MDP bone scans are a good screening test for bone and joint abnormalities where a positive scan indicates affection of the wrist. Negative scans indicate that the problem probably lies in the soft tissues rather than in the skeleton.
- An arthrogram can be used for determining if there is a tear or perforation in the ligamentous structures in the wrist.
- Ultrasound can be used for locating cystic lesions or other soft-tissue abnormalities such as tendon or pulley ruptures.
- Arthroscopy is done in patients where there is a need to directly see the state of the articular cartilage, the intercarpal ligaments, or the TFCC. Arthroscopy may be used to make or to confirm a diagnosis and should be considered the gold standard for investigation and diagnosis of intra-articular wrist conditions. Very often the treatment could be carried out at the same time as an arthroscopically assisted procedure.
- MRI is highly dependant of the equipment and the radiologist interpreting (reading) the images. MRI has excellent sensitivity and specificity; it should not be used, however, as a screening tool for determining the cause of a patient's wrist pain.

Common Injuries

Wrist Sprain

Wrist pain may be caused by a fall on an extended hand, a direct blow to, or twisting of, the wrist, in combination with an extension or flexion motion. Most people who fall and injure themselves do not seek medical assistance because the subjective symptoms are moderate and temporary. Generally, there is a contusion of the soft-tissue or a joint-capsule injury. The accompanying swelling and pain subside after a few days.

Wrist sprain is an exclusion diagnosis when the X-rays do not demonstrate direct signs of a fracture or indirect signs of a ligament injury (dislocation of intact bones). Pain caused by a capsule injury is subjective and varies from patient to patient.

- Symptoms and signs: Patients experience pain, tenderness, swelling, and limited range of motion.
- Diagnosis: If there are signs of discoloration, swelling, malalignment, or instability, the patient *should* be referred for a radiographic examination. Likewise if no objective signs of a fracture or a ligament injury are found during the clinical examination; however, if the patient indicates that he has a great deal of pain, he *should* be given a radiographic examination. If pain and swelling do not improve within a week, the patient *should* be referred for radiographic examinations. A clinical examination may demonstrate swelling and reduced range of movement, but a sprain is often an exclusion diagnosis after additional examinations have excluded other injuries.
- Treatment by physician: The recommended treatment is PRICE, nonsteroidal anti-inflammatory drugs (NSAIDs), and a possible immobilization in a cast for a few days. Gradual retraining and possibly taping or use of a brace when resuming sport activities are also recommended.
- Treatment by physical therapist: A physical therapist may tape the patient or create special custom made splint(s) to facilitate gradual return to sports activities (Figure 9.4).
- Prognosis: The prognosis for a simple sprain is good, and if other injuries have been excluded, sport activities may be resumed within 1–2 weeks.

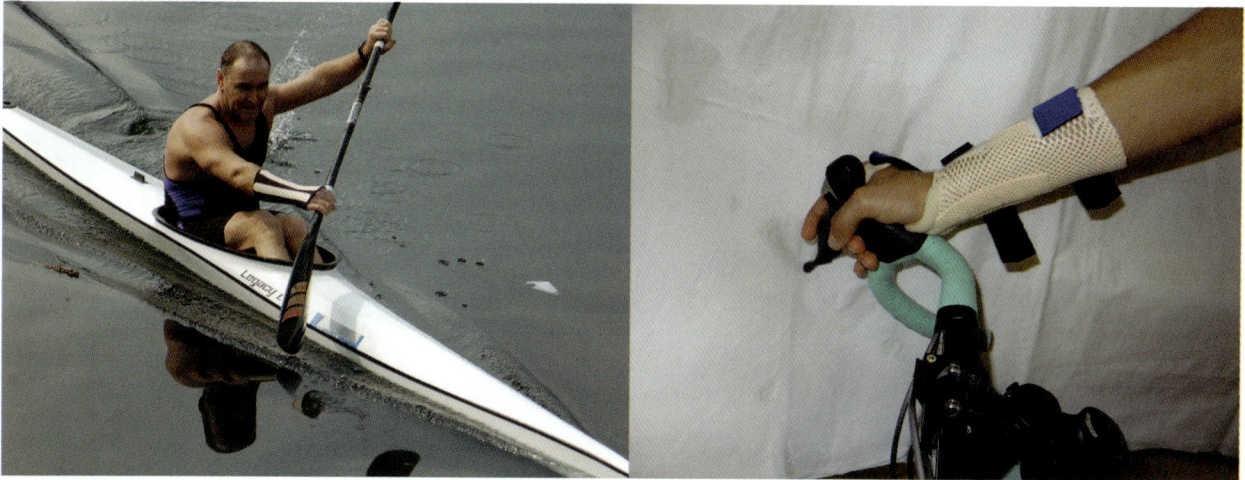

Figure 9.4 Splints are custom made in order to facilitate early return to sports activities. (Reproduced with permission from the Norwegian Sports Medicine Association.)

Other Injuries

Distal Radius Fracture—*Fracture Through the Lower Portion of the Radius*

A fall on an extended hand may cause a fracture through the distal radius. The type of injury caused by a fall depends on (1) the position of the hand at the time of the fall, (2) the direction and magnitude of the force, and (3) the age of the person who falls (related to bone quality). The most common type of fracture (a Colles fracture) runs through the distal metaphysis of the radius, causing a dorsal angular deformity known as a "dinner fork" deformity (Figures 9.5a and 9.5b). A palmar angulated fracture of the distal radius is known as a Smith fracture (or a reverse Colles fracture)(Figures 9.6a and 9.6b). Young people participating in different sports activities often sustain high-energy fractures of the distal radius. These fractures may be highly comminuted displaced fractures.

A Colles fracture (or Colles-type fracture) often causes shortening of the radius, dorsal angulation of the distal articular surface (normally 10°–12° of palmar tilt), reduction of the radioulnar inclination (measured on an PA view as the angle between a line running through the distal radial and ulnar corner of the radius and another line that is perpendicular to the longitudinal axis of the radius; normally 22°), or a combination of these malalignments. Normally, nearly 80% of the force from the wrist is transferred to the forearm over the radiocarpal joint, whereas more than 20% is transferred over the ulnocarpal joint. Changes in normal anatomy alter the transfer of force in the wrist, and the cartilage will undergo wear and tear in various locations. If there is shortening of 5 mm (or more), a change occurs in the DRUJ and the TFCC. If dorsal angulation in the radiocarpal joint increases, there is a transfer of force in the ulnar direction. Major portions of the remaining force transferred between the radius and the wrist will be between the dorsal side of the scaphoid and the radius, causing cartilage degeneration in that location. To prevent this, correction of malalignment caused by a fracture should be obtained.

- Symptoms and signs: The patient has pain from the wrist, where a classic deformity (Figures 9.5 and 9.6) is often found. The hand may be held in a slightly flexed and pronated position, while the distal ulna seems to protrude somewhat. There is swelling and tenderness, and palpation will cause pain. Attempts to use the hand cause pain and difficulties, and symptoms of compression of the median nerve and/or the ulnar nerve may exist. There may be tenderness and possibly instability of the distal end of the ulna.

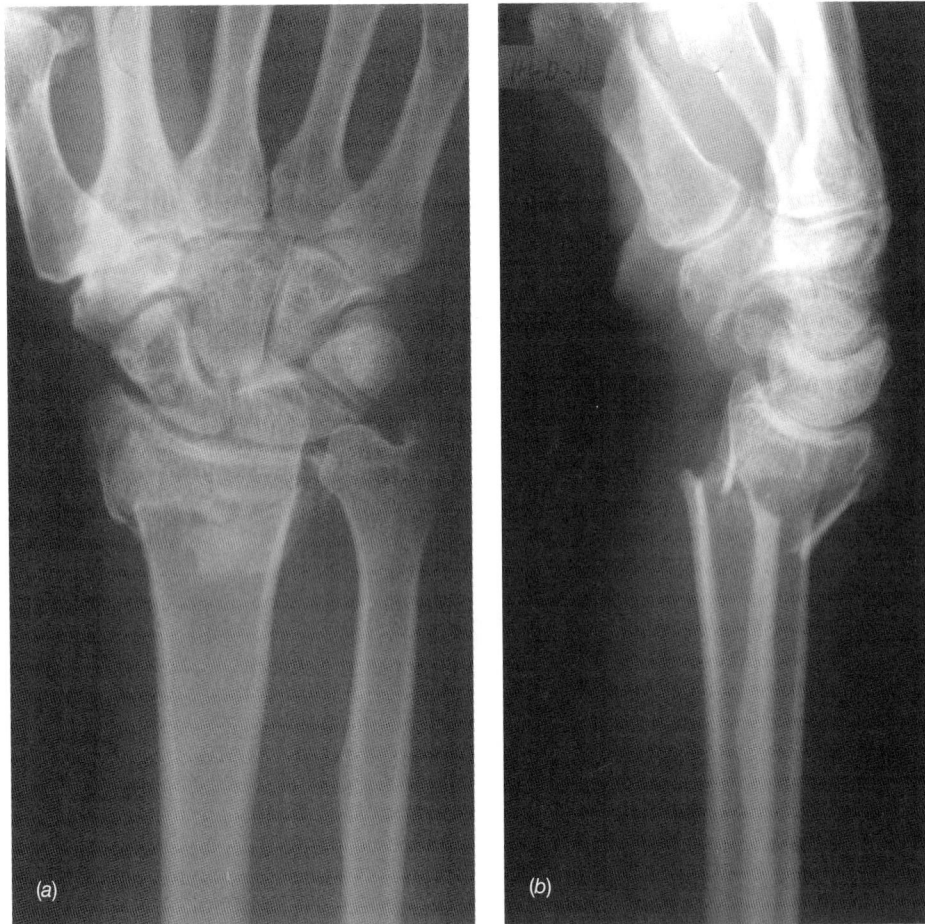

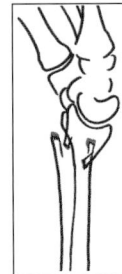

Figure 9.5 Colles fracture ("fractura radii typica"). Shortening of the radius (*a*) and dorsal displacement of the distal articular fragment (*b*). (© Medical Illustrator Tommy Bolic, Sweden.)

• Diagnosis: Diagnosis is often made based on clinical examination, but patients experiencing wrist pain and having a deformity in their wrist, should be referred for a radiographic examination to have the diagnosis confirmed and for the fracture type and severity to be classified. A radiographic examination should likewise be performed if there is any doubt about the presence of a fracture. One PA and one lateral view often suffice, but the physician may need to request various additional views and possibly a CT scan if the first views are difficult to read.

• Treatment: The goal of the treatment is to restore the alignment to as close to normal as possible. If there is any angulation, the fracture must be reduced. It is difficult to provide definite guidelines for the angulation that can be accepted. This depends on the age of the patient and to some degree the attitude of the physician treating the patient. For patients younger than 25–30 years of age, only anatomic position (i.e., a palmar tilt of 10°–12° on a lateral view) should be accepted. The radius should not be shortened. If an X-ray taken during a check-up 1 week later demonstrates that the fracture has been redisplaced, the patient should be referred for surgical evaluation. The same applies if there is a radial shortening of 3–5 mm. In any older patient, 10°–15° of dorsal tilting and a shortening of 3–5 mm is generally accepted. Even greater displacement is tolerated in patients older than 75 years. If the physician is inexperienced in treating fractures of the distal radius, the patient should be referred to an orthopedic or hand surgeon. If reposition succeeds, a well-molded cast is applied to prevent the fracture from redislocating. Check-up X-rays should be taken after reposition and application of the cast, as well as 1, 2, 4, and 6 weeks after the initial treatment. If the wrist redislocates while

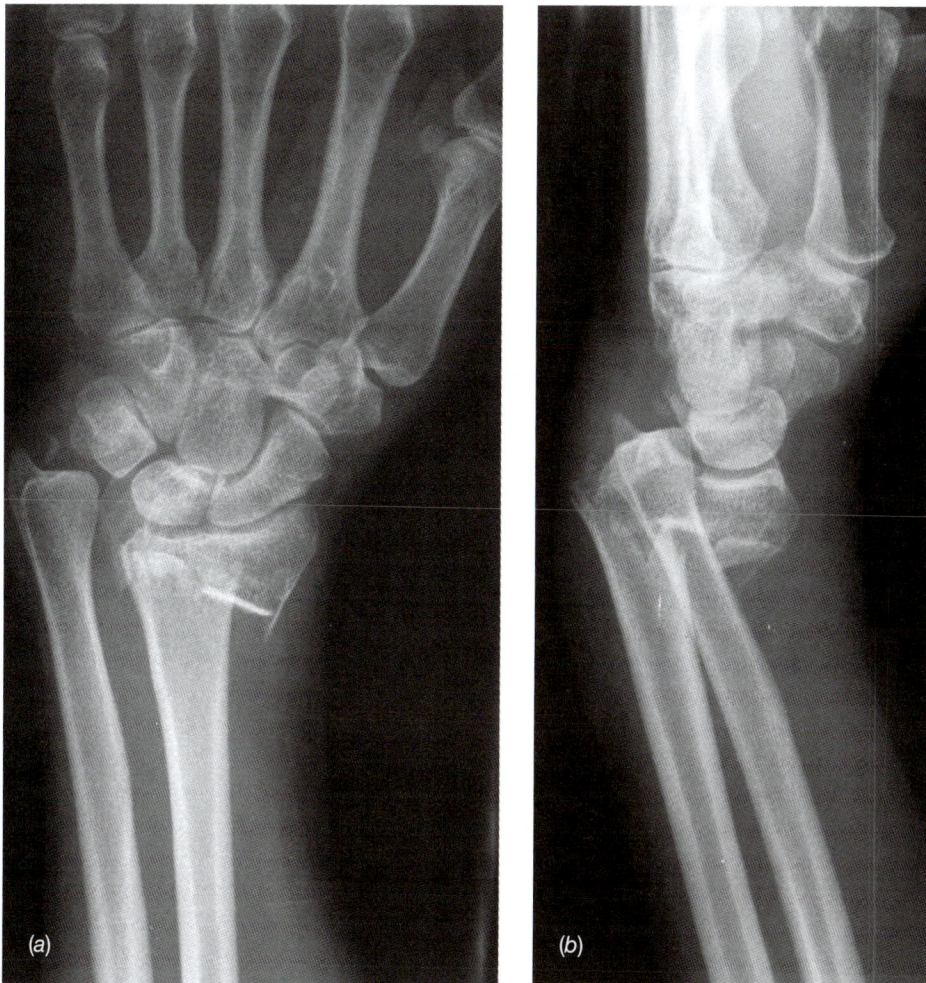

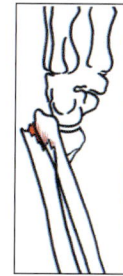

Figure 9.6 Smith fracture ("fractura radii atypica"). Shortening of the radius (a) and palmar displacement of the distal articular fragment (b). (© Medical Illustrator Tommy Bolic, Sweden.)

in a cast, rereduction may be attempted, but this often fails and surgery should be considered. Many fractures return to the initial position (shortening and angular displacement) during the period when the patient is wearing a cast. As a consequence, some authors consider surgery as the treatment of choice if shortening and dorsal angulation of the radius occur. Whenever in doubt, a hand surgeon should be consulted. Operating on displaced or angulated distal radius fractures, especially in young active people, has become more popular. Using newly designed plates and screws there is a trend toward early mobilization even in comminuted fractures. Even if the bone heals it is yet to be shown that early mobilization is beneficial for the concomitant soft-tissue injuries; be cautious when there is a potentially extensive ligament injury. If an intra-articular fracture with incongruity of the articular surface and/or a major displacement that cannot be reduced has occurred, surgery is mandatory. Surgical options include closed, open, or arthroscopic-assisted reduction in combination with some type of osteosynthesis such as percutaneous pinning, use of an external fixator or screws and plate. The choice of surgical treatment depends on the age of the patient, the type of fracture and the demands of the sport. Depending on age, fracture type, and the type of treatment that is used, the wrist has to be immobilized from 4 to 6 weeks. External fixation devices should be removed earlier. A feared complication is reflex sympathetic dystrophy, which causes intense pain and swelling and reduced function in the hand and fingers. Patients with this complication should immediately be referred to a hand therapist with experience in treating reflex sympathetic dystrophy.

WRIST, HAND, AND FINGERS

• Prognosis: Fractures of the distal radius where normal alignment and bone length are reestablished usually result in a pain-free and well-functioning wrist. However, many patients experience pain and discomfort in the wrist for up to 1 year after the injury, and they should be so informed. If normal anatomy is not reestablished, reduced range of motion and pain in the radiocarpal joint and in the DRUJ (rotation) may occur. A corrective osteotomy of the malpositioned bone may be performed. After many years of malalignment, osteoarthritis may develop, making a salvage procedure such as a partial or a total artrodesis, or a wrist arthroplasty, a possible treatment alternative. However, the best treatment and the best prognosis result from optimal initial care, restoring normal wrist anatomy.

Scaphoid Fracture !

A fracture of the scaphoid is the most common carpal fracture (Figure 9.7). As in the case of a fracture of the distal radius, the mechanism of injury is a fall on an extended, radially deviated hand. Most athletes who sustain a scaphoid fracture by this mechanism are young, active men, but children and the elderly may also sustain this type of fracture. The blood supply to the scaphoid comes from branches of the radial artery that enter the bone on its distal and palmar aspect and run proximally. Healing can be a problem with scaphoid fractures because of (a) its retrograde blood flow and (b) its anatomical position spanning the two rows of carpal bones. Fractures in the distal half of the bone usually heal without problems, but healing in the waist is only about 40% and in the proximal pole only about 10%. A fracture of the scaphoid is often associated with wrist ligament injuries.

• Symptoms and signs: The patient complains of pain and weakness in the hand and may refer to a major or minor trauma that occurred in the past. This may have been considered to be a sprain, but the symptoms have not gone away. Tenderness and pain in the anatomic snuffbox or at the palpable distal pole on the volar radial aspect of the wrist are common.

• Diagnosis: If there is tenderness in the anatomic snuffbox or at the level of the scaphoid tubercle immediately after the injury a scaphoid fracture should be suspected. A distal radius fracture can be excluded by means of a radiographic examination, but a scaphoid fracture may not. If a scaphoid fracture is suspected on clinical examination (i.e., tenderness in the anatomic snuffbox), a cast should be applied, even if the radiographic examination is normal. The patient should be seen for a follow-up within 5–10 days. If a fracture is still suspected, the patient is given another radiographic examination including an additional examination such as CT scan or MRI to demonstrate the pathology in the scaphoid.

• Treatment: If the fracture is not displaced more than 1 mm and there is no axial angulation, the fracture can be treated with a cast. A short arm cast is used for this injury, immobilizing the thumb to the IP joint and leaving the other fingers free from the MCP joint level. Because the

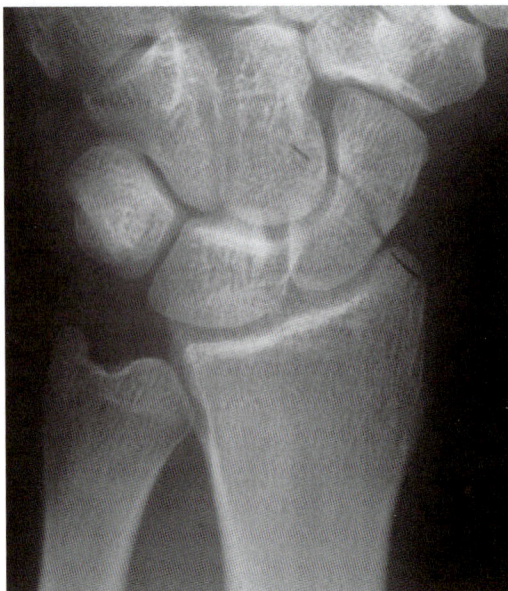

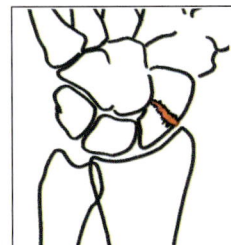

Figure 9.7 Scaphoid fracture, the most common fracture in a carpal bone. (© Medical Illustrator Tommy Bolic, Sweden.)

circulation in the scaphoid is poor, it takes a long time for the fracture to heal. The cast should, therefore, be worn for 6–12 weeks. A CT scan should confirm healing of the bone or to determine whether the patient needs further casting (until the fracture is shown to have healed, both clinically and radiographically). Premature removal of the cast may result in delayed union or development of a pseudoarthrosis. Delay in starting treatment for more than 4 weeks is also associated with increased risk of pseudoarthrosis. There is an increasing move toward screw fixation of scaphoid fractures. Although union rates are similar to those treated in a cast, screw fixation allows for earlier rehabilitation to maintain movement and reduce morbidity. Therefore, active athletes with scaphoid fractures should consider having surgical treatment to allow them to return to the sport activity as soon as possible. Displaced (>1 mm) and angulated scaphoid fractures should always be referred for surgical evaluation. If a pseudoarthrosis develops, surgery may be attempted even several years after the primary fracture. When this surgery is performed, malalignment should be corrected, and bone should be transplanted and fixed using pins or screws. The patient will have to wear a splint or cast for a minimum of 6–12 weeks after surgery.

• Prognosis: The prognosis is good if initial patient care is adequate. The fracture must be confirmed to be healed clinically and radiographically before the athlete is allowed to return to sport activity. A CT scan is highly recommended for the evaluation of healing of a scaphoid fracture. Surgically treated pseudoarthrosis also has a relatively good prognosis. Post-traumatic arthritis may result from scaphoid nonunion; however, the onset of the changes and the symptoms could develop as late as 15–30 years after the primary injury. If secondary changes develop in the wrist the patient should be referred to a specialist for surgical evaluation.

Carpal Bone Fracture

If a patient has wrist pain after trauma, the possibility of a fracture in a carpal bone should be considered. The most common fractures have already been discussed. During the clinical examination, the most tender area can be demonstrated, as can any areas with contusion marks and swelling. This information may be important in helping the radiologist determine what views to take for a fracture to be demonstrated. An isolated fracture of a carpal bone (other than the scaphoid) is rare. Avulsion fractures from dorsal radiotriquetral or LT ligament injuries or an occasional transverse fracture within the body may be seen in the triquetrum. If this occurs, the patient will have maximum soreness on the dorsal and ulnar side of the wrist. A golfer or another athlete (baseball batter) who hits hard with a racket or club may injure the hook of the hamate (which projects into the palm of the hand). This causes distinct soreness on the ulnar side of the palm. Direct blows to the ulnar side of the hand may cause a pisiform fracture. If a carpal bone fracture is demonstrated, the patient should be referred to a specialist for further diagnostics and treatment.

• Symptoms and signs: Symptoms are pain, soreness, and swelling, possibly combined with reduced function.
• Diagnosis: Fractures should be suspected when the clinical examination reveals localized tenderness, swelling, and possibly bruising. The diagnosis is confirmed radiographically. If a fracture in the wrist is suspected, several views are needed. Additional CT, MRI, or other examinations are commonly used. If the hook of the hamate is injured, a carpal tunnel view should be asked for to demonstrate a freely projected hamulus (hook), or a CT scan should be requested to evaluate the specific carpal bone (or all carpal bones) in question.
• Treatment: An isolated, nondisplaced fracture through the triquetrum, the hamate, or the pisiform may be treated with a cast or splint for 4–6 weeks. Patients with

displaced fractures, or fractures through other bones in the wrist, should be referred for appropriate evaluation and treatment. Some fractures are part of a serious fracture-dislocation injury, and the treatment alternatives include open reposition of displaced bones, repair of ligaments, osteosynthesis using pins or screws, and a cast for 8–12 weeks. If there are late symptoms from a hamate or pisiform fracture, the hook of the hamate or the pisiform can be surgically removed without any noticeable loss of function.

• Prognosis: The prognosis depends completely on the type of fracture, when the injury is diagnosed and treated, and especially on the type of treatment that is given. Most patients recover fully; however, some end up with persistent pain and should be investigated for treatable nonunions or post-traumatic arthritis from displaced carpal bones that may eventually make some type of arthrodesis necessary. The patient, the physical therapist, and the physician will need to discuss every case individually as to when the athlete may resume sport activity.

Ligament Injury in the Wrist

A number of ligaments stabilize the various carpal bones to each other and to the radius, ulna, and metacarpal bones. Some of the interosseous ligament connections have the strongest part on the palmar side, whereas others have greater dorsal strength. If there is a strong blow to the hand, usually caused by a fall on a hyperextended, ulnar-deviated, and somewhat rotated hand, then a fracture, a ligament injury, or a combination of the two may occur. Ligament injuries, with or without dislocation of the carpal bones, may be difficult to diagnose. The most common injuries are to the SL or LT ligaments (Figures 9.8a and 9.8b).

Figure 9.8 Scapholunar (SL) and lunotriquetral (LT) ligament injuries. When both ligaments are injured, the lunate bone becomes unstable and may become dislocated. Most commonly, only one of the ligaments ruptures. The wrist and carpus are seen from the dorsal side, with intact ligaments (a). If an athlete falls on an extended hand, the ligaments in the carpus may rupture (as seen from the palmar side) (b). (© Medical Illustrator Tommy Bolic, Sweden.)

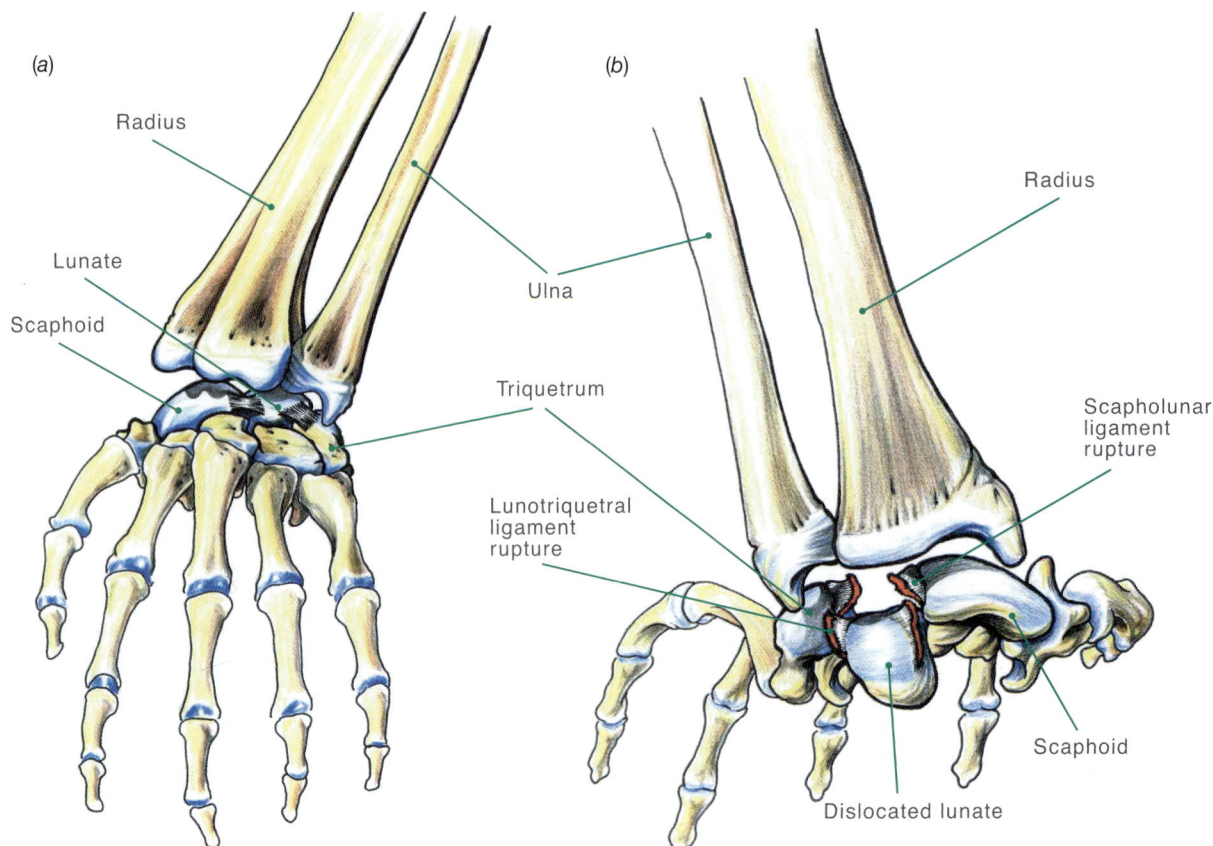

- Symptoms and signs: Pain, swelling, tenderness, and reduced range of motion are symptoms of ligament injuries in the wrist.
- Diagnosis: Diagnosis is based on radial or ulnar (depending on what ligament is injured) instability and tenderness in the wrist. During the acute phase it is difficult to do a clinical test of the various carpal ligaments ("everything hurts"), but this is often possible later on. Therefore, reports of a strong force as the mechanism of injury, and a great deal of swelling and pain during the examination may cause the suspicion of a ligament injury, and the patient should be referred to a hand surgeon for further examinations. There are numerous examples of radiologists, even experienced ones, who have overlooked obvious deformities in the wrist. Therefore, patients who seek medical attention after several weeks of pain, discomfort, clicking, and the feeling that "something gives away" in the wrist should be referred. Radiographs including several additional imaging studies may demonstrate increased distance between carpal bones as a sign of ligament disruption. Views of the wrist with the hand in a maximum radial- and ulnar-deviated position as well as fist views under stress (Figure 9.9) may demonstrate increased distance between the scaphoid and the lunate, whereas views of a supinated hand may demonstrate increased distance between the carpal bones in the ulnar side of the carpus (always compare with the noninjured side).

  However, a partial ligament rupture often occurs. If that is the case, a dynamic instability may be present. The patient experiences pain, clicking, and feeling of something giving away when he rotates his hand. In this situation, a radiograph (PA and lateral views) will not show anything wrong, and additional examinations, such as MRI and CT, are of limited help. An arthrography or a fluoroscopic visualization of the wrist while the patient's hand is being rotated may demonstrate instability. However, an arthroscopic examination is the only method of visualizing the various ligaments and performing stability testing of the carpal bones at the same time. Arthroscopy is the only possible way to diagnose the extent of the ligament injury.

- Treatment: The patient should be referred to a hand surgeon. Generally, surgical treatment includes reposition and fixation of the bones and repairing of the ligaments. In case of an old injury with established instability and damage to adjacent cartilaginous surfaces, reconstruction of the ligaments or other procedures

Figure 9.9 Having the patient make clenched fists and compare the injured (left side) to the noninjured (right) wrist reveals a widening (arrow) of the interval between the scaphoid and the lunate indicating a scapholunate (SL) ligament injury. (Reproduced with permission from the Norwegian Sports Medicine Association.)

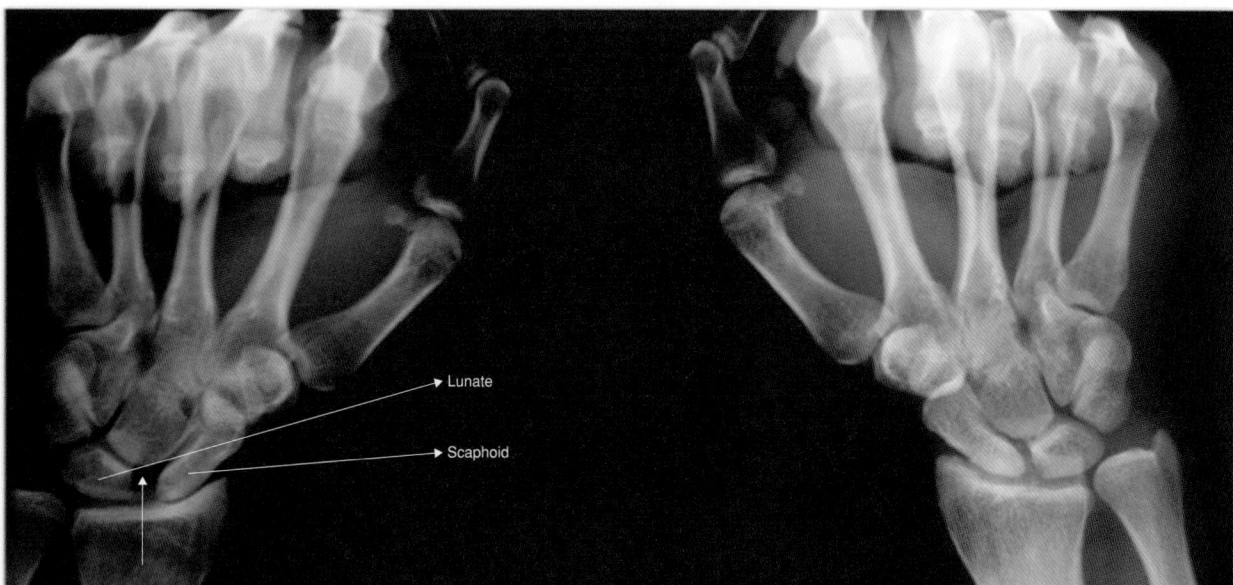

Lunate

Scaphoid

(capsulodesis, tenodesis, or arthrodesis) may be indicated. The wrist should be immobilized in a cast for 6–12 weeks.
• Prognosis: With early treatment, normal anatomy can be reestablished with a good outcome. Usually, the consequences for the athlete will be limited range of motion (flexion) and sometimes pain in the wrist. Sport activity should be restricted for at least 3 months.

Carpal Dislocation

The practitioner should recognize the possibility of carpal dislocations with or without a simultaneous fracture through the carpus (Figures 9.10 and 9.11). A perilunar (fracture-) dislocation can be divided into a midcarpal, a transscaphoid perilunate, a palmar, an axial, or a radiocarpal dislocation. The mechanism of injury and symptoms are the same as for an isolated carpal fracture or ligament injury. A carpal dislocation is rare, and it is often overlooked at first. Therefore, if a carpal dislocation is suspected, the patient should be referred to a hand surgeon for further diagnostics and treatment.

The prognosis is best with early diagnostics and treatment; late treatment often makes surgical intervention necessary that will limit wrist motion. If there are large deformities having existed for a long time and caused osteoarthritis in several joints, the patient may end up with some type of a limited carpal arthrodesis or even a total wrist fusion.

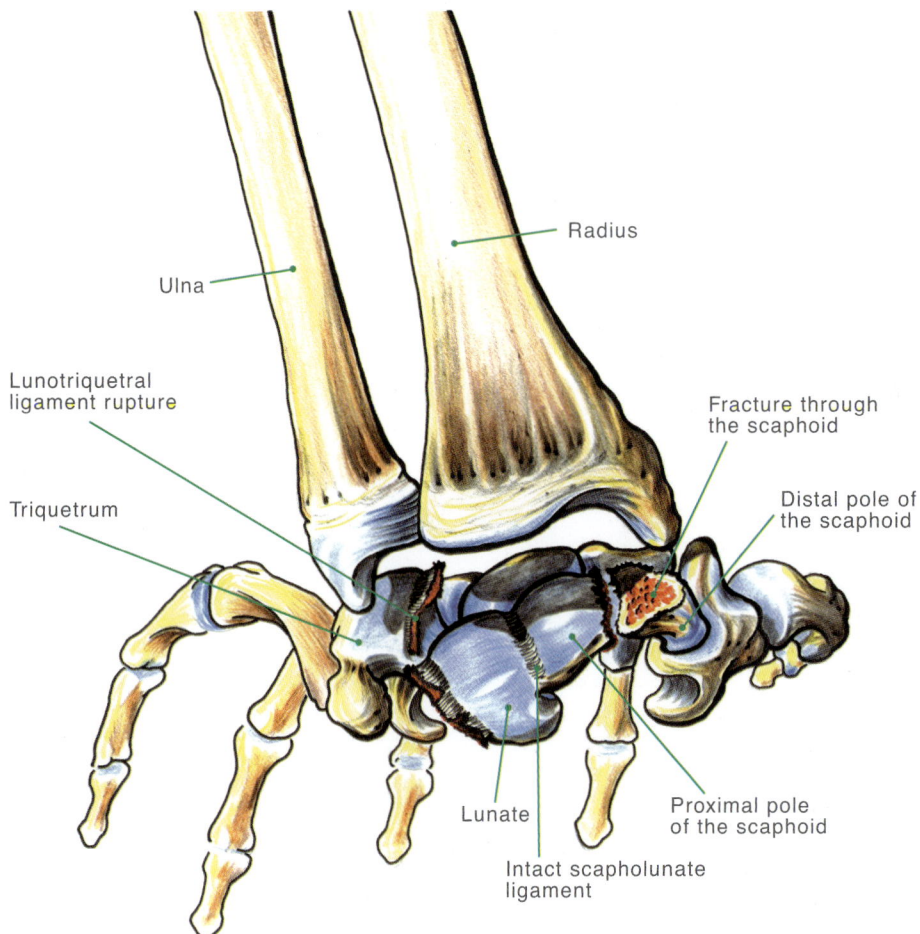

Figure 9.10 Carpal dislocation. Forceful trauma to the carpus can cause various types of fractures, dislocations, or combinations thereof. In the transscaphoid perilunar dislocation shown, a fracture through the scaphoid and a rupture in the lunotriquetral (LT) ligament have occurred. However, the scapholunate (SL) ligament is intact, so that the proximal part of the scaphoid is dislocated at the same time as the lunate. (© Medical Illustrator Tommy Bolic, Sweden.)

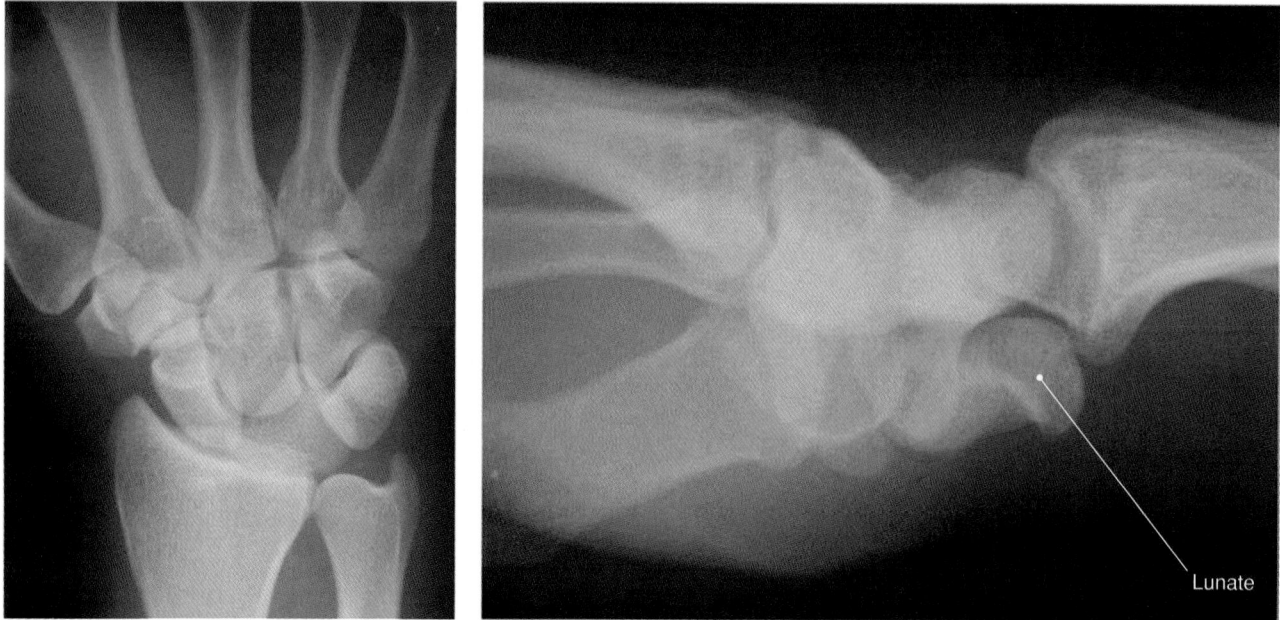

Lunate

Distal Radioulnar Joint Injury—*Injury of the Lower Joint between the Radius and the Ulna*

Forearm rotation takes place in the proximal and distal radioulnar joint (DRUJ). There is a concave articular surface (the sigmoid notch) on the distal radius, where the head of the ulna (which is convex toward the radius) fits. Motion in the DRUJ is a combination of rotation and translation. Stability in the same joint depends partly on the skeleton and partly on the soft tissues (i.e., the TFCC, the ulnocarpal ligaments, the ECU tendon, the pronator quadratus musculature, the interosseous membrane, and the capsule). Trauma to the wrist may cause a DRUJ injury. This could be a soft-tissue injury or a soft-tissue injury combined with a fracture (Figures 9.12a and 9.12b). The fracture may be an intra-articular radius fracture that engages the sigmoid notch or a fracture through the styloid process of the ulna.

- Symptoms and signs: Symptoms and signs are pain and sometimes clicking in the wrist, particularly from the ulnar side, and reduced forearm rotation in combination with instability or increased motion of the head of the ulna.
- Diagnosis: Patients suspected to have a DRUJ injury should be referred for an X-ray or a CT scan of the wrist (which provides the best overview of the joint). A CT scan directly demonstrates the congruence in the DRUJ and any dislocation of the radius relative to the ulna. (The uninjured side should be taken for comparison). An isolated soft-tissue ligament injury that causes instability in the DRUJ is diagnosed by clinical examination. Stability should be examined for in a neutral rotational position and at maximum supinated and pronated positions. These tests also need to be compared to the uninjured side. If instability or dislocation is suspected or demonstrated, the patient should be seen by a hand surgeon.
- Treatment: The physician should refer the patient to a hand surgeon for treatment. Surgery is performed on a fracture to ensure congruence in the DRUJ, whereas a ligament injury is repaired by open or closed repositioning of the joint, followed by possibly suturing the ligament, and immobilization for 6 weeks with a high cast (above elbow level to prevent rotation of the forearm). For an old injury, an

Figure 9.11
Posteroanterior (PA) and lateral views of the wrist show a dislocated lunate. (Reproduced with permission from the Norwegian Sports Medicine Association.)

WRIST, HAND, AND FINGERS

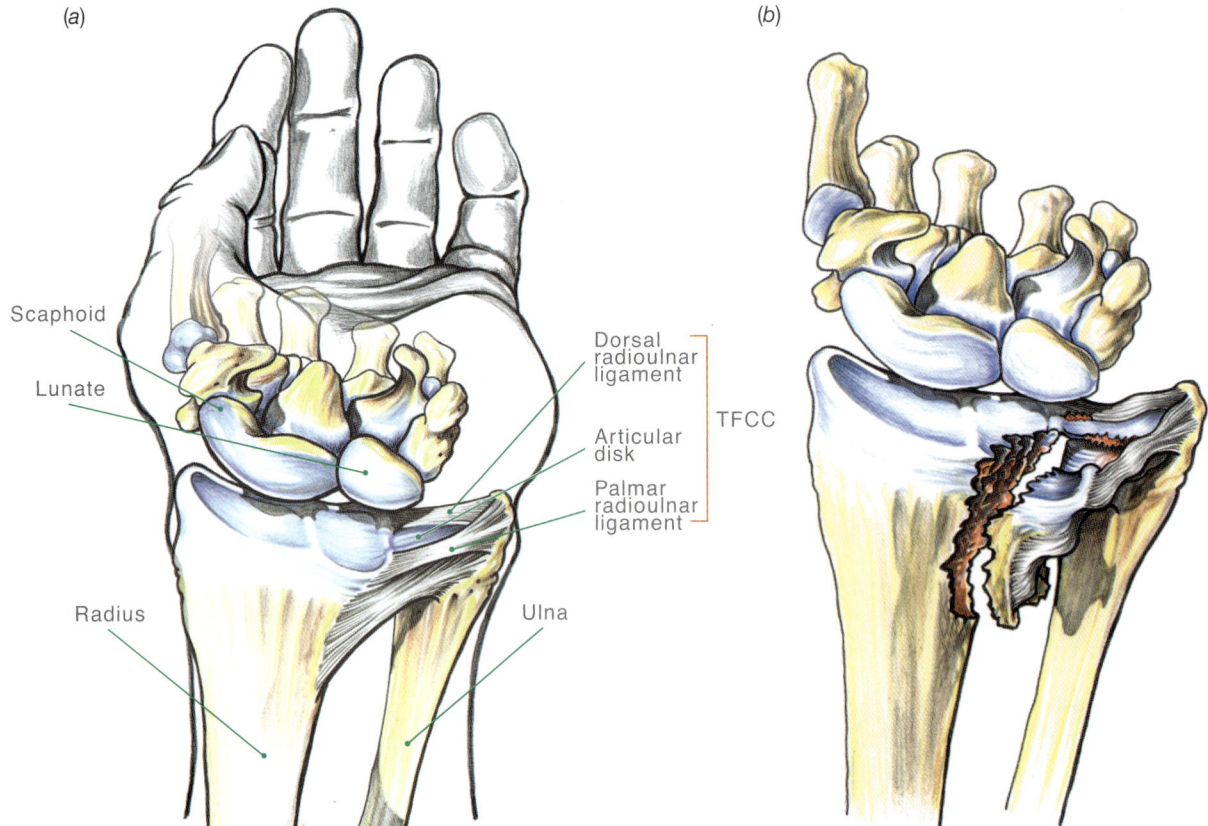

(a)

Scaphoid

Lunate

Radius

Ulna

Dorsal
radioulnar
ligament

Articular
disk

Palmar
radioulnar
ligament

TFCC

(b)

Figure 9.12 Distal radioulnar joint injury. The wrist, seen from the palmar side, with an intact triangular fibrocartilage complex (TFCC) (*a*) Intra-articular radial fracture that engages the articular surface of the distal radioulnar joint, and the TFCC (*b*). (© Medical Illustrator Tommy Bolic, Sweden.)

attempt may be made to reconstruct the skeletal structure in the DRUJ. Other options include, in a small group of patients, a limited resection of the distal end of the ulna, a reconstruction of the ligaments using a free tendon graft, or an arthroplasty.

• Prognosis: Results are good when acute injuries are treated, and the athlete may resume sport activity after about 12 weeks. If the patient has an old injury, function (forearm rotation) and pain will determine the need for surgical intervention. If so performed, the situation may be improved but the prognosis is less predictable and poor results are not uncommon.

Triangular Fibrocartilage Complex Rupture

Several structures contribute to stability in the DRUJ and in the ulnocarpal joint. A key structure is the TFCC. It consists of a meniscus-like structure, the articular disk, and the palmar and dorsal radioulnar ligaments. Hyperextension and rotation of the wrist may often injure the TFCC (Figure 9.13). This also occurs in combination with a radius fracture. In addition, degenerative changes occur in the central part of the TFCC as the patient ages, or in cases when the ulna is longer that the radius, a so-called ulna plus. Traumatic ruptures are often peripheral.

• Symptoms and signs: Symptoms and signs are ulnar-sided pain in the wrist, particularly in forearm rotation and ulnar deviation of the wrist in combination with power grip function. A slightly flexed wrist is often tender to palpation around the tendon sheath of the flexor carpi ulnaris tendon. The patient may experience clicking, but real locking is less common.

• Diagnosis: An injury of the TFCC may be suspected based on the mechanism of injury and the clinical examination. Patients with indefinite ulnar-sided wrist pain especially during pronation and supination, possibly accompanied by clicking or a clicking sensation, should be further evaluated. An MRI examination is highly dependent on the radiologist interpreting the different views, and different findings from MRI and surgery are often reported. A negative MRI does not exclude a TFCC injury, and wrist arthroscopy should be considered the gold standard for diagnosing pathology. A positive fovea sign; tenderness upon pressure distally and deep into the "soft spot" between the ulnar styloid process, flexor carpi ulnaris tendon, volar surface of the ulnar head, and the pisiform is indicative of an injury of the foveal attachment of the TFCC (the DRUJ unstable) or a split tear of the ulnalunate (UL) and ulnatriquetral (UT) ligaments (the DRUJ stable).

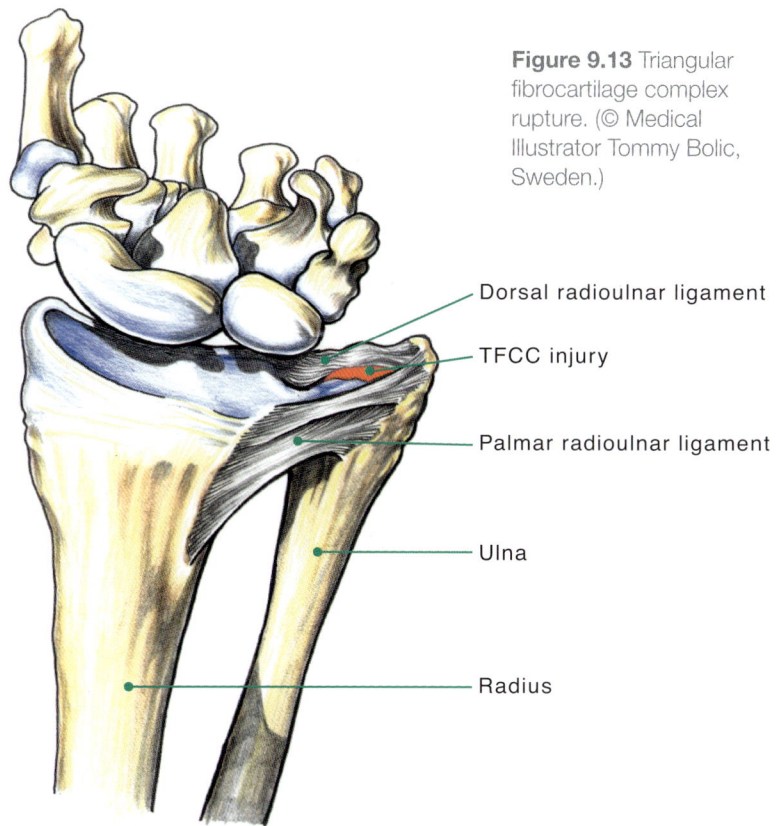

Figure 9.13 Triangular fibrocartilage complex rupture. (© Medical Illustrator Tommy Bolic, Sweden.)

Dorsal radioulnar ligament

TFCC injury

Palmar radioulnar ligament

Ulna

Radius

• Treatment: Degenerative changes with central defects in the TFCC may be arthroscopically resected so that a loose flap does not interpose in the joint and cause pain. An ulnarimpaction syndrome with degenerative changes in the proximal carpal row as well as on the distal ulna including degenerative changes of the TFCC could be treated with an arthroscopic resection of the ulna or an ulnar shortening osteotomy. Avulsion from the radius is seldom repaired (because of a lack of blood vessels in this part of the cartilage, making the chances of healing slight), whereas a peripheral ulnar avulsion may be sutured using an arthroscopic-assisted suture technique. A foveal detachment of the TFCC is repaired using an open or an arthroscopically assisted technique. A resection of a central injury does not require immobilization, while a repair requires 4–8 weeks of immobilization in a splint or a cast.

• Prognosis: Studies have shown that patients with central (usually degenerative) ruptures that are resected and peripheral ruptures that are repaired are pain free and satisfied. Patients with central injuries may resume sport activities immediately. Athletes who have undergone a repair of the TFCC should not return to sports for 12 weeks after surgery.

Tendon Injury

Tendon injuries at the wrist level are rare without a simultaneous open wound. One exception, which is not uncommon, is rupture of the EPL tendon in connection with a radius fracture (Figures 9.14a and 9.14b). This is due to increased pressure within the tendon sheath of the tendon where it curves around Lister's tubercle (a bony prominence on the dorsal side of the radius just proximal to the wrist). This creates an area with reduced circulation, and consequently, a tendon rupture. The use of a volar plate for fixation of a radial fracture may also cause impingement of tendons due to long screws.

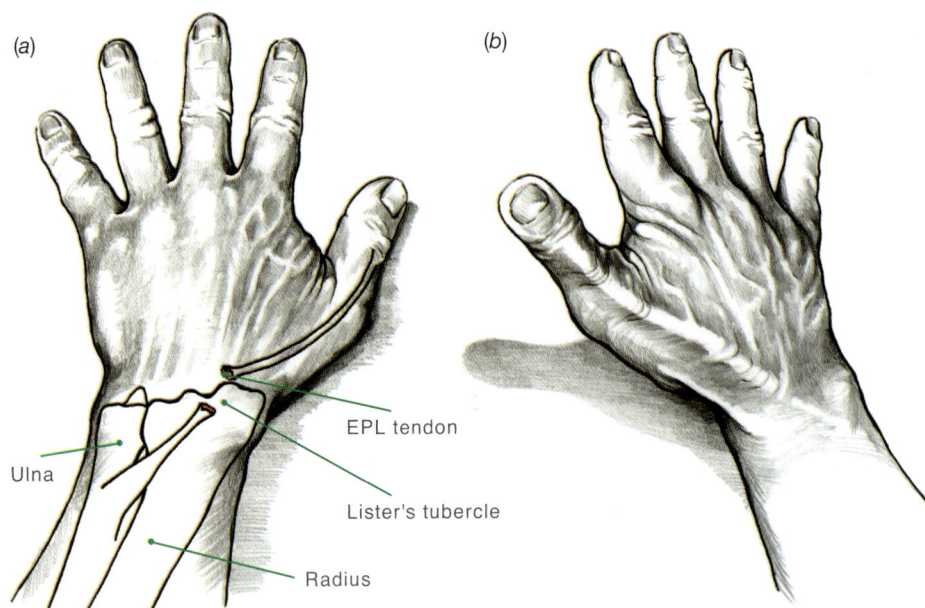

Figure 9.14 Extensor pollicis longus (EPL) rupture. To test for EPL tendon function, the patient places the palms of both hands on a tabletop and lifts his thumbs off the surface. If the EPL tendon is ruptured, he will not be able to do this (a). If the tendon is intact, the contours of the tendon can be observed and palpated (b). (© Medical Illustrator Tommy Bolic, Sweden.)

- Symptoms and signs: Tenderness, swelling, and reduced strength and range of motion.
- Diagnosis: The best way to test for EPL function is to have the patient place the palm of her hand on a surface and ask her to lift her thumb off that surface. She cannot do this if her tendon is injured.
- Treatment: If there is a suspected or a diagnosed tendon injury, the patient should be referred for surgical treatment. It may be difficult to suture an EPL tendon rupture directly. If so, one option is transposition of one of the index finger's extensor tendons (the extensor indicis proprius tendon) to the thumb's extensor tendon. Flexor tendons are put in a dynamic casting for 4 weeks, while extensor tendons are immobilized for 5 weeks after surgery.
- Prognosis: Prognosis is good after surgical treatment. A flexor tendon does not have normal strength for active grip until 12 weeks after the injury. If an injury of the extensor tendons has occurred, sport activity may be resumed after 8 weeks.

Nerve Entrapment

The median and ulnar nerves may both be subjected to pressure at the wrist level (Figure 9.15). In sports, the most common nerve compression is on the ulnar nerve, such as that caused when a cyclist holds onto the handlebars, exercising pressure on the ulnar side of the wrist. This may cause reduction of sensation in the little finger and the ulnar half of the ring finger, but it may also reduce the intrinsic muscle function in the hand (Figure 9.3, p. 260). The patient will experience difficulties with fine motor activity in his hand. Carpal tunnel syndrome is caused by pressure on the median nerve and can also occur in cyclists. It is also seen as an acute complication of serious wrist injuries where prompt diagnosis and treatment is needed. Carpal tunnel syndrome produces numbness and tingling ("the fingers feel asleep") in the thumb, index finger, middle finger, and the radial half of the ring finger (Figure 9.3, p. 260).

- Symptoms and signs: The patient may experience tingling and numbness radiating into various fingers and reduced hand function. The patient may report that "the hand is clumsy," and that he drops objects.
- Diagnosis: Mild tapping (with a finger) over the affected nerve could cause radiating pain, discomfort, or paresthesia corresponding to the course of the affected

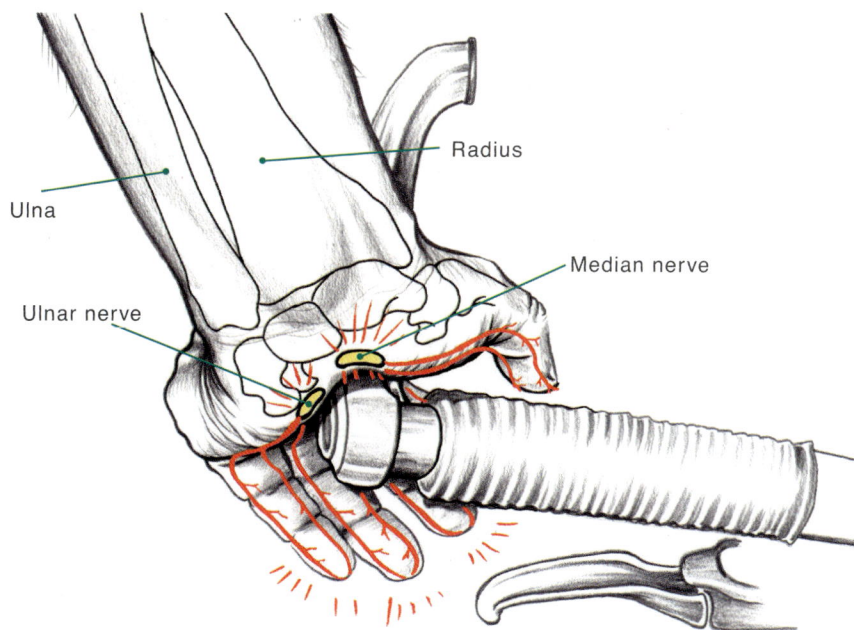

Figure 9.15 Nerve compression. Long-term pressure on the flexor side of the wrist/carpus can cause pressure injuries to the ulnar nerve or the median nerve. (© Medical Illustrator Tommy Bolic, Sweden.)

nerve (positive Tinel sign). Compression of the median nerve at the wrist level will not significantly reduce muscle function. Longstanding compression of the ulnar nerve may reduce the patient's ability to abduct and adduct her fingers and may cause atrophy in the hypothenar area and in the area between the first and second fingers; the hand appears "flat."

- Treatment: The most important precaution is, if possible, to avoid putting pressure on the nerve. The symptoms may gradually disappear on their own or with splinting. Alternatively, a surgical procedure releasing the ligament compressing the nerve may be performed.
- Prognosis: The prognosis is good if the nerve compression has not existed for a long time, the results of the median nerve treatment being better than ulnar nerve treatment.

Finger Injuries

Jan-Ragnar Haugstvedt[1], Vaughan Bowen[2], and Loris Pegoli[3]

[1]Østfold Hospital Trust, Moss, Norway
[2]University of Calgary, Calgary, AB, Canada
[3]University of Milan, Milano, Italy

Incidence

Finger injuries frequently occur as a result of various types of sport activities, particularly in ball sports such as volleyball, basketball, and handball. The most common injury is a sprain (strain), which usually only requires symptomatic treatment. Sometimes the patient sustains a major injury, such as a dislocation, a ligament injury, or a fracture, which requires referral to an orthopedic or hand surgeon for exact diagnostics and specific treatment.

Differential Diagnoses

Table 9.2 shows various types of finger injuries. The most common are sprains, but fractures, dislocations, and ligament injuries are not uncommon sport injuries. Tendon injuries are less common. Although diagnosing and treating finger injuries could be done by simple means, some cases require additional examinations or special treatment.

Diagnostic Thinking

The physician should examine a finger for an open wound (for possible tendon and nerve disturbance), swelling and discoloration of the skin (for bleeding, as in the

Most common	Less common	Must not be overlooked !
Sprain, p. 280	Finger fracture, p. 281	Interposed soft tissue after dislocations
	Metacarpal fracture	Rotary malalignment with finger fractures
	Bennett fracture	
	Reversed Bennett fracture	
	Collateral ligament ruptures in the PIP and MCP joints, p. 284	
	Collateral ligament ruptures in the MCP joint of the thumb, p. 285	
	Mallet finger (drop finger)	
	Tendon rupture, p. 286	
	Pulley rupture, p. 287	
	Finger joint dislocation, p. 288	
	Nerve injury, p. 289	

Table 9.2 Overview of differential diagnoses of finger injuries. (Reproduced with permission from the Norwegian Sports Medicine Association.)

case of ligament injuries, dislocations, and fractures), malalignment (for fractures and/or dislocations), or reduced muscle tone (for tendon injury). If reduced sensation in a finger is found, the patient should be referred to a hand surgeon. Injury of a dorsal digital nerve (especially to the radial nerve) may not need to be repaired as this injury causes minor discomfort for the patient. However, whenever an injury to the digital nerve on the palmar side of the finger is diagnosed, the patient *should* be referred for surgical treatment as soon as possible, at the latest by 1–2 weeks. There is no need for further observation. A compression (closed) injury, however, may be observed for 2 weeks before referring the patient for surgical evaluation. The patient should also be referred to a hand surgeon if absence of flexion or extension of the fingers is found.

If a patient exhibits swelling and discoloration, function of the affected digit should be tested. The easiest way to do this is to ask the patient make a fist and extend her fingers. Tenderness and stability are examined for. If finger motion causes pain, and if instability is definite or suspected, the patient should be referred for radiographic examination. Likewise, if the patient has a malalignment, a fracture, or a dislocation, he should be referred for a radiographic examination. A dislocated joint may be reduced immediately, after which the patient should be referred for a radiographic examination to verify the reduction and to rule out a fracture combination. Depending on the results of the radiographic examination, a finger fracture may be treated by immobilization alone, protected mobilization, or the patient may be referred for surgery.

History

In most cases, information about the mechanism of injury reveals a great deal about the type of injury involved. A direct trauma to one or more fingers or a force in the axial direction may cause an avulsion of a tendon insertion or a dislocation of a finger joint. The patient probably suffers from a dislocation or a fracture if there is a side-to-side trauma leading to malalignment and a finger pointing in a wrong direction. If a dislocation was reduced, information on how the reduction was made should be included. For example, in a hyperextension trauma of the PIP joint with a tear of the volar tendon plate, the finger will be dorsally dislocated, and a flexion maneuver will be required to reduce the finger. Did the athlete (or others) hear a crack or other sounds indicating tearing of soft tissue or fracturing of bone? Did the swelling or discoloration occur immediately, indicating a ligament injury or a fracture?

Clinical Examination

Inspection. Discoloration of the skin and swelling may indicate bleeding, such as that caused by ligament injuries, dislocations, and fractures. This may also be suspected if there is a deformity with malalignment or rotary deviation (Figure 9.16).

A single finger observed in a flexed position may indicate the finger's extensor apparatus being injured, whereas a finger observed in an extended position (the dorsum of the hand against the surface) with a lack of tension on the flexor side of the finger may indicate injured flexor tendons. If there is an open wound, the possibilities of nerve and tendon injuries should always be considered.

Palpation. The physician should examine for the most sore point and determine whether the swelling is soft (as in the case of a hematoma)

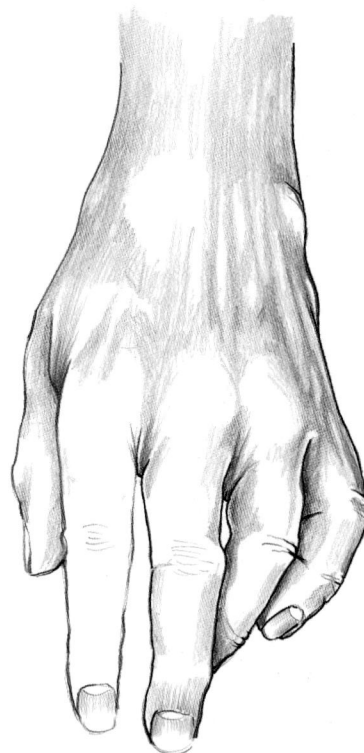

Figure 9.16 Inspection of the hand reveals malrotation of the fingers suffering from a fracture. (© Medical Illustrator Tommy Bolic, Sweden.)

WRIST, HAND, AND FINGERS

or hard (as in the case of a displaced bone). Exercising pressure on an injured finger makes it possible to verify instability from fractures or ligament injuries.

Nerve function. An open wound or a compression injury of a finger may cause a loss of sensation. The motor nerve branches originate in a more proximal location on the hand and forearm and will not cause a loss of muscle/tendon function when there are finger-level injuries. The easiest way of examining for sensation is by touching one side of the finger with a cotton ball, the ends of a paper clip or simply by using a pen. Compare this to the other side of the same finger, an adjacent finger, or a finger on the other hand. The median nerve innervates the thumb, index finger, middle finger, and the radial side of the ring finger, whereas the ulnar nerve innervates the ulnar side of the ring finger and the entire little finger (Figure 9.3, p. 260).

Range of motion. The normal range of motion in the four ulnar fingers is full extension, that is, to 0° in the metacarpo phalangeal joint (MCP), the proximal interphalangeal (PIP) and the distal interphalangeal (DIP) joints. It should be possible to flex all three joints on the individual fingers to 90°. A somewhat simplified examination of the motion is to ask the patient make a fist to see whether the pulp of the fingers can reach the distal crease in the palm. The IP joint of the thumb is extended to 0° and flexed to 90°, whereas the MCP joint is extended to 0° and flexed to 50°–60°. In some people, hyperextension of some finger joints is normal. In others, hyperextension may be a sign of an injury (e.g., avulsion of the volar tendon plate in the PIP joints). The physician should compare motion to that of the other fingers and to ask if motion has changed after the injury.

Tendon function. Findings by inspection may indicate a tendon injury. If the patient can flex the IP joint of his thumb, the long flexor tendon of his thumb is intact. The flexor tendons of the four ulnar fingers need to be tested individually (Figures 9.17a and 9.17b). The attachment of the flexor digitorum superficialis is palmar and proximal on the middle phalanx, and the function is tested by holding the other three fingers locked in an extended position while asking the patient to bend the PIP joint of the examined finger. The attachment of the flexor digitorum profundus is palmar and proximal on the distal phalanx, and the function is tested by fixing the middle phalanx (keeping the PIP joint in an extended position) of the finger to be examined and asking the patient to flex the DIP joint. If an extensor tendon injury is suspected, ask the athlete to fully extend the injured finger. When the long extensor tendon of the thumb (EPL) is involved, the best way to test it is by asking the patient to place the palm of her hand on a surface and to lift her thumb off that surface. This is not possible if this tendon is injured (Figure 9.14, p. 274).

Testing of stability. When examining the stability of the collateral ligaments, one should remember that the ligaments of the four ulnar fingers have different origins and insertions in the MCP joints as compared to the PIP joints. In the MCP joints, the lateral ligaments are tight when the fingers are flexed to 90°, whereas they are relaxed when the fingers are extended. For this reason, the lateral ligaments of the MCP joints should be tested with the MCP joints in a flexed position. The opposite is true of the PIP joints, where the lateral ligaments are tight when the fingers are extended (0°) and more relaxed when the PIP joints are flexed. Therefore, the lateral ligaments of the PIP joints should be tested with the PIP joints in the extended position. The collateral ligaments of the MCP joint in the thumb should be tested in a fully extended position and in a slightly flexed (20°–30°) position (Figure 9.18).

All testing of stability may reveal a great deal of individual variation. Therefore, comparison with the adjacent fingers, or best of all, with the corresponding finger on the opposite, uninjured hand, is important. The best tests are usually given immediately

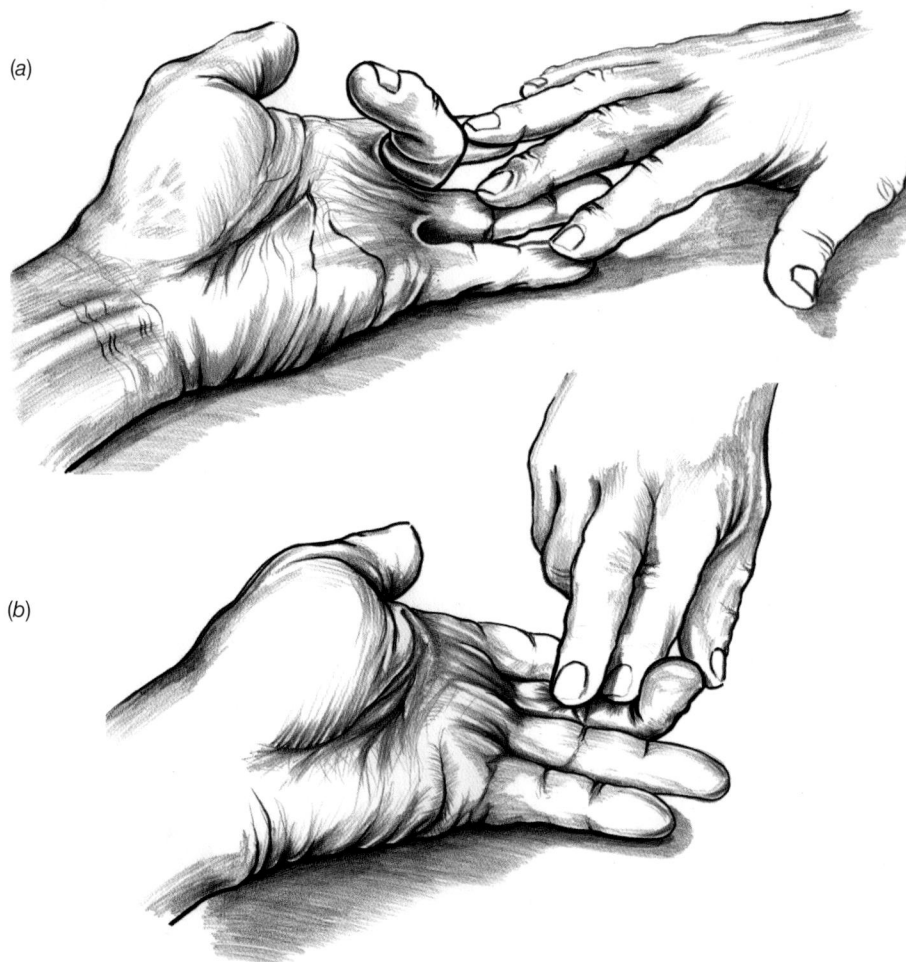

Figure 9.17 Function test of the deep and superficial flexor tendons. During testing of one of the superficial flexor tendons, the adjacent fingers are locked in full extension while the patient flexes the proximal interphalangeal (PIP) joint (a). When testing the deep flexor tendons, the proximal part of the finger is immobilized in the extended position while the patient flexes the distal interphalangeal (DIP) joint (b). (© Medical Illustrator Tommy Bolic, Sweden.)

after the injury occurs. The patient does not feel the same pain as she would later on, when it may be necessary to use local anesthesia for adequate testing.

Additional Examinations

Radiographic examination. Even if the patient has been given a thorough clinical examination, it is not always possible to exclude a skeletal injury without additional examinations. It may be very important to the future hand function of the patient to recognize a skeletal injury (e.g., avulsion of a tendon insertion, ligament insertion, or the insertion of the volar tendon plate of the finger joints) as early as possible so that proper treatment can be started. If there is doubt, the patient should be referred for an additional examination. No one benefits from a wait-and-see attitude. In children, a fracture may begin to heal after 2 weeks, and delaying the diagnostic examination may result in the need to reopen a fracture line so that it can be properly reduced. Generally, routine radiographic examinations, using several views (always a minimum of two), will confirm a suspected fracture. If there is doubt, additional oblique views should be requested. The use of radiographs taken while stressing the finger (static force or tension is applied to determine if a ligament is torn or ruptured) makes it possible to expose instability. Corresponding views of the other (uninjured) hand should always be taken for comparison.

Other examinations, such as MRI, CT scans, and bone scan, are not commonly used for suspected finger injuries. MRI may provide information about interposed soft

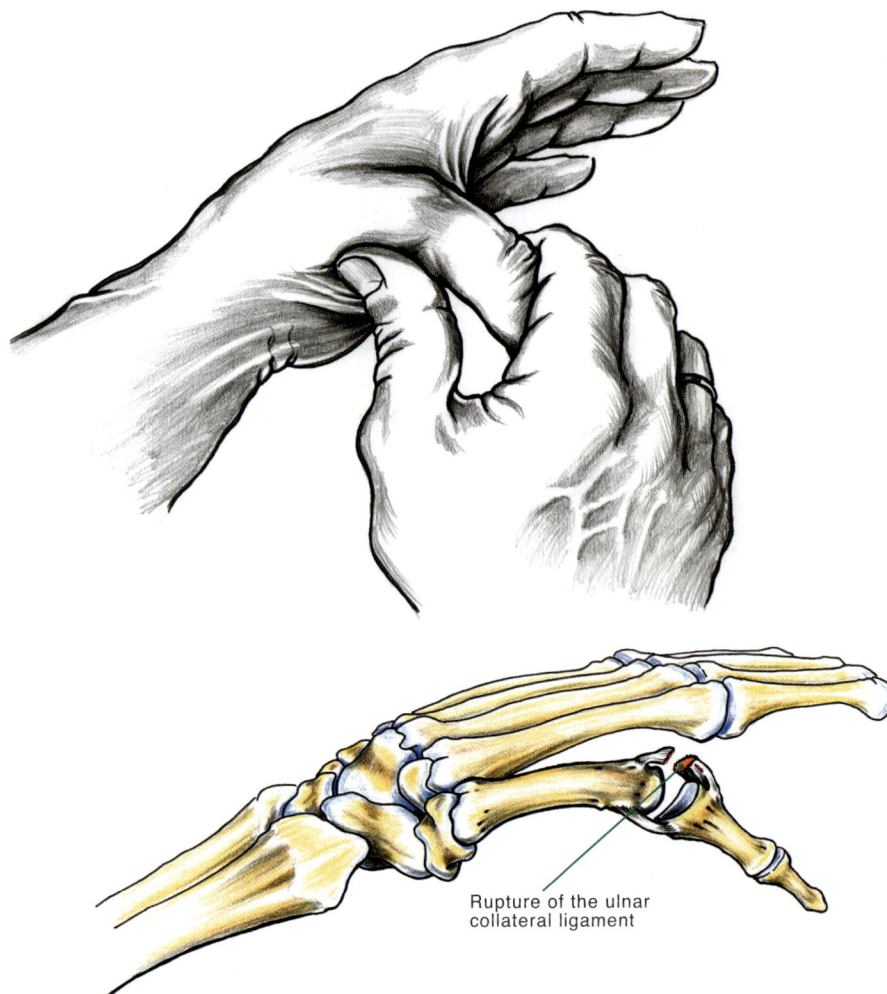

Figure 9.18 Stress test of the thumb's metacarpophalangeal (MCP) joint. When the ulnar collateral ligament is ruptured, lateral instability increases in comparison with the noninjured hand. (© Medical Illustrator Tommy Bolic, Sweden.)

Rupture of the ulnar collateral ligament

tissue in a joint after a dislocation, but usually these examinations are unnecessary at the finger level and should only be requested by a hand surgeon. Ultrasound, preferably dynamic ultrasonography examinations, may be useful in diagnosing a suspected tendon or a pulley rupture.

Common Injuries

Sprains

The most common finger injuries are caused by a blow to a finger because of a fall, a ball or puck hitting the finger; a finger getting stuck in equipment; or a finger attempting to grab the jersey of a teammate or opponent. The finger is swollen, becomes painful and sore on palpation, and range of motion is limited due to a partial lesion of the joint capsule or a ligament.

- Symptoms and signs: Symptoms are pain, swelling, and tenderness, no instability, but often limited range of motion (particularly flexion).
- Diagnosis: If there is malalignment and palpation causes pain, a fracture is suspected and the patient should be referred for a radiographic examination. If the

radiographic examination is normal and the finger is stable in flexion and extension, the patient could be considered having a sprain. A sprain is an exclusion diagnosis with normal radiographic views, a stable finger with intact sensation and tendon function, but with mild swelling and some soreness. The diagnosis is based on the clinical examination, but a radiographic examination is necessary to exclude a fracture.

• Treatment by physician: The recommended treatment by a physician is PRICE treatment, NSAIDs, and possibly immobilization in a cast, brace, or tape for a few days for pain relief and prevention of edema. It is often useful to buddy tape the injured finger to an adjacent finger when resuming activity. Active movement should be initiated as soon as possible in order to reduce or minimize stiffness.

• Prognosis: The prognosis is good. However, it may be a long time before motion (particularly flexion) in a sprained PIP joint has returned to normal. The PIP joint may look swollen for a long time (up to a year) without anyone finding anything wrong or being able to give any specific treatment. Sport activity that is within the limits of pain can normally be resumed within a couple of weeks with the finger being buddy taped to an adjacent finger for support. If reduced motion and stiffness resumes for weeks, hand therapy including splinting of the finger(s) might become necessary.

Other Injuries

Finger Fracture

Direct or indirect force to a finger may cause ligament injury, fractures, or a combination of the two. In this section, we discuss all finger fractures. In fractures at the base of the first and fifth metacarpals, Bennett's fracture and reversed Bennett's fracture (Figures 9.19a and 9.19b), a small fragment on the base of the metacarpal

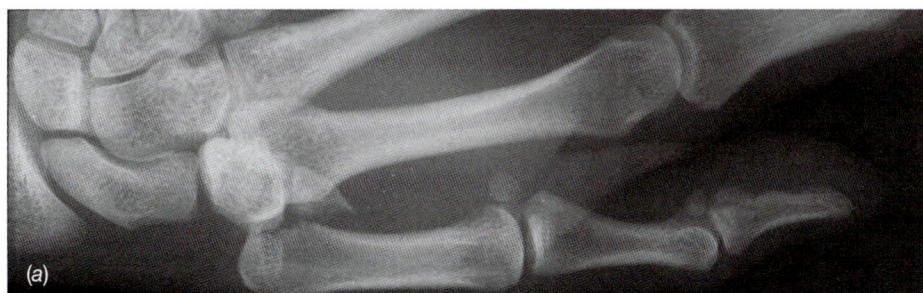

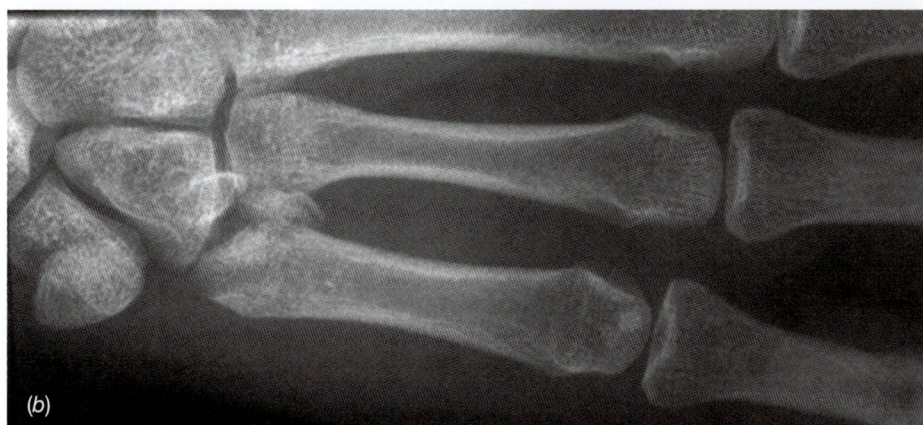

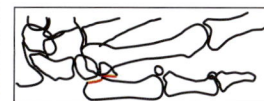

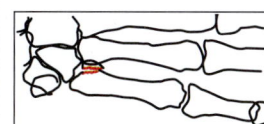

Figure 9.19 Bennett fracture (a): Avulsion fracture of the base of the first metacarpal. Reversed Bennett fracture (b): Avulsion fracture of the base of the fifth metacarpal. The small triangular bone fragments are "in place" while the body of the metacarpal bones is dislocated and must be reduced. (© Medical Illustrator Tommy Bolic, Sweden.)

is avulsed, while this fragment represents an important ligament insertion. The bone fragment remains in place, while the remainder of the bone (finger) is out of position and must be reduced. The athlete may also sustain other transverse, oblique, spiral, intra-articular, or multifragment finger fractures (Figures 9.20a and 9.20b).

- **Symptoms and signs:** Symptoms are pain, tenderness, swelling, and malalignment.
- **Diagnosis:** Radiographs only can verify a suspected fracture. For individual fractures (such as a reversed Bennett's fracture) a CT scan may be helpful in demonstrating the fracture dislocation. To examine the finger for possible malrotation, the patient should be asked to make a fist. The nails on the four ulnar fingers are normally in the same plane, the fingertips merging toward the scaphoid.
- **Treatment of transverse fractures (Figure 9.20):** These are usually stable fractures that can be treated by immobilizing the finger by buddy taping it to an adjacent finger. However, these fractures (e.g., on the middle phalanx) can be greatly displaced because of pulling from tendons (the flexor digitorum superficialis muscle). If a displacement is found, the fracture must be reduced and immobilized in a cast for 3–4 weeks before mobilization. If reduction fails, surgery is necessary. Surgery would also be an option when a rigid fixation is possible enabling early motion and return to sport.
- **Treatment of oblique and spiral fractures (Figures 9.21a and 9.21b):** These are often shortened and involve malrotation. The position cannot be maintained after reduction, and as a consequence, these fractures should be treated surgically—for example, by percutaneous pinning, or open surgery using plates and/or screws. When the reduction and stable osteosynthesis are performed, the athlete can resume training more quickly. Fractures that are not treated surgically should be checked by a second radiographic examination after 1 week.

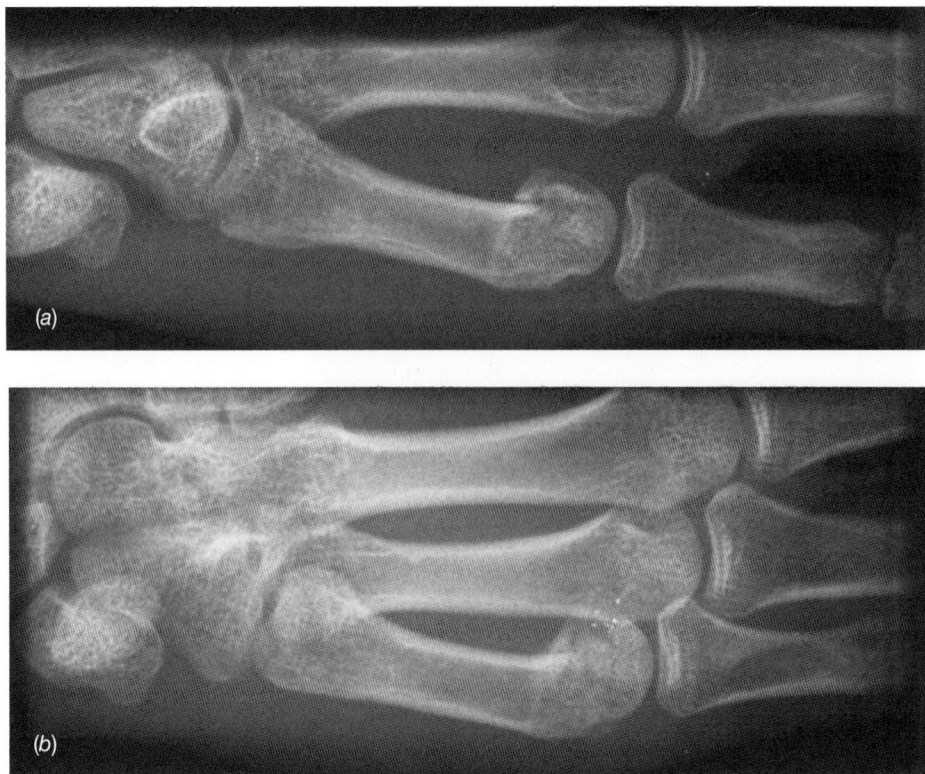

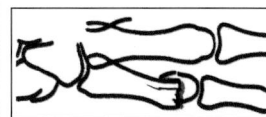

Figure 9.20 Transverse fracture of the fifth metacarpal. Frontal (a) and oblique lateral (b) views demonstrate a distal subcapital fracture. However, it is difficult to obtain a direct lateral view of these fractures. Therefore, it must be noted that malalignment could be significantly greater than what is revealed by the lateral views. (© Medical Illustrator Tommy Bolic, Sweden.)

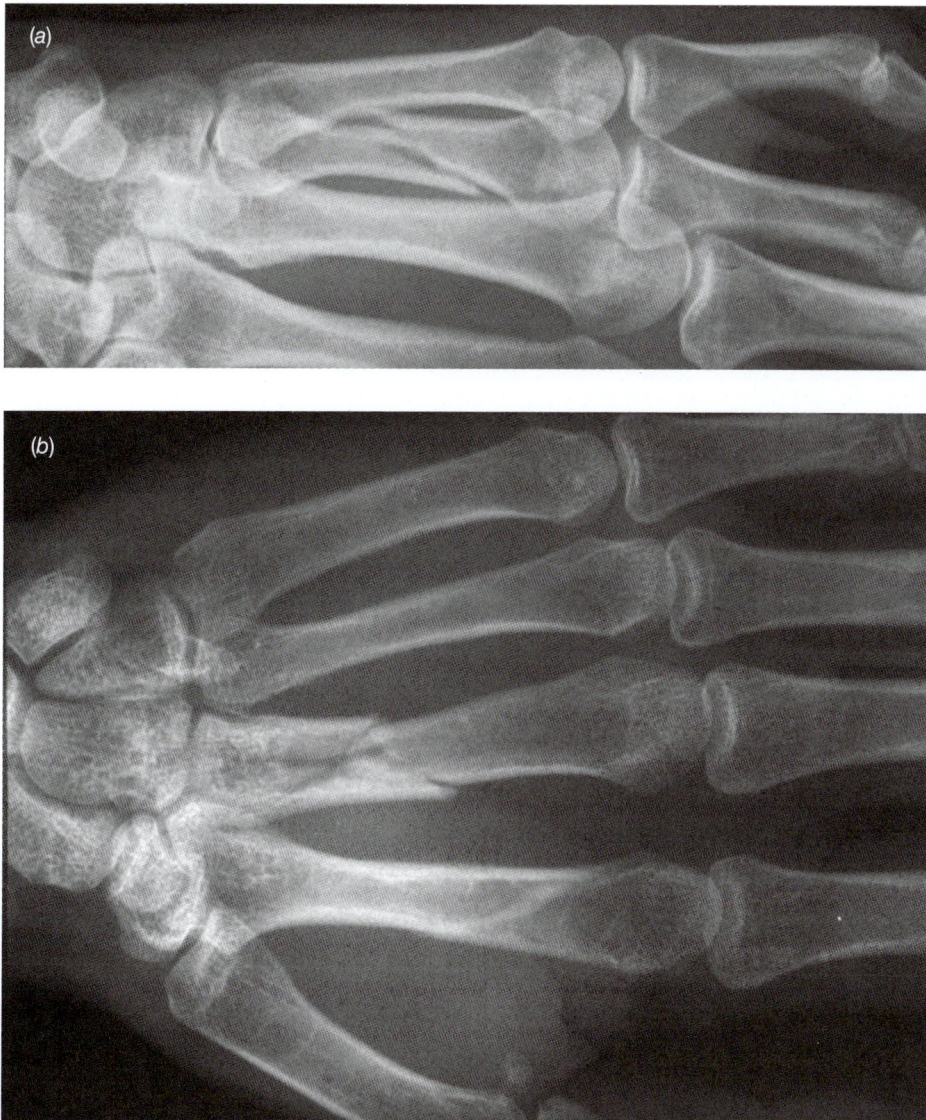

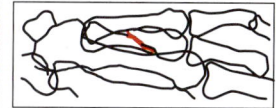

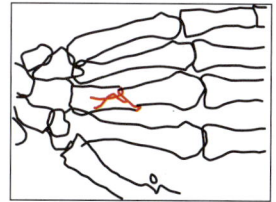

Figure 9.21 Oblique (a) and shaft fractures (b). These fractures often cause shortening and/or malrotation of the finger and, therefore, require surgery. (© Medical Illustrator Tommy Bolic, Sweden.)

- Treatment of intra-articular fractures (Figures 9.22a and 9.22b): Comminuted fractures and intra-articular fractures, compromising joint congruity, should be referred to a hand surgeon for consideration of surgical treatment.
- Treatment of Bennett's fracture and reversed Bennett's fracture: These fractures require surgery.
- Prognosis: Usually short-term immobilization and early retraining are prioritized to achieve good functional results. If the fracture is properly reduced and stabilized, retraining may begin after 3–4 weeks of immobilization, and the prognosis is good. If initial treatment is inadequate, there may be a prolonged rehabilitation period keeping the athlete from participating in sports activities. Surgery may eventually be required to correct any deformity that has occurred. The combination of tendon injuries and fractures is challenging due to adhesions between the skeleton and the tendon. This may require long-term retraining by a hand therapist. Depending on the type of fracture, the treatment, and the sport involved, the patient may usually return to sport activity after 4–6 weeks.

WRIST, HAND, AND FINGERS

283

(a)

(b)

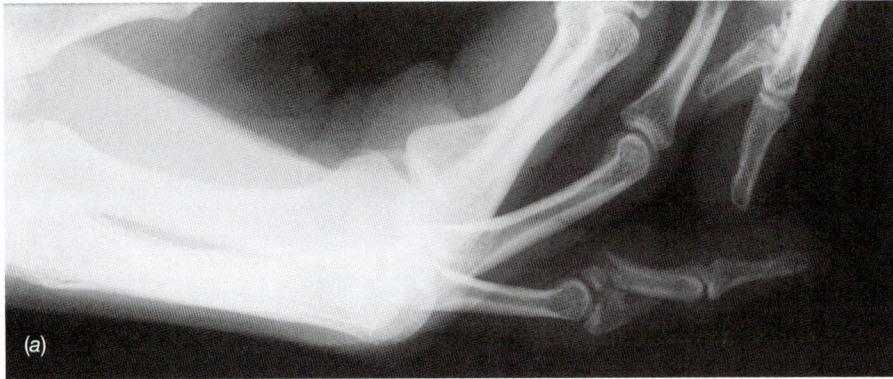

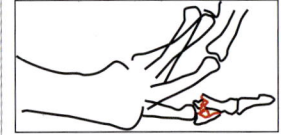

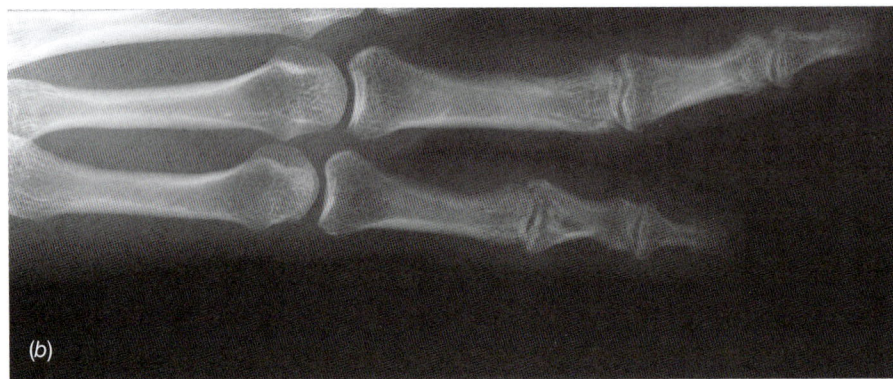

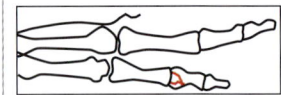

Figure 9.22 Intraarticular Fracture, lateral (*a*) and PA (*b*) view. These fractures require exact repositioning to provide good function and to prevent the development of osteoarthritis. Surgery is usually necessary. (© Medical Illustrator Tommy Bolic, Sweden.)

Rupture of the Collateral Ligament in the PIP Joint and the MCP Joint—*Injury of the Lateral Ligaments in the Finger*

The collateral ligaments in the finger's PIP and MCP joints are injured by direct side-to-side trauma or by a finger getting caught on an object.

- Symptoms and signs: Patients experience pain, tenderness, and swelling, as well as reduced flexion-motion.
- Diagnosis: The diagnosis is based on soreness and pain by palpating and stability testing the injured ligament. A complete rupture may cause instability. A radiographic examination is indicated to diagnose avulsed bone fragments. This rarely occurs in the PIP joint but is somewhat more common in the MCP joint.
- Treatment: The injured finger is immobilized to an adjacent finger for 1–3 weeks, and then free exercise is allowed. If much swelling and pain occur, immobilization in a cast may be indicated for a few days: 90° in MCP and fully extension of the PIP and DIP joints. One should aim for early motion in order to minimize stiffness. A fracture may be an indication for open reduction for fixation of a large bony fragment followed by immobilization for 3–4 weeks.
- Prognosis: The prognosis is generally good, but, as in the case of a sprain, it may take a long time to return to normal range of motion, and the PIP joint may be swollen for as long as a year. Buddy taping it to an adjacent finger for a few more weeks is a good prophylactic, particularly in ball sports such as team handball or volleyball, where there is a risk of another injury.

Rupture of the Collateral Ligament in the MCP Joint of the Thumb—*Skier's Thumb*

The most common mechanism of injury is falling while skiing, causing trauma to the thumb with increasing stress leading to a possible rupture of the ulnar collateral ligament (Figure 9.23).

- Symptoms and signs: Symptoms and signs are pain when the thumb is being moved, as well as swelling (bleeding) and soreness to palpation corresponding to the injured collateral ligament. Soreness is often also present on the palmar side of the thumb's MCP joint (simultaneous injury of the palmar tendon plate).
- Diagnosis: It is best to examine the injury immediately after the accident occurs, when the proper diagnosis can be made on the basis of the clinical examination alone. By moving the thumb away in a radial direction from the rest of a stabilized hand, the ulnar collateral ligament is being tested for stability (Figure 9.18, p. 280). The thumb should be examined both fully extended and at 20° of flexion in the MCP joint. Slightly increased laxity followed by a *distinct stop* is often interpreted as a partial (incomplete) ligament injury. If there is increased laxity without a distinct stop, the patient *should* be referred for a radiographic examination and evaluation by a hand surgeon. A radiographic examination should be performed with tension on the injured ligament. Similar views of the other, uninjured thumb should be taken for comparison. Correspondingly, the patient should also be examined in a similar way for a possible rupture of the radial collateral ligament.
- Treatment: A partial injury (distinct stop while testing) may be treated by immobilization in a cast for 4–6 weeks. If there is an avulsion and displacement of the ligament insertion (fracture), surgery is required. If there is no fracture, but a definite instability is found, surgery is required as well. This is particularly true of the ulnar collateral ligament, where the mechanism of injury may involve the ruptured ligament becoming "caught" by the aponeurosis of the adductor pollicis longus, preventing the ligament ends from healing without surgery. After surgery, the patient needs to be in a cast for 5–6 weeks. Injuries to the radial collateral ligament are less common and have traditionally been treated conservatively (with a cast for 5–6 weeks). There is often a combination of injury to the radial collateral ligament and the volar tendon plate. The current tendency is to perform surgery on these injuries (as in the case of the ulnar collateral ligament).

WRIST, HAND, AND FINGERS

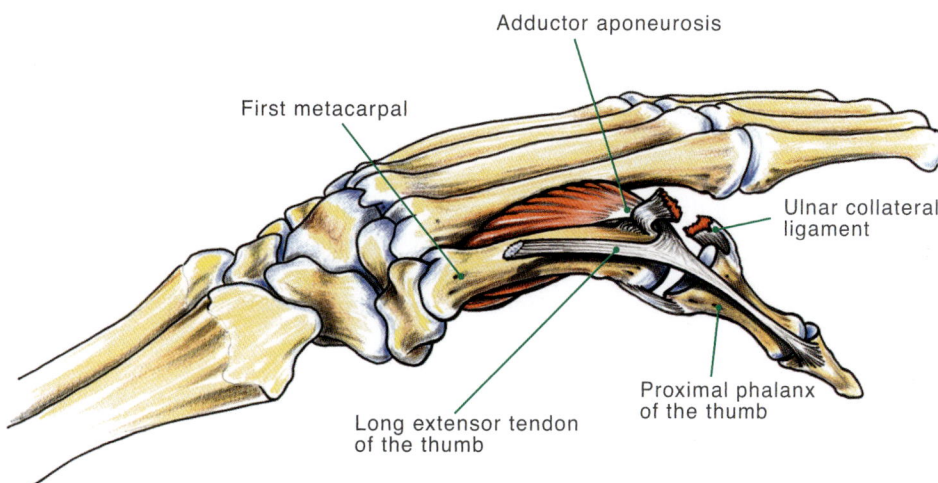

Figure 9.23 Rupture of the ulnar collateral ligament in the thumb's MCP joint (skier's thumb). The ulnar collateral ligament usually ruptures at the insertion to the proximal phalanx, sometimes with a bone fragment that is avulsed. The proximal part of the ligament becomes displaced by the adductor aponeurosis (as shown). These ruptures will not heal without surgery. (© Medical Illustrator Tommy Bolic, Sweden.)

Labels in figure: Adductor aponeurosis · First metacarpal · Ulnar collateral ligament · Proximal phalanx of the thumb · Long extensor tendon of the thumb

• Prognosis: Prognosis is good with proper treatment. When treatment in a cast is completed, the patient may benefit from a brace when resuming sport activity after about 8 weeks.

Tendon Rupture

If there is a wound, a rupture of the extensor or flexor tendons should be suspected, depending on the localization of the injury. A tendon rupture without an open wound is rare, but a flexor tendon rupture may result from strong pulling on the finger (the curling of a finger against resistance, a "jersey finger") or from extreme loading, as in the case of mountain climbing. The EPL tendon of the thumb may rupture after a radius fracture (Figure 9.14, p. 274).

• Symptoms and signs: Symptoms include pain, tenderness, mild swelling, reduced tone in the injured tendon, and a finger in an extended or flexed position without the capacity to be moved in the opposite direction (depending on which tendon is injured).
• Diagnosis: A clinical examination provides a basis for making the diagnosis. Ultrasound may help, and a radiographic examination may demonstrate an avulsed bone fragment. A retracted proximal end of a ruptured tendon may be palpable as a tender soft lump proximally in the digit or in the palm.
• Treatment: Surgery is the recommended treatment.
• Prognosis: The prognosis is good if surgery is performed. The athlete may return to sport activity 8 weeks after an extensor tendon injury, but full loading is not allowed until 12 weeks after a flexor tendon injury.

Mallet Finger—*Drop Finger*

If a ball (e.g., handball, basketball, or volleyball) hits the very tip of a finger, or if it is necessary to pull on tight boots, subjecting the finger to sudden external force that forces the extended finger into a flexed position, the extensor tendon insertion, with or without a bony fragment, to the dorsal side of the distal phalanx (Figures 9.24a and 9.24b) may be injured.

• Symptoms and signs: Symptoms are tenderness, mild swelling, possibly discoloration as a sign of bleeding, and pain. The finger's DIP joint is in a flexed position and may be extended passively, but not actively.
• Diagnosis: The diagnosis is made clinically, but a radiographic examination should be provided to exclude a fracture or a subluxation of the DIP joint.
• Treatment: If there is an avulsion fracture of the extensor tendon insertion involving 1/4–1/6 of the articular surface, surgery should be performed on the finger within a few days. Otherwise, a drop finger can be treated with a splint that immobilizes the DIP joint in an extended (slightly hyperextended) position, while allowing free motion in the PIP and MCP joints. The splint should be worn day and night for 6–8 weeks (8 weeks with no fracture), and from then it should be worn as a night splint for a few more weeks. If there is no fracture, surgery does not provide better results.
• Prognosis: The prognosis is good. Improvement is gradual, it may, however, take from 6 to 12 months before the DIP joint can be fully extended. Even a several months old drop finger injury may be treated as described with a good result. Sport activity may be resumed after about 10 weeks, but it is recommended that the finger be protected with tape or a brace.

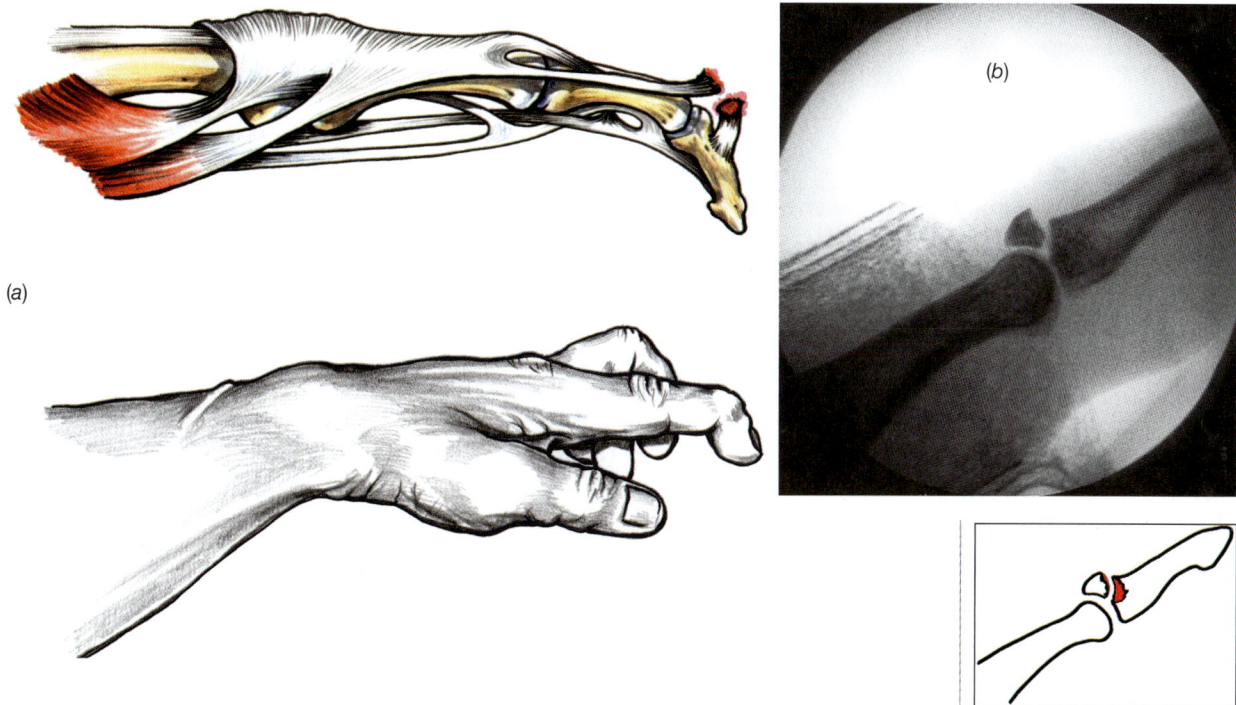

(a)

(b)

Pulley Rupture—*Tendon Sheath Injury*

Pulleys are thickened areas within the flexor tendon sheath, located in specific spots along the course of the tendon. They serve the purpose of keeping the tendons in place next to the skeleton preventing bowstringing and maximizing flexor tendon efficiency (Figure 9.25). The finger's flexor tendons may rupture as a result of extreme loading (such as mountain climbers impose on their fingers), the ruptures usually occur at the A2 pulley.

Figure 9.24 Mallet finger. Mallet finger can be treated conservatively in case of a torn tendon insertion, if the skeleton is intact (*a*). Always take an X-ray to exclude skeletal injury. If there is a fracture, the patient must be evaluated for surgery (*b*). (© Medical Illustrator Tommy Bolic, Sweden.)

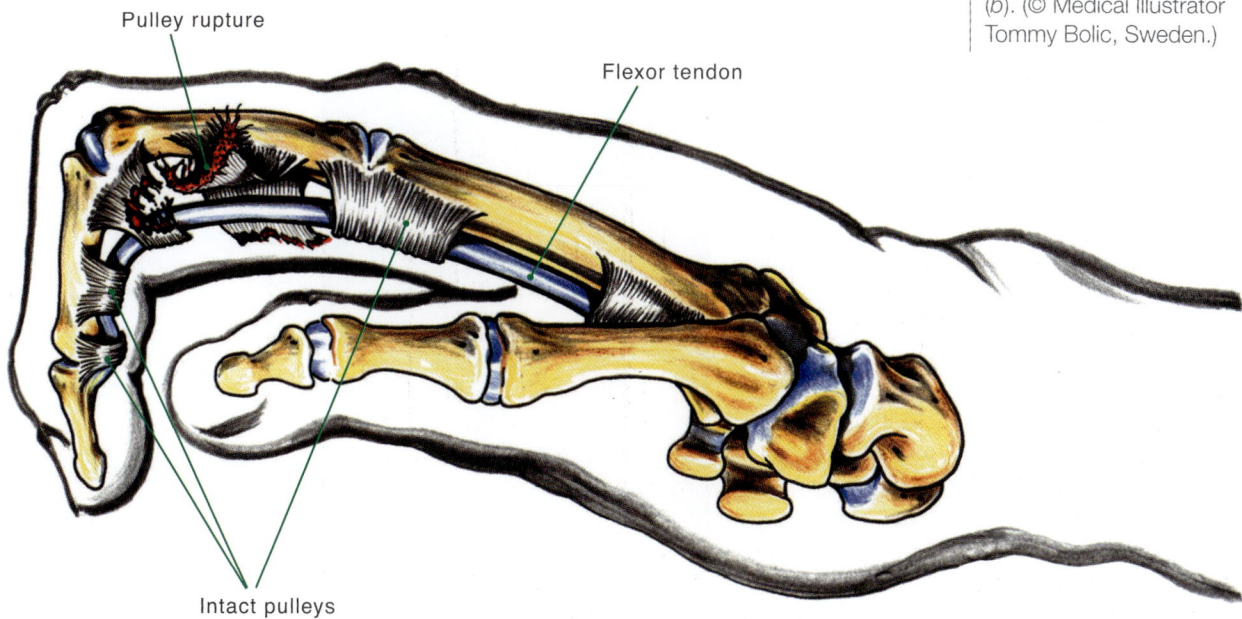

Pulley rupture

Flexor tendon

Intact pulleys

Figure 9.25 Pulley rupture. Extreme pulling of the flexor tendons of the finger, such as when mountain climbing, may cause the sheath of the flexor tendons to rupture. (© Medical Illustrator Tommy Bolic, Sweden.)

- Symptoms and signs: Pain, tenderness, and swelling on the palmar side of the finger are the symptoms, while in severe cases bowstringing may be seen.
- Diagnosis: Diagnosis is based on soreness to palpation over the pulley and to flexion motion in the affected finger. If several pulleys are torn, the flexor tendon may be palpated as a bowstring in the subcutaneous tissue. A trained radiologist should be able to see the ruptured pulleys by performing an ultrasound examination.
- Treatment: If a bowstring is palpated, the patient should be referred to surgery for suturing or reconstruction of the pulleys. There is no good treatment for cases that do not have bowstringing. The patient should be informed about what causes the condition and should use caution when returning to rock climbing after symptoms have subsided.
- Prognosis: The prognosis is good. When the pulleys are reconstructed, adhesions may develop that might reduce the flexion of the affected finger. The patient should wait 8–10 weeks after surgical intervention before resuming sport activity.

Finger Joint Dislocation

Dislocation of a finger joint (Figure 9.26) is a relatively common injury resulting from playing various types of ball sports. Dislocations of the little finger or thumb are the most common injuries, but dislocation of any joint on any finger is reported.

- Symptoms and signs: Symptoms are swelling, tenderness, deformity, and limited range of motion.
- Diagnosis: Diagnosis is based on the presence of malalignment and instability, or history of the same. Radiographic examination is necessary to see if there are any associated fractures.
- Treatment: Reduction of a dislocated finger by pulling the finger in axial direction is usually easy to do immediately after the injury has occurred. A *radiographic examination should be performed to confirm the reduction* and to rule out any fracture while relocating the joint. The finger is immobilized or fixed to an adjacent finger with a cast or tape for 3–4 weeks, after which exercises may begin. The injured finger should be buddy taped to an adjacent finger for a few more weeks during sport activity. The PIP joints, in particular, but also the MCP joints may be dorsally dislocated as a result of hyperextension trauma. *Interposition of the* patient's *volar tendon plate or flexor tendons* may also occur, making closed reduction impossible and surgery necessary. In cases of a fracture dislocation the athlete should be referred to a hand surgeon for evaluation of surgical treatment.
- Prognosis: The prognosis is good, but there is often reduced motion (particularly in PIP joints) for several months after the injury occurs. Swelling in the joint may last for up to a year. Sport activity may be resumed 5–6 weeks after the injury occurs, but the finger should be protected by a buddy tape.

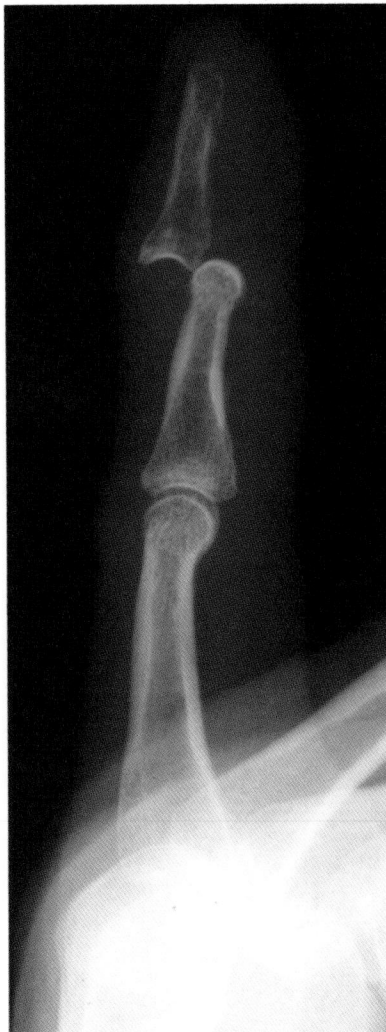

Figure 9.26 Dislocation. Forceful trauma to a finger may cause dislocation of a finger joint, as shown in the DIP joint of this little finger. (Reproduced with permission from the Norwegian Sports Medicine Association.)

Nerve Injury

Digital nerve laceration may occur in an open wound injury. A compression of a nerve may cause reduced sensation, but the continuity is intact. Dorsal finger nerves (primarily from the radial nerve) are usually not repaired, as this injury causes minor discomfort for the patient. However, an injured digital nerve on the palmar side of the finger *should* be referred for surgical treatment as soon as the injury is diagnosed, or no later than 1–2 weeks after injury. There is no reason for "observation" after this injury. The patient may indicate whether sensation is any different on different sides of each finger when the radial and ulnar sides of each finger are examined as previously described. (The physician should compare it to the other hand if that hand is uninjured.) If the patient indicates reduced sensation in all or part of his hand, he *should* be referred for surgery.

Rehabilitation of Hand and Finger Injuries

Oddvar Knutsen[1] and Jan-Ragnar Haugstvedt[2]

[1]*Lia Terapi Trysil, Trysil, Norway*
[2]*Østfold Hospital Trust, Moss, Norway*

Goals and Principles

Table 9.3 lists the goals of acute hand and finger injury rehabilitation.

A combination of several measures is needed to rehabilitate major hand and finger injuries. It is preferable for an experienced hand therapist to administer or direct this therapy. A well-functioning hand must have motion, stability, strength, and sensation, and must be pain free. In cases in which stabilizing surgery is necessary, systematic conservative rehabilitation must follow, with the goal of achieving good long-term results.

During the acute phase, it is important to gain control over pain and inflammation by cooling with ice, elevation, compression, and rest from activities that cause pain.

During the rehabilitation phase, braces, splints, or taping to an adjacent finger are often used to ease resumption of active assisted mobilization of joints with the greatest possible joint motion. If a joint is stable, early mobilization is recommended. If there is much swelling, compression treatment is used. This can be accomplished by having the patient wear fitted compression gloves, individually adjusted finger stockings (or Coban), or Tubigrip on his hand or wrist. Elastic bandages about 2.5 cm wide are well suited to fingers.

	Goals	Measures
Acute phase	Reduce pain and inflammation	PRICE
Rehabilitation phase	Normalize movement and strength in the hand and finger joint	Strength and stretching exercises
	Normalize endurance and coordination	
Training phase	Complete healing of injured ligaments without the loss of mechanical stability or movement	Functional exercises
		Sport-specific exercises
	Practice training in sport activity while gradually increasing loading	
	Reduce the risk of reinjury	

Table 9.3 Goals and measures for rehabilitation of acute hand and finger injuries. (Reproduced with permission from the Norwegian Sports Medicine Association.)

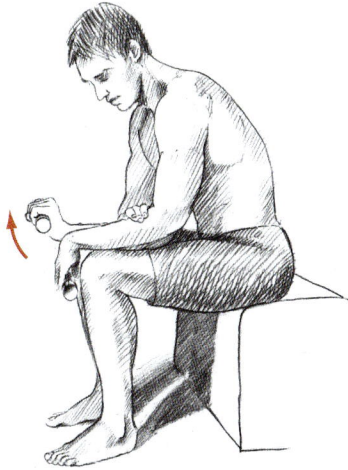

Figure 9.27 Strengthening the extensor muscles of the wrist

- Lift your hand gently, as shown in the figure.
- Hold for 1 second.
- Lower your hand.

(Reproduced with permission from the Norwegian Sports Medicine Association.)

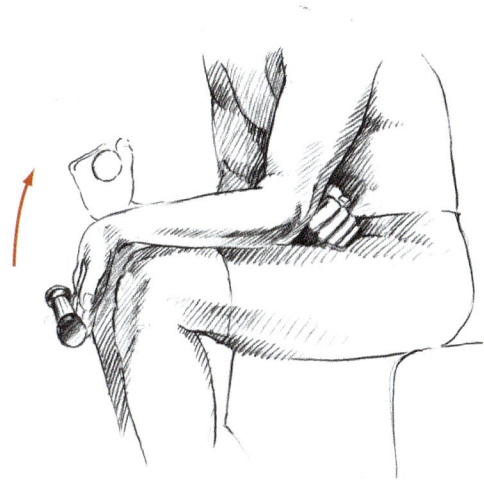

Figure 9.28 Strengthening the flexor muscles of the wrist

- Lift your hand gently, as shown in the figure.
- Hold for 1 second.
- Lower your hand.

(Reproduced with permission from the Norwegian Sports Medicine Association.)

Several people benefit from a contrast bath before mobilization because this reduces discomfort during passive mobilization. Two bowls of water, one with ice and the other with hot water, should be used. The hand or fingers should be moved around for 45 seconds in the hot water and then for 15 seconds in the cold water. This should be repeated 10–15 times. Electrotherapy may also be used to mobilize intra-articular fluid. If pain increases during activity, the activity must be stopped immediately and ice applied locally to the painful area for 15–20 minutes.

To avoid overloading the tendons, isometric or concentric exercises are recommended for strength training during the initial training phase (e.g., Figures 9.27 and 9.28). Toward the end of the training phase, the exercises are increased to eccentric loading, so that the athlete is ready to meet the requirements of the sport. Progressive loading of the tendons is achieved in this manner. In addition to the general warm-up, warming the injured muscles and tendons well is necessary during the training phase before starting specific functional exercises. After training, ice may be applied locally, to prevent the recurrence of symptoms.

For the fingers, the function of the thumb is the most important thing to normalize because it provides a backup for the other fingers. A "rubber sponge" can be used to ease the gripping function during the start-up phase (Figure 9.29). Rubber tension bands can also be used (Figure 9.30).

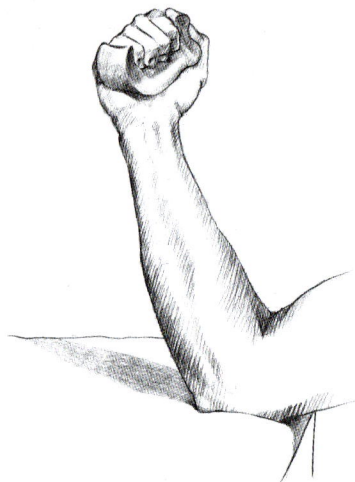

Figure 9.29 Strengthening the flexor muscles of the fingers

• Grasp a foam rubber grip.
• Hold for 3–5 seconds.
(Reproduced with permission from the Norwegian Sports Medicine Association.)

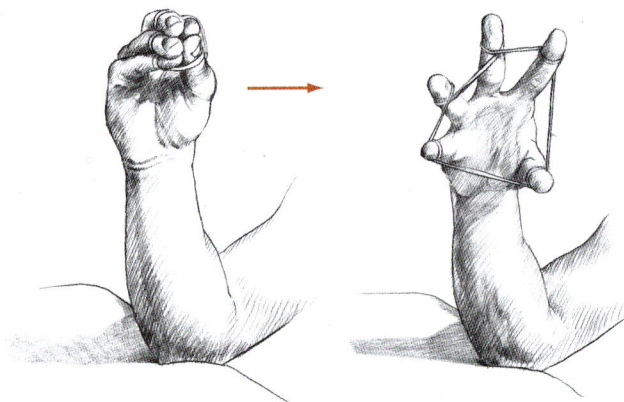

Figure 9.30 Strengthening extensor muscles of the fingers

• Wrap a tension band around each finger once, and spread your fingers.
• Hold for 3–5 seconds.
(Reproduced with permission from the Norwegian Sports Medicine Association.)

10 Pelvis, Groin, and Hips

Acute Injuries to the Pelvis, Groin, and Hips

Marc J. Philippon[1,2,3], Éanna Falvey[4], Geoffrey M. Verrall[5], and Karen K. Briggs[1]

[1]*Steadman Philippon Research Institute, Vail, CO, USA*
[2]*McMaster University, Hamilton, ON, Canada*
[3]*University of Pittsburgh Medical Center, Pittsburgh, PA, USA*
[4]*Sports Surgery Clinic, Dublin, Ireland*
[5]*Sportsmed SA, Sports Medicine Centre, Adelaide, SA, Australia*

Occurrence

Athletes frequently sustain acute injuries in the pelvic, inguinal, and hip regions. Athletes who participate in soccer, ice hockey, tennis, downhill skiing, cross-country skiing (especially freestyle), speed skating, hurdling, high jumping, and horseback riding are particularly vulnerable. In a study of college athletes in the United States, the hip was the second most common area for injury, with 17% of all injuries being in the hip region. Hip injuries often occur in contact sports and athletes who do repeated rotational maneuvers such as adduction, abduction, internal rotation, and external rotation. Falls and lateral impact injuries are also common causes of acute injuries. Sports with a high incidence of groin injury often involve kicking and twisting movements while actions that place strain on fascial and musculoskeletal structures that are fixed to a number of bony anatomical points in very close proximity. The resultant tissue damage and/or entrapment of anatomical structures may cause hip or groin pain, thereby resulting in time lost participating in the athlete's sport of choice. Groin injury is the fourth most common time-loss injury in professional soccer.

Differential Diagnoses

The most frequent acute injuries to athletes in the pelvic, inguinal, and hip region are groin injuries and labral tears (Table 10.1). Acute groin injury is most often

Most common	Less common	Must not be overlooked !
Rectus abdominis strain, p. 162	Hip fracture, p. 305	Hip joint dislocation, p. 304
Adductor longus muscle rupture, p. 297	Other muscle ruptures, p. 305	Slipped capital femoral epiphysis (SCFE), p. 308
Rectus femoris muscle injury, p. 300	Avulsion fractures, p. 306	Avascular necrosis
Iliopsoas muscle injury, p. 301	Pelvic fracture, p. 306	
Femoroacetabular impingement, p. 302	Acute trochanteric bursitis, p. 308	

Table 10.1 Overview of differential diagnoses of acute injuries in the pelvic, inguinal, and hip region. (Reproduced with permission from the Norwegian Sports Medicine Association.)

The IOC Manual of Sports Injuries, First Edition. Edited by Roald Bahr.
©2012 International Olympic Committee. Published 2012 by John Wiley & Sons, Ltd.

soft tissue in nature affecting the adductors, hip flexor muscles, gluteal muscles, and lower abdominal and oblique muscle aponeuroses. In the younger population traction injury at the apophysis (growth plate) may lead to pain and dysfunction, apophysitis, or more significantly disruption of the apophysis in an avulsion fracture. Hip fractures occur for a number of reasons across age groups. Fractures in the hip are common in the elderly, usually people with osteoporosis who are physically inactive, although traumatic pelvic fracture is seen in collision and high speed sports. Stress fracture, secondary to increased training load, may cause acute onset groin pain. Bursitis is described at the greater trochanter but is accompanied by tendinosis of the gluteal muscles in proximity to the bursa and an acute manifestation of a more chronic problem.

An injury that cannot be overlooked is hip dislocation or subluxation. A forceful traumatic event can cause the hip joint to dislocate. Fractures requiring surgery may be associated with these dislocations. In addition, femoral head avascular necrosis can be a serious complication that must be evaluated early. These injuries are often accompanied by other intra-articular pathologies such as labral tears, torn ligamentum teres, torn capsule, and chondral injuries.

Diagnostic Thinking

The first step in the diagnosis is to obtain a detailed history from the patient. This will assist in ruling out metabolic disorders, as well as infectious and inflammatory diseases. The patient's description of injury or when pain is experienced can be helpful in the diagnosis. The case history often provides direction for proper diagnosis, for muscle tears, fractures, dislocations, and intra-articular injuries. Radiographs can provide immediate diagnosis of fractures and dislocation that are not reduced. Dislocations and fractures typically elicit pain that is distinct and severe. Physical examination will determine, in most cases, whether the pain has an intra- or extra-articular source. It will also provide more information on the exact location of the injury. The athlete should be observed at rest, while standing, if possible, structures palpated, range of motion and strength tested, and pulses checked. Determining the areas of pain, tenderness and decreased movement or movement with symptoms is critical in determining the correct diagnosis.

Muscle injury is seen most often in the adductor musculature, particularly the adductor longus. These muscles adduct (and to some degree flex and medially rotate) the thigh, a function that is particularly important in soccer. They are also important pelvic stabilizers during locomotion and movement. The combination of kicking a ball with the inside of the foot, multiple, rapid changes in direction, and tackling with an abducted leg causes major loading and a high frequency of injuries. Injury to the adductor muscles is common in kicking sports and often reported as "simple" groin strain. Familiarity of both athletes and coaches with this injury may lead to under-treatment and continued sporting activity. This often results in a gradual transition to a chronic disorder that may be much more difficult to treat than the original muscle injury. Therefore, early diagnosis and early adequate treatment are crucial. This pathogenesis may be more important for tendon injuries rather than for muscle injuries.

Traumatic fracture such as pelvic fracture usually results in so much pain that the diagnosis is made early, for example, in the emergency department setting. Stress fracture of the inferior pubic ramus should be considered in individuals involved in long-distance endurance events, high-frequency training and those who have significantly increased their workload. It is appreciated as exercise-related groin pain. Apophyseal reaction with avulsion fracture may have a more insidious onset and a less clear cut presentation. In such cases, the practitioner must be aware of this diagnosis and test the muscle group involved by loading the painful area during clinical examination. Intra-articular pathologies are also seen acutely in patients following a traumatic event.

Case History

In a traumatic injury, location of pain and presence of radiating symptoms should be determined. In addition, mechanical symptoms of catching, clicking, or locking and symptoms of instability can be helpful in the diagnosis. Hip joint dislocation is often described by the patient at the time of major trauma or impact. A careful injury history allows the clinician to narrow the differential diagnosis. A history of forceful abduction of the hip during contraction of the adductors, such as tackling, causing sudden onset medial thigh pain, is strongly suggestive of adductor pathology. This is further reinforced by pain on attempted active adduction, such as side stepping or kicking a ball. Similarly, injury to the iliopsoas, the rectus femoris, the gluteal muscles and the abdominal muscles (rectus abdominis, internal and external oblique and transversus abdominis) are seen when contraction against load exceeds the energy required to cause fiber tear and muscle injury. Active muscle testing of the group will recreate pain. For the iliopsoas, climbing stairs is painful in the anterior thigh, for the gluteal muscles rising from a chair recreates posterolateral pain and sit-up movements engage the abdominal muscles.

The same mechanism applies to avulsion fractures and apophyseal injuries. The apophysis is often less able to tolerate load than the musculotendinous junction or muscle belly. In adolescents who are undergoing a growth spurt, muscle tension raises the strain on this area. Pain localization indicates that growth plate may be injured, that is, at the anterior inferior iliac spine for the rectus femoris.

Direct trauma to the greater trochanter region, such as a fall, may cause a fracture in the upper end of the femur or in the pubic rami. However, a much stronger injury mechanism is required to cause a stable or unstable pelvic girdle fracture, such as high-energy trauma caused by downhill skiing or motocross accidents. Acute onset pain, unrelated to trauma, may be seen in athletes with a stress fracture. These athletes often have increased their training load; for example, runners preparing for their first marathon will significantly increase mileage in the last few weeks of their training program.

Clinical Examination

Inspection. The patient's morphology, gait, and posture should be assessed. Shortening of the stance phased and shortening of the length of step should be noted. In addition, pelvic obliquity, limb length, muscle contractures, and scoliosis should be identified. The skin should be inspected for bruising, swelling, or cuts. Muscle atrophy should be noted. If the patient has an acute injury, muscle defects during contraction or swelling over a tear may be present. However, this is an uncommon finding. Discoloration of the skin over and distal to the location of the injury may also be present if there is an intramuscular injury due to torn muscle fascia and bleeding into the subcutaneous tissue. This type of discoloration appears about 3 days following the injury. If the patient sustains a major injury of the gluteal musculature, the Trendelenburg test may be positive. The back, especially the lumbar section, should also be examined in any suspected hip or groin injury. However, the most common examination finding in acute injuries is pain on resisted contraction.

In the case of displaced fractures in the upper end of the femur, the affected lower extremity will be somewhat externally rotated and shortened, whereas a fracture in the pelvic girdle usually does not cause any outer visible signs of injury other than possible contusion marks. Weight bearing will be altered in these injuries.

Traumatic hip joint dislocation is usually posterior. It causes the hip to be held in a flexed, adducted, and internally rotated position. At the same time, incongruence above the hip joint is clearly visible in thin people. Slipped capital femoral epiphysis (SCFE) that has significantly progressed will also make incongruence visible.

Palpation. Palpation will assist in differentiating hip injuries from spine and knee issues. It is important to determine length of symptoms for each patient. Caution should be used when palpating around the hip, pelvis and groin. We suggest that an assistant should always be in the room when palpating around the hip, pelvis, and groin to avoid any misunderstanding by the athlete as to the purpose of the palpation. On lateral exam, the greater trochanter, pubic cleft, and the anterior superior iliac spine (ASIS) are palpated. If a stress fracture of the pubic ramus is suspected, palpate for a feeling of crepitus; however, always have an assistant in the room regardless of the gender of the patient. For pelvic obliquity, palpate the iliac crest. Palpation of soft tissue can assist with diagnosis of piriformis syndrome, lipoma, tumor, myositis ossificans, and hernia.

If the patient has an acute muscle injury, thorough palpation of the affected muscle shortly after injury may reveal a tender defect in the muscle belly that corresponds to the site of injury. Eventually, this defect will fill with blood and edema fluid, which gradually changes to scar tissue. This may feel like a somewhat sensitive, firm area (infiltrate) in the muscle belly.

If the patient has a fracture, palpation may indicate major or minor hematoma in the area of the fracture. Unstable pelvic fractures may be demonstrated by gently pressing on both anterior superior iliac crests at the same time.

Specific Tests

Range of motion. Motion of the hip should be assessed in several planes. Supine flexion is often decreased in the presence of injury, as is supine abduction. The range for normal flexion is 125°–135° and normal abduction is 45°. Adduction is also measured in the supine position. The normal value for adduction ranges from 25° to 35°. Abduction and adduction can also be measured in the lateral position. Internal rotation and external rotation are measured in the prone position. The normal value range for internal rotation is 35°–45° and external rotation normal value is 45°–50°.

Modified Tomas test. For this test, the patient is in the supine position. The patient is placed at the end of the table until their knees are approximately 10 cm over the edge of the table. The patient then flexes both hips and brings their knees to their chest. The patient then holds one leg to the chest and the other leg is let down to the starting position. If the thigh rises off the table, flex the knee on that side. If the knee flexes easily then the tight hip flexor is the iliopsoas. If the knee is unable to flex or resistance is felt, the rectus femoris is tight.

Functional testing. If a muscle has been injured, testing of the indicated muscle against resistance will cause pain generally corresponding to the area of injury. With simultaneous palpation, the defect or infiltrate can be localized, and it may be possible to determine the size of the muscle injury. In professional/elite athletes, MRI is often used to more accurately assess the size and site of the muscle/tendon injury. A partial or total tear will appear as asymmetrical bulging of the muscle during contraction and may be present for an extended period of time even after full recovery has ensued.

Pain at the muscle insertion of young patients who are not fully developed/skeletally mature may indicate an avulsion fracture/apophysitis. Other types of fractures in the area usually cause so much pain that specific testing is impossible. However, impacted fractures of the femoral neck and simple fractures of the pubic rami may cause only a few symptoms. Passive hip joint movement, particularly internal and external rotation, will cause pain if there is femoral neck fracture, and bimanual pressure over the greater trochanter will cause groin pain when there is a fracture of the pubic bone.

Supplemental Examinations

Radiographic examination. If major trauma to the pelvic region is present, particularly from a high-energy injury (e.g., from motor sports or downhill skiing), radiographs should be taken to exclude fractures or dislocations. If an avulsion fracture is suspected in a young athlete, radiographs will usually confirm this. If there is even the slightest indication of a slipped cap femoral epiphysis of the femoral head, the patient must immediately undergo radiographic examination and further evaluation and treatment by an orthopedic surgeon.

Magnetic resonance imaging (MRI). MRI is the diagnostic tool of choice for soft-tissue and intra-articular hip injuries. Muscle injuries, location, and size can be clearly demonstrated, both during the acute phase and during the scar-tissue phase. With respect to prognosis, there is a lack of published literature regarding size of muscle and tendon injures about the hip and groin being useful to predict timing and successful return to athletic activity. MRI is particularly useful for deep-lying muscle groups, such as the iliopsoas.

Computer tomography (CT). CT scans of the pelvic, inguinal, and hip region are often performed in case of major trauma, to define the injuries in more detail. Otherwise, CT scans are rarely useful for routine evaluation of sport injuries in this area.

Skeletal scintigraphy. This examination is seldom used in diagnosing acute injuries in the pelvic, inguinal, and hip region. Radiation exposure is quite high and means this modality is now replaced by MRI.

Ultrasound examination. In experienced hands, ultrasound is an excellent aid in diagnosing muscle tears. It provides a good estimate of the size of the tear and hematoma, and it helps with localization, particularly of deep injuries. In chronic injuries, changes can be seen in the muscle belly, and it will also be possible to demonstrate beginning calcium deposition (myositis ossificans). It has the advantage of being less expensive than MRI but is highly dependent on operator experience.

Common Injuries

Adductor Injury—*Acute Groin Strain*

The most common soft-tissue injury in the pelvic, inguinal, and hip region is a tear in the adductor group of muscles (pectineus, brevis, longus, magnus, and gracilis).

Strains occur primarily in the proximal portion of the adductor longus, at the muscle tendon junction, or at the insertion of the pubic bone itself (Figure 10.1). The injury mechanism is usually a strong hip abduction movement, simultaneous with contraction of the adductors, such as, tackling in soccer. Overloading of this muscle group, such as from repeated strong abduction and adduction movements in skating or freestyle in cross-country skiing or hurdling in athletics, may also result in minor tears of the affected area. This pattern of microtearing is more often related to the development of chronic groin pain but may predate complete rupture. Adductor magnus ruptures can usually be diagnosed by the large amount of ecchymosis demonstrated 3 days after injury.

- Symptoms and signs: Intense pain in the groin or, if the injury is large, the pain is slightly more distal on the inside of the thigh is often reported by the athlete. Attempts at continued activity cause the pain to return. Eventually, swelling over the tear will be present, and if intramuscular bleeding occurs where blood comes out of the muscle belly via a tear in the muscle, the skin above and distal to the tear becomes discolored (Figure 10.2). This will not occur until 2 or 3 days after the injury. When a complete rupture or avulsion injury occurs, the pain may be paradoxically less than a less severe injury. A greater degree of ecchymosis is noted; however, the retracted muscle may often be palpated distally in the leg.
- Diagnosis: History and clinical examination produces the diagnosis. When adductors are contracted against resistance, the patient will indicate pain corresponding to the tear area, and strength will be reduced. MRI or ultrasound, in the hands of a skilled sonographer, are worthwhile to determine the extent or derangement that will direct rehabilitation and prognosis.

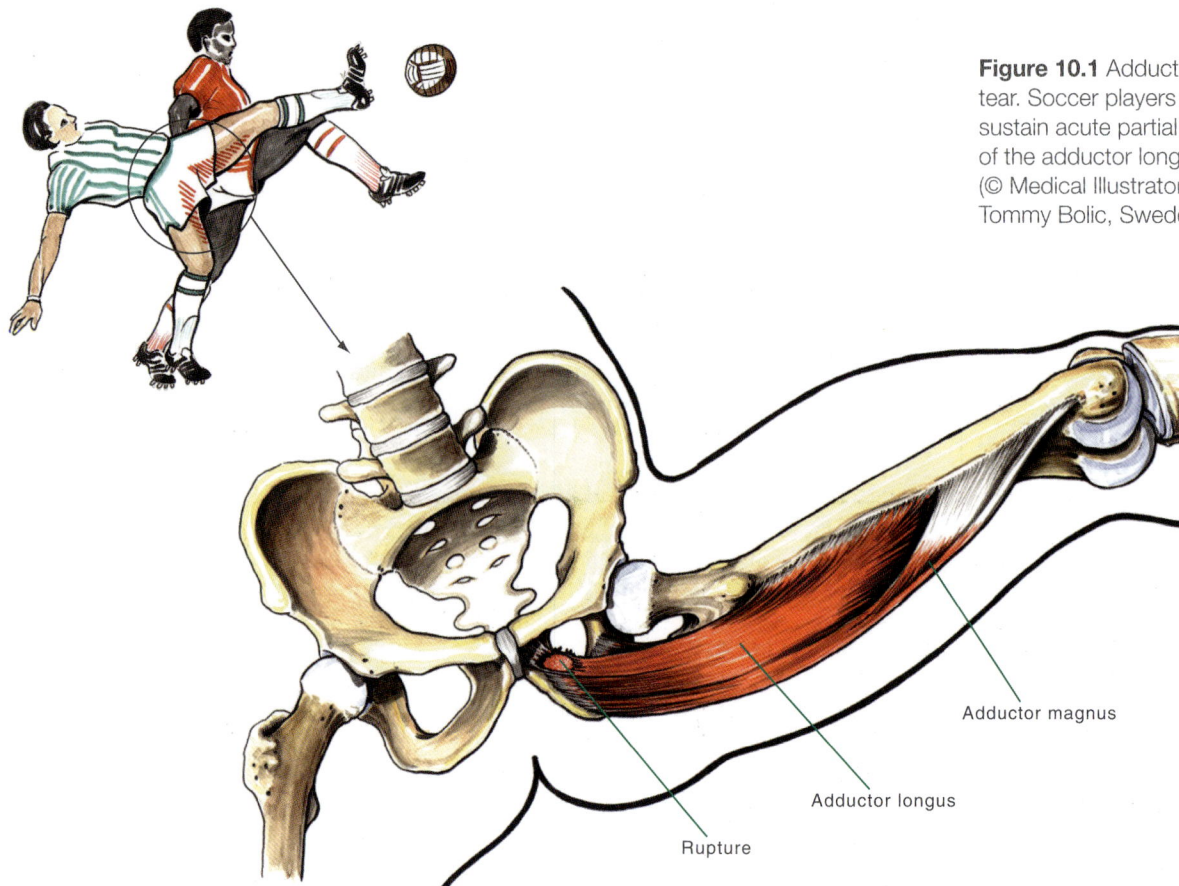

Figure 10.1 Adductor tear. Soccer players often sustain acute partial tears of the adductor longus. (© Medical Illustrator Tommy Bolic, Sweden.)

Adductor magnus

Adductor longus

Rupture

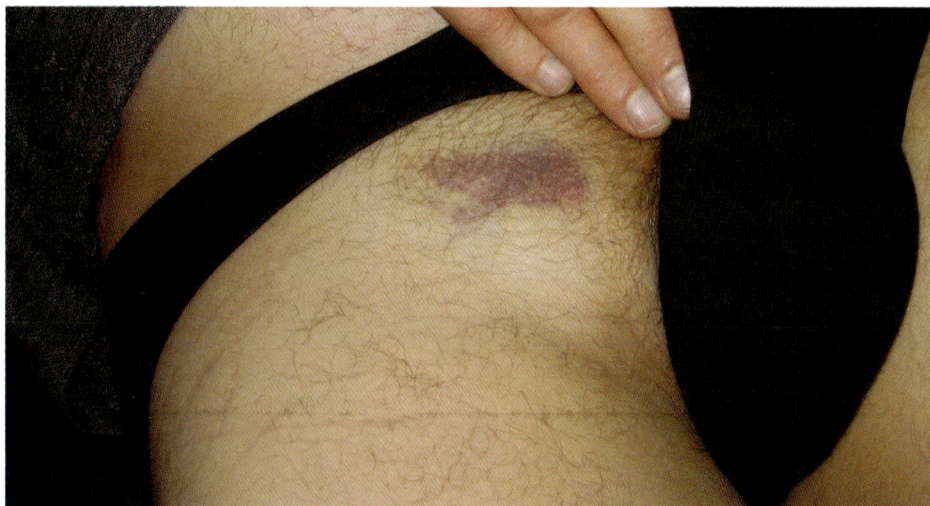

Figure 10.2 Bruising seen following an acute adductor tear.

- Treatment by physician: During the acute stage, the injury is treated according to the PRICE principle. In the past, nonsteroidal anti-inflammatory drugs (NSAIDs) were prescribed in this setting, but it is now well established that the inflammatory process that occurs postinjury is an important initial phase of the healing response and to interfere with this may delay the healing process. Instead, efforts are made to ensure that further injury does not occur. When complete rupture occurs surgical reattachment is not indicated. The postinjury hematoma quickly begins the process of organization and pseudo-tendon is seen at the 4-month mark. Any residual weakness is compensated for by the remainder of the muscle group. Physicians should encourage athletes to participate in early mobilization and rehabilitation as this helps in proper muscle healing.
- Treatment by therapist: As soon as the pain begins to abate, the athlete must begin to actively exercise the injured musculature. A graduated progression in return to activity is also required. Hence, the athlete must be followed up closely and must train the entire time without, or with only minimal, pain. If rehabilitation is too fast, this injury may reoccur or in some cases become chronic. Initially, careful isometric exercises for the adductors are sometimes recommended. However, our experience is that after 3 or 4 days the athlete may begin careful, active strength training, accompanied by careful stretching. If flexibility of the muscle groups on both sides is full and pain free, strength training can be increased to full loading. The goal is for the patient to have normal muscle length and strength before returning to his sport. Sensory motor training (balance training) of the hip and groin musculature may begin as soon as pain allows it. In addition, the patient must undergo a period of controlled functional training in the relevant sport before returning to full training and competition. If long-term stiffness and moderate pain in the inguinal region are present, applying heat packs locally before training may have a good effect. To maintain the best possible general strength and condition during injury recovery, the athlete must be instructed in alternative types of training. Bicycling and swimming (not breaststroke) are normally tolerated well, as is the elliptical trainer and straight line running can be started as soon as pain diminishes. General strength training for the rest of the body is started as soon as the patient is able to do it without local pain. Total tears may be treated conservatively in the same manner as acute proximal injuries, with stretching and strength training. Functional loss of strength in the adductors will usually be insignificant after adequate rehabilitation.

- Prognosis: There are great differences in the amount of time needed for rehabilitation, depending on whether intramuscular or intramuscular bleeding occurred at the time of injury. As for all muscle injuries, patience and caution are key in retraining. If the athlete ignores pain, the likelihood that this injury will become a chronic, painful, difficult-to-treat condition is high. The development of myositis ossificans tends to increase when the rehabilitation of more distal tears with intramuscular bleeding is too active. This calcification may cause chronic pain in the area and may make surgical extirpation of the changes necessary.

Rectus Femoris Muscle Injury—*Tearing in the Muscle Belly of the Thigh*

The rectus femoris muscle originates at the anterior inferior iliac spine and from a reflected head arising from the acetabulum and its insertion is via the quadriceps tendon of the patella. The rectus femoris muscle crosses two joints, flexing the hip and extending the knee, so it must be differentiated from iliopsoas, as a hip flexor and the other three heads of the quadriceps as a knee extensor. It is commonly injured in sports where forceful quadriceps contraction is combined with extension of the hip such as kicking a ball or sprinting (Figure 10.3a and b). Total ruptures are usually located mid-thigh or distal, and commonly occur at the muscle tendon junction to the knee joint. Partial tears (strains) usually occur proximally or mid-thigh, but in both cases always at the musculotendinous junction. The injury normally occurs when the athlete has his hip extended and the knee-joint flexed and flexes his hip and while extending the knee with great force–for example, when kicking the soccer ball. The rectus femoris muscle may tear, especially if there is unexpected resistance (the shot is blocked) to this movement. In the adolescent acute pain proximally at the muscle origin on kicking a ball with explosive force indicates an apophyseal injury and must be high on the clinicians list of differential diagnosis.

- Symptoms and signs: If there is a proximal partial tear, the athlete experiences acute intense pain up toward the groin. When function is affected, the athlete will often report an ability to jog but not sprint.

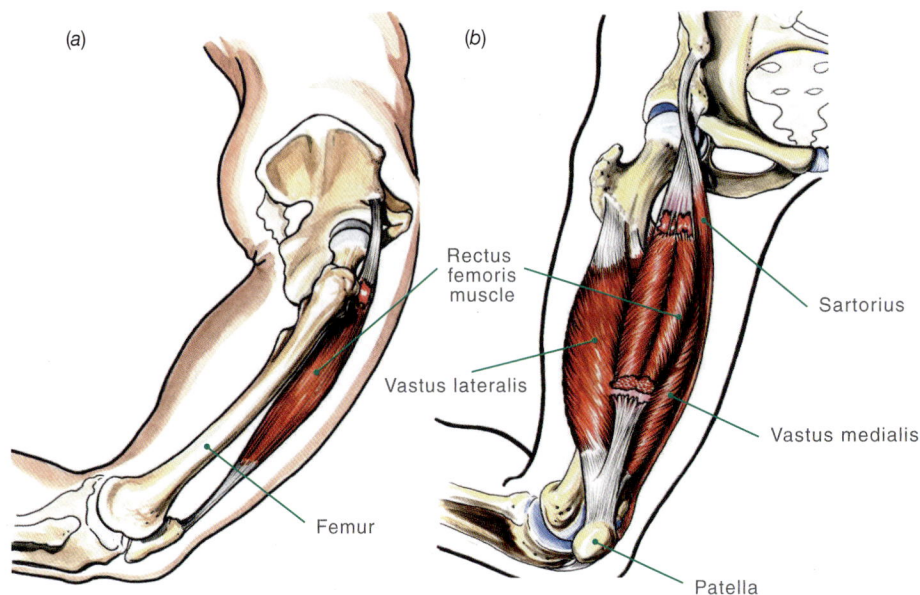

(a)

(b)

Rectus femoris muscle

Sartorius

Vastus lateralis

Vastus medialis

Femur

Patella

Figure 10.3 Tear of the rectus femoris. These types of tears may be partial or total. Partial tears usually occur in the proximal muscle–tendon junction (*a* and *b*), whereas the less common total tears usually occur distally (*b*). (© Medical Illustrator Tommy Bolic, Sweden.)

- Diagnosis: Depending on size of the injury, it may be possible to palpate a tender defect in the muscle belly during the acute phase. Extension strength in the knee will be reduced and painful. If the tear causes intramuscular bleeding, the skin above and distal to the site of the injury will become discolored within 2 or 3 days. The modified Tomas test or the rectus femoris contracture tests are the clinical tests of choice. If there is a total tear, it should be possible to palpate the end of the muscle belly distally, and it can be moved a few centimeters proximally and distally. Minor tears, particularly those that are at the muscle tendon junction, may be difficult to palpate. Ultrasound or MRI is useful in such cases. When presentation is delayed the athlete will often complain of a "lump" in their muscle. On examination, this in fact corresponds to retracted muscle and a defect will be palpable either proximally or distally depending on the injury site. Injuries also occur in the rectus femoris muscle belly rather than at the musculotendinous junction. It has been demonstrated that this is due to injury to the reflected head of the rectus femoris arising from the acetabular ridge and denotes a longer period of rehabilitation (4 weeks instead of 2).
- Treatment: Treatment for partial tears is the same as tears of the adductor longus. If a total tear of the muscle-tendon junction has occurred, the athlete may be offered surgical treatment. More commonly, conservative treatment is generally the treatment of choice.
- Prognosis: Prognosis for partial tears is good, provided the patient receives adequate conservative therapy. However, these injuries have a high recurrence rate particularly in kicking sports such as football. The athlete is usually able to return to full sport activity after 4–6 weeks, but care must be taken in rehabilitation. Particularly later in the rehabilitation process (weeks 3–6) care must be taken to stress the rectus femoris rather than the rest of the quadriceps muscles. However, the player will often feel 100% on adding explosive sports-specific movements such as sprinting or kicking a ball at full strength off of the ground reinjury may occur as the rectus femoris is recruited when not fully rehabilitated. If activity starts too early, and particularly if the tear is close to the muscle-tendon junction, the injury can develop into chronic tendinosis. After surgical treatment for a total tear, the patient can normally participate in his sport again after about 8–12 weeks. Stretching and strength training of the quadriceps is used to rehabilitate overlooked total tears. There is surprisingly little function loss once retraining has been completed.

Iliopsoas Muscle Tear

The iliopsoas muscle consists of three muscles (the psoas major, the psoas minor, and the iliacus), and has a broad origin from the L1 to L5 transverse processes and the inside of the ilium. The muscles are retroperitoneal and collect in a joint insertion on the lesser trochanter of the femur. It is the hip's strongest flexor muscle. Tears in this muscle (Figure 10.4) typically occur as a result of forced flexion of the hip against resistance, generally as a result of significant force. These injuries are much less common than adductor or rectus femoris injuries. Far more common than a tear is pain, weakness and "shortening" of the muscle. This dysfunction is often anticipated in the anterior groin and due to the medial position of the lesser trochanter may be clinically difficult to differentiate form adductor pathology.

- Symptoms and signs: Tears in the muscle belly are uncommon; however, if sustained, pain is deep in the abdomen, radiating down toward the inguinal ligament. A large hematoma may develop causing pressure on the surrounding nerves (the lateral cutaneous nerve of the thigh, ilioinguinal, genitofemoral, and femoral nerves) with sensory deficit and possibly weakening of the quadriceps. These symptoms are usually short-term and disappear when the hematoma is resorbed. If the tear is localized to the muscle tendon junction, pain is more central in the groin. Total tears of the il-iopsoas seldom occur. In the adolescent partial avul-sion of the apophysis at the common insertion at the lesser trochanter may occur.

- Diagnosis: The patient indicates pain correspond-ing to the area of the tear when she flexes her hip against resistance or when she lifts her leg with the knee extended while sitting on a chair. Pain may also be felt in the anterior groin in the FABER (flexion, abduction and external rotation) position. Patients with proximal tears indicate tenderness to pressure but not rebound tenderness to palpation of the lower portion of the abdomen (i.e., there is no peritoneal irritation). If there is a partial distal tear, bimanual palpation over the lesser trochan-ter may trigger significant pain. The most critical differential diagnoses that need to be excluded are appendicitis, diverticulitis, strangulated hernia, kidney stones, and a tear in the rectus abdominis muscle.
- Treatment: Treatment is conservative, as in the case of a tear of the adductor longus. If rehabilitation is too aggressive or return to sport activity is too early, a partial distal tear can develop into chronic tendinosis. This is particularly impor-tant in the case of the iliopsoas as it has been shown to play a pivotal role in the development and aggravation of other groin conditions.
- Prognosis: The prognosis is good with proper rehabilitation.
- Prevention: Regular stretching and strength training of the hip flexors is particu-larly important in specific sports in which athletes are vulnerable, including soccer, high jumping, hurdle jumping, and rowing.

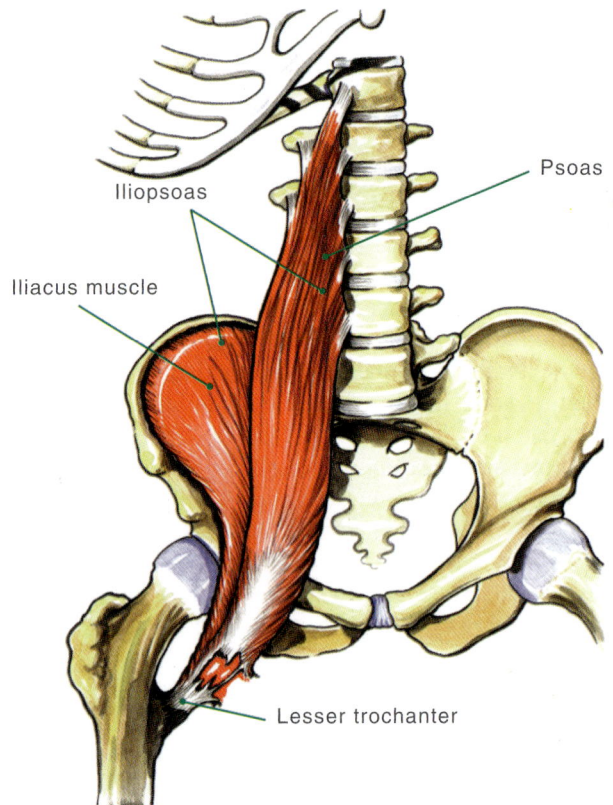

Figure 10.4 Partial tear in the distal part of the iliopsoas. (© Medical Illustrator Tommy Bolic, Sweden.)

Injury to the Acetabular Labrum—*Femoroacetabular Impingement* !

Almost all labral tears (Figure 10.5) that present for arthroscopic treatment are as-sociated with femoroacetabular impingement (FAI). Cam-type FAI is the result of abnormal morphology of the femoral head-neck junction (Figure 10.6). In this case, the aspherical bony anomaly of the femur is jammed into the acetabulum during flexion or internal rotation. This results in shear forces that stress the junction be-tween the acetabular articular cartilage and the labrum. The labrum may then de-tach and the articular cartilage may peel away from the subchondral bone (Figure 10.7). Pincer-type FAI is a consequence of abnormal acetabular morphology (Figure 10.6). It can be a result of either global acetabular over-coverage in the setting of coxa profunda or protrusio acetabuli, or focal anterior over-coverage in the setting of acetabular retroversion. This results in atypical contact between the acetabular rim and the femoral head-neck junction, crushing the labrum. Loss of labral func-tion can lead to overloading of the articular cartilage of the hip and may be a pre-cursor of osteoarthritis in the hip. Associations between labral tearing and articular cartilage damage have been reported.

• Symptoms and signs: The onset of symptoms in a hip with a labral tear may be associated with a traumatic incident or may be insidious. In order of frequency, patients complain of pain in the groin, anterior thigh or knee, lateral hip, and buttock. Pain while walking, pain while pivoting, pain during impact activities, or pain while sitting may also be reported. Mechanical symptoms may include snapping or locking.

• Diagnosis: Radiograph will demonstrate the bony abnormalities associated with FAI. MRI is the preferred tool for diagnosis of a labral tear.

• Treatment: Initial treatment for labral tears is usually conservative, consisting of physical therapy, anti-inflammatory medication, and activity modification. The goal of physical therapy is to restore pain free range of motion, normal gait and prevent muscle atrophy. With pain free motion, the patient may move on to regaining pelvic and trunk stabilization. It is important that the patient regain pain free movement before moving forward with rehabilitation. If patients have persistent pain after 4 weeks of treatment, they are candidates for hip arthroscopy. Recent data suggest that early intervention in labral pathology leads to better results; hockey players with labral tears who underwent arthroscopic treatment within 1 year from time of injury returned to sports earlier than patients who had surgery more than 1 year after injury. Arthroscopic repair, preserving as much labral tissue as possible, is the preferred method to treat labral tears and must be accompanied by correction of the bony abnormalities to protect the labrum from new injuries.

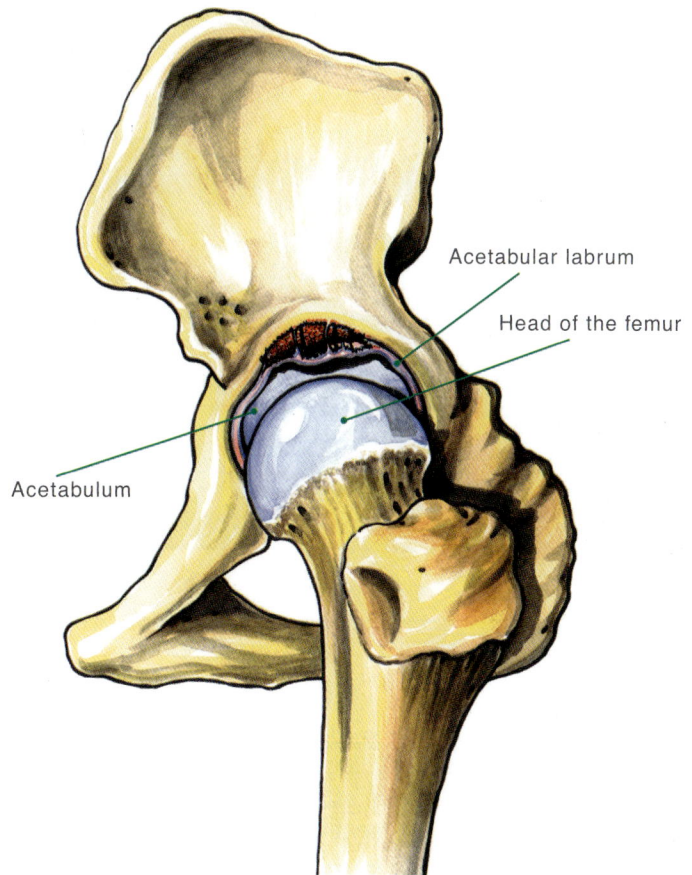

Figure 10.5 Injury to the acetabular labrum. (© Medical Illustrator Tommy Bolic, Sweden.)

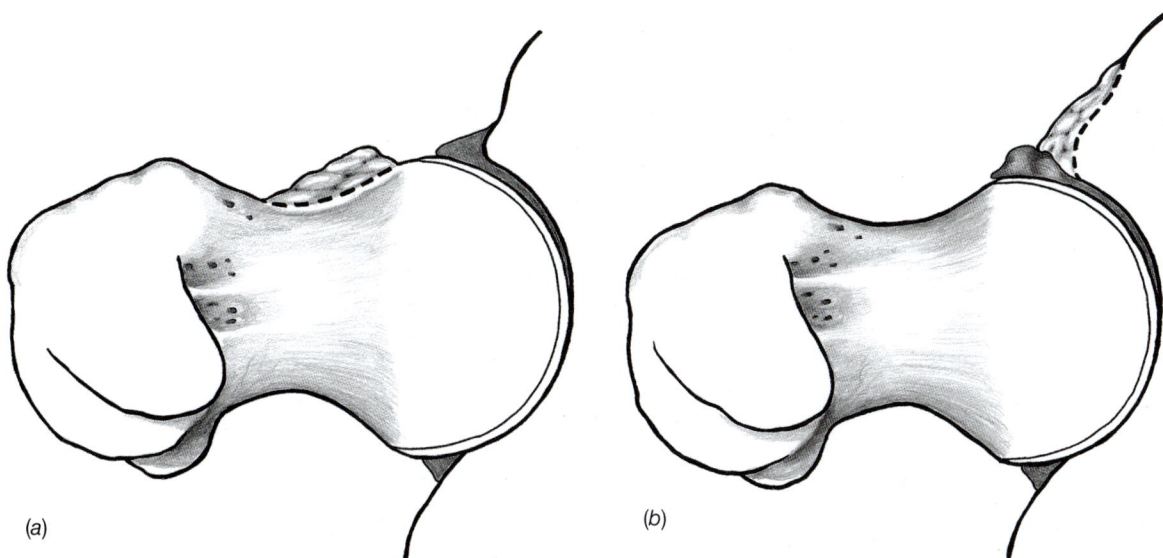

Figure 10.6 Illustration of femoroacetabular impingement (FAI) etiologies. Cam impingement (a) shows abnormal bone growth at the femoral head–neck junction. Pincer impingement (b) results from abnormal bone growth of the acetabular rim. (© Medical Illustrator Tommy Bolic, Sweden.)

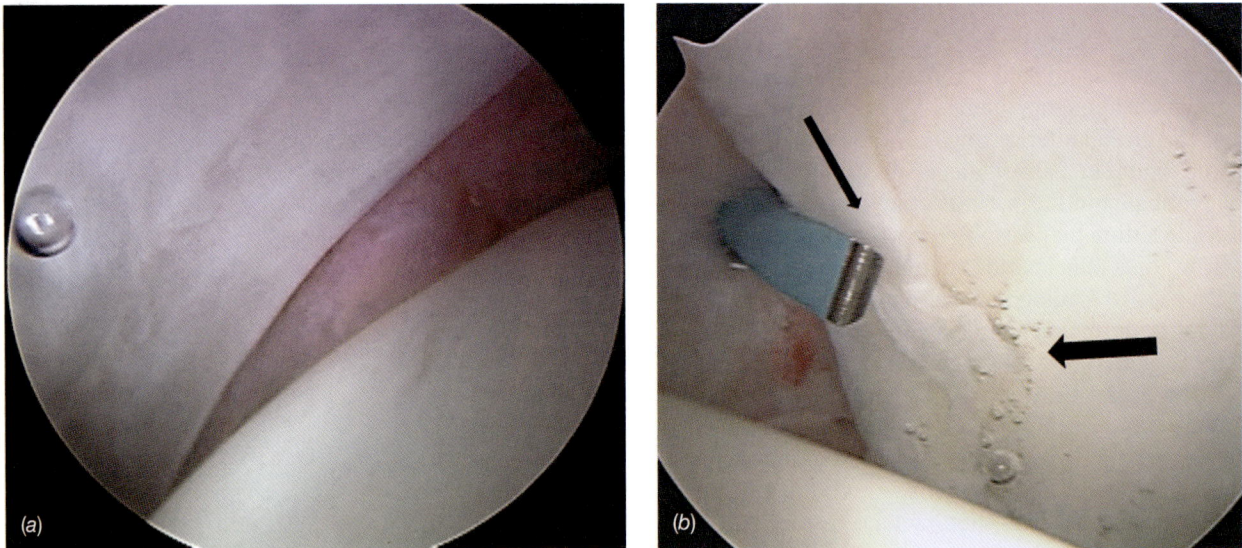

Figure 10.7 Arthroscopic view of a normal labrum (*a*). Arthroscopic view of a torn labrum (*b*) that is detached (small arrow) with damage to acetabular articular cartilage (large arrow). (Reproduced with permission from the Norwegian Sports Medicine Association.)

- Prognosis: The prognosis is good if there are limited degenerative changes in the hip joint. After surgery, the athlete is usually back to full activity after 4–6 weeks. Several reports have shown excellent functional outcomes and return to sport following arthroscopic treatment of labral pathology.

Other Injuries

Hip Joint Dislocation !

Hip joint dislocations are caused by high-energy trauma resulting from accidents (e.g., motor sports and downhill skiing accidents) or impact sports. Hip dislocations are commonly associated with acetabular fractures, femoral head and neck fractures, and significant intra-articular hip injuries.

- Symptoms and signs: If posterior dislocation has occurred, the patient has an adducted, internally rotated, and flexed lower extremity with a great deal of pain, even when the hip is at rest.
- Diagnosis: Attempts at hip joint movement trigger significant pain, and elastic resistance may be felt. The dislocation may injure the sciatic nerve, and its function always must be examined before reduction. A radiograph confirms the diagnosis.
- Treatment by physician: Early evaluation and treatment has been advocated as the best prevention for osteonecrosis. A dislocation must be reduced as quickly as possible, but not at the site of the injury. When no fracture is present, nonoperative treatment is widely accepted as long as blood flow to the femoral head has been assessed. Athletes who sustain a dislocation, continue to have persistent disabling hip pain, and are unable to participate at a high level. If patients have a successful closed reduction, physical therapy protocol is recommended in patients without fractures. If they cannot return to their sport, they are referred for arthroscopic evaluation. In these cases, patients usually undergo treatment of labral damage and chondral defects. In addition, many patients have treatment of the bony abnormalities associated with FAI. Patients may also have ligamentum teres ruptures

and tears in the hip capsule. Following arthroscopic treatment patients are recommended physical therapy that commences on postoperative day 1.

- Treatment by therapist: This is focused on protecting the repaired tissue. Initially, the goal is to reduce inflammation and pain. In addition, motion of the hip must be maintained to avoid the development of contractures. The patient rides a stationary bike to maintain motion. As pain dimishes and range of motion returns, the focus shifts to weight-bearing gait and pelvic and trunk stabilization. Once this is accomplished, the patient moves on to regaining strength, endurance and fitness. Following this, the patient is allowed to begin sport-specific training.
- Prognosis: Blood supply to the femoral head may be damaged as a result of dislocation, and segmental collapse of the femoral head may occur. The risk of this happening increases significantly if the dislocation remains unreduced for more than 6 hours. Prognosis is good if reduction occurs quickly and the blood supply is maintained. The hip should not bear weight for 4–6 weeks, and the patient may not return to full activity until about 3 months following the injury. Osteonecrosis of the femoral head following hip dislocation has been reported in 6–40% of hip dislocations.

Injuries to Other Muscles in the Inguinal and Hip Region

Other muscles, such as gracilis, sartorius, tensor fasciae latae, and gluteal muscles, may also tear. The physician performs a thorough examination, including palpation and specific tests, to determine which muscle or muscle group has been injured. The principles for treatment and prophylactic measures are the same as those for the treatment of an adductor longus muscle injuries.

Fractures in the Proximal End of the Femur—*Hip Fracture*

Fractures in the upper end of the femur (the neck of the femur and the trochanter region) occur frequently in the elderly and seldom in young people. Nevertheless, young athletes may also sustain a fracture in this area, but are usually stress fractures in runners. The injury mechanism of an acute fracture is often a fall that causes direct strong trauma to the trochanter area–for example, on the skating rink, during downhill skiing, or cycling. With the increase in cycling as a recreational sport, these fractures are becoming more common in the sporting population, where the athlete's feet are locked in the pedals when crashing to the ground. Stress fracture is discussed in the next section but may present as an acute onset pain, in the proximal femur this usually presents as exercise-related groin pain occurring with significant loading such as long distance running.

- Symptoms and signs: Patients feel intense pain when attempting movement or loading of the hip.
- Diagnosis: If a displaced fracture has occurred, the lower extremity is shortened and externally rotated, and the patient experiences great pain caused by pressure over the trochanter region and when attempting hip movement. A radiographic examination confirms the diagnosis.
- Treatment: Treatment is always surgery, except for stress fractures, at a hospital with preoperative reduction and often internal fixation.
- Prognosis: The prognosis is guarded in the athlete, particularly for displaced fractures. About 20% of the patients develop osteonecrosis of the femoral head with segmental collapse of the articular head, and 10–20% of the fractures do not heal. In such cases, treatment will either be arthrodesis (immobilization of the joint) or total prosthesis. In recent years, total prosthesis has been used more and more for

younger patients, because the long-term results are improving. Caution should be demonstrated in the use of hip replacements in younger athletes.

Pelvic Fractures

Pelvic fractures or acetabular fractures are rare in athletes but can occur after high-energy injuries, such as those caused by motor sports or downhill skiing accidents. Dislocated hip joints are often accompanied by acetabular fractures. Pelvic fractures are divided into stable and unstable fractures. Stable fractures affect only part of the pelvic girdle, usually the inferior and superior pubic rami on one side. In unstable fractures, the entire pelvic girdle is broken. This either results from an anterior fracture and posterior dislocation of the sacroiliac joint or when the pelvic girdle is fractured in two places. The stable fractures are the most common type. As with stress fractures of the femur stress fracture of the pubic ramus (inferior or superior) may present as acute onset groin pain on prolonged exercise.

- Symptoms and signs: The symptom is pain in the pelvic area.
- Diagnosis: Bimanual pressure on the crest triggers pain in the pelvis. This type of pressure makes it possible to get an impression of whether the fracture is unstable or not. X-rays and CT scans are mandatory for making the diagnosis and demonstrating which type of fracture is involved.
- Treatment: The only treatment required for a stable fracture is a brief period without weight bearing whenever pain makes it necessary. Prognosis for these fractures is very good. Because the pelvic area has a good blood supply, these fractures heal quickly. The athlete is usually training again within 12 weeks. Unstable fractures are potentially life threatening because of major bleeding (usually retroperitoneal). These fractures require rapid surgical treatment, either by external fixation with screws fixed in the pelvic crest and attached to a solid frame or by internal fixation with plates and screws. Pelvic fractures that affect the acetabulum require surgical reposition and fixation if the articular surface is significantly incongruent or a large posterior edge fragment has been knocked off. Prognosis for these fractures is less definite, and major injuries of the acetabulum often result in the early development of osteoarthritis in the hip.

Avulsion Fractures—*Apophyseal Injury*

An avulsion fracture is a tearing (avulsion) of an apophysis, and an apophysis is a secondary ossification center that contributes to peripheral growth in a bone. The apophysis is separated from the rest of the bone by a growth plate and is always the origin or insertion for muscles or tendons. Patients (usually boys) between the ages of 13 and 17 years sustain most avulsion fractures. During this period of rapid growth, high levels of muscle tension exert supraphysiological forces on the growth plate, which is the weakest point. A strong contraction in a muscle group may cause the related apophysis to sever through the growth plate (Figure 10.8).

Avulsion fractures may occur in six different locations in each half of the pelvic and hip area (the affected muscle or muscle group is indicated in parenthesis): the iliac crest (abdominal musculature), ASIS (sartorius muscle), the anterior inferior iliac spine (rectus femoris muscle), the ischial tuberosity (hamstring musculature) (Figure 10.9), the lesser trochanter (iliopsoas muscle), and the greater trochanter (gluteus medius and gluteus minimus muscles). There will be slight displacement of the iliac crest and the anterior inferior iliac spine because the surrounding soft tissue holds the fragment in place, whereas the other apophyses may be significantly displaced.

- **Symptoms and signs:** The patient will have pain with acute onset that corresponds to the avulsion site. Slight dislocation causes relatively little expressed pain. A major dislocation causes intense pain, such as the pain caused by a fracture. The athlete usually cannot move the affected area.
- **Diagnosis:** Diagnosis of an avulsion fracture is based on case history combined with palpation of painful area and specific muscle testing. Radiographic examination usually produces the diagnosis, but it is necessary to compare it with the healthy side, and oblique images are often needed to adequately demonstrate the affected apophysis. MRI with inversion recovery or fat suppressed sequences through the affected area are also helpful.

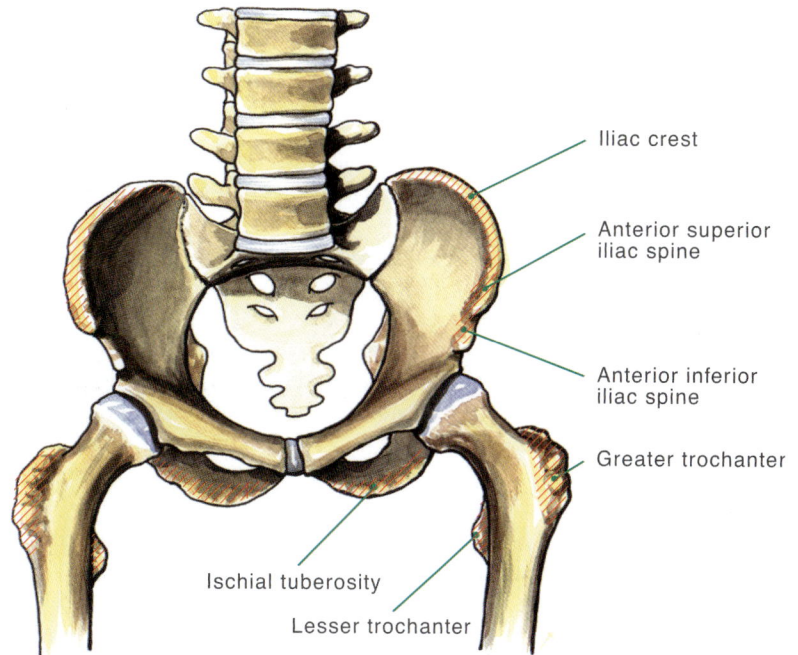

Figure 10.8 Location of avulsion fractures in the pelvic and hip areas. (© Medical Illustrator Tommy Bolic, Sweden.)

- **Treatment:** Treatment is usually conservative with a period of not bearing weight and analgesics. Major dislocations (of more than approximately 2 cm) of the apophysis fragment may be an indication for surgical reduction and fixation. This is particularly true of the greater trochanter, to avoid gluteal failure and the ischial tuberosity for hamstring musculature injuries.
- **Prognosis:** Prognosis is good in most cases. Normally, the apophysis heals within 4–6 weeks and the athlete can return to his sport again after a few more weeks of stretching and strength training the affected muscles. Painful pseudoarthrosis

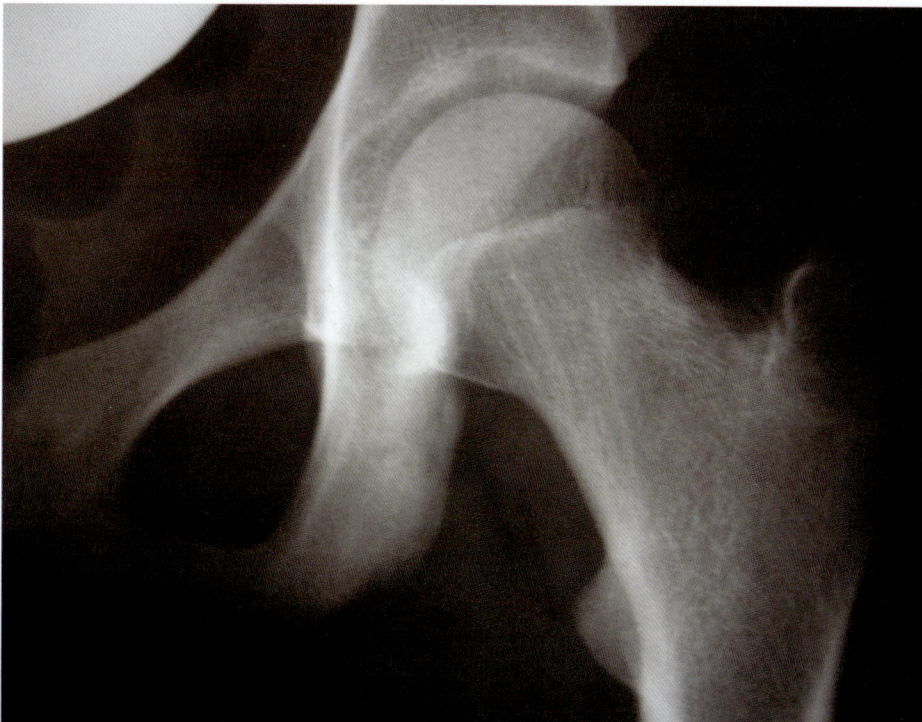

Figure 10.9 Radiograph of an ischial tuberosity avulsion fracture. (Reproduced with permission from the Norwegian Sports Medicine Association.)

occasionally develops between the apophysis and the rest of the bone. If pseudoarthrosis does develop, surgery with fixation of the apophysis is necessary. It is important in athletes, especially young athletes, that the progress through rehabilitation is at a steady pace rather than rapid pace. Young athletes commonly experience reinjury with rapid rehabilitation and loss of confidence is common.

Slipped Capital Femoral Epiphysis (SCFE)—*Slipping of the Femoral Neck Growth Plate*

SCFE is described as the posterior slip of the proximal femoral epiphysis (Figure 10.10) caused by a shearing force with external rotation of the femoral neck and shaft. Again this occurs more commonly in males with a peak incidence at 13 years, in females the peak occurs earlier at 11.5 years. The major risk factor appears to be increased BMI, whether primary or secondary to endocrine or metabolic causes.

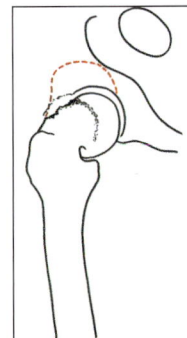

- **Symptoms and signs:** Pain is localized to the groin or more often to the inside of the knee, particularly with weight bearing. Presentation is insidious but associated with exercise. Altered gait, with an everted, externally rotated hip is described.
- **Diagnosis:** Findings from the clinical examination are limited rotational hip movement, leg length shortening measured from anterior superior iliac spine to medial malleolus but also pain and limitation in flexion and external rotation is noted. Radiographic examinations on two planes will demonstrate slipping. If there is the slightest indication of epiphyseolysis, the patient is sent for radiographs rays and evaluation by an orthopedic surgeon as soon as possible.
- **Treatment:** Treatment is always surgical fixation of the head as soon as possible. The less slipping in the epiphysis, the better the prognosis. Some orthopedists routinely perform prophylactic fixation of the femoral head on the opposite side because of the significantly increased risk of epiphyseolysis there as well. However, it is more common to provide the patient and her parents with detailed information so that they can seek medical assistance as soon as symptoms appear.
- **Prognosis:** Prognosis is good with minimal slippage and early fixation. If there is major slippage, the head and neck of the femur often become deformed, causing risk of early osteoarthritis development in the joint.

Acute Trochanteric Bursitis—*Acute Inflammation of the Bursa of the Hip*

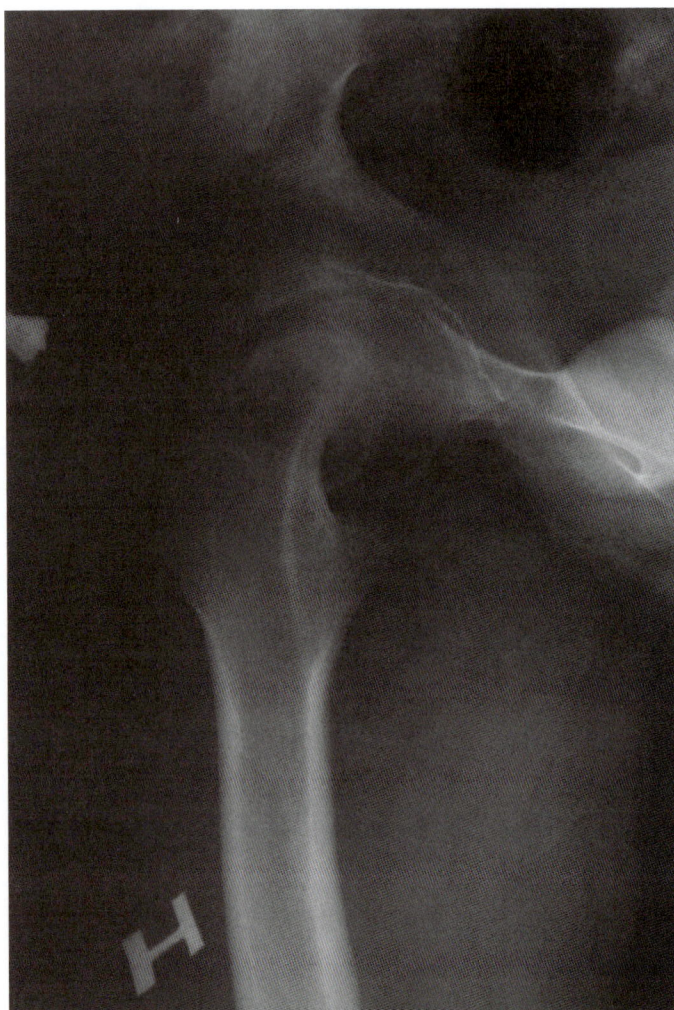

Figure 10.10 Epiphysiolysis of the femoral head. (© Medical Illustrator Tommy Bolic, Sweden.)

The trochanteric bursa is the only superficial bursa in the pelvic and hip region. Therefore, the bursa may be subjected to direct trauma, such as that caused when a handball player falls on her hip. This may cause crushing of part of the mucous membrane in the bursa, resulting in bleeding and an inflammatory reaction (hemobursitis).

- Symptoms and signs: The patient experiences pain and possibly swelling over the greater trochanter, sometimes radiating down along the lateral side of the thigh. This may be confused with sciatica.
- Diagnosis: Diagnosis is based on tenderness and swelling over the greater trochanter. Adduction and rotation of the hip when the knee is extended will trigger pain. Ultrasound and MRI examinations may demonstrate a thickened wall and an increased amount of fluid in the bursa.
- Treatment: Recommended treatment is nonweight bearing for pain control, NSAIDs, and alternative training. If this regimen is not carried out thoroughly, the symptoms may become chronic.

Pain in the Pelvic, Inguinal, and Hip Region

Marc J. Philippon[1,2,3], Éanna Falvey[4], Geoffrey M. Verrall[5], and Karen K. Briggs[1]

[1]*Steadman Philippon Research Institute, Vail, CO, USA*
[2]*McMaster University, Hamilton, ON, Canada*
[3]*University of Pittsburgh Medical Center, Pittsburgh, PA, USA*
[4]*Sports Surgery Clinic, Dublin, Ireland*
[5]*Sportsmed SA, Sports Medicine Centre, Adelaide, SA, Australia*

Occurrence

In sport traumatology, chronic painful conditions in the pelvic, inguinal, and hip region are among the most difficult injuries to deal with, both with respect to diagnosis and treatment. In many cases, athletes continue to perform with groin pain with no diagnosis or a misdiagnosis. Studies in professional sports have found groin injury the fourth most common injury affecting soccer players, the third most common injury in Australian rules football. It also has a high prevalence in ice hockey and rugby, and is increasingly diagnosed in American football. The symptoms caused by chronic groin injuries are often diffuse and uncharacteristic and usually appear in several areas at the same time. For example, pain that primarily originates from a particular muscle group will often trigger secondary pain from other areas because of improper loading. Therefore, these injuries are a big diagnostic challenge. A good outcome to treatment requires a proper initial diagnosis.

Differential Diagnoses

Table 10.2 provides an overview of the current differential diagnoses that cause chronic painful conditions in the pelvic, inguinal, and hip region. The most common

Most common	Less common	Must not be overlooked ⚠
Adductor tendinopathy, p. 320	Iliopsoas tendinopathy/bursitis, p. 322	Myositis ossificans, p. 329
Rectus femoris tendinopathy, p. 321	External snapping hip, p. 329	Internal snapping hip, p. 330
Rectus abdominis tendinopathy, p. 322	Other muscle/tendon injuries, p. 329	Gluteal tendinopathy/bursitis, p. 330
Stress fractures in the femur/femoral neck, p. 323	Inguinal insufficiency, p. 331	
Public bone stress injury, p. 324	Nerve entrapment, p. 332	
Trochanteric pain syndrome, p. 326		
Labral injuries, p. 327		
Hip joint chondral injuries, p. 328		

Table 10.2 Overview of diagnoses of chronic injuries in the pelvic, inguinal, and hip region. (Reproduced with permission from the Norwegian Sports Medicine Association.)

source of pain is the tendon insertion of the adductor longus, the rectus femoris, the rectus abdominis, the iliopsoas, and the gluteus medius muscles. Formerly, these symptoms were described as tendinitis. However, examinations have not demonstrated obvious inflammatory changes in the tendons, other than possibly at the very beginning of the process. Histological examinations later on demonstrate degenerative changes in the tendinous tissue. Therefore, the designation tendinopathy is used instead of tendinitis. At this point in time, the causes of the pain during and after loading are unclear.

While traditional approaches have focused on the trochanteric bursa, "greater trochanter pain syndrome" is an umbrella term for pathology arising from the "rotator cuff of the hip," the insertion of the gluteus medius tendon insertion to the greater trochanter and the bursae that separate the gluteals tendons from each other and the underlying bone. While a classical bursitis often exists, treating this in isolation is rarely successful if the concomitant tendinosis is neglected.

Painful snapping of the hip often occurs where excessive gluteal tension causes irritation of the proximal iliotibial band at the greater trochanter; this is termed external snapping hip. In many dancers a tight iliopsoas muscle may lead to painful snapping of the common tendon over the iliopectineal eminence in the pelvis; this is termed internal snapping hip. Diagnosis and treatment in these cases can be difficult.

Stress fractures in the upper end of the femur and in the pubic rami, particularly the inferior branch, often occur in athletes who primarily train and compete on hard surfaces, especially runners. Osteitis pubis, more appropriately termed pubic bone stress injury, is generally due to overuse and overload in athletes where the muscular control around the pelvis is poorly coordinated or imbalanced. Deficiencies in hip flexor, gluteal and abdominal muscle strength lead to abnormal/excessive forces across the pubic symphysis leading to chronic pain, loss of function and ultimately inability to train and play. It is most common in soccer players. The same is true of inguinal insufficiency. Here, the athlete complains of acute onset pain at the junction of the external oblique aponeurosis and the rectus abdominis at the superficial inguinal ring.

Hip disorders, in particular FAI, are a common cause of activity-related chronic groin injury. Overuse and abnormal hip morphology are considered to precipitate the injury and subsequent pain Hip and groin pain in the athlete has long been associated with structural abnormalities of the femoral neck and labral pathology. Labral tears are commonly seen in athletes in association with FAI. Repetitive rotation with adduction, abduction, internal rotation and external rotation with hip flexion may attribute to the development of impingement and subsequent chondrolabral lesions. A labral tear alone may cause progression of osteoarthritis in the hip. The role of the labrum is as a sealant of the joint, enhancing stability and proprioception. Labral tears typically do not respond to nonoperative care and result in significant loss of playing time in athletes.

Diagnostic Thinking

Injuries to the hip and groin region can cause significant disability in any level of athlete. Hip injuries can result from both sudden, traumatic episodes and repetitive stress and strain. Subtle hip subluxation injuries may often go unrecognized and undertreated. When witnessed or reported, traumatic hip subluxations warrant a careful exam and consideration for an urgent MRI to evaluate the extent of injury and resultant bleeding, which may require surgical evacuation. Repetitive stress to the hip occurs across a wide variety of athletic pursuits. Dancers, skiers, hockey, soccer, football and basketball players frequently place supraphysiologic demands on their hips. The repetitive nature of these stresses over the course of time may contribute to the wide spectrum of hip injuries seen in these athletes. Tendon injuries are commonly seen as a cause of pain; however, there is considerable overlap in symptoms with intra-articular injuries. Tendon injuries should be ruled out before moving on to other pathologies. In addition, injuries to the spine should also be ruled out as the symptoms may be similar. Other extra-articular pathologies, such as stress fractures and pubic bone injury can be identified on supplementary exams such as radiographs or MRI. For intra-articular pathology, the most common problem seen is FAI. The bony abnormalities associated with FAI cause labral tear and cartilage injuries of the hip. Capsular injuries are less common; however, they can occur with subluxation that has gone untreated. If FAI is suspected, then an MRI will identify other intra-articular pathologies. If diagnostic testing is inconclusive then systematic causes should be considered.

As in acute injuries, a thorough description of the patient's symptoms is necessary. The patient must describe when the symptoms are most notable and if certain positions aggravate the symptoms. The patients gait must also be assessed. The gait should be evaluated for a limp, stride length, stance phase, foot rotation, and pelvic rotation. We then assess range of motion as described earlier. Specific tests are performed to narrow the diagnosis, followed by supplementary exams.

Case History

Several differential diagnoses can initially be excluded by means of a thorough case history, in which the conditions surrounding the onset of the symptoms of chronic painful conditions are recorded. Chronic groin injury is often of insidious onset. The relatively mild nature of the injury means that it may not be noticed, or if it is, that it is minor enough so as not to stop the player from training and participating in their sport. By this mechanism it may develop/worsen into a more significant problem.

If the patient has a stress fracture in the pubic rami, the pain will also have a relatively acute onset, but in this case the triggering cause is often running a long distance on a hard surface. Pubic bone stress injury and posterior inguinal wall deficiency result in gradually increasing diffuse pain in the groin region, during and after weight bearing and sports activity. Gradually, performance is affected and pain the next day after exercise is more severe. But pain in the ischial tuberosity, which occurs when the patient sits with his hips slightly hyperflexed (e.g., when driving a car for a long time), may represent hamstring tendinopathy, piriformis syndrome or in rare situations ischiofemoral impingement.

With FAI and chondrolabral dysfunction, the majority of patients report groin pain with no inciting event. When patients do have an injury, studies have shown that many wait 3–4 years before seeking treatment. Most patients have severe limitations in activities of daily living and sporting activities.

Intra-articular injuries are common with repetitive rotational movements with adduction, abduction, internal rotation and external rotation with hip flexion. Athletes will frequently complain of sport limitation due to hip pain. Patients are unable to perform sports, and have difficulty running or jumping and with quick starts and stops. Patients with labral tears typically complain of anterior groin pain, but pain also can be referred to the buttock, greater trochanter, thigh, or medial knee. Other symptoms include clicking, locking, catching, instability, giving way, and stiffness.

In the pediatric patient, limp or groin pain may indicate SCFE or Perthe's disease (osteochondritis of the femoral head) in which case radiographic imaging of the femoral head is mandatory.

Referred pain is typical of several disorders in the pelvic and inguinal region—which means that the patient feels pain in an area other than where the pain originated. This is particularly true of pain originating from the sacroiliac joint and the sacroiliac ligaments.

Clinical Examination

Inspection. The position of, and the mobility in, the pelvis and hips are examined from the front and from the back while the patient is standing and walking. A patient who walks pigeon-toed may have increased femoral neck anteversion. If a stress fracture has occurred in the pubic rami or in the neck of the femur, the patient will be able to localize the pain from weight bearing exactly to the groin or to the medial side of the thigh. By hopping on the affected lower extremity, the patient will provoke the pain further, making it easier to localize (positive hop test). Anisomelia (leg-length discrepancy) can be roughly measured while the patient is standing with his knees extended and bearing weight equally on both lower extremities. The pelvis must not be rotated when this measurement is taken.

Palpation. If the patient has lumbosacral back pain, the physician should palpate the insertion of erector muscles of the spine on the sacrum and the crest. The spinous processes of L4 and L5 should be palpated to check for spondylolisthesis between L5 and the sacrum. If spondylolisthesis is found in that location, the spinous process of L4 will be displaced in a position that is anterior to L5. Sacroiliac joint arthritis or overuse of the posterior sacroiliac ligaments will trigger pain from palpation above the joint or ligaments. Weight bearing on one leg, or a compression test of the sacroiliac joints (pressing the crests of the iliac bones hard against each other), may also trigger pain from the sacroiliac joints when they are affected.

If a groin hernia or posterior inguinal wall deficiency is suspected, the superficial inguinal opening is palpated while the patient is coughing. If the patient has manifest hernia, it will be possible to palpate the hernial sac. A patient with groin insufficiency will indicate more pain on the affected than on the opposite, nonaffected side. Palpation of the superficial inguinal ring reveals dilation and tenderness but usually no overt hernia or hernial sac. It will be possible to palpate a femoral hernia immediately distal to the inguinal ligament beside the vessel/nerve stem. However, positive physical findings for sports hernia, apart from localized tenderness, are uncommon.

With the patient in the supine position, the physician should palpate the various muscles and muscle insertions while the suspected muscle group is loaded. Pain may be a sign of tendinopathy at the insertion, and a defect or tender infiltrate in the muscle belly indicates a tear, possibly with scar tissue formation. With a pubic bone stress injury often the pubic symphysis and parasymphyseal bone region are tender.

Palpation over the greater trochanter will trigger pain if the patient has trochanteric bursitis, gluteus medius tendinopathy or snapping hip. Pressure over the lateral cutaneous nerve of the thigh where it passes under the inguinal ligament immediately medial to the ASIS may increase the symptoms of meralgia paresthetica.

Femoral anteversion. The concept of femur anteversion refers to the angle that the femoral neck forms to the condyle plane of the femur (Figure 10.11). Normally, this angle is about 15°. Increased anteversion will increase internal rotation of the femur, and the patella will be too far in the medial direction. Walking and running pigeon-toed is the most characteristic clinical finding, in addition to reduced external rotation of the hips. This is considered an important cause of chronic overuse disorders in the lower extremities.

Specific Tests

Hip examination must address motor strength, range of motion, points of tenderness, presence of limping, and Trendelenburg test. The shape of the hip joint (ball-and-socket joint) enables it to move in every direction. The joint capsule is relatively loose to allow great mobility, but three solid ligaments–the iliofemoral, the pubofemoral, and the ischiofemoral ligaments–strengthen it. These three ligaments prevent (in order) extension, abduction, and internal rotation from becoming too great. Hip joint stability is due primarily to the depth of the acetabulum and the strength of the muscles that control articular movement.

Figure 10.11 Femoral anteversion (anteversion of the femoral neck). (© Medical Illustrator Tommy Bolic, Sweden.)

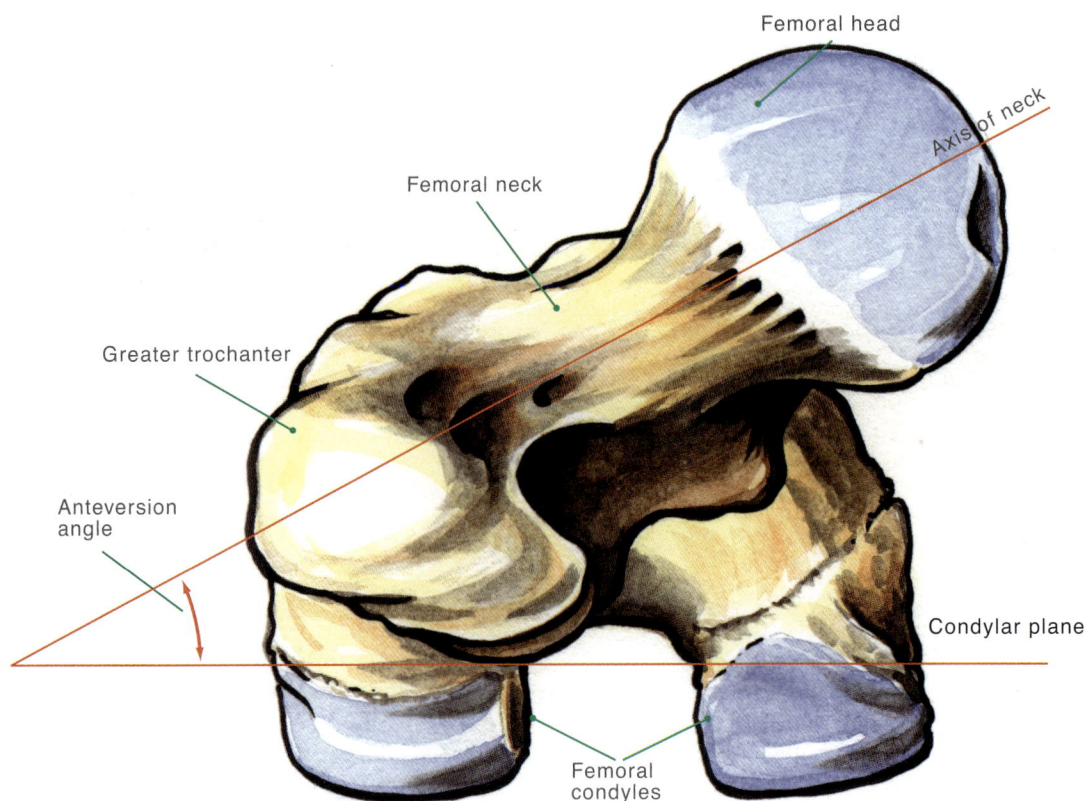

Range of motion. Range of motion should be assessed as previously described. Pain with specific motion or excessive motion is important to the diagnosis. Supine flexion is often decreased in the presence of impingement, as is supine abduction. Adduction is also measured in the supine position. Abduction and adduction can also be measured in the lateral position. Internal rotation and external rotation are measured in the prone position. Increased anteversion of the neck of the femur causes increased internal rotation in the hip joints (often up to 90°), whereas external rotation is correspondingly reduced or discontinued. Normally, internal and external rotation are about equal and depend on joint laxity.

Strength testing. Specific muscle groups, such as the hip flexors (iliopsoas and the rectus femoris), the abductors (gluteal muscles), the adductors, the internal and external rotators in the hip, and the abdominal muscles, are tested against resistance. Pain at the muscle insertion indicates tendinopathy and possibly an avulsion fracture in adolescent patients. Measurement of hip strength can also play an important role in diagnosis. Isometric tests are commonly performed to minimize risk of injury and muscle soreness. Studies have recommended ipsilateraleral hip strength measurements as a test to determine strength deficits associated with hip injuries. The quadriceps and hamstring are tested against resistance while the patient is in the prone position. Tears or scar tissue in the hamstring can often be palpated by contraction against loading. Strength in the short rotator muscles of the hip is tested with the hip extended and the knee joint flexed to 90°.

Squeeze test. The most evidence-based test for adductor pathology is guarding to passive adduction but in practice the "squeeze test" is an excellent clinical test for adductor dysfunction (Figure 10.12).

Ludloff test. The Ludloff test is a specific test for the iliopsoas muscle (Figure 10.13a). It is done by flexing the patient's hip about 90° and internally rotating the femur against resistance or by lifting her leg with her knee extended while she is sitting on a chair. In this position, the iliopsoas is the only active hip flexor, and pain deep in the groin during this test indicates that the muscle's tendon insertion to the lesser trochanter (the Ludloff sign is positive) is affected.

Thomas test. The Thomas test (Figure 10.13b) may be used to check for flexibility in the iliopsoas, and to determine whether stretching triggers pain. The test is done with the patient supine, with his buttocks close to the edge of the examination table. Both lower extremities are flexed to the maximum in the hip and knee, and one lower extremity is held back while the other one is extended. Incomplete extension is a sign of a short iliopsoas. Pressing on the patient's thigh and passively extending the hip further will trigger pain that affects the iliopsoas.

FABER test. The FABER (flexion, abduction and external rotation) distance test (Figure 10.14) is used to determine presence of impingement. The affected leg is placed in a figure of four position so that the ipsilateral ankle is positioned proximal to the contralateral knee. The clinician should evaluate presence of anterior hip pain, as well as vertical distance between the

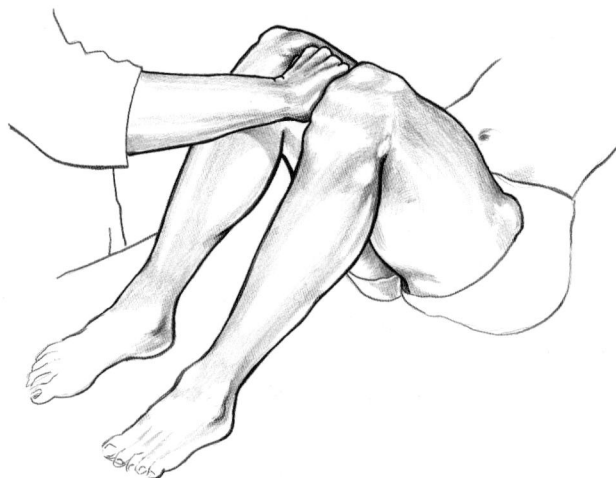

Figure 10.12 Squeeze test for groin examination. (© Medical Illustrator Tommy Bolic, Sweden.)

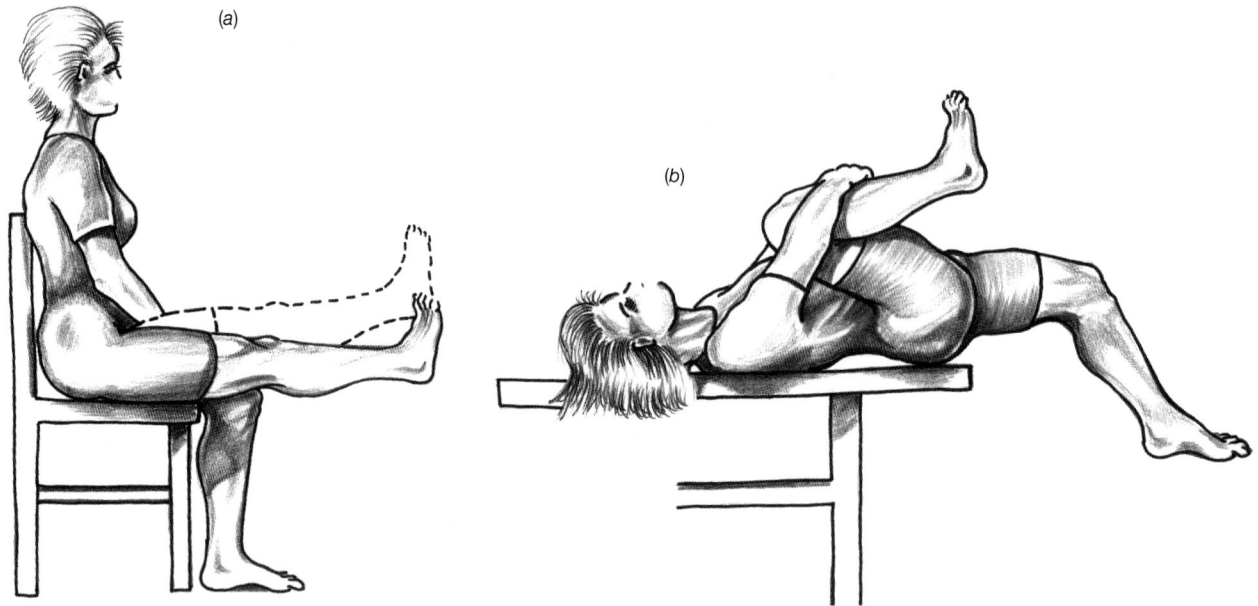

Figure 10.13 Specific tests: Ludloff test for the iliopsoas muscle (*a*) and Thomas test to evaluate range of motion in the iliopsoas muscle (*b*). (© Medical Illustrator Tommy Bolic, Sweden.)

lateral genicular line and the examination table, which is typically increased compared with the contralateral side in patients with FAI. This exam is integral part of a screening program to identify young athletes who may be at risk of chondrolabral pathologies due to FAI.

Anterior impingement test. An anterior impingement test (Figure 10.15) is performed to assist with the diagnosis of FAI. To perform the anterior impingement test, the patient is placed supine on the examination table. The hip is passively flexed to 90°, followed by forced adduction and internal rotation. In this position, the anterior femoral neck approximates the anterosuperior acetabulum, the most frequent region of chondral and labral injury. Forced external rotation with extension can also trigger hip pain related to acetabular labral tears.

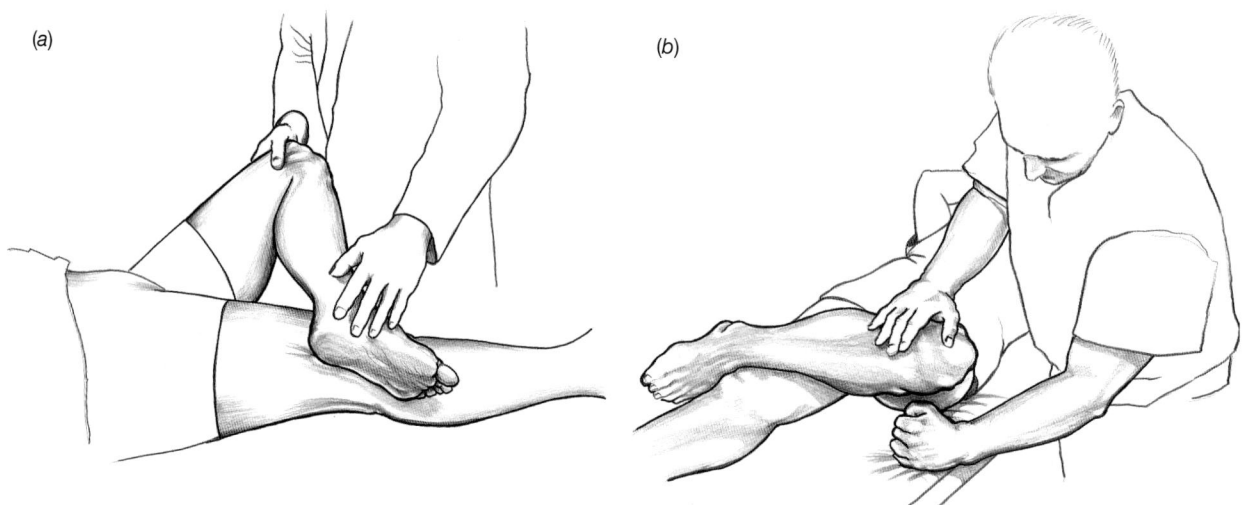

Figure 10.14 FABER (flexion, abduction and external rotation) test, Foot placement (*a*) and distance measurement (*b*). (© Medical Illustrator Tommy Bolic, Sweden.)

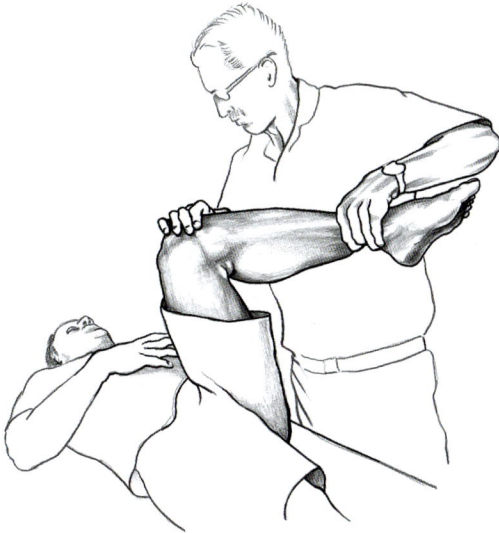

Figure 10.15 Anterior impingement test.
(© Medical Illustrator Tommy Bolic, Sweden.)

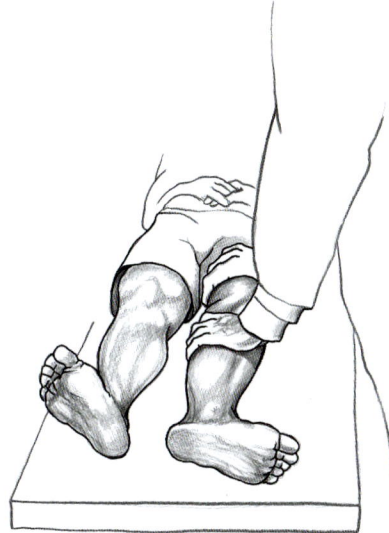

Figure 10.16 The hip dial test is performed with the patient in the supine position. The femur is grasped just above the knee and the other hand is used to grasp just below the knee. A gentle external rotation force is applied and if an end point is not felt within 45°, the test is positive. (© Medical Illustrator Tommy Bolic, Sweden.)

Hip dial test. To test for capsular laxity of the hip, the hip dial test is performed with the patient in the supine position. The leg is grasped just above and below the knee while a gentle external rotation force is applied (Figure 10.16). The amount of external rotation allowed is noted along with the presence and type of end point felt (Table 10.3). A cutoff point of 45° is used to delineate normal from abnormal.

Sacroiliac joint testing. The practitioner should test the sacroiliac joint by applying strong pressure posteriorly (toward the ASIS), bilaterally, or by forceful passive abduction of a flexed hip. If the joints or the surrounding ligaments are affected, these tests may trigger sacroiliac pain. However, they are somewhat nonspecific, and it is difficult to make a good clinical examination of the sacroiliac joint region.

Supplemental Examinations

Radiographic examination. Stress fractures can be diagnosed by means of a radiographic examination but often not until sometime after the fracture occurred,

Grade	Laxity on axial distraction	Clinical feel
1 (mild)	None (negative pain on axial distraction test	Soft end point
2 (moderate)	Yes (positive pain)	Laxity at 45°
3 (severe)	Yes (pistoning and pain)	Patient can demonstrate subluxation/dislocation (history of previous dislocation)
		No end point at 45°
4 (collagen disease)	Ehlers–Danlos syndrome, Down syndrome, Marfan syndrome	Upper extremities and lower extremity joint laxity

Table 10.3 Classification of hip laxity from the hip dial test. Acetabular and femoral neck version must be taken into account. (Reproduced with permission from the Norwegian Sports Medicine Association.)

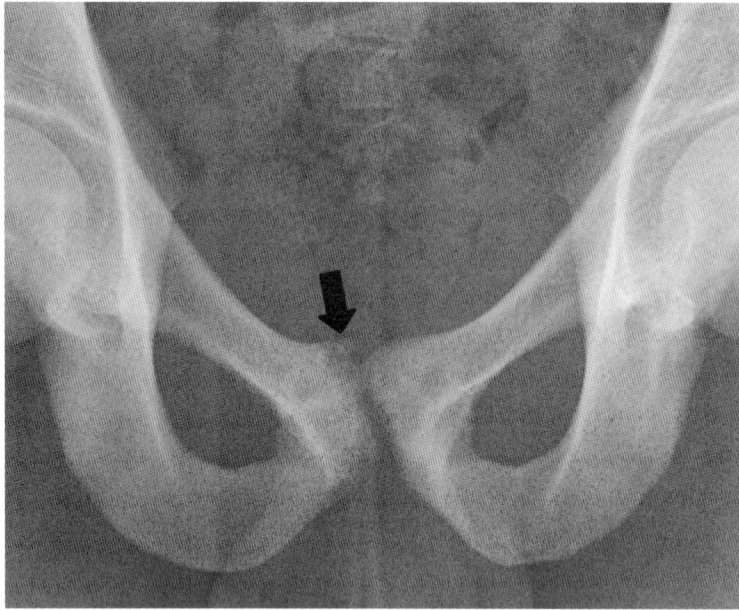

Figure 10.17 Radiograph of patient with severe pubic bone stress reaction. The bone appears moth-eaten at the pubic symphysis (arrow).

when callus begins to form around the narrow fracture cleft. If the patient has pubic bone stress, the bone at the pubic symphysis can look moth-eaten on the radiograph (Figure 10.17). If they remain long enough, chronic tendinopathy and bursitis may cause calcium deposition at the muscle insertion or in the bursa. These calcium deposits often look like gray shadows on the radiographs of the affected area. This is also true for myositis ossificans. Indefinite painful conditions in the pelvic, inguinal, and hip regions are general indicators for radiographs to be taken, especially to exclude bone tumors or other differential diagnoses (e.g., hip joint osteoarthritis, osteochondritis dissecans coxae, and Bekhterev disease (rheumatoid spondylitis)).

In the case of FAI, bone abnormalities can be demonstrated on radiographs. It is crucial to assess proper patient positioning during radiographs to correctly determine osseous anatomy, especially acetabular rim morphology.

In addition, factors associated with degenerative change should be determined. Specifically, presence of significant joint space narrowing, acetabular sclerosis, or medial acetabular osteophyte formation (fossa or floor) are suggestive of degenerative changes (Figure 10.18).

CT. If spondylolysis is suspected without radiographically demonstrable spondylolisthesis, a CT scan can clearly demonstrate the fracture cleft. Otherwise, indefinite disorders in the pelvic area may be present, and CT scanning of the entire area may be indicated, particularly when a tumor is suspected.

MRI. Tendinopathy, particularly bursitis, may be demonstrated by an MRI examination. If a patient has pubic bone stress or a stress fracture, MRI will demonstrate edema and changes in the bone structure of the affected area. MRI is the standard examination for evaluating tumors. MRI provides the most detailed images of intra-articular hip pathology, showing with great details of labral anatomy and femoral and acetabular cartilage. MRI can also be used to assess the presence of acetabular labral injury and chondral defects in the hip. Alpha angle is measured in the axial oblique sequences to evaluate the femoral head–neck junction (Figure 10.19).

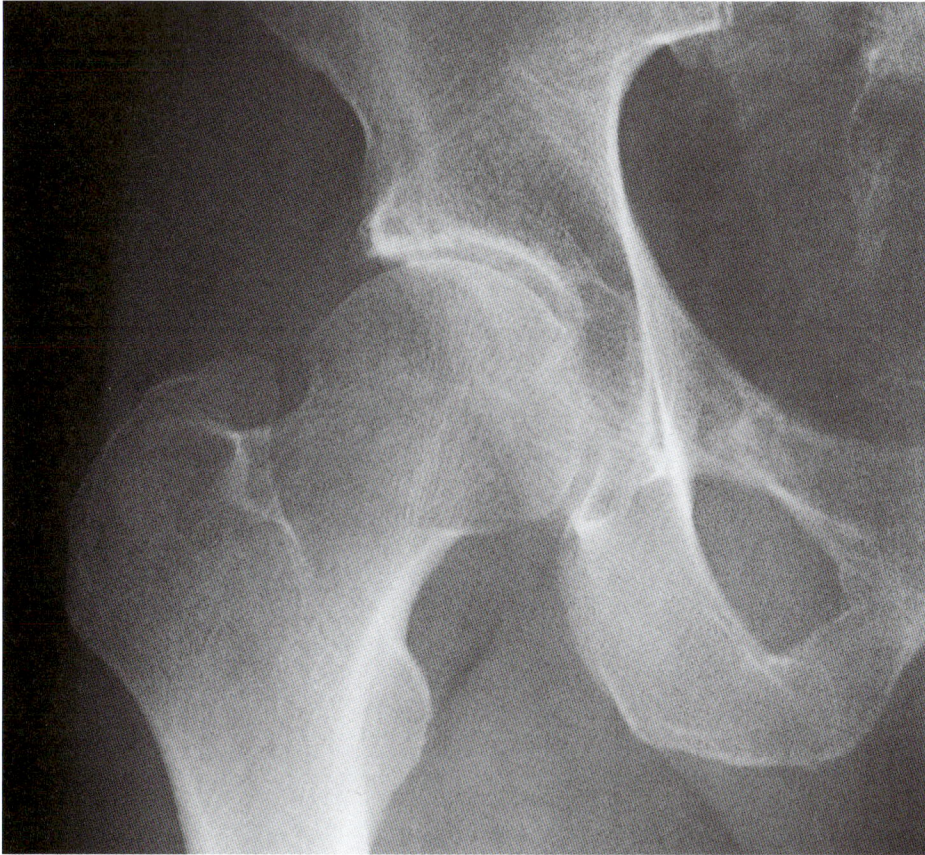

Figure 10.18 Radiograph demonstrating joint space narrowing with osteophyte formation.

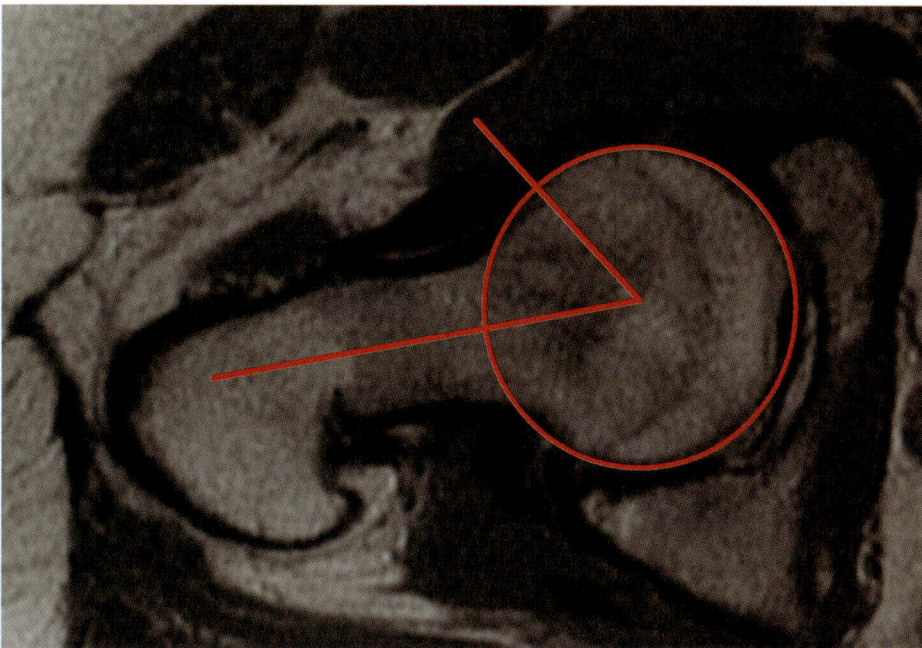

Figure 10.19 The alpha angle of the hip is determined by drawing a line from the middle of the femoral head to the midpoint of the femoral neck, and then a second line is drawn from the center of the femoral head to the anterior point when the neck of the femoral head deviates from the circle. The angle formed by the lines is the alpha angle.

Skeletal scintigraphy. Skeletal scintigraphy is almost immediately positive in the case of stress fractures, and it is the best diagnostic aid for demonstrating these fractures. Scintigraphy will produce the diagnosis for pubic bone stress injury with small changes and for spondylolysis without listhesis. Scintigraphic findings are positive for bone tumors (malignant and some benign, such as osteoid osteoma). This test is being replaced by MRI to reduce radiation exposure to young athletic patients.

Ultrasound examination. Ultrasound may be used to diagnose myositis ossificans and bursitis and to demonstrate the localization and extent of scar tissue changes after muscle tears. It is also commonly used to assist in the diagnosis of posterior inguinal wall deficiency though the diagnostic criteria that constitute a positive test remain disputable.

Common Injuries

Adductor Tendinopathy—*Chronic Groin Strain*

Chronic adductor tendinopathy is often seen when an acute proximal adductor tear is poorly rehabilitated or neglected and the patient returns to sport activity too soon. This type of overuse is relatively common among horseback riders, skaters (particularly ice hockey), cross-country skiers who ski freestyle and soccer players. The exact pathogenesis is unknown.

- Symptoms and signs: The initial symptoms are often slightly diffuse in the inguinal region or localized over the tendon to the adductor longus. As the disorder gradually becomes more chronic and the pain more expressed, it may radiate downward on the inside of the thigh and upward toward the rectus abdominis (the adductor longus origin and rectus abdominis insertion are part of a conjoint aponeurosis). Other muscles in the area may also trigger pain because they will be subjected to improper loading when the patient unconsciously attempts to protect and unload the painful area. The pain is often accompanied by stiffness, particularly in the morning and when starting a training session. As the athlete gradually warms up, the stiffness disappears while pain increases.
- Diagnosis: The examination of a patient with long-term, chronic groin pain must be very thorough. Several differential diagnoses for adductor tendinopathy in this region exist, and the diagnosis can only be made with any certainty by means of a good case history and clinical examination. When the tendon insertion of the adductor longus is affected, flexibility is often reduced in comparison to the opposite side, and stretching against resistance triggers pain corresponding to the muscle tendon junction or at the tendon insertion to the pubic bone. Passive hip abduction will also trigger pain in this area, and the patient will often indicate significant pain from palpation. The remainder of the groin area must be palpated carefully, particularly the lymph nodes, the scrotum, and the symphysis. Squeeze test is a useful means of assessing strength of adduction. A neurological examination of the lower extremities should be completed. A rectal exploration may be included if the patient has long-term chronic groin pain. Supplemental examinations are usually necessary; radiographs of the pelvis and hips should be done first. If the patient has long-term adductor tendinopathy, radiographs will sometimes demonstrate calcium precipitation that corresponds to the tendon insertion. An MRI examination may demonstrate changes proximally in the adductor muscles.
- Treatment by physician: Like all groin injuries, the patient must be made aware immediately that conservative treatment of chronic adductor tendinopathy can take a considerable length of time, often 4–6 months or longer. Treatment

primarily consists of various types of training. Steroid injections usually have only a temporary effect but may be used in the short term to advance rehabilitation by removing painful negative feedback allowing strengthening of the adductor group. Steroid injections should never be used in the short term to allow a player with a painful groin to return to play/competition due to the increased risk of tendon rupture. If conservative treatment does not produce satisfactory results within 6 months, the patient should be thoroughly reexamined to exclude other causes for the pain such as iliopsoas pain or hip labral pathology. If these are excluded, the patient should be given the option of surgery. Surgery is usually performed under local anesthesia with tenotomy, because either only the adductor longus tendon or all adductor tendon structures in the area are released from the periosteum. This procedure normally causes mild bleeding and small reactive changes in the area of the surgery. Postoperatively, the patient avoids weight bearing by using crutches for a few days until full loading can be tolerated. Active and passive stretching and strength training of the adductors begins early, and after 2–3 weeks the patient may bicycle with some weight bearing. Running training is allowed after about 6 weeks, and the athlete can normally return to full sport activity after 10–12 weeks. In some cases, the patient may have mild pain in the area where the surgery was performed for a long time after the intervention, but the pain is usually not so expressed that it hinders full activity. A good surgical outcome depends on a proper initial diagnosis, an atraumatic surgical technique, and optimal postoperative rehabilitation.

- Treatment by physical therapist: The physical therapist should begin treatment by instructing the patient in careful stretching and circulation training. As soon as the patient can tolerate it, strength training of the adductors is emphasized. Both stretching and strength training must be done with minimum provocation of pain! Eccentric strength training is gradually emphasized more. Sensory motor training of the inguinal and hip musculature is included in the training program as soon as pain allows. Once the patient has achieved full pain-free mobility that is the same on both sides, with normal strength in the adductor muscles, controlled functional training that is related to the relevant sport may begin. The return to full sport activity must be gradual and must take place under the care of physical therapists and trainers or coaches.

Rectus Femoris Tendinopathy—*Pain at the Proximal Insertion of the Straight Muscle of the Thigh*

This disorder may occur during intense shooting training in soccer or in sprinters who perform repetitive high intensity kicking or sprinting sessions. It may also be caused by returning to sport activity too early after a partial proximal tear occurs (Figure 10.3).

- Symptoms and signs: Pain is experienced centrally in the groin during weight bearing, especially when attempting fast sprints or kicking a ball, or when the rectus femoris muscle is forcefully contracted with the lumbar spine extended.
- Diagnosis: Flexion of the hip with extension of the knee against resistance causes pain up toward the anterior inferior iliac spine (modified Thomas test). Palpation causes significant tenderness over the proximal portion of the muscle toward the tendon insertion, about 8 cm distal to the ASIS. Intramuscular bleeding proximally in the muscle may cause calcium precipitation that is demonstrated on a lateral radiograph of the area. However, MRI is the investigation of choice.
- Treatment: The main element in treatment is the same strength and motion training (with gradually increasing weight bearing) as for adductor tendinosis. In

treatment-resistant cases in which the patient does not begin training because of pain, an injection of cortisone and local anesthesia can be administered. Surgical treatment to remove granulation tissue from the tendon is very seldom indicated. Tenotomy must not be performed on the rectus femoris tendon.

- Prognosis: The prognosis is good with adequate conservative treatment. This disorder is significantly easier to treat than chronic adductor tendinopathy. Care must be taken in rehabilitation as mentioned previously for acute injury that return to activity must be preceded by sports specific high intensity activity. This injury has a high recurrence rate if the athlete is returned to sport too quickly.

Iliopsoas Tendinopathy/Bursitis—*Pain at the Distal Insertion of the Large Hip Flexors*

Tendon pain and inflammation of the bursa are seen in this disorder. This disorder occurs with overuse, especially with hip flexion, such as running, dancing, rowing. The iliopectineal bursa is between the anterior side of the hip joint and the iliopsoas muscle (Figure 10.24). It is the largest bursa in the body, and in 15% of adults, communication between the bursa and the hip joint is present. Inflammation in this bursa may occur in isolation or in combination with a disorder (tear or tendinitis) in the iliopsoas muscle. The most common triggering cause is intense periods of running training, particularly in hurdlers and marathon runners.

- Symptoms and signs: The patient feels pain centrally in the groin, possibly directly over the inguinal ligament and directly lateral to the rectus abdominis from loading, such as running uphill. Pain may occur when sitting with a flexed hip for a long time in cases of bursitis.
- Diagnosis: Bimanual palpation of the tendon insertion of the lesser trochanter may also trigger significant pain, particularly in thin patients. The Ludloff test is positive when the iliopsoas muscle tendon insertion to the lesser trochanter is affected. The Thomas test can be used to check for flexibility of the iliopsoas and also reveal pain associated with the iliopsoas. If iliopsoas is suspected, ultrasound or MRI examination will demonstrate the thickened and possibly fluid-filled bursa.
- Treatment: The main element of treatment is the same strength and motion training (with gradually increasing loading) as for adductor tendinosis. In cases that are resistant to treatment when the patient does not begin training because of pain, an injection of cortisone and local anesthesia can be administered using fluoroscopy, 2–3 cm proximal to the lesser trochanter. The bursa can also be treated with aspiration of as much fluid as possible. After 1 or 2 weeks of rest, the patient can resume rehabilitation with systematic stretching and strength training of the iliopsoas.

Rectus Abdominis Tendinopathy—*Pain at the Insertion of the Straight Abdominal Muscle on the Pubic Bone*

Long-term overuse of the distal tendon insertion of the rectus abdominis, such as in rowing and tennis, or beginning activity too soon after a distal partial tear may cause chronic tendon changes to develop in this area. The distance between the tendon insertion of the rectus abdominis and the adductor longus is short, which often causes an irritation and pain in chronic cases, as well as when the adductors are loaded.

- Symptoms and signs: The patient has pain down toward the symphysis from loading and contraction of the rectus abdominis. Pain may become fully disabling, and eventually the adductors may also be affected, particularly the adductor longus.
- Treatment: The main element of treatment is the same strength and motion training (with gradually increasing weight bearing, as for adductor tendinosis). In

treatment-resistant cases in which the patient does not begin training because of pain, an injection of cortisone and local anesthesia can be made into the tendon insertion on the pubic bone, followed by 1–2 weeks of rest before active rehabilitation is resumed. If the patient does not make progress with conservative treatment, surgical treatment with extirpation of the granulation tissue from the tendon may be indicated.

- Prognosis: The prognosis is good with early and adequate treatment. Some chronic injuries do not heal regardless of what is done and have resulted in the end of the sport career of a number of top athletes.

Stress Fractures in the Femur/Femoral Neck

Stress fractures are relatively common in the neck of the femur and less common in the proximal portion of the femur or in the pubic rami (usually the inferior ramus) (Figure 10.20). Stress fractures in the neck of the femur constitute 7% of all stress fractures sustained by long-distance runners. Precipitating causes are usually too rapid an increase in the amount and intensity of training or switching from a soft to a hard training surface. Running on only asphalt on one side of a road predisposes the athlete to this injury. Anatomic axial deviation such as that caused by leg-length discrepancy may also predispose the athlete to stress fractures in the pelvis and hips. Stress fractures occur most frequently in female athletes and may be related to eating disorders and irregular menses.

- Symptoms and signs: The patient has pain in the hip region (usually in the groin), which worsens with ongoing training. Eventually, the athlete will have pain with normal weight bearing. The pain disappears at rest, but recurs as soon as training is resumed. Stress fracture of the inferior pubic ramus should be considered in those involved in long distance endurance events, high frequency training, and those who have significantly increased their workload. It is appreciated as exercise-related groin pain often in the medial proximal thigh (adductor) area.

- Diagnosis: The case history indicates a stress fracture. The diagnosis is suspected clinically with a positive clinical sign being the athlete sitting on the end of the examination table and downward pressure applied at the knee and pain felt in the upper thigh. Strong passive movement in the hip joint often triggers pain as well. Radiographic examinations are often not positive until 3–4 weeks after the fracture occurred, when callus begins to form in the area. However, MRI or isotope bone scan will show increased bone signal consistent with the site of injury. MRI has the distinct advantage of showing early stress reaction prior to a fracture developing and is now the preferred investigation of choice due to its zero radiation dose profile.

- Treatment by physician: Treatment is unloading with crutches for 4–6 weeks. Fractures in the pubic bone usually heal quickly and without complications. If the neck of the femur is fractured, patient follow-up must include several radiographs. If a continuous fracture is indicated, or signs of dislocation are present, the fracture must be surgically fixed. Care must be taken to ascertain the site of stress fracture of neck of femur as fracture on the superior surface is termed a "tension" injury and may lead to catastrophic fracture-tension stress fracture requires immediate immobilization and orthopedic review.

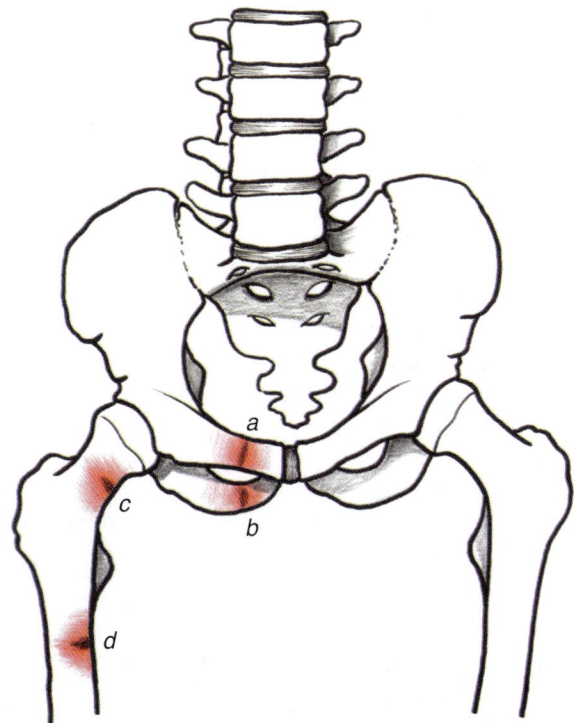

Figure 10.20 Stress fracture. Location of the most commonly occurring stress fractures in the pelvic and hip area: superior ramus of the pubis (a), inferior ramus of the pubis (b), femoral neck (c), and proximally on the femur shaft (d). (© Medical Illustrator Tommy Bolic, Sweden.)

PELVIS, GROIN, AND HIPS

- Treatment by physical therapist: During the nonweight-bearing period, the patient must have an alternative exercise program, such as swimming, running in water, bicycling, and general strength training. Running training must be resumed gradually, with a careful progression that does not cause pain. Any triggering causes, such as malalignment or training surfaces, must also be corrected if possible.
- Prevention: The use of appropriate equipment, good running shoes, soft or varied surfaces, and a well-monitored training program should make it possible to avoid stress fractures in this region.
- Prognosis: The prognosis is good as long as no bone displacement has occurred, but the athlete often misses a season. If there is a displaced fracture in the femoral neck, the prognosis is indefinite and some risk exists for osteonecrosis of the femoral head and segmental collapse.

Pubic Bone Stress Injury

Formerly, descriptions of this disorder were associated with chronic urinary tract or prostate infection and given the designation of osteitis. However, more recent studies have shown that the disorder is not conditional on infection. The injury results from pubic bone stress. Individual studies have shown a high correlation between disorders in the back, the sacroiliac joint, and the hips (increased collum anteversion, coxa vara), and pubic bone stress injury; the condition in athletes is almost exclusively a reaction to overuse. However, reduced hip joint movement, which is usually caused by short and strong muscles in the area, is frequently found in these patients. In practice soft tissue contracture around the hip, such as hip flexor pathology, limitation of hip range of motion (FAI) or primary adductor/rectus abdominis dysfunction, is the cause of this problem that is very much a "symptom" rather than a disease entity as it is often portrayed. The disorder is three to five times more common in men than in women. It is most common in long-distance runners and in soccer, ice hockey, and tennis players, but may be found in athletes in all sports where running with rapid changes of direction are a large part of the activity. Of a group

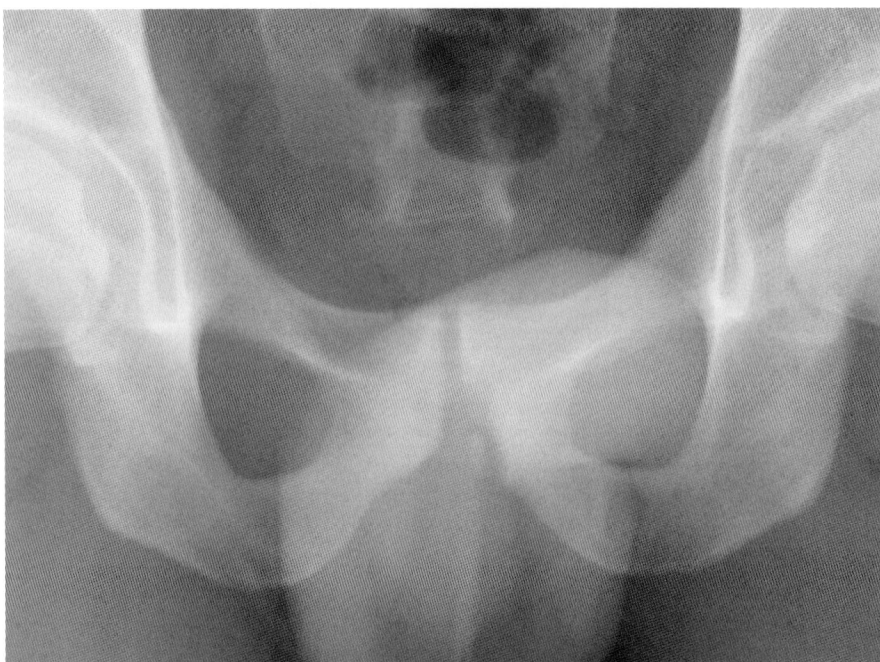

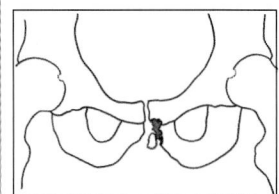

Figure 10.21 Pubic bone stress injury. The "moth-eaten" appearance of the inferior ramus of the pubis medially on the left side should be noted. (© Medical Illustrator Tommy Bolic, Sweden.)

of professional soccer players, 76% were found to have radiographic changes that are consistent with pubic bone stress injury (Figure 10.21).

- Symptoms and signs: The symptom is pain localized to the lower abdomen and the inside of the thighs during and for a while after loading. The symptoms gradually increase with activity and may become so expressed that they make running training completely impossible. The pain is usually unilateral but can be bilateral.
- Diagnosis: As with any stress injury, a thorough case history with a review of the patient's training program is key, particularly with respect to loading of the pelvic rim. Clinical examination findings are tenderness when both the rectus abdominis muscle insertion, pubic symphysis, superior pubic ramus bone, and the adductor muscles bony insertion. Maximum tenderness is usually found over the pubic symphysis and surrounding parasymphyseal pubic bone. Pain is triggered with contraction of the abdominal and adductor musculature against resistance. Internal rotation of the hip is decreased. In cases in which the patient has had pain for a long time, the radiograph of the pubic bone toward the symphysis has a typically moth-eaten and partially sclerotic appearance, often with an overweight of changes on one side (Figure 10.21). Shortly after the onset of symptoms, the radiograph may be negative. If it is, isotope scintigraphy will demonstrate intensive uptake, usually in both pubic bones (Figure 10.22). Radiographic changes remain for a long time after the symptoms disappear, and in some cases the radiographic can demonstrate the typical changes without the athlete having had special symptoms. MRI examinations demonstrate edema in the bone marrow of the pubic bone (Figure 10.23a and b).
- Treatment: The only effective treatment is to avoid activities that cause pain for at least 6–8 weeks. Abdominal and hip muscle stretching is recommended, especially for patients with reduced hip joint movement. The athlete needs an alternative training program for maintaining strength and condition during the unloading period. Treatment in the high-pressure chamber (hyperbaric therapy) may decrease the time needed for healing. It cannot be emphasized enough, but unloading is the cornerstone of treatment.
- Prognosis: The prognosis is good with adequate unloading, but it often takes 6–12 months before the patient becomes completely asymptomatic. Imaging does not help with return to sport prognosis so is not needed.

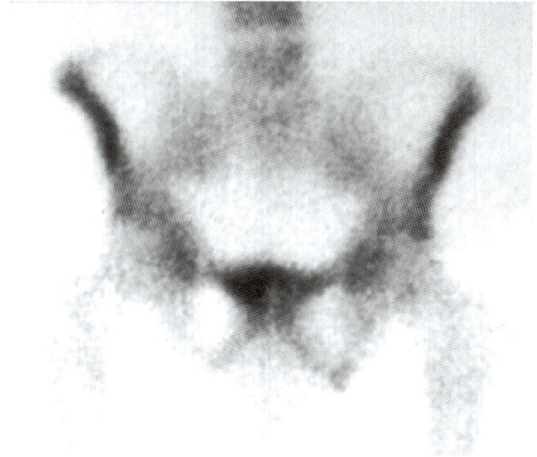

Figure 10.22 Positive scintigraphy finding of pubic bone stress injury.

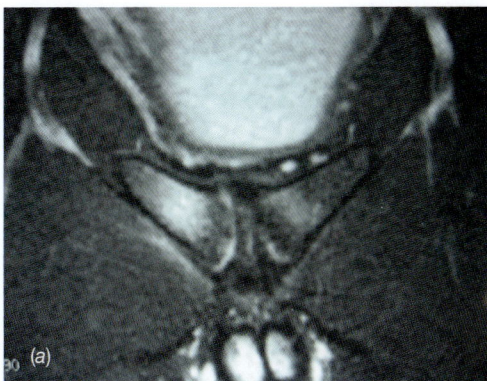

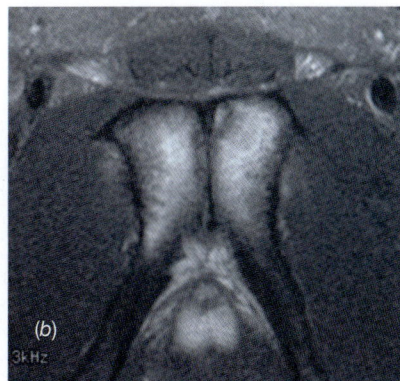

Figure 10.23 Positive MRI finding of pubic bone stress injury. The image shows bone marrow edema of the pubic bone bilaterally (*a*). Image shows adductor tendinosis with pubic bone edema with extrusion of the disc, all signs of remodeling due to stress (*b*).

PELVIS, GROIN, AND HIPS

Trochanteric Pain Syndrome

Several bursae exist in the pelvic, inguinal, and hip region. The most important ones to athletes are the trochanteric, the iliopectineal, and the gluteal bursae (Figure 10.24). An inflammatory reaction may occur in all of these as (1) bursitis triggered by friction, (2) a chemical bursitis, or (3) an infectious (purulent) bursitis. In athletes, bursitis is almost exclusively caused by mechanical irritation, usually from a muscle or tendon that frequently slips back and forth over the bursa. The trochanteric bursa is located between the iliotibial tract/tensor fascia lata and the greater trochanter (Figure 10.24). Because of its relatively superficial location over the bone, it is subject to direct trauma with bleeding and acute inflammation. The blood may coagulate and form fibrin deposits in the bursa, which in turn will cause chronic irritation. Eventually, these fibrin lumps calcify, and when the bursa is palpated they may feel like small movable rice bodies. Key triggering causes of chronic friction bursitis are anatomic axial deviation, such as anisomelia, increased column anteversion, a broad pelvis, a rigid iliotibial tract, and pronation foot with compensatory internal rotation of the tibia. Another cause is frequent running on one side (usually the left) of the road. This causes functional anisomelia with overuse of the iliotibial tract and the tensor fascia lata on the leg that is closest to the edge of the road, as well as the risk of developing trochanteric bursitis in this location.

Gluteal tendinopathy is often classified as trochanteric pain syndrome. This is a chronic, painful condition at the insertion of the gluteus medius and minimus, on the posterior margin of the greater trochanter (Figure 10.25). The cause is often simple overloading, and it is most frequently found in long-distance runners and orienteering runners. Running on only asphalt on the same side of a road (usually the left), which slants down toward the ditch, causes functional leg-length discrepancy, which may trigger the symptoms. Endogenous causes, such as true anisomelia, increased femoral neck anteversion, being knock-kneed, and pronation foot, are important triggering factors.

- Symptoms and signs: Pain and possibly swelling occur over the greater trochanter, sometimes radiating down along the lateral side of the thigh. This may be confused with sciatica. Pain may become so strong that running training becomes impossible.
- Diagnosis: The diagnosis is made on the basis of tenderness, swelling, and possibly crepitation with, in chronic cases, the rice body feeling over the greater trochanter. Adduction and rotation in the hip with an extended knee will also trigger pain. It is possible to demonstrate the thickening of the wall and an increased amount of fluid in the bursa by using ultrasound and MRI.

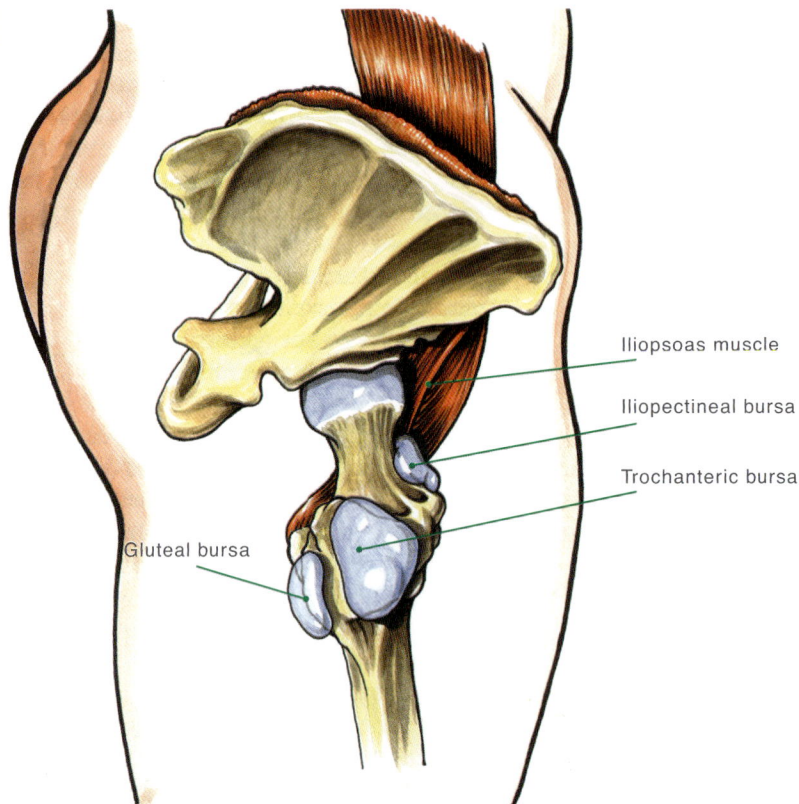

Iliopsoas muscle

Iliopectineal bursa

Trochanteric bursa

Gluteal bursa

Figure 10.24 Bursae in the hip area. Bursitis may occur in several of the bursae of the hips, the iliopectineal bursa, the trochanteric bursa, and the gluteal bursa. (© Medical Illustrator Tommy Bolic, Sweden.)

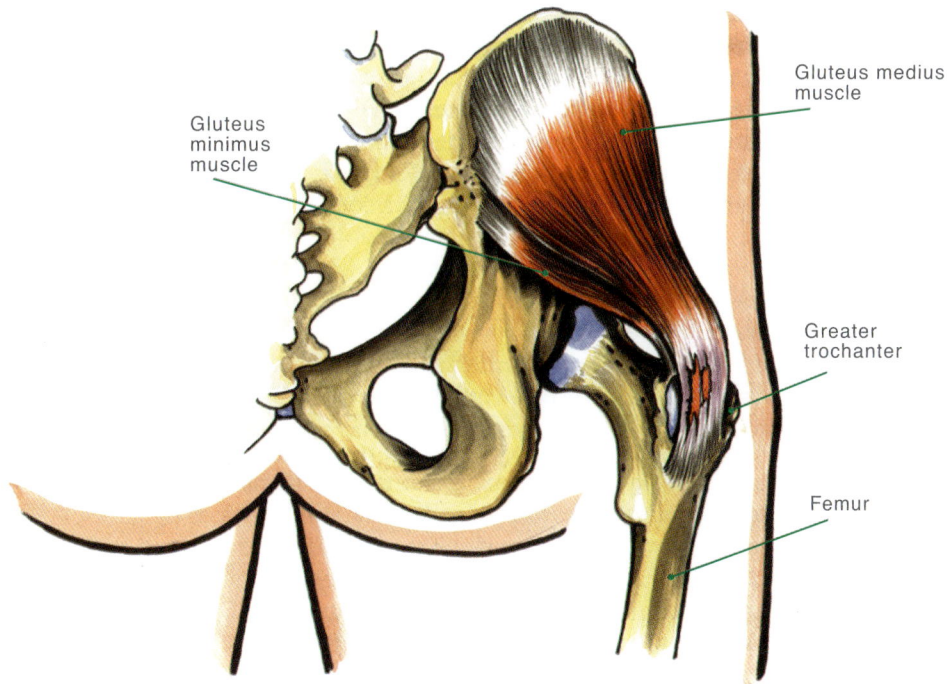

Figure 10.25 Trochanteric pain syndrome. (© Medical Illustrator Tommy Bolic, Sweden.)

- Treatment: Unloading, NSAIDs, and alternative training are recommended treatments in acute cases. If symptoms are long term or recurring, treatment includes puncture, tapping of fluid, and possibly steroid injection, as well as intense stretching of the iliotibial tract and the tensor fascia lata. At the same time, any axial deviation and training errors are corrected as much as possible. The use of hip protectors may be helpful to athletes who often fall on their hip, including handball players and goalies. Occasionally, a patient requires surgery with extirpation of the bursa and excision of an oval "window" in the fascia lata over the greater trochanter. This "window" must be large enough for the trochanter to be moved freely during flexion and extension, without the edges getting pinched.
- Prognosis: The symptoms have a tendency to recur if triggering causes are not corrected.

Labral Injuries

In our experience, many patients present following many years of FAI and a degenerative labrum is seen at hip arthroscopy. This can also result in cartilage loss and other sign of osteoarthritis in the hip. The relationship between osteoarthritis and FAI is well established through clinical studies, radiographic studies, and computer simulations.

Symptoms and signs: Patients often present with ongoing hip pain with no specific traumatic incident. Symptoms have interfered with activities of daily living and this has caused them to seek treatment. Many athletes following their professional career also present with chronic hip injuries. These symptoms are often accompanied by loss of motion of the hip or pain with motion. As with acute injuries, the impingement test, and FABER distance test are positive from the bony abnormalities that have caused the labral damage.

PELVIS, GROIN, AND HIPS

Diagnosis: Bony abnormalities associated with FAI are seen on radiographs and labral and chondral injury are diagnosed on MRI.

Treatment: For resolution of symptoms, patients are treated with hip arthroscopy. Treatment is dependent on the quality of the labral tissue and the amount of labral tissue. Labral repair is the preferred treatment; however, in many cases of chronic injuries, there is inadequate tissue or the longitudinal fibers have been disrupted. In these cases, the area of damage or deficiency is reconstructed with an iliotibial band graft. Clinical studies have shown excellent early outcomes following labral reconstruction. As with the acute injury, the bony abnormalities that cause impingement must be addressed to protect the repairs or reconstruction.

Prognosis: The prognosis is good if there is adequate joint space and limited degenerative changes in the hip joint. After surgery, the patient can return to full activity after 6 weeks. Studies have shown that a longer recovery and slower return to full activity are seen in patients who wait over 1 year to have surgical intervention.

Injury to the Acetabular or Femoral Head Articular Cartilage

Articular cartilage defects rarely heal spontaneously. They commonly occur in the presence of FAI. Acetabular defects commonly occur at the area of labral tears. The most common location of acetabular defects is the anterior acetabulum. Cartilage injuries are often seen as cartilage flaps and watershed lesions. Acetabular cysts and femoral head cysts are also associated with chondral injuries. Cartilage defects of the femoral head are common in patients with hip dislocation. Articular cartilage defects in the chronic hip are often more diffuse and less well defined. This damage often occurs with FAI and when the bony impingement is removed, cartilage lesions respond well to treatment. The presence of a joint space narrower than 2 mm on any part of the weight-bearing surface has been shown to be a negative predictor of outcome in patients with cartilage defects.

- Symptoms and signs: Clicking, catching, or other mechanical symptoms during the examination are common findings associated with the diagnosis of a labral tear. Unfortunately, there is no specific examination maneuver to assess for chondral injuries.
- Diagnosis: Plain radiographs are essential for the initial workup to determine joint space narrowing and other signs of degenerative changes in the joint. MRI can provide reliable information on the diagnosis of cartilage defects in the hip with a 3T MRI.
- Treatment: Many techniques have been used to treat cartilage injuries of the hip. These include chondroplasty, osteoarticular autograft or allograft transplants, autologous chondrocyte implantation and microfracture. In a patient with an acute injury with a lesion less than 800 mm^2, with adequate surrounding cartilage to provide a rim to hold the clot, microfracture is the procedure of choice. Microfracture provides an enriched environment for tissue regeneration by taking advantage of the body's own healing abilities. The lesion is prepared by removing any unstable cartilage around the rim of the defect and the calcified cartilage layer is removed using a curette. Small holes are made in the defect about 3–4 mm apart at a depth of 2–4 mm. Fat droplets and blood can be visualized coming from the holes. It is critical that any sclerotic bone be removed along with the calcified cartilage layer. This will allow for the repair cartilage to adhere to the surface. For cartilage defects of the acetabulum, when trimming the acetabular rim for a pincer impingement, the size of the lesion can be significantly reduced by trimming the edge. In cases of bone loss, mosaic plasty or bone plugs can be used. As with all procedures, proper technique and rehabilitation are critical to the success of the procedure.

Postoperative management includes the use of a continuous passive motion and nonweight bearing for 8 weeks.

- Prognosis: With adequate joint space and patient compliance with postoperative protocol, cartilage defects of the hip generally respond well to treatment with microfracture. In patients with chronic changes within the joint, less than optimal results will be seen if these factors are not considered prior to surgery.

Other Injuries

Injuries to Other Muscles and Tendons in the Inguinal and Hip Region

Other muscles, such as the gracilis, the sartorius, the tensor fascia lata, and the gluteal muscles (particularly the gluteus medius), may also be subjected to tears or tendinosis. A thorough examination, including palpation and specific testing of the relevant muscle, is key in the determination of what has been injured. The guidelines for treatment and prophylactics are the same as for an adductor longus tear or tendinosis.

Myositis Ossificans—*Ossification in the Injured Muscle* !

Myositis ossificans is calcification and eventually ossification of a deep intramuscular hematoma. It is most commonly seen in post-traumatic injury to the quadriceps muscle (vastus intermedius) but in the groin it is seen with distal tears in the adductor group. The etiology is unclear. Some authors believe that calcification results from torn-off periosteal cells, whereas others maintain that undifferentiated fibroblasts in the hematoma are converted into osteoblasts. In any case, it is typical for the disorder to appear when activity begins too early after an injury, with hemorrhaging and a long-term inflammatory reaction.

- Symptoms and signs: Symptoms are pain and reduced function corresponding to the affected muscle group.
- Diagnosis: Sometimes a solid tumor can be palpated in the muscle belly. Ultrasound and X-rays demonstrate calcium deposition.
- Treatment: The primary treatments are prophylactic, in the form of adequate unloading and gradual, careful training after a muscle tear. Avoidance of deep tissue massage in the first 10 days post-injury is essential. Compressing the area to prevent further bleeding is helpful and maintenance of muscle length by regular stretching is essential. For extremely long-term recalcitrant symptoms, it may be necessary to surgically excise the new bone formation. However, this may not be done before calcification in the area is complete and, at the earliest, about 1 year after injury. The risk of new bone formation in the muscle is high if surgery is performed too early.

External Snapping Hip

The most common cause of snapping hip is irritation of the posterior margin of the iliotibial tract, which passes over the top of the greater trochanter (Figure 10.26). A mound-shaped prominence, consisting of fibrous tissue, eventually forms here. Secondary trochanter bursitis develops at the same time. When the hip is bent and stretched, the mound-shaped prominence slips back and forth over the trochanter, often with an audible click and visible and palpable "slipping." The disorder is most common in thin, flexible women, such as ballet dancers and gymnasts.

- Symptoms and signs: Aching pain is felt over the greater trochanter during loading with flexion and extension movements of the hip. Discomfort is experienced from the often very audible click.

- Treatment: The recommended treatments are stretching of the iliotibial tract and the tensor fascia lata and possibly steroid injection in the trochanteric bursa. Persistent pain often results in the need for surgical treatment, as is the case for patients with chronic trochanteric bursitis.

Internal Snapping Hip

Intra-articular snapping can be caused by several conditions, including loose bodies and labral pathology. In addition, internal snapping can occur when the iliopsoas tendon moves over a bony prominence (Figure 10.26).

- Symptoms and signs: Pain deep in the groin is accompanied by a click in the same place when the hip is extended from a flexed, externally rotated, and abducted position. Internal snapping of the iliopsoas tendon over the iliopectineal eminence, femoral head, or lesser trochanter may or may not be painful. Pain or discomfort associated with internal snapping is an indication of associated iliopsoas tendinopathy.
- Diagnosis: The chief component to diagnosis of snapping hip is reproduction of the audible snapping over the hip.
- Treatment: Initial management of painful iliopsoas tendonitis consists of rehabilitation. If symptoms persist, an ultrasound-guided injection can provide relief and predict the response to surgical release. A tenotomy of the iliopsoas tendon can be performed with an intra-articular approach. The tendon is visualized through an anterior capsulotomy made during arthroscopy. The tendon is divided away from the muscle and the tenotomy is completed.
- Prognosis: Most patient respond well to rehabilitation. In those patients who require surgical intervention, complete relief of symptoms with arthroscopic release of the iliopsoas has been reported.

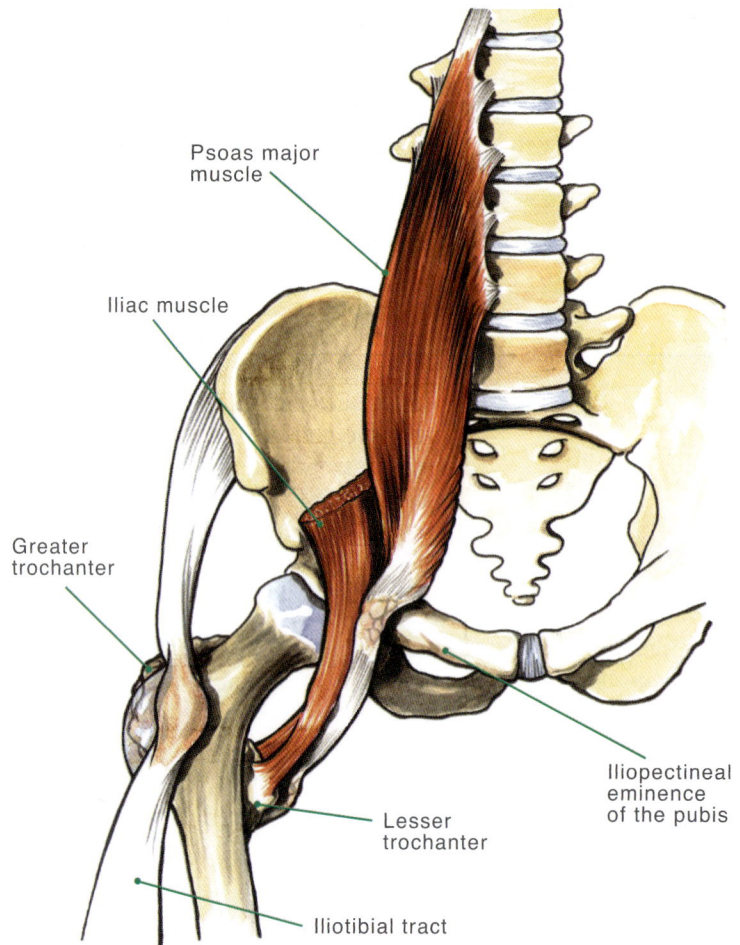

Figure 10.26 Snapping hip. External ("typical") snapping hip is caused by the iliotibial tract gliding over the greater trochanter, whereas internal ("atypical") snapping hip is caused by the greater psoas tendon gliding over the iliopectineal eminence of the pubis proximally or a bony eminence at the lesser trochanter distally. (© Medical Illustrator Tommy Bolic, Sweden.)

Gluteal Tendinopathy/Bursitis—*Pain in the Trochanter Insertion of the Gluteal Musculature*

This is a chronic, painful condition at the insertion of the gluteus medius and minimus, on the posterior margin of the greater trochanter (Figure 10.25). The cause is often simple overloading, and it is most frequently found in long-distance runners and orienteering runners. Running on only asphalt on the same side of a road (usually the left), which slants down toward the ditch, causes functional leg-length discrepancy, which may trigger the symptoms. Endogenous causes, such as true anisomelia, increased femoral neck anteversion, being knock-kneed, and pronation foot, are important triggering factors. The gluteal bursa is located between the tendon of the gluteus medius and the tensor fascia lata, behind the greater trochanter

(Figure 10.24). Inflammation in this bursa is usually caused by overuse and is most common in long-distance runners. Axial deviation is another important contributing factor in this case.

- **Symptoms and signs:** The patient feels pain in the gluteal region that sometimes radiates down into the back side of the thigh. Sitting for a long time may cause significant pain.
- **Diagnosis:** The diagnosis is made on the basis of pain from palpation behind the greater trochanter and from passive flexion of the hip. It is difficult to clinically differentiate these symptoms from those of gluteal tendinopathy, but ultrasound and MRI examinations will demonstrate the inflamed bursa.
- **Treatment:** The treatment is essentially the same as for iliopsoas bursitis, but includes stretching of the gluteal musculature and the tensor fascia lata.

Inguinal Insufficiency

This disorder is thought to be caused by an overuse injury of the lower portion of the abdominal musculature, particularly the lower fibers of the external oblique muscle and the aponeurosis of the transverse muscle of the abdomen (Figure 10.27). This causes weakness, a defect, or tearing in the wall of the inguinal canal. The disorder is most common among soccer players but may also occur in athletes in other sports, such as long-distance running, football, and rugby.

- **Symptoms and signs:** Loading causes gradually increasing pain in the inguinal region that has the character of an aching toothache, and the symptoms often remain for a while after the activity has ended. Pain worsens significantly from quick spurts, hitting balls hard, or impulse pain is often present (pain on coughing and sneezing). Eventually, pain begins earlier and earlier during activity; ultimately, both training and competition become impossible. It may be difficult for the patient to localize the pain, and if the disorder becomes long term, secondary pain often develops at the insertions of the adductor muscles and the rectus abdominis on the pubic bone. Pain frequently radiates to the scrotum, the perineum, and the lumbar area of the back.
- **Diagnosis:** The physician must perform a thorough case history and clinical examination, particularly with respect to differential diagnoses such as adductor tendinopathy, pubic bone stress injury, FAI, and rectus abdominis tendinopathy. Many patients with chronic

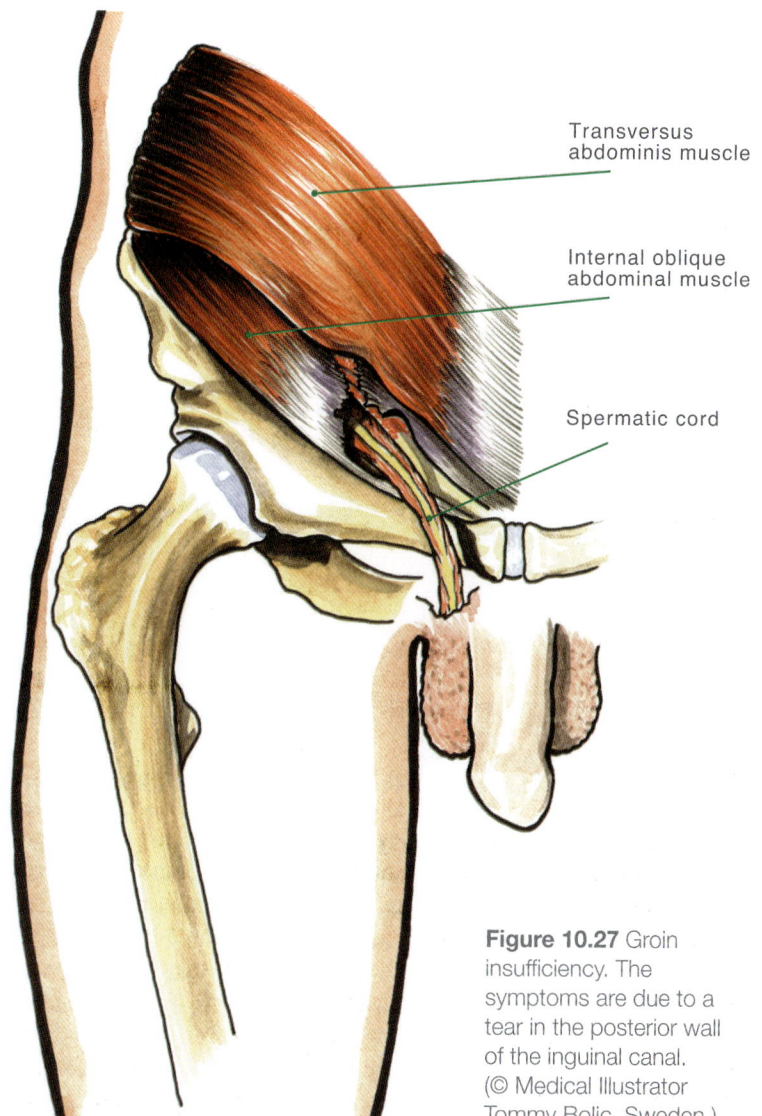

Transversus abdominis muscle

Internal oblique abdominal muscle

Spermatic cord

Figure 10.27 Groin insufficiency. The symptoms are due to a tear in the posterior wall of the inguinal canal. (© Medical Illustrator Tommy Bolic, Sweden.)

PELVIS, GROIN, AND HIPS

symptoms will indicate tenderness when the pubic bone's adductor and rectus abdominis insertions are palpated, and loading of these against resistance will also trigger pain. With the patient standing up and coughing, the external inguinal opening is palpated via the scrotum. This, as well as palpation over the middle portion of the inguinal canal, will trigger the patient's typical pain. The external inguinal opening may be slightly expanded in contrast with the unaffected side, but it rarely receives an impact as in the case of a regular hernia. Herniography (with radiographic contrast in the abdominal cavity) and ultrasound examinations are sometimes recommended, but both radiographic and ultrasound images may be difficult to see and are often negative during the early stage when changes are small. There are some clinicians who do not consider inguinal insufficiency a credible diagnosis in activity-related chronic groin injury.

- Treatment: Conservative treatment includes unloading and careful strength training of the abdominal musculature. This rarely brings about permanent improvement. Several studies have shown that surgical treatment using hernioplasty to reinforce the posterior wall in the inguinal canal has a very good effect on the disorder. Most reports indicate that more than 90% of patients return to sport activity after adequate postoperative training. Postoperative training consists of unloading the muscles of the abdominal wall for 4–6 weeks, after which strength training is carefully and gradually increased.

- Prognosis: Normally, the athlete may resume full sport activity after about 3 months. With surgical repair, return to sport has been seen in 3–4 weeks. Return to sport or recurrence may be complicated by co-existing pathologies, such as labral pathology.

Nerve Entrapment

The following nerves in the inguinal and hip region may be subjected to pressure injuries: the sciatic, the lateral femoral cutaneous, the ilioinguinal, the genitofemoral, and the obturator nerves (Figure 10.28a and b). The ilioinguinal, the genitofemoral, and the lateral femoral cutaneous nerves may become caught in scar tissue from changes after trauma and surgery or may be subjected to pressure from long-term and intense training of the abdominal musculature. Wearing tight belts or jeans may also irritate the lateral femoral cutaneous nerve (also called meralgia paresthetica). Piriformis syndrome occurs when the sciatic nerve is irritated, where it goes out of the pelvis on the anterior side of the piriformis muscle. The disorder occurs most often in well-trained people with short, strong, and poorly stretched musculature. Athletes, particularly those in strength sports and bodybuilding, may have irritation of the obturator nerve where it extends into the obturator canal.

- Symptoms and signs: The ilioinguinal nerve innervates the base of the penis and scrotum and of the labium major, as well as the medial side of the thigh proximally. The genitofemoral nerve also innervates the scrotum and the labium major, as well as the anterior side of the thigh immediately below the inguinal ligament. The lateral femoral cutaneous nerve supplies an anterior and lateral skin area on the thigh, and the obturator nerve innervates the adductor muscles and an area of skin that corresponds to the distal portion of the inside of the thigh down toward the popliteal space (Figure 10.28). Affection of these nerves causes parenthesis and pain corresponding to their area of innervation, particularly with hard use of the musculature, which is near the area of the nerve to which pressure is applied. When the piriformis muscle puts pressure on the sciatic nerve, aching pain from the ischial tuberosity occurs, possibly radiating down into the back side of the thigh. Patients often have the sensation that the hamstring muscles are too short, and they do not reach maximum speed during spurts because of the disorder.

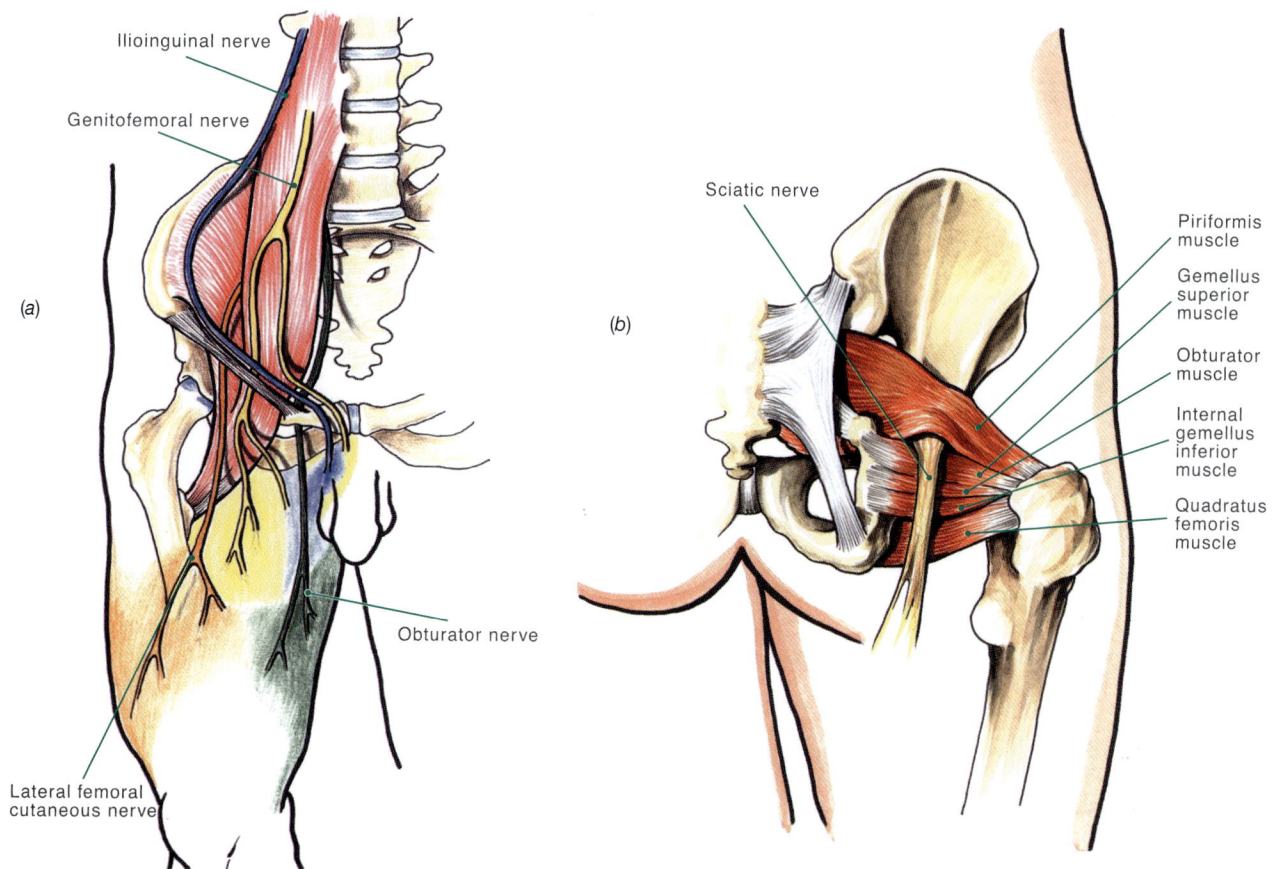

Figure 10.28 Entrapment syndromes. The distribution of symptoms is shown, when various nerves in the inguinal area (a) become entrapped, as well as entrapment of the sciatic nerve (b). (© Medical Illustrator Tommy Bolic, Sweden.)

Typically, pain also increases when the patient is sitting with slightly flexed hips for a long time, such as when driving a car. The patient should stop often, get out, and stretch her legs before continuing to drive.

- Diagnosis: The patient often indicates reduced sensibility, pain, and parenthesis in the skin area that is innervated by the indicated nerve. Blockage of the nerve by injecting local anesthesia confirms the diagnosis. Piriformis syndrome is an exclusion diagnosis. All other possible causes of pain in the affected region must be eliminated before this diagnosis can be made with certainty. When the piriformis muscle is loaded, the patient typically has pain from the ischial tuberosity down on the posterior side of the thigh, and in a few cases all the way down in the calf.
- Treatment: In some cases, modification of training routines, particularly reduction of intense strength training combined with stretching of neighboring muscles, may make the patient asymptomatic from nerve compression. NSAIDs given at an early stage may also be effective. In some cases, particularly if the patient has meralgia paresthetica, the nerve must be surgically released in the affected area. Piriformis syndrome must be treated conservatively at the source by stretching the piriformis muscle. The best type of stretching the athlete can do alone involves maximum flexion, adduction, and external rotation of the hip. A few patients do not become asymptomatic from conservative treatment, and if there are numerous symptoms, surgical release of the tendon of the piriformis muscle is indicated.

Rehabilitation of Injuries to the Pelvis, Groin, and Hips

Marc J. Philippon[1,2,3], Éanna Falvey[4], Geoffrey M. Verrall[5], and Karen K. Briggs[1]

[1]*Steadman Philippon Research Institute, Vail, CO, USA*
[2]*McMaster University, Hamilton, ON, Canada*
[3]*University of Pittsburgh Medical Center, Pittsburgh, PA, USA*
[4]*Sports Surgery Clinic, Dublin, Ireland*
[5]*Sportsmed SA, Sports Medicine Centre, Adelaide, SA, Australia*

Goals and Principles for Treating Acute Injuries

The goals of conservative treatment using rehabilitation of acute injuries in the pelvic, inguinal, and hip region are listed in Table 10.4. For acute injuries that have been treated arthroscopically, the most important factor of the postsurgical rehabilitation process is that it is specific to the procedure performed, the patient's healing time, discomfort tolerance, desired sport-specific activities and postoperative athletic participation goals. Weight-bearing progression and range of motion limitations in the immediate postoperative period are specific to the surgery performed and differ between types of procedures.

Rehabilitation of Nonsurgically Treated Injuries

As soon as the muscle can be activated without pain, the patient may begin doing mild dynamic exercises. The patient should begin with mild weight-bearing and numerous repetitions. The exercises may be repeated several times during the day. The muscle must be completely relaxed between contractions. The goal is improved circulation and improved relaxation in the portion of the musculature that is not injured, which speeds up the healing process.

Active stretching of the muscles begins as soon as possible. There is no stretching in the usual sense of the word. Only the mobility that exists should be used; the patient

	Goals	Measures
Acute phase	Reduce swelling	PRICE principle
Rehabilitation phase	Reduce pain	Dynamic exercises with gradually increasing intensity
	Normalize movement, strength, and sensory motor function	Sensory motor training
Training phase	As a minimum, achieve the same sensory motor function, strength, and mobility as before the injury	Functional training
		Sport-specific training
	Reduce the risk of reinjury	Recuperate fully before returning to maximum activity

Table 10.4 Goals and measures for rehabilitation of injuries in the pelvic, inguinal, and hip region. (Reproduced with permission from the Norwegian Sports Medicine Association.)

should not stretch further and should stay within the limits of pain. The exercises must always be done without, or with only minimal, pain.

Exercises are of primary importance during the rehabilitation phase, but other physical therapy treatment may be useful in removing bleeding residue and avoiding scar tissue in the injured area. Massage, stretching, and various types of electrotherapy may be indicated. Eventually, the patient will have to train actively in the entire path of motion to regain the flexibility that is the same as the flexibility on the healthy side. The patient must also achieve the greatest possible functional scar tissue, thereby preventing recurrence. He must always follow up increased flexibility with control and strength training (e.g., Figure 10.29). He must also protect the stabilizing function of the muscles through exercises that stabilize the pelvis. Various sensory motor exercises are important for this purpose. The progression of exercise is controlled by pain and function in the patient. If the progression is too rapid, chronic painful conditions may result.

Good alternatives for maintaining general condition during the nonweight-bearing period in connection with acute injuries are bicycling, running in water (while wearing a wet vest), and swimming (although breast stroke should be avoided if there are adductor injuries).

Rehabilitation of Surgically Treated Injuries

There are 4 stages and levels for the rehabilitation protocol treatment of the injured hip. The first stage is mobility and maximum protection. This stage is dependent on soft-tissue and osseous healing. The other stages include controlled stability of movement, reclamation of strength, and return to sport. The timing for the first stage covers approximately the initial 6–9 weeks, while the following stages have a variable timeline and are dependent on the athlete's ability to meet specific criteria to advance. It is critical for the success of the intervention that each program is individualized to the athlete and his or her progress, with careful monitoring of their progress.

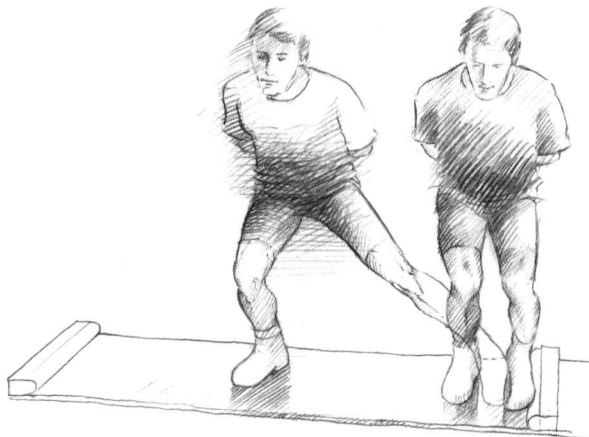

Figure 10.29 Functional abductor muscle training:

- Wear wool socks outside your shoes. Stand on a slide board and push from side to side.
- Make sure that your weight is over the leg that will stop the movement.
- Use slight hip flexion to train the abductor muscles and greater hip flexion (more of a proper skating position) to train your quadriceps coxae.
- Progression: Increase speed.
(© Lill-Ann Prøis.)

The first stage of the protocol protects the integrity of the repaired or healing tissue. The goal is to diminish inflammation, prevent muscular atrophy, contraction and inhibition, and restore passive range of motion. Depending on the treatment, the patient may be limited to flat foot weight bearing. To maintain motion, the athlete rides a stationary bike with no resistance and uses a continuous passive motion machine. A key rehabilitation exercise that research has shown reduces the prevalence of scar tissue following hip arthroscopy is hip circumduction. With the knee bent at 70°, the leg is moved in a circular motion with the patella always facing upward. The requirements to progress are experiencing minimal pain or pinching with all exercise and achieving ROM of ≥75% of the nonoperative side. Excessive hip flexion, internal rotation, and abduction should be avoided initially, as it may cause increased tissue inflammation around the joint.

The second stage of the protocol focuses on regaining pelvic and trunk stabilization and weight-bearing gait. Exercises (e.g.,Figure 10.30) in the second phase include standing or prone resisted internal and external rotation, 1/3 knee bends, wall sits with an abductor band for resistance, sidesteps with an abductor band for resistance and two-legged bridging for core strength. When all treatment-specific restrictions are lifted, functional movements, such as light jogging for field and court sports, skating for ice sports and dance movements for dancers, can be started. Aquatic therapy may be useful in the progression of weight bearing and ambulation, as the buoyant environment allows for controlled gait training. Treadmill use is not recommended at any time.

The goal of the third phase is to restore muscular strength, endurance, and cardiovascular fitness, and continue improving neuromuscular control, balance and proprioception. Exercises include standing resisted hip external rotation, walking lunges, lunges with trunk rotation, plyometric bounding in water, cord-resisted walking in the forward, backward or sideways direction, and progressive exercise ball work for increasing core strength. For athletes, passing a sport test (see Table 10.5) is required to progress to the fourth phase of rehabilitation. The fourth phase consists of sport-specific training to restore the athlete's prior level of power, explosiveness and agility to enable return to play.

Iliopsoas pain or tendinitis has been reported following hip arthroscopy. This may be due to gluteus medius weakness. Research has shown that specific exercises can maximize the ratio between gluteus medius activation compared with iliopsoas

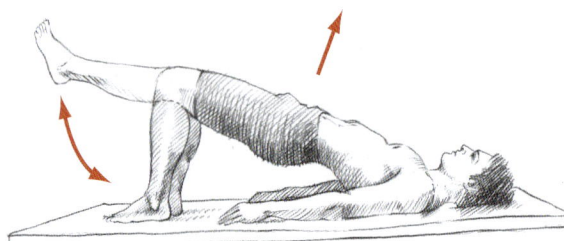

Figure 10.30 Hip lifts while lying on your back:
- Stabilize your back by pulling in your abdomen and stretching deep in your lumbar region. Lift your buttocks until your hip is fully extended. Maintain this position and extend one knee. Make sure that your knee and hip are at the same height on both sides. Switch legs.
- Progression: Place legs on a balance pad.

(Reproduced with permission from the Norwegian Sports Medicine Association.)

activation. For the first phase of rehabilitation, resisted terminal knee extension and resisted knee flexion are recommended. For the second phase, resisted hip extension stool hip rotations and later in the second phase, side-lying hip abduction exercises with wall sliding are recommended. For hip flexor tendinitis, hip clam exercises with hip extension can be used with caution. In the third phase, prone heel squeezes and side-lying abduction with internal hip rotation are recommended.

Rehabilitation of Chronic Painful Conditions

The main elements of rehabilitation of muscle injuries and tendinopathy in the groin, inguinal, and hip region are strength and stability training. Training initially begins with light loading and numerous repetitions (usually 30 repetitions in each series), and if pain does not worsen, usually several sessions a day as well. The load is gradually increased while the number of repetitions is correspondingly reduced.

If pain in the area has lasted for a while, it may result in a change in the movement pattern, which can easily result in overloading in other places. Therefore, when the patient is being rehabilitated for injuries in this area, he must train the muscles as stabilizers. The quadriceps coxae (external rotators), adductors, and abductors balance and stabilize the pelvis on the femoral head. Therefore, sensory motor training in this area should be emphasized, as is true for the knee and ankle area. Therefore, weight transfer and training on a balance or wobble board should be encouraged (e.g.,Figure 10.31). The transverse abdominal muscle and the multifidus muscles contribute to stabilization of the lumbar region and the pelvis as a whole. Therefore, this musculature should be activated before doing the exercises outlined in this chapter. The significance of the pelvic floor must also be remembered.

If the patient has chronic pain in this area, axial deviation (such as leg-length discrepancy and overpronation) may be present, and it may be possible to correct this by wearing insoles, both as a basis for rehabilitation and to prevent new injuries.

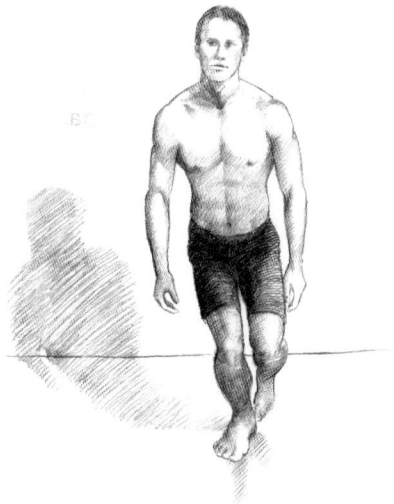

Figure 10.31 Single-leg knee bends:

- Make sure that your hips and shoulders are at the same height on both sides and that your knee points over your toes.
- Progression: Use a wobble board or a balance board.

(Reproduced with permission from the Norwegian Sports Medicine Association.)

Test	Goal	Score
Single knee bends	3 min	1 point earned for each 30 s completed
Lateral agility	100 s	1 point earned for each 20 s completed
Diagonal agility	100 s	1 point earned for each 20 s completed
Forward lunge on box	2 min	1 point earned for each 30 s completed

Table 10.5 Scoring of the hip functional test. (Reproduced with permission from the Norwegian Sports Medicine Association.)

Return to Sport

Athletes in explosive sports must not load at maximum before the injury is completely healed, which may take up to 3 months after an acute groin injury. They should not compete before they have trained at maximum intensity, and athletes in team sports must have trained in practice game situations before they should play in a game.

For return to sport following treatment of hip injuries, passing a functional test is a requirement for an athlete to progress on to sport specific training. The hip functional test is a test comprised of four exercises with a 20-point scoring system. It tests the patient's pelvic stability, endurance, functional strength in the lower extremity, good explosion off and absorption onto the involved lower extremity in both a lateral and a rotational direction, and ability to flex and extend into a lunge position without pain, fatigue or compensation. These are tested through single knee bends, lateral and diagonal agility exercises, and box lunges. A test is stopped and considered a failure if the athlete experiences pain. A test is also a failure if the athlete cannot do the specific exercise for the given amount of time. A point total of 17 or higher indicates passing and allows progression of the rehab to intensifying sport-specific exercises (Table 10.5).

Preventing Reinjury

Because injuries in the pelvic and inguinal region have a tendency to become chronic or to recur, prevention is key. Athletes may continue with some of the exercises that place the greatest demand on sensory motor activity and stabilization once or twice a week for at least 1 year after they have been fully rehabilitated and have returned to their sport. Any malalignment must also be corrected.

11 Thigh

Acute Thigh Injuries

Geoffrey M. Verrall[1], Juan-Manuel Alonso Martín[2], Lars Engebretsen[3],
Toru Fukubayashi[4], William E. Garrett[5], Grethe Myklebust[3], Gil Rodas[6], and
Per Renström[7]

[1]Sportsmed SA, Sport Medicine Centre, Adelaide, SA, Australia
[2]Real Federación Española de Atletismo, International Association of Athletics
Federation (IAAF), Madrid, Spain
[3]Oslo Sports Trauma Research Center, Norwegian School of Sport Sciences, Oslo, Norway
[4]University of Waseda, Tokorozawa, Saitama, Japan
[5]Duke University Medical Center, Durham, NC, USA
[6]Medical Services, Futbol Club Barcelona, Barcelona, Spain
[7]Center for Sports Trauma Research and Education, Karolinska Institutet,
Stockholm, Sweden

Occurrence

Acute sports injuries are common both in the anterior and posterior thigh. Contusions and more often strains of the hamstrings and quadriceps occur frequently in sports requiring repeated sprint ability such as soccer or individual sports such as track and field athletics and all contact sports. Studies show that up to 30% of all soccer injuries are thigh muscle injuries. The muscles can be injured by direct contact, as well as by muscle strain mechanism where the muscle-tendon apparatus is acutely stretched beyond the limits of tolerance, causing injury to the muscle fibers resulting in pain. Other parts of the thigh, including the nerves, vessels, and bone, may be injured in acute situations, but these types of injuries are usually caused by high-energy trauma, such as falls during downhill skiing or motor biking.

Differential Diagnoses

Table 11.1 provides an overview of the differential diagnoses. The most common injury is hamstring muscle strains and there is usually not too much difficulty in making this diagnosis. Contusions also occur frequently in contact sports like soccer.

Most common	Less common	Must not be overlooked ❗
Thigh contusion, p. 342	Posterior thigh pain secondary to neural compression of the lower back (sciatica), p. 135	Acute compartment syndrome, p. 347
Hamstrings muscle strain injury, p. 344		Femur fracture including stress fracture
Quadriceps muscle strain injury, p. 346	Femoroacetabular impingement, p. 302	Bone and soft-tissue tumors
Muscle cramps	Adductor muscle strain injury, p. 347	Vascular and nerve abnormalities

Table 11.1 Overview of the differential diagnoses of acute thigh injuries. (Reproduced with permission from the Norwegian Sports Medicine Association.)

The IOC Manual of Sports Injuries, First Edition. Edited by Roald Bahr.
©2012 International Olympic Committee. Published 2012 by John Wiley & Sons, Ltd.

In rare cases, hamstring avulsion in children may cause painful conditions that result in a long-term absence from sport activity.

Diagnostic Thinking

Acute thigh injuries are usually not serious and generally should not be treated surgically. In most cases, they can be treated at the primary-care level and are a good example of using a multidisciplinary team for rehabilitation. Three major aspects to evaluate are (1) the exact site, (2) the mechanism of injury, and (3) the severity. The clinician should perform the necessary exams to set the appropriate diagnose: a proper history and examination to determine the site and injury mechanism so that the exact etiology of the thigh pain is recognized after considering the most common conditions without missing others less commonly seen injuries and conditions (Table 11.1). In the high-performance professional athlete the use of imaging such as diagnostic musculoskeletal ultrasound or MRI could be considered to help determine the etiology and extent of the injury. It is difficult to make a prognosis or diagnosis during the initial examination on the field or in the medical setting within the first hour. Prescribing PRICE treatment for 24–48 hours and performing a new physical evaluation with the possible use of imaging at this time can help the clinician to formulate the correct diagnosis. An important clinical challenge is to distinguish between intramuscular and intermuscular injuries (Figure 11.1), as well as between hamstring strains, hamstring avulsions, and total hamstring ruptures as these have distinctly different outcomes with respect to time lost from sport and recurrence injury rate. Occasionally, a contusion may be so severe that the differential diagnosis of fracture is indicated, or pressure in the anterior thigh muscle compartment becomes so great that acute compartment syndrome is suspected. In such cases, the patient must be sent to a hospital for additional examinations.

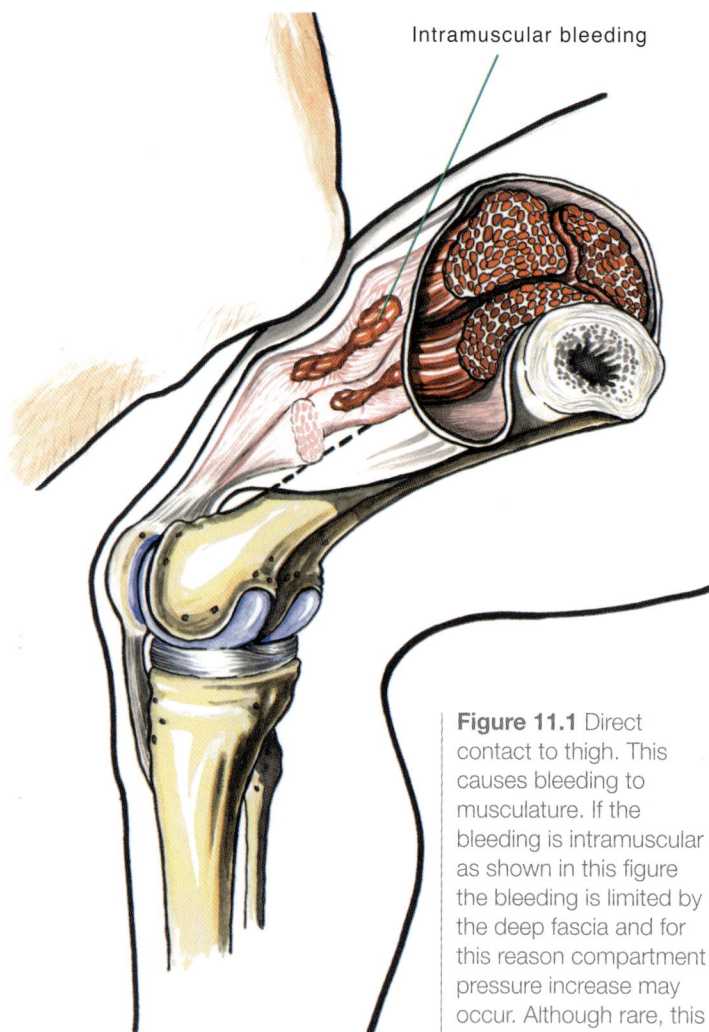

Intramuscular bleeding

Figure 11.1 Direct contact to thigh. This causes bleeding to musculature. If the bleeding is intramuscular as shown in this figure the bleeding is limited by the deep fascia and for this reason compartment pressure increase may occur. Although rare, this can constitute a medical emergency. (© Medical Illustrator Tommy Bolic, Sweden.)

Case History

Although the injury site can initially be pinpointed by the patient, the clinician should perform muscle functional tests and may require imaging (ultrasound or MRI) to assess the exact muscle involved. If a contusion is present, the patient usually states that he received a direct blow to the front or side of the thigh (Figure 11.1). This causes pain immediately, and the diagnosis is usually simple. If the patient's thigh has a deformity, the diagnosis of fracture (which is confirmed by radiographs) is normally obvious. The anterior compartments of the thigh may be affected by acute compartment syndrome after strong direct trauma. For acute thigh injuries the pain can vary markedly with an acute compartment syndrome being extremely painful and this can vary to a hamstring muscle strain where the pain may be no more than what is experienced in a simple cramp. In hamstring muscle strains it has been shown that the more pain experienced upon injury the larger the strain is and the more match playing time the athlete will subsequently miss before being adequately rehabilitated to return to sport.

Strains are normally located in the muscle-tendon junction. Generally, though not always, the free tendons at the origin and insertion of the muscles are not affected in isolation but can occur in conjunction with a musculotendinous strain. When a strain has occurred, the patient has sudden, stabbing "like a knife" or "pointing" pain, usually on the posterior side of the thigh. The diagnostic challenge is whether to classify the injury as a strain (and the magnitude of the strain), as a total rupture, or as an avulsion. Imaging may be required to determine this as it is often difficult to distinguish between strains and cramps (defined as a reversible spasm of muscle where the fibers are not damaged) and difficult to assess clinically the exact extent or magnitude of the injury.

Clinical Examination

The diagnosis of muscular injuries is mainly clinical with only limited cases requiring imaging modalities to assist in the determining the diagnosis.

History. Important aspects of history are the mechanism of injury, for example, contact, running, stretching, the timing of injury with muscle strains more common when the muscle is fatigued and the timing of injury—acute, chronic, intermittent, or recurrent. The level of immediate dysfunction can be a clue to the underlying cause.

Inspection. If a significant injury has occurred, the involved thigh can be swollen when compared to the normal side on inspection (Figure 11.2). A major contusion may leave a mark on the thigh, leaving no doubt whether the patient sustained high-energy trauma or not. If the patient has a completely ruptured muscle or tendon, a depression may be visible at the site of the injury (this is most common in mid-thigh quadriceps injuries), and ecchymosis will gradually appear distal to the location of the rupture (Figure 11.3).

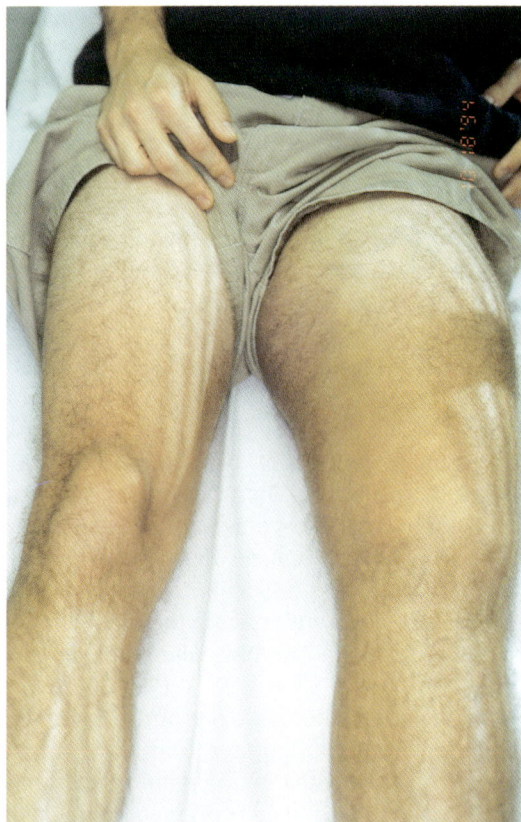

Figure 11.2 Muscle contusion, with the resultant obvious swelling on the left side. A contusion often causes bleeding and swelling in the compartments on the anterior and lateral side of the thigh. (Reproduced with permission from the Norwegian Sports Medicine Association.)

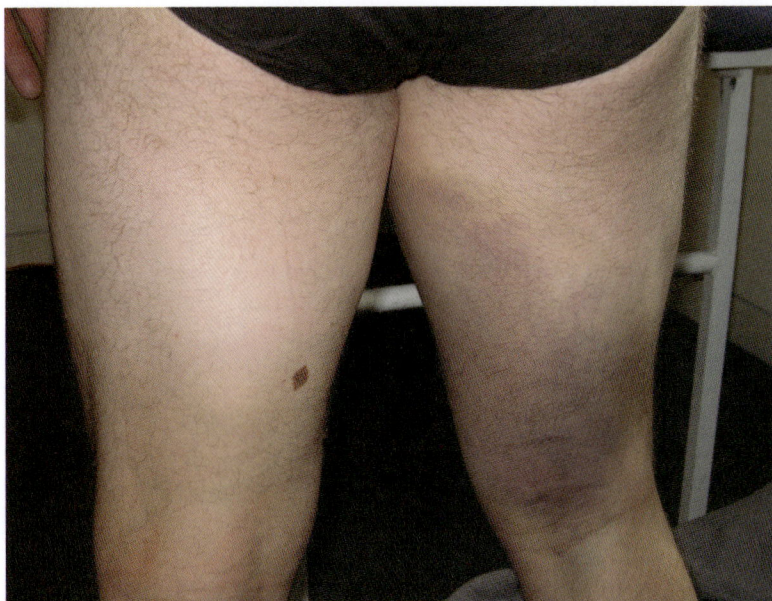

Figure 11.3 Posterior thigh ecchymosis after a severe hamstring muscle strain injury on the right side.

THIGH

A few days after the patient sustain an intermuscular injury; bruises will usually be visible in the skin (often distal to the location of the injury). This does not occur after an intramuscular injury. Most thigh injuries of the strain variety do not demonstrate bruising on the skin.

Palpation. The goal of the palpation is to try and locate the exact muscle that has been injured by finding the points of pain or muscle spasms. The anterior and posterior aspects of the thigh are palpated for defects of the tendon or muscle indicative of ruptures. The thigh will feel rigid if the patient has compartment syndrome. Palpation a few days after injury may be completely normal.

Functional tests. In the case of thigh contusions evaluating the degree of reduced knee flexion can help distinguish between an intramuscular and an intermuscular injury, thus making it easier to predict when the athlete can return to sport. If the compartments are intact, bleeding (usually in the vastus intermedius or rectus) is limited by the fascia. Therefore, an intramuscular hematoma forms, leading to increased intramuscular volume and increased pressure, which reduces muscular flexibility. This in turn reduces flexion in the knee joint. An intermuscular hematoma generally causes less restriction of range of motion when compared to intramuscular hemorrhage, and consequently the rehabilitation period tends to be shorter than for injuries resulting in intermuscular bleeding.

Functional muscle tests are performed to try and distinguish between partial and total tendon or muscle ruptures. Both the quadriceps and the hamstring apparatus can be tested isometrically and dynamically to obtain information about the degree of the injury. Pain on resisted contraction is a common finding with most thigh injuries especially in the acute phase of the injury.

Supplemental Examinations

For a history and examination that suggests a strain injury has occurred there may not be any requirement for imaging. Athletes in professional sports often use the imaging modalities of ultrasound or MRI to determine nature of injury and severity of the thigh injuries. Radiographs in acute thigh injuries are only required when a fracture needs to be excluded.

Common Injuries

Thigh Contusion

Muscle contusions (Figure 11.1) and strains make up the majority of all sports-related injuries with thigh contusions being among the most common acute thigh injuries in sports. It most commonly results from a direct blow to the extremity and is frequently situated in the anterior medial or lateral thigh in the area of the muscle belly of the quadriceps femoris. Sports where the injury occurs are generally contact sports such as tackle football, rugby, martial arts, and soccer. Thigh contusions can be complicated in the immediate setting with acute compartment syndrome or in the subacute setting with myositis ossificans (Figure 11.4).

• Symptoms and signs: Athletes typically report a direct blow to the extremity followed by pain and swelling, decreased range of motion in the injured muscles, and occasionally a palpable mass. Animal studies have shown that a muscle contusion usually causes a partial rupture of the muscle fibers with infiltrative bleeding leading to hematoma formation.

- Diagnosis: Often evident from an athlete reporting a direct blow to the thigh followed by pain, swelling, and impaired athletic performance. Ultrasound has been used successfully to distinguish swelling and edema from a localized circumscribed hematoma and has been advocated as a relatively inexpensive noninvasive aid in determining when to consider surgical evacuation of the hematoma. In athletes the clinician must always have a high index for suspicion for a developing compartment syndrome, as this is an orthopedic emergency.
- Treatment by physician: Mild injuries can be treated by relative rest and compression. For more severe injuries we recommend immobilizing the thigh with the muscles held in a stretched position for a short duration (<24 hours). The knee is held in a hyper-flexed position with a compression dressing (Figure 11.5). It should be noted that this can be a very painful position for the athlete to hold their leg following contusion injury. Initial pain relief should be simple analgesia—the need for opiates and stronger analgesia should be a signal to the clinician for reassessment of the problem and consideration of acute compartment syndrome. Nonsteroidal anti-inflammatory drugs (NSAIDs) can be used after 48 hours.
- Treatment by therapist: Following the period of immobilization, early mobilization should be the focus with passive range of motion and stretching progressing to concentric active range of motion and strengthening as tolerated. Finally, a progression to functional rehabilitation with gradual increased eccentric range of motion is warranted.
- Prognosis: The average disability that can be expected is 14–21 days depending on the severity of the contusion. For the majority of injuries recovery ensues with very few athletes developing long-term problems. In practical terms, players with these injuries either miss no time (i.e., they are able to play the following week) or 2 weeks (i.e., they are unable to play until the third week following injury).

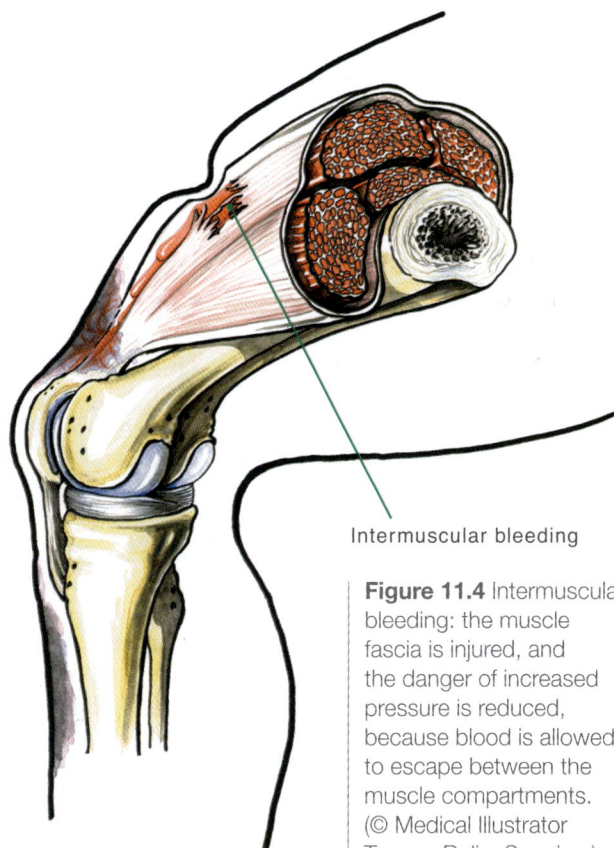

Intermuscular bleeding

Figure 11.4 Intermuscular bleeding: the muscle fascia is injured, and the danger of increased pressure is reduced, because blood is allowed to escape between the muscle compartments. (© Medical Illustrator Tommy Bolic, Sweden.)

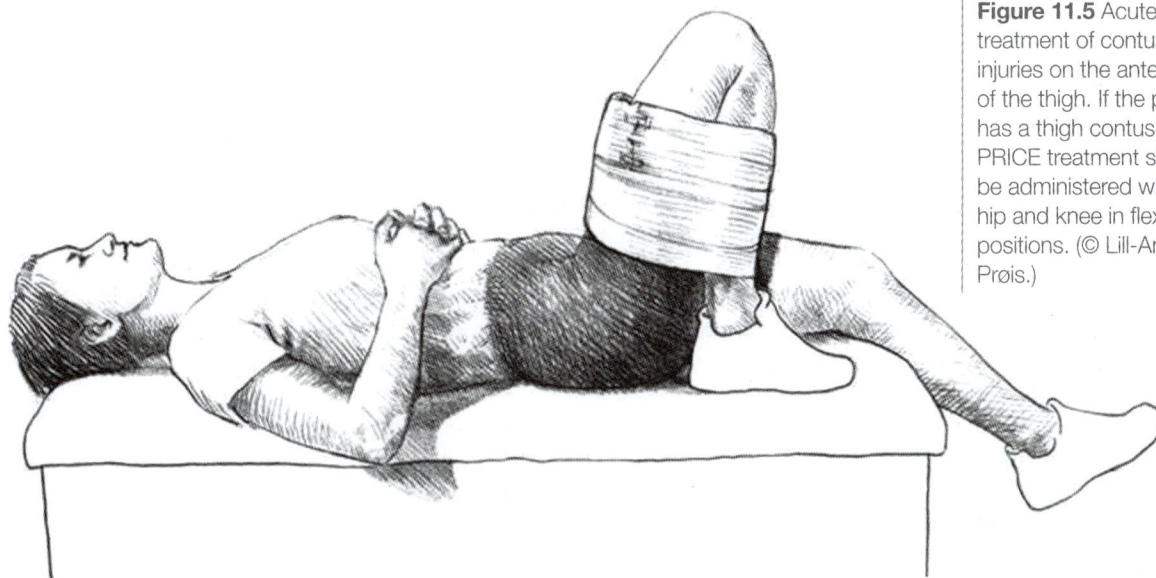

Figure 11.5 Acute treatment of contusion injuries on the anterior side of the thigh. If the patient has a thigh contusion, PRICE treatment should be administered with the hip and knee in flexed positions. (© Lill-Ann Prøis.)

THIGH

Hamstring Muscle Strain Injury

A hamstring muscle strain injury is the most common of all the muscle strains in sport and with athletes in sports with repeated high-intensity sprinting such as the football codes and athletics being the most vulnerable. The injury occurs at the muscle-tendon junction of the muscle. In sprinters and footballers it is most commonly located in the biceps femoris muscle (Figure 11.6). Injuries to other hamstring muscles can also occur with overstretch injuries, for example, in ballet dancers; in this case they are most often located in the semimembranosus muscle. The semitendinosus muscle can also be injured though its mechanism of injury is not as apparent. The hamstring muscles are characterized by long muscle-tendon junctions, and an injury may occur at any location along them though generally not in the free tendon ends.

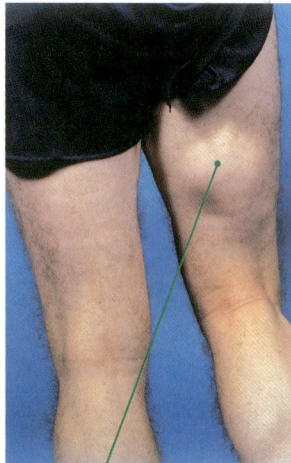

The major risk factor for hamstring muscle strain injuries is the athlete having a previous injury. A previous injury increases the risk to athletes by between five and ten times when compared to an athlete without previous injury. Other risks such as increasing age, decreased flexibility, having decreased posterior thigh strength compared to the anterior thigh have also been indicated in some studies as being risk factors for sustaining a hamstring muscle strain injury. To prevent these injuries and to optimize the rehabilitation it is important to analyze in what situations they occur. It is important to know the mechanism of injury to understand how the muscles are injured. For example, the semimembranosus muscle usually injures with hyperstretching and biceps femoris injuries occur with an eccentric contraction in the course of a sprint. Other factors are also thought to influence the nature and significance of hamstring muscle injuries, including the biomechanics of the hamstring, muscle microarchitecture histology, the physiology of the muscle itself (i.e., fatigue conditions or overtraining), changes in the anatomical axis of the lower extremity, and external factors such as the type of training, sport, the surface, and the equipment used.

- Symptoms and signs: A hamstring muscle strain injury in almost all cases is characterized by acute pain, almost as if someone struck the back of the thigh, and the athlete has to stop activity. Strength is significantly reduced. The athlete can no longer run at maximal speed.
- Diagnosis: Functional test findings are reduced isometric and dynamic strength. Sometimes a torn tendon or muscle can be palpated. MRI (Figure 11.7a through d) and ultrasound can be used to determine the extent and severity of the injury and whether the patient has a total tendon rupture or avulsion. Injury type, palpation of maximal pain, and ultrasound and MRI findings (tissues involved) can give

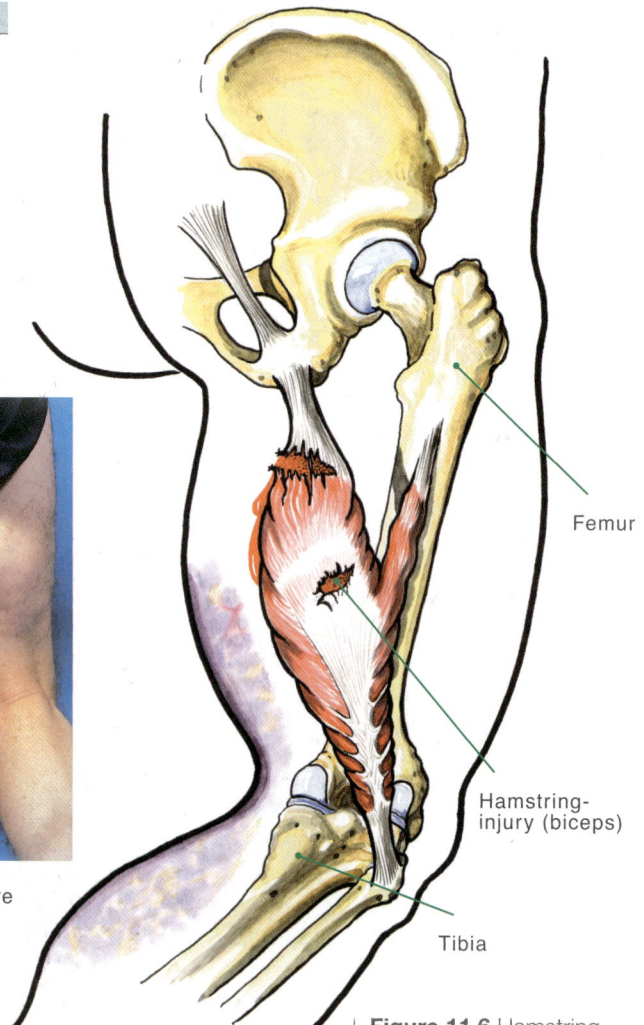

Hamstring rupture

Femur

Hamstring-injury (biceps)

Tibia

Figure 11.6 Hamstring strains are predominately in the biceps femoris muscle and occur in the intramuscular segment of the muscle (the free tendon ends are generally, but not always, spared) and located at the musculotendinous junction. The biceps femoris muscle has an intramuscular tendon from proximal to distal, and strains can occur anywhere along the region where the muscle attaches to the tendon. (© Medical Illustrator Tommy Bolic, Sweden.)

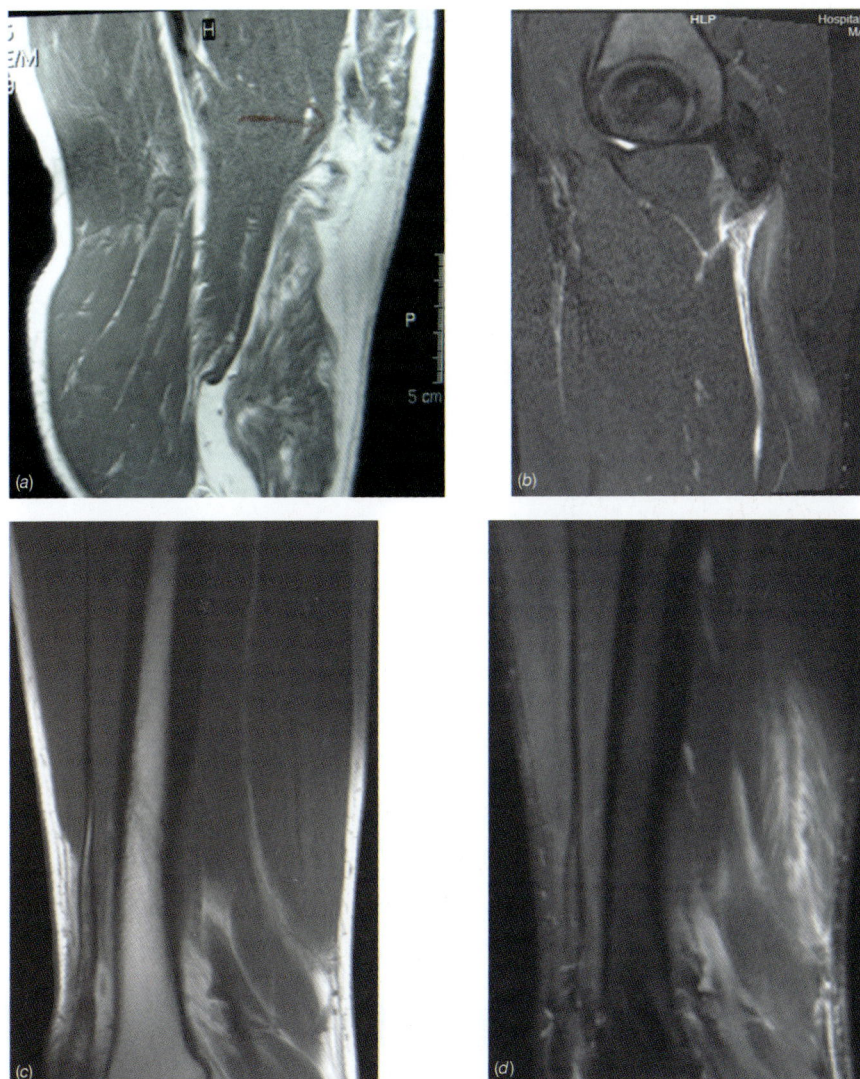

Figure 11.7 MRI can be used to determine location and extent of hamstring strains. Semimembranosus muscle injury (*a*) at ischial tuberosity bony origin following an overstretch injury. Complete hamstring muscle rupture (*b*). Coronal MRI T1 view (*c*) of hamstring injury demonstrating very little anatomical changes and coronal MRI T2 view (*d*) of hamstring injury of same patient as (*c*) demonstrating the fenestrated appearance of a large hamstring strain injury.

important information about diagnosis and prognosis. The relationship between injury situations, muscle-tendon involvement with regard to recovery time of the hamstring injuries is becoming more widely known. This is probably one of the areas where most progress in muscle strain injuries has been made. Knowledge of the exact location of the injury (relation with the connective tissue, number of muscles affected, impact area, volume of injury) that is provided by the use of MRI and ultrasound imaging have allowed us to more accurately identify the injury and predict return-to-play.

- Treatment: Treatment follows the PRICE principle and the standard rehabilitation process for muscle injuries, which is described on pp. 354–356. Acute rupture of all three hamstring tendons, an uncommon injury, from the ischial tuberosity can be surgically fixed with good results. For the best results the surgery should be performed within 2 weeks of the injury. The majority of hamstring muscle strain injuries do not require surgical intervention.

- Prognosis: The long-term prognosis is good. In usual cases the athlete can return to training after 1–8 weeks, but the injury can result in a long absence from sports that require explosive use of the muscles. Accurately determining prognosis just using clinical parameters can be difficult as the principal measure used is the amount of pain and this is highly subjective. The use of MRI, and to a lesser extent ultrasound, allows the clinician to determine the exact site and size of the injury with a biceps femoris injury and a larger size of hamstring injury having a worse prognosis with respect to return to sport when compared to another muscle injury and a smaller size of hamstring muscle injury. If the athlete returns to sport activity too soon, the danger of recurrence is great and in this manner makes the short-term prognosis more questionable. Recurrence rates for all football codes are high, ranging between 10% and 40%.

Quadriceps Muscle Strain Injury

A quadriceps muscle strain injury is less common than its posterior thigh counterpart the hamstring but is common in sports requiring kicking such as the football codes. The injury like all muscle strain injuries occurs at the muscle-tendon junction of the muscle. The major risk factors for quadriceps injury are in the kicking sports with muscle inflexibility; overuse and fatigue have been implicated in the pathogenesis.

• Symptoms and signs: A quadriceps muscle strain injury in most cases is characterized by acute pain and the athlete has to stop activity. However, in many cases it presents as chronic pain associated with kicking.
• Diagnosis: Functional test findings are reduced isometric and dynamic strength. Sometimes a torn tendon or muscle can be palpated particularly in the mid-thigh injuries. MRI (Figure 11.8) and ultrasound can be used to determine the extent and severity of the injury and whether the patient has a total tendon rupture or avulsion.
• Treatment: Treatment follows the PRICE principle and the standard rehabilitation process for muscle injuries, which is described later in the chapter. Quadriceps strain injuries generally do not require surgical intervention.
• Prognosis: The long-term prognosis is good. However, like for hamstring muscle strain injuries, there is a high recurrence injury rate generally as a consequence of the athlete returning to sport prior to adequate healing and complete rehabilitation of the injury.

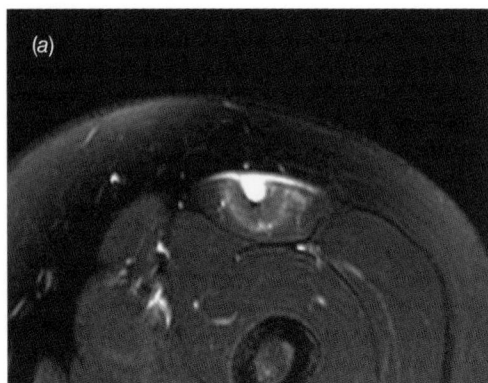

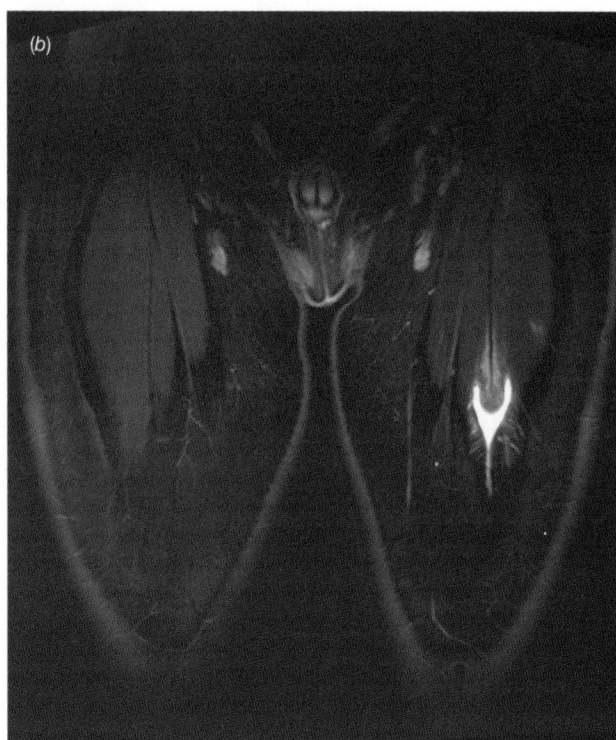

Figure 11.8 Axial MRI T2 view (a) and coronal MRI T2 view (b) of a typical quadriceps muscle strain demonstrating injury to the musculotendinous junction.

Other Injuries

Adductor Muscle Strain Injury

An adductor muscle strain injury is less common than its anterior and posterior thigh counterparts but is common in sports requiring rapid change in direction. The injury, like all muscle strain injuries, occurs at the muscle-tendon junction of the muscle. There is an association with groin injuries so it is very difficult to be precise about risk factors, but relative abductor weakness compared to adductor strength has been implicated as a risk factor for adductor muscle injuries.

- Symptoms and signs: An adductor muscle strain injury in most cases is characterized by acute pain and the athlete has to stop activity.
- Diagnosis: This injury is generally determined by clinical history and examination. Again as for all muscle injuries imaging may be useful in confirming the diagnosis and its extent.
- Treatment: Treatment follows the PRICE principle and the standard rehabilitation process for muscle injuries, which is described later in the chapter. Adductor muscle strain injuries do not require surgical intervention.
- Prognosis: The long-term prognosis is good. However as with all muscle strain injuries they also have a high recurrence injury rate.

Acute Compartment Syndrome !

Acute compartment syndromes of the thigh after trauma are rare; however, it is an injury with potentially significant consequences for the athlete and should be considered an orthopedic emergency. Athletes in sports with body contact are the most vulnerable such as ice hockey and the majority of the football codes. The pathophysiological mechanism that causes compartment syndrome is an increased tissue pressure that prevents muscle blood flow with the resulting development of ischemia, which can lead to irreversible muscle damage.

- Symptoms and signs: It is critical to have a high index of suspicion and perform serial examinations in patients at risk after blunt trauma to the thigh. The classic diagnosis encompasses the six Ps: (1) pain, (2) pressure, (3) pulselessness, (4) paralysis, (5) paresthesiae, and (6) pallor. Pain out of proportion to the injury, aggregated by pain with passive stretch of the affected muscles, is one of the earliest and clinically most sensitive signs. Symptoms are muscle that is rigid on palpation and pain if knee flexion or extension is attempted.
- Treatment by physician: Historically it was thought that compartment syndromes necessitate a decompressive fasciotomy to avoid devastating sequelae of missed compartment syndromes. However, elevated tissue pressures in the thigh usually do not lead to a compartment syndrome due in part to the large muscle volume and the relatively elastic fascia. Therefore, high pressures in the thigh are usually treated nonoperatively with conservative treatment options such as rest and leg elevation.
- Prognosis: The prognosis is good, but occasionally myositis ossificans develops, resulting in a long absence from sport.

THIGH

Chronic Thigh Pain

Geoffrey M. Verrall[1], Juan-Manuel Alonso Martín[2], Lars Engebretsen[3], Toru Fukubayashi[4], William E. Garrett[5], Grethe Myklebust[3], Gil Rodas[6], and Per Renström[7]

[1]*Sportsmed SA, Sports Medicine Centre, Adelaide, SA, Australia*
[2]*Real Federación Española de Atletismo, International Association of Athletics Federation (IAAF), Madrid, Spain*
[3]*Oslo Sports Trauma Research Center, Norwegian School of Sport Sciences, Oslo, Norway*
[4]*University of Waseda, Tokorozawa, Saitama, Japan*
[5]*Duke University Medical Center, Durham, NC, USA*
[6]*Medical Services, Futbol Club Barcelona, Barcelona, Spain*
[7]*Center for Sports Trauma Research and Education, Karolinska Institutet, Stockholm, Sweden*

Occurrence

Chronic thigh pain is relatively uncommon in athletes. However, a few athletes have posterior thigh pain in connection with back problems and also with sequelae following proximal hamstring muscle injuries. Chronic compartment pain has been described in long-distance runners during periods of hard exercise. Impingement of the femoral nerve with accompanying muscle atrophy is seen primarily in weight training athletes.

Differential Diagnoses

Table 11.2 provides an overview of the differential diagnoses. Referred pain from the lumbar spine is probably the most common diagnosis. Damage to the sciatic nerve following hamstring injuries/ruptures is probably the most common local diagnosis. Myositis ossificans that occurs after a muscle contusion in a soccer player is also seen with some frequency. As rehabilitation has improved with an earlier emphasis on movement and return to function, fewer injuries of this nature are now seen. Stress fractures in the ramus of both the superior and inferior pubis, as well as in the femur, have been reported in female cross-country skiers. Tumors and vascular malformations must also be considered. Finally, the pain from the hip such as in femoroacetabular impingement can give rise to chronic pain of the anterior or posterior thigh.

Most common	Less common	Must not be overlooked !
Sciatic nerve irritation	Stress fracture in the femur/femoral neck, p. 323	Bone and soft-tissue tumors, p. 352
Hamstring muscle strain recurrences	Myositis ossificans, p. 351	
Sequelae from hamstring ruptures, p. 349	Chronic compartment syndrome, p. 351	
Thigh pain, p. 350	Vascular malformations, p. 352	
Osteoarthritis of the hip	Nerve entrapment, p. 352	
Femoracetabular impingement		

Table 11.2 Overview of current differential diagnoses of thigh pain. (Reproduced with permission from the Norwegian Sports Medicine Association.)

Diagnostic Thinking

Patients with long-term thigh pain are a diagnostic challenge. Previous injuries in the hamstrings and quadriceps are the most common causes of thigh pain and can be become chronic due to failure to heal and/or recurrences. However, the less common conditions listed in Table 11.2 are more difficult to diagnose and treat. At any age the back needs to be considered in the differential diagnosis and pain arising from the hip joint can also afflict a wide range group. In athletes older than 50 years, referred pain from osteoarthritis may be a possible diagnosis, whereas younger athletes may have radiating pain from the pelvis and back. In this connection, the physician should remember that young, active athletes may also have rare vascular and malignant diseases. It is always necessary to X-ray the pelvis (including the hips and thigh) to uncover any stress fractures, myositis ossificans, or tumors. However, the perhaps most common presentation is an endurance athlete (cycling, cross-country skiing, cycling) with thigh pain of unknown etiology, even after extensive investigations.

Case History

The clinical history must include any acute trauma that may have occurred. Due to the possibility of conditions that have the potential to cause long-term morbidity, and although rarely mortality, chronic thigh pain should be assessed until the clinician is confident of the diagnosis so that treatment can be appropriately directed.

Clinical Examination

Examination findings may be unremarkable in many cases. However, findings can include muscle atrophy, swelling (myositis ossificans or tumors), or sequelae from a tendon rupture in the hamstring or extensor apparatus. Neurological status must be included in the exam because thigh pain often originates from a back problem. Although circulatory disorders that cause thigh pain in young athletes are rare and difficult to find by clinical examination, the pulse in the lower extremity should be checked routinely.

Supplemental Examinations

Imaging should be used to diagnose the etiology of chronic thigh pain if clinical examination does not lead to a reasonable explanation for the pain. Radiographs of the thigh and pelvis (which include the hips) must always be taken to exclude hip disorders, stress fractures, myositis ossificans, or tumors. MRI examination (which is a useful examination for labral hip disorders, chronic muscle injuries and ruptures, suspected stress fractures, myositis ossificans, and tumors) is often indicated. A CT scan is helpful for bony abnormalities. Ultrasound examinations may demonstrate ruptures in the muscles but is dependent on the skills of the operator. Scintigraphy is highly sensitive to stress fractures but is a nonspecific examination, and generally, it must be followed up with an MRI or CT examination if positive.

Common Conditions

Sequelae From Hamstring Ruptures—*Hamstring Syndrome*

This is usually a problem in sprinters, soccer players, and others involved in intense, hard, eccentric muscle work. A pulled muscle causes scar tissue to form presumably in the muscle-tendon junction although exact location upon imaging can

THIGH

be difficult to ascertain. This scar tissue may also form around the sciatic nerve; this can add to the irritation felt in the posterior thigh. Muscle range of motion can be reduced with a principal finding being the athlete is unable to train at full capacity because maximum muscle use causes pain. Pain can in some athletes is considered to be due to irritation on the sciatic nerve in the lumbar region or more distally.

- Diagnosis: An accurate examination is key in making the diagnosis. The diagnosis is based on pain on palpation, occasionally reduced range of motion and pain from isometric and dynamic testing. During isokinetic testing, strength can be reduced compared with the healthy side. Imaging (MRI or CT) may or may not be helpful in establishing the diagnosis.
- Treatment by physician: The key to treatment is recognizing the condition. There is no evidence that NSAIDs or cortisone injection have any long-term positive effects. Surgery can be considered if identification of the condition leads to a conclusion that the free tendon ends (proximal or distal) have been disrupted.
- Treatment by therapist: Supervised rehabilitation is necessary with the athlete in many cases needing to be commenced at a very low level of activity to prevent the onset of the pain. The exact diagnosis of hamstring syndrome is often difficult to establish, and subsequently verify, making rehabilitation frustrating for the athlete and the clinician.
- Prognosis: The prognosis over time for hamstring syndrome is good, but the athlete should plan on prolonged retraining, often as long as 6 months.

Thigh Pain—Undetermined Etiology

With the increasing popularity of some sports that are now a recreational phenomenon all over the world such as cycling and cross-country skiing, that have to some extent replaced recreational running, there has been an increase in injuries that are associated with these sports. In particular thigh pain, especially anterior thigh pain, during and after exercise is a common presentation to the sports medicine clinician. The exact etiology of this thigh pain has not as yet been determined with vascular, muscular, and compartment pressure in isolation or in combination considered as factors in causing the condition.

- Diagnosis: In cases of thigh pain of undetermined etiology it is important that this diagnosis is considered a diagnosis of exclusion with other more important conditions being ruled out. Thus, in many cases radiographs to exclude stress fractures and tumors and sometimes MRI may be necessary to ensure that the not to be missed diagnoses are excluded.
- Treatment by physician: When making the diagnosis it is important to determine the fitness level of the athlete and also look at the biomechanical factors of the sport, for example, cycling, cross-country skiing, as these can be important in the genesis and treatment of this troublesome condition. After exclusion of not to be missed diagnoses some physical therapy may be helpful, but often the athlete is reassured there are no sinister findings and manage by changing/modifying activity levels.
- Treatment by therapist: Local mobilization of thigh tissues maybe helpful as may be structures proximal to the thigh such as the mobilization of the back, pelvis, and hip.
- Prognosis: If the cause is readily apparent and easily correctable the prognosis is excellent. In some cases this condition is frustrating for the athlete and the clinician.

Other Conditions

Myositis Ossificans

Myositis ossificans, bone formation in the femoral muscles, is sometimes seen as a consequence of major bleeding in the deep thigh muscles (Figure 11.9). The process often begins with thigh contusion that causes swelling and pain with hematoma formation. Usually the hematoma is absorbed after a few weeks, but occasionally it calcifies. At the beginning of the calcification process, the area is still swollen and often very tender (warm phase). Pain and swelling result in long-term reduced range of motion, which usually restricts knee joint flexion. The calcification eventually stabilizes (cold phase).

- Symptoms and signs: Symptoms are swelling and pain, followed by reduced mobility for knee joint flexion.
- Diagnosis: Radiographs, MRI, or ultrasound produces the diagnosis.
- Treatment: The patient can engage in stretching and exercise therapy to the extent that pain allows. Usually, the calcification and hematoma are resorbed without surgical treatment, but if more than 6 months pass without signs of resorption surgery maybe an option to be considered.
- Prognosis: Prognosis is good but recovery can be prolonged.

Chronic Compartment Syndrome

Chronic compartment syndrome in the thigh is rare. Usually, acute compartment syndrome is caused by high-energy trauma resulting from a motor vehicle accident or a fall from a great height. However, the same type of syndrome is also described in the chronic phase as a consequence of chronic overuse. Therefore, the syndrome is often described as a stress problem in the musculature. We have seen the syndrome in the lateral compartment of long-distance runners, bicyclists, skaters, and cross-country skiers (see Section Thigh pain–Undetermined Etiology).

- Symptoms and signs: Patients experience thigh pain after strenuous exercises such as after a cross-country skiing and road cycling.
- Diagnosis: Patients suspected of having compartment syndrome are referred to a specialist for evaluation. There are no clinically valid methods of making the diagnosis, with thigh pressure with exercise being measured. However, this method is controversial.
- Treatment: The patient should reduce the intensity and amount of training so that the training routine does not cause pain. Fasciotomy can be considered in some cases.
- Prognosis: The prognosis is usually good.

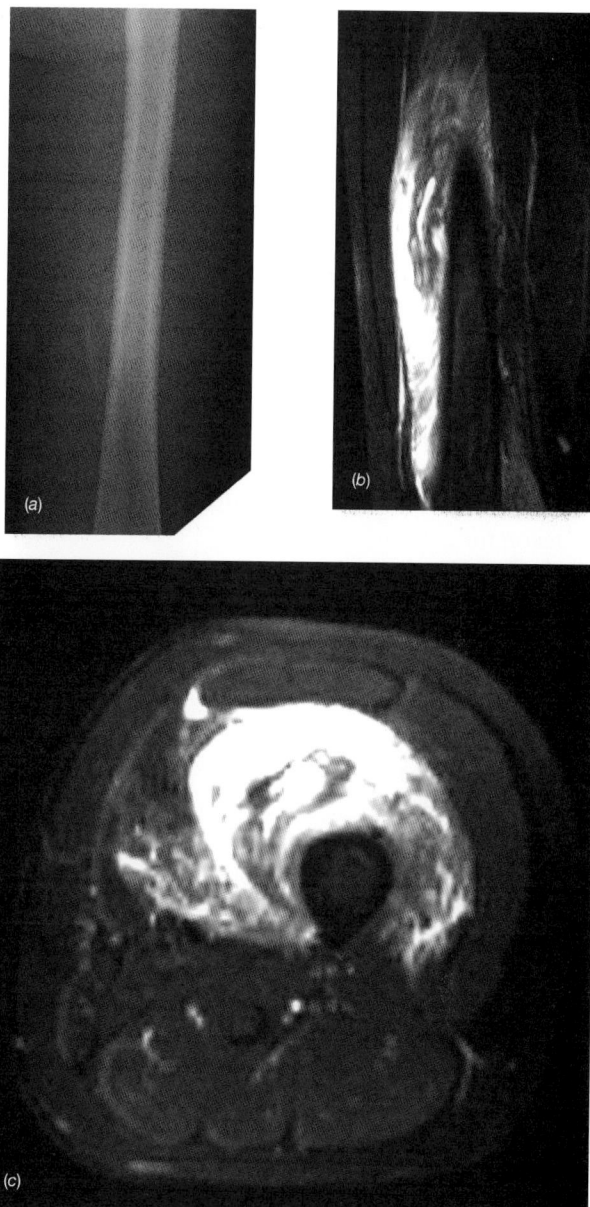

Figure 11.9 Myositis ossificans in a 20-year-old female basketball player, 1 month following contusion of the thigh. Radiograph (a) of left femur shows faint calcification shadow at the anteromedial portion of the femur. MRI (STIR) anterioposterior (b) and axial (c) views demonstrate large intramuscular bleeding and hematoma in vastus intermedius muscle. (Reproduced with permission from the Norwegian Sports Medicine Association.)

THIGH

351

Vascular Malformations

Vascular malformations are rare but may lead to reduced circulation in the lower extremities and cause symptoms similar to the symptoms of intermittent claudication. However the clinical picture can vary considerably. The most common vascular malformation described is an endofibrosis of the external iliac artery primarily seen in cyclists, but has also been described in cross-country skiers.

- Symptoms and signs: Pain occurs during activity. Generally to elicit symptoms the activity needs to be maximal with the athlete complaining of vague leg and thigh pains, cramps, and decreased performance. Normal conditions prevail when the athlete does not train or compete.
- Diagnosis: The diagnosis is made by having an index of suspicion and provocative exercise testing with vascular imaging such as digital subtraction angiography, magnetic resonance angiography, and color Doppler ultrasound. Patients suspected of having vascular malformations/iliac artery stenosis should be referred to a vascular surgeon for evaluation.
- Treatment: The treatment is interventional radiology (endovascular surgery) or less commonly surgery.
- Prognosis: The prognosis is good if the diagnosis is correct and the condition readily treatable. This is not always the case though with controversy in diagnosis and preferred treatment remaining.

Nerve Entrapment

Nerve entrapments include the ilioinguinal nerve, obturator nerve, and lateral femoral cutaneous nerve of the thigh (meralgia paresthetica). Compression can result from muscle hypertrophy or injury.

- Symptoms and signs: The clinical picture varies and is usually related to the nerve that is entrapped. Nerve conduction studies may be helpful.
- Treatment: Generally, the treatment for nerve entrapment is modification of activity, biomechanical assessment, and correction and mobilization of soft tissues, but occasionally surgical release may be necessary.
- Prognosis: Prognosis is good, but can take up to 12 months before resolution of symptoms occurs.

Bone and Soft-Tissue Tumors !

Soft-tissue tumors in the thigh are typically sarcomas. There are two main types of sarcoma: osteosarcoma, which develops from bone, and soft-tissue sarcomas, which can develop from soft tissues like fat, muscle, nerves, fibrous tissues, blood vessels, or deep skin tissues. Although they can be found in any part of the body most of them develop in the extremities. When there is a sarcoma the tumor is malignant. It should be pointed out that most soft-tissue tumors are benign tumors and they are much more common than malignant ones.

A benign tumor in fat tissue is called lipoma and is the most common benign soft-tissue tumor. Liposarcoma is a malignant fat-tissue tumor with several types. A rare type is myxoid liposarcoma, which may be seen in the deep thigh muscles in young patients. Tumors of muscle and nerves are not common. A synovial sarcoma can be seen in the thigh in young males in their 30s. The risk of spread to the lungs can be high over an extended period of time.

• Diagnosis: In general it can be said that if a tumor is large, that is, bigger than 5 cm and located deep in the tissues, then it is more likely to be a cancer. If the tumor is fixed to bone a plain X-ray may be taken. MRI can be used to identify a tumor's size and depth, and its relationship to normal muscle, fat, nerves, and blood vessels. A biopsy is used to determine the grade and this assist in prognosis evaluation and treatment. Positron emission tomography (PET scan) is a recently developed scan to detect and monitor a tumor's response to treatment.

• Treatment: May include radiation therapy, which often is combined with surgery to lower the risk of recurrence. Radiation can be given before or after the tumor is surgically removed. There may be some improvement in survival by using chemotherapy, but its exact role is debated.

• Prognosis: The chance for survival depends on age and gender, but also of size and grade of the tumor when it first was identified.

THIGH

Rehabilitation of Thigh Injuries

*Geoffrey M. Verrall[1], Juan-Manuel Alonso Martin[2], Lars Engebretsen[3],
Toru Fukubayashi[4], William E. Garrett[5], Grethe Myklebust[3], Gil Rodas[6], and
Per Renström[7]*

[1]*Sportsmed SA, Sports Medicine Centre, Adelaide, SA, Australia*
[2]*Real Federación Española de Atletismo, International Association of Athletics
Federations (IAAF), Madrid, Spain*
[3]*Oslo Sports Trauma Research Center, Norwegian School of Sport Sciences, Oslo, Norway*
[4]*University of Waseda, Tokorozawa, Saitama, Japan*
[5]*Duke University Medical Center, Durham, NC, USA*
[6]*Medical Services, Futbol Club Barcelona, Barcelona, Spain*
[7]*Center for Sports Trauma, Research, Karolinska Institutet, Stockholm, Sweden*

Goals and Principles

The goals for the rehabilitation of acute thigh injuries are listed in Table 11.3.

Compression for 48 hours should be used for all acute thigh injuries. As soon as tolerated after swelling/bleeding has been controlled, the athlete should do some slow circulation and range of motion exercises. This is to minimize, or if possible avoid secondary effects like muscle and leg stiffness, with these exercises being done several times every day. After a major thigh injury, strain, and/or contusion, it is recommended to wait 3–5 days before starting more active exercises. The patient should then start with gentle stretching of the relevant muscle and joint (e.g., Figure 11.10), letting the pain guide the intensity and frequency. External force/loads should not be applied during the first phase. The use of an ergometer bicycle and/or water exercises are gentle and effective methods of increasing function in the first rehabilitation phase.

Exercises are of primary importance during the rehabilitation phase, but other types of physical therapy may be useful in removing the hematoma and avoiding scartissue formation in the injured area. Massage, stretching, and gentle mobilization may be indicated.

As recovery ensues the exercise program should include various types of exercise including strength (e.g., Figures 11.11 and 11.12), range of motion, neuromuscular, and

	Goals	Measures
Acute phase	Minimize or reduce swelling	PRICE principle with emphasis on proper compression,
Rehabilitation phase	Normalize range of motion, strength, and neuromuscular function	Dynamic exercises, massage, stretching
Training phase	As a minimum, achieve previous range of motion, strength, and neuromuscular function	Functional exercises—sport-specific training
		Recover fully before engaging in maximum activity
	Reduce the risk of reinjury	

Table 11.3 Goals and measures for rehabilitation of acute thigh injuries. (Reproduced with permission from the Norwegian Sports Medicine Association.)

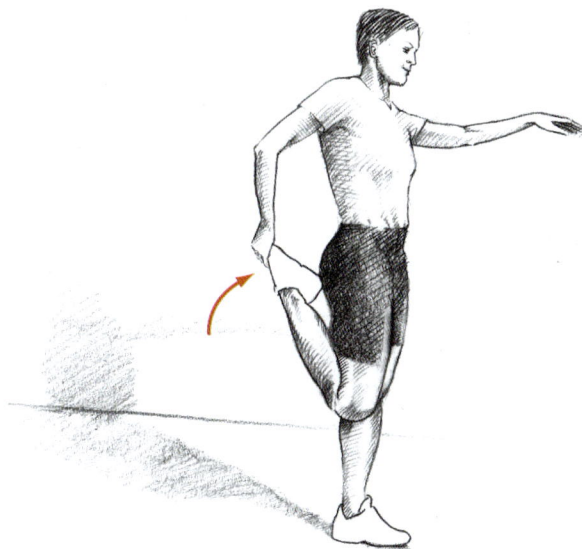

Figure 11.10 Stretching the anterior side of the thigh

- Stand on one leg. Support yourself so that you can maintain your balance. Hold your ankle using your hand on the same side, then press your hip forward and your knee backward. Your knee should point straight down. Do not allow your thigh to slide out to the side. Feel to make sure that you are stretching the anterior side of your thigh. Do not use much force. Hold about 30 seconds, release gently, and then go a little farther in the path of motion.
- Early in the rehabilitation stage, knee flexion can be reduced so much that you cannot hold your ankle. In that case, put your leg on a bench or low stool at a height that allows you to stretch the anterior side of your thigh.

(Reproduced with permission from the Norwegian Sports Medicine Association.)

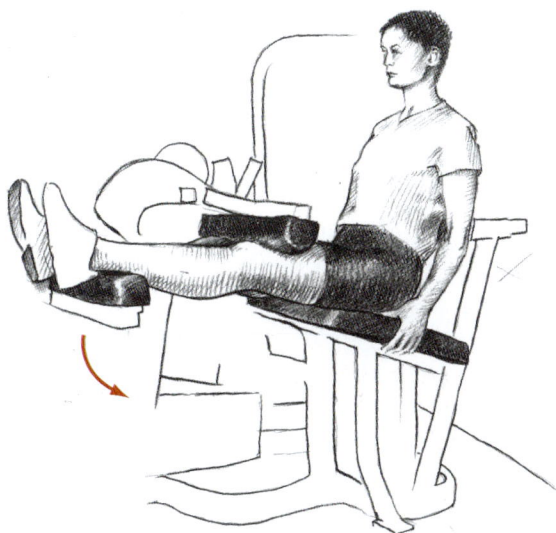

Figure 11.11 Hamstring strength while sitting in apparatus

- Press both legs down gently as far as you can without pain.
- Work with both legs or with the injured leg alone.
- Gradually increase knee flexion.

(Reproduced with permission from the Norwegian Sports Medicine Association.)

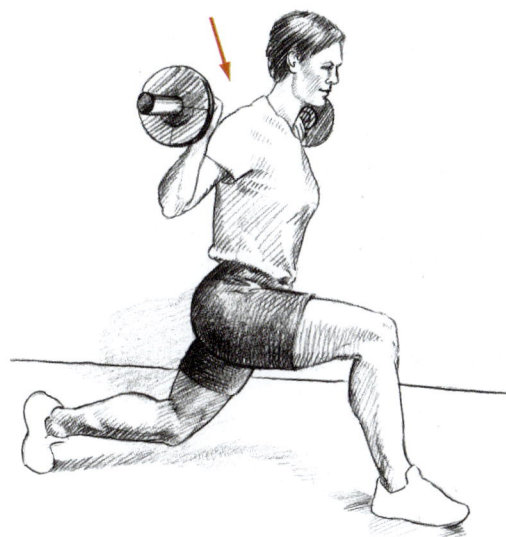

Figure 11.12 Hamstring strength while lowering yourself from a standing position

- Begin by lowering yourself a short distance, then gradually lower yourself longer and deeper (as shown in the figure).
- Keep knees over toes.
- Keep hips level.
- The same movement may be done straight, or at an angle, out to the side.

(Reproduced with permission from the Norwegian Sports Medicine Association.)

THIGH

exercises replicating function, all aimed at the sport that the athlete is returning to. The progression of the exercises is controlled by pain and function. In general, numerous repetitions and light loads (such as four series repeated 20–30 times) are emphasized early in the rehabilitation phase. Loads are then gradually increased, and the number of repetitions decreased as function improves. Exercises are done with light resistance during the start-up phase, and then the speed and degree of explosiveness are gradually increased.

Athletes in explosive sports with muscle strain injuries must not run at their maximum pace during training until the injury is completely healed. This can take as long as 6–8 weeks before the muscles will tolerate maximum sprints or turns. Light running training in a relaxed running style may begin as soon as pain allows. A neoprene sleeve might be useful during the retraining phase to keep the muscles warm, especially if the athlete trains outside in a cold environment. A proper warm-up and stretching of the muscles must be routine. The athlete should train without symptoms at a competitive intensity level before participating in games or competition. The athlete must perform sport-specific conditioning, particularly with regard to muscle strengthening and full-velocity sprinting. In addition, athletes should test their muscle strength and jumping performance compared to the opposite leg before returning to competitions.

Rehabilitation of Painful Conditions in the Thigh

Athletes with chronic thigh pain are rehabilitated according to the diagnosis made. In many cases, this diagnosis is a result of sequelae from a strain injury or because they are bothered by cramps during exercise and competition. If there is a muscle strain, the goal is to loosen up any scar tissue and achieve maximum range of motion and strength in the affected area. The athlete should be informed that these injuries may take a long time to heal, so that they have realistic expectations when rehabilitation begins.

A patient who struggles with cramp-like pain in the thigh should be examined for possible trigger points in the affected area including muscles around the painful area. The practitioner must also examine the lumbar spine, since various problems in this area may make the patient feel like he/she has cramps in the thigh musculature. It is important to detect possible involvement of the sciatic nerve at the site of a proximal hamstrings injury by doing the ordinary nerve tests. Making a correct diagnosis is most important.

Preventing Reinjury

Athletes with muscle strain injuries often experience recurrent injuries. The most common cause is that they have not fully recovered before they begin maximum training and competition. It should also be remembered that reinjury risk also occurs after the athlete has seemingly successfully returned to sport.

The practitioner should convey the following points to the patient about reducing the risk of reinjury:

• Allow injured tissue time to heal.
• Achieve sufficient strength, including eccentric training.
• Regain, and possibly improve, range of motion through stretching.
• Improve neuromuscular function, coordination, and balance.
• Do sport-specific training, including maximum speed and explosiveness.
• Let the body recover between training and competitions. Avoid fatigue.
• Listen to your body, and be aware of mild symptoms and cramping in the area.

12 Knee

Acute Knee Injuries

Robert F. LaPrade[1, 2], Casey M. Pierce[2], Roald Bahr[3], Lars Engebretsen[3], Jill Cook[4], Elizabeth Arendt[5], and Nicholas Mohtadi[6]

[1]The Steadman Clinic, Vail, CO, USA
[2]Steadman Philippon Research Institute, Vail, CO, USA
[3]Norwegian School of Sport Sciences, Oslo, Norway
[4]Monash University, Frankston, VIC, Australia
[5]University of Minnesota, Minneapolis, MN, USA
[6]University of Calgary Sport Medicine Centre, Calgary, AB, Canada

Occurrence

The knee is the most commonly injured joint in the body, likely due to the functional demands placed on the joint and its complex anatomy. Knee injuries constitute nearly 5% of all acute injuries treated in physicians' offices, emergency rooms, and outpatient clinics. However, only 10% of these represent the most severe soft-tissue injuries, with meniscus tears and anterior cruciate ligament (ACL) tears being the most common. Half of all meniscus and knee ligament injuries are related to sports. The annual incidence of ACL and meniscus tears due to sports related injuries is 2 to 5/10,000 and 1/1000, respectively; however, in certain countries, nearly 50% of ACL injuries are treated non-operatively so the annual incidence is likely higher than previously reported.

The sports where ACL tears most commonly occur are soccer, skiing, basketball, team handball, and American football. Three out of every four ACL injuries are sports related. The incidence of ACL tears is generally higher in males than females; however, female athletes between the ages of 15 and 20 years old have a 2–8 times higher risk of suffering an ACL injury when participating in sports. The annual

Most common	Less common	Must not be overlooked !
Injuries that usually cause hemarthrosis:		
Anterior cruciate ligament rupture, p. 370	Fibular collateral ligament tear, p. 368	Knee dislocation, p. 377
Peripheral meniscus tear, p. 371	Femoral condyle/tibial plateau fracture, p. 375	Extensor mechanism rupture, p. 378
Tibial plateau or other fracture	Osteochondral injuries, p. 378	
Dislocated patella, p. 373	Patellar fracture, p. 379	
Injuries that usually do not usually cause hemarthrosis:		
Medial collateral ligament tear, p. 368	Posterior cruciate ligament tear, p. 375	
Central meniscus tear, p. 371	Cartilage injury, p. 378	

Table 12.1 Overview of the differential diagnoses of acute knee injuries. (Reproduced with permission from the Norwegian Sports Medicine Association.)

The IOC Manual of Sports Injuries, First Edition. Edited by Roald Bahr.
©2012 International Olympic Committee. Published 2012 by John Wiley & Sons, Ltd.

incidence of cruciate ligament tears among American female collegiate soccer players is approximately 8%. Hence, every team typically loses one to two players per year to this type of injury. The higher risk observed in female athletes is likely due to a interaction of multiple intrinsic and extrinsic factors, which include muscle strength, conditioning, skill level, ligament size, limb alignment (knee valgus, wider pelvis, and foot pronation), joint mobility, and intercondylar notch variation.

Diagnostic Thinking

Swelling of the knee within 12 hours following the initial injury denotes bleeding into the joint (hemarthrosis). Knee injuries that create a bleed into the joint should be immediately evaluated by an orthopedic surgeon and usually require acute surgical intervention. Injuries without hemarthrosis generally do not require acute surgery and can be evaluated and initially treated at the primary-care level. Identifying mechanisms of specific injuries that cause hemarthrosis (Table 12.1) is important to allow physicians to assess a patient's surgical need.

Intra-articular bleeding will usually occur within the first 12–24 hours following an injury; therefore, if a patient has a swollen knee within 12 hours of an accident, it may be assumed to contain blood. Subsequently, aspiration of the swollen knee is rarely indicated in the setting of an acutely injured knee, but if necessary, it must be performed under sterile conditions Athletes with a hemarthrosis, in the setting of an acute knee injury, will have an ACL tear in approximately 75% of the cases. In the remaining 25%, the differential diagnosis should include a posterior cruciate ligament tear, chondral and intra-articular fracture, patellar dislocation, meniscal tear, and joint capsule tear.

Peripheral bucket-handle meniscus injuries and significant osteochondral injuries should be repaired if diagnosed in the acute phase (typically less than 2 weeks) of the injury. In addition, a major injury of the lateral or posterolateral side of the knee is much easier to repair or reconstruct during the first 2 weeks following the injury. When surgery is delayed, a reconstruction usually will be required. Injuries that are considered orthopedic emergencies and require immediate treatment include fractures and major knee injuries (such as a dislocation), or any injury with signs of vascular and/or nerve injuries.

Therefore, the goal of the clinical examination of an acutely injured knee is to identify injuries that will require acute treatment such as meniscus cartilage injuries, dislocations, and fractures. Routine anteroposterior and lateral view radiographs will usually verify or rule out a fracture, whereas clinical examination will identify possible ligament tears, meniscus injuries, dislocation, or osteochondral injuries. Because many patients do not have access to magnetic resonance imaging (MRI), it is comforting to know that there is usually sufficient time to treat these types of injuries. Acute cruciate ligament injuries and patellar dislocations may be diagnosed clinically without the help of MRI. If a patient has dislocated knee their knee, clinical examination will reveal such a degree of instability that there will be no doubt that the patient has a severe knee injury. This type of patient must be rapidly transported to an orthopedic department that has experience treating these types of injuries. MRI should only be required in the minority of patients. Indications for an MRI in the acutely injured knee would include one or more of the following: acute hemarthrosis in a skeletally immature individual, multiple ligament injury, inability to distinguish between a knee that is mechanically locked from one which is stiff, characterization the size of an osteochondral fracture, discordance between the history and physical examination, and situations where an associated comorbidity compromises the interpretation of the history, physical examination, and x-rays.

Commonly, fractures in children may clinically resemble ligament injuries in adults, but radiographs will often reveal a physeal or avulsion fracture. Practitioners should be mindful when examining children and young adolescents because they have growth zones at both the ends of the femur and tibia as well as an apophysis at the tibial tuberosity. These growth zones make the knee a particularly vulnerable area to fractures in this age group, which usually require emergency treatment. *A qualified professional must examine a child with an extension deficit within a few days to look for growth pate injuries.* Practitioners should be aware that common knee injuries in children often have to be immobilized to prevent further damage, whereas fully grown patients will only require active rehabilitation within a few days of the injury to promote healing.

Case History

Knowledge regarding the injury mechanism often produces a diagnosis prior to the patient being physically examined. Therefore, a thorough history of the mechanism of injury is extremely important and, whenever possible should include comparative information from trainers/physical therapists, coaches, or teammates. Performing a plant-and-cut movement or landing after a jump on a nearly extended and slightly valgus knee is typical of an ACL tear in team sports like basketball, handball, and soccer (Figure 12.1). This type of injury frequently results in subchondral bruising of the lateral femoral condyle and tibial plateau, which usually coincides with the patient hearing a pop as the injury occurred. Meniscus injuries have been reported to occur in more than 70% of ACL tears, while bone bruises have been reported in greater than 80%. Hyperextension trauma causing an ACL tear is not an uncommon mechanism of injury (Figure 12.2) in basketball or soccer players. ACL tears can also be the result of contact mechanisms, such as when an opponent falls over the athlete's knee and forces it to bend backward into hyperextension. Direct trauma to the lateral aspect of the knee often injures the medial structures and may, in addition, cause a tear of the ACL (Figure 12.2).

Recreational skiers are most commonly injured when the tip of their ski gets stuck in the snow, causing a valgus and external rotational trauma to the knee (Figure 12.3a). This primarily results in a tear of the medial collateral ligament and occasionally of the ACL as well. In addition, these patients often have bone bruises of the lateral compartment. The most common mechanism of injury leading to ACL tears among recreational skiers can occur even at low speeds. While traveling downhill, the skier falls backward, shifting all of his or her weight onto the outer ski. This is known as the "phantom foot" and it allows the back edge of the ski to catch, forcing the ski to cut inward, causing internal rotational trauma to the knee while it is fully flexed (Figure 12.3b). In the same situation, the ski can also cut outward, producing external rotational trauma, which can also tear the ACL. The internal joint motion causing the ACL to tear in skiing injuries appears to be the same as that seen in noncontact injuries. A study among World Cup skiers showed that professional skiers are likely to suffer an acute knee injury due to three distinct mechanisms. The first, known as the "slip-catch" mechanism, is the most common and is set up when the outer ski *slips* and loses contact with the snow. The injury occurs when the ski edge then *catches* the surface again. This sudden return of contact causes the knee to internally rotate while being stressed in a valgus manner with abrupt compression loading (Figure 12.4a) and tears the ACL. The second mechanism of injury that regularly affects downhill skiers is known as the "dynamic snowplow." This takes place when skiers lose their balance backward with most of their weight distributed on only one ski. The unweighted ski drifts outward, spreading the skier's legs apart. As the legs continue to spread, the weighted ski catches

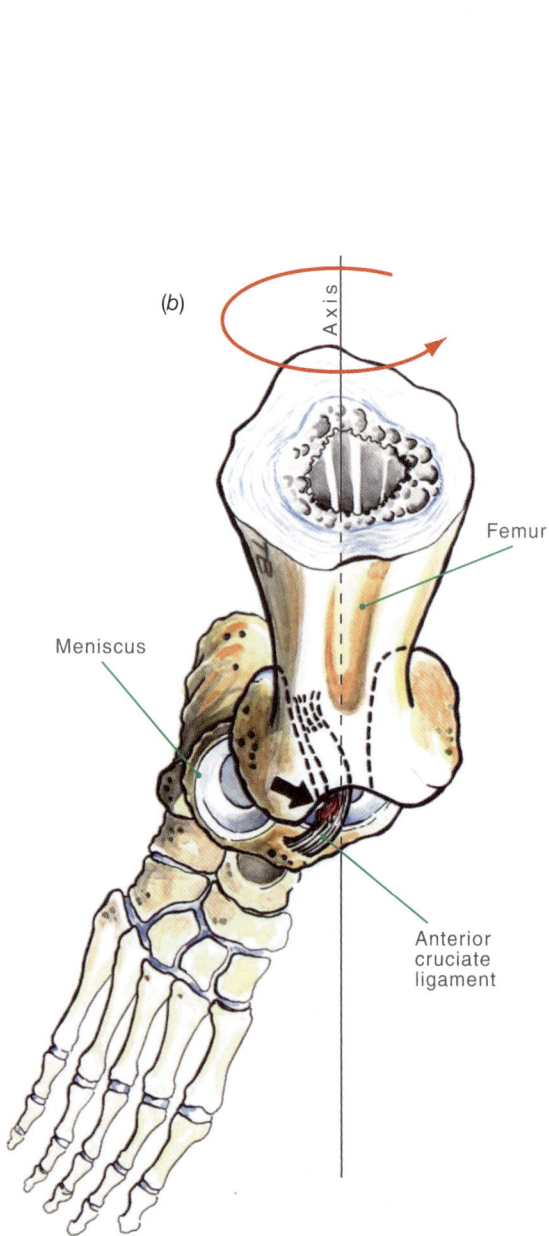

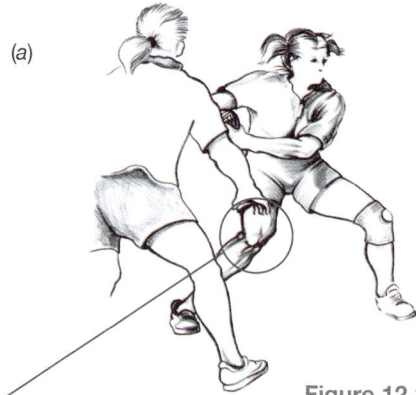

Figure 12.1 Noncontact anterior cruciate ligament (ACL) injury mechanism. This is the most common mechanism for ACL injuries in team handball, soccer, and basketball. The foot is planted on the ground (a) while the lower leg rotates in valgus (b), with the knee nearly straight at ground contact. (© Medical Illustrator Tommy Bolic, Sweden.)

Figure 12.2 Anterior cruciate ligament (ACL) injury mechanism involving contact. This is a common contact injury. In this case, both players injured an ACL. The ACL of the player on the left is injured by hyperextension. The player on the right suffers a valgus trauma that causes injuries to the following structures in the order listed: the medial collateral ligament, the ACL, the lateral meniscus, and the lateral compartment articular cartilage. (Reproduced with permission from the Norwegian Sports Medicine Association.)

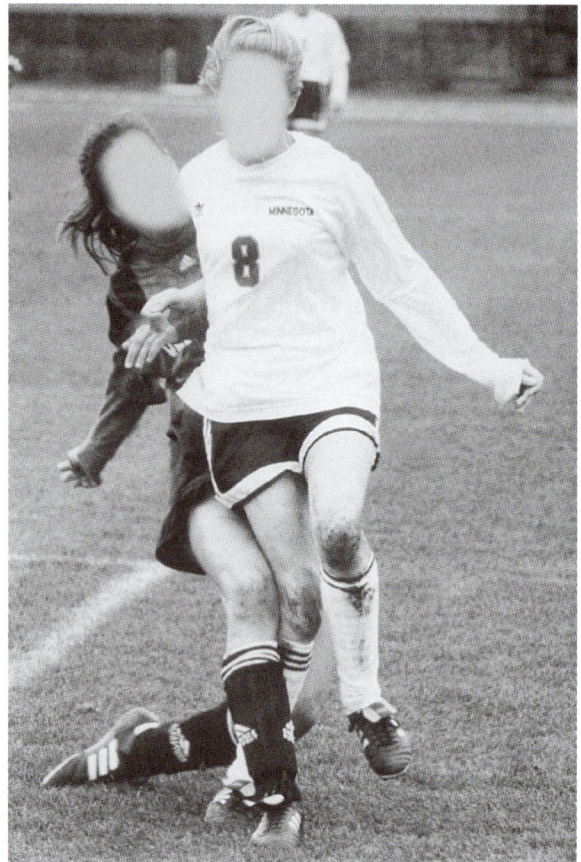

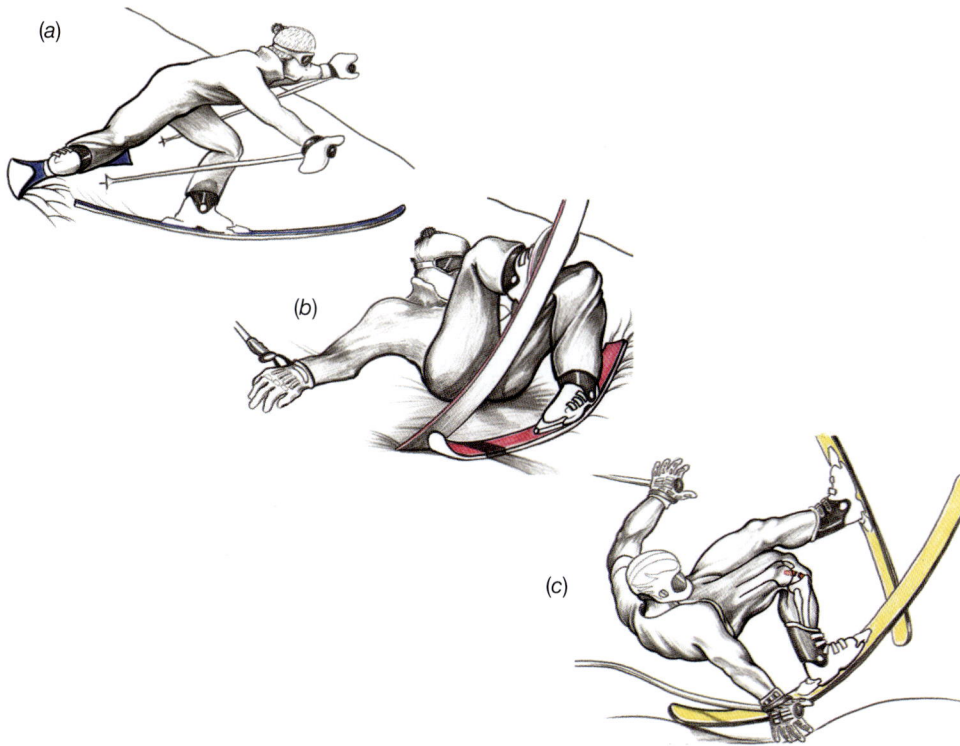

Figure 12.3 Injury mechanisms in downhill skiing. Valgus external rotation injury commonly seen in recreational skiers (a). Phantom-foot injury occurring as a skier loses balance backward and the weighted outer ski catches (b). Top-level downhill skiers may sustain this injury when they jump and land with their weight too far to the rear (c). (© Medical Illustrator Tommy Bolic, Sweden.)

its inside edge, forcing the knee to internally rotate (with or without a valgus stress) and causing injury (Figure 12.4b). Finally, top professional skiers may sustain ACL tears due to a combined blow to the rear ski, concentric contraction of the quadriceps muscle, and slight valgus stress in the knee when the athlete lands with his or her weight too far back after a jump (Figure 12.3c). The skier's boot, along with the contraction of the quadriceps muscles, causes an anterior drawer force that tears the ligament. This injury mechanism is also likely to cause a bone bruise in the medial compartment due to tibial femoral compression. The same mechanism of injury, especially in men and women over 40 years old, may cause a tibial plateau fracture and leave the ligaments intact.

Posterior cruciate ligament injuries usually occur from a direct blow to the anterior tibia while the knee is flexed. Half of these injuries result from traffic accidents (such as when the knee hits the dashboard), while the other half are sports-related injuries, for example, an athlete falling onto their knee in soccer or football, or a player crashing into the sideboard while playing ice hockey. Approximately 20% of complete posterior cruciate ligament tears are isolated (i.e., only the posterior cruciate ligament is injured), whereas the remainders are combined injuries in which the fibular collateral ligament, the popliteus tendon, or both are injured at the same time.

Patellar dislocations are most often a noncontact injury sustained when twisting the knee in early flexion. The patella dislocates laterally, injuring or tearing the medial soft tissue restraints. Most often the patella self reduces as the athlete extends their knee. A less typical mechanism is a direct blow to the medial patellar margin, with the knee slightly flexed (a classic example is an injury caused by running into a slalom gate). Patients with patellar dislocations can show signs of hemarthrosis, often quite large, and usually complain of pain along the medial patellar retinaculum.

KNEE

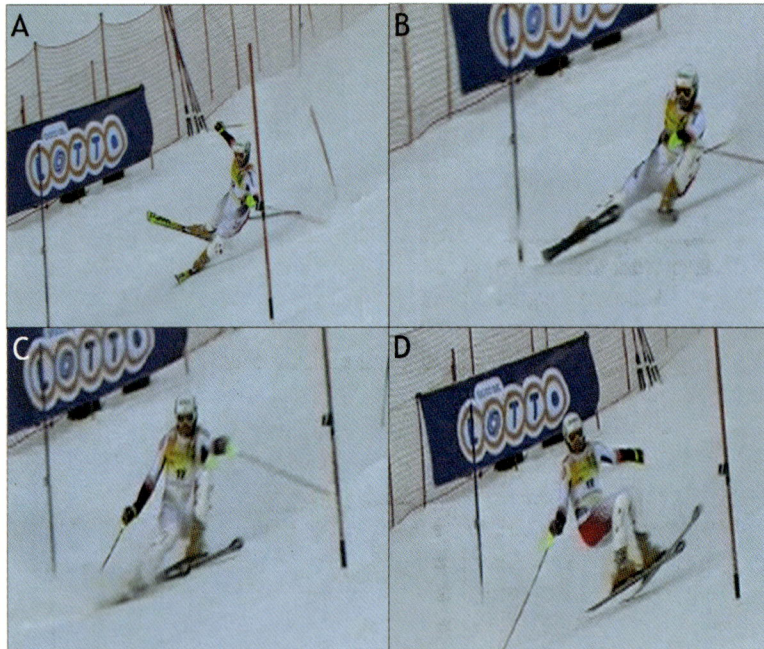

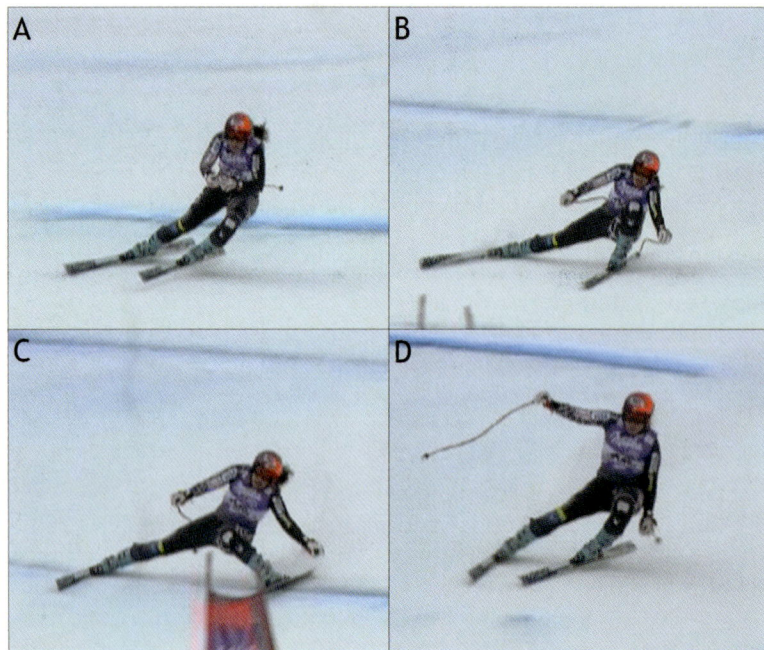

Figure 12.4 Sequence of injury mechanisms in elite downhill skiing. Upper panel (A through D) shows slip-catch mechanism: The ski drifts backward before catching the snow again, causing internal rotation and valgus stress. Lower panel (A through D) shows dynamic snowplow: as the legs drift apart, the weighted ski catches leading to forceful internal rotation (B). (© Oslo Sports Trauma Research Center.)

Clinical Examinations

Inspection. With the patient's knee at rest on the examining table, the practitioner inspects both knees. Usually, there is no doubt as to whether a knee contains intra-articular fluid (Figure 12.5). A knee ligament injury seen on the field or in the training room immediately after injury may not demonstrate an effusion; however, after several hours, swelling and pain will typically make an examination difficult. The patella may be laterally displaced or sitting high or low, indicating that a patella dislocation or rupture of the patellar or quadriceps tendon, respectively, has occurred; however, examiners should be mindful of the fact that the patella often spontaneously relocates making the diagnosis less obvious.

Palpation. The patellar tendon, the patellar retinaculum, medial patellofemoral ligament, and the quadriceps tendon are all palpated for pain and discontinuity. The medial ligaments may be directly palpated, and painful points at their origins on the femoral condyle and tibia are typical for these injuries. Both the fibular collateral ligament and biceps femoris tendon can also easily be palpated, and the practitioner should compare them to the healthy side. If a major lateral injury has occurred, the fibular collateral ligament and the biceps tendon are often more difficult to recognize by palpation than the structures on the healthy side. The joint spaces can be palpated and a meniscus injury will usually cause pain along the joint line.

Movement. Normal range of motion for the knee is 0°–10° of extension and approximately 135°–140° of flexion; however, considerable variability exists between individuals with respect to what is a normal range of motion for the knee. Therefore, examiners should always compare the injured side with the contralateral healthy side to determine normality. If a patient has suffered an acute knee injury, both flexion and extension will often be limited. The challenge lies in determining whether there is true locking or pseudolocking. With true locking, the meniscus typically has become impinged, and the joint is mechanically blocked. This is frequently due to a rupture, such as a bucket handle tear, but there are often pieces of the ACL or cartilage between the femur and the tibia, which cause the joint to lock. Seen just as often, a pseudolocked knee has no structures mechanically limiting joint mobility, but movement is prevented by intense pain. The most important clinical sign of a locked knee is limitation of passive terminal extension while flexion is essentially normal.

Neurovascular function. The practitioner palpates the dorsalis pedis pulse on the dorsum of the foot and the posterior tibial artery behind the medial malleolus, and then compares them to the healthy side. Strength and sensation should be evaluated; the musculature innervated by the common peroneal nerve is frequently weakened with a posterolateral knee injury. This nerve is particularly vulnerable with varus trauma or in a knee dislocation. In such cases, the patient will demonstrate a reproducible weakness of great toe extension and possibly ankle dorsiflexors and toe extensors. In addition, loss of sensation occurs between the first and second toes and on the lateral aspect of the foot on the involved side.

Special Tests

When a patient has suffered an acute knee injury, a series of special tests are performed to evaluate the integrity of the cruciate ligaments, the collateral ligaments, and the menisci. It is always necessary to compare the clinical tests on the injured side with those on the healthy side.

Lachman test at 30°. This clinical test (Figure 12.6) is used to evaluate the integrity of the ACL. At 30° of knee flexion, the examiner stabilizes the femur and applies an anterior directed force to the tibia. In an ACL-deficient knee, the tibia will "slip" forward in relation to the femur, resulting in an absent or soft end point. It is especially important for this test to have the patient completely relax. If the patient is not completely relaxed, a false negative Lachman test may occur.

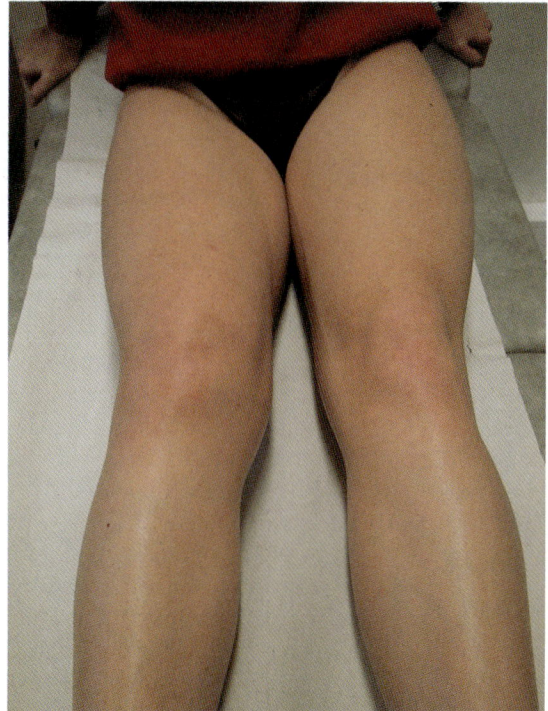

Figure 12.5
Hemarthrosis. When a patient sustains an intra-articular injury, the joint can fill with 60–70 mL of fresh blood within a few hours (<12). The blood arises from injuries to the cruciate ligament, meniscus, capsule, or bone. The best way to evaluate for hemarthrosis is to compare the patient's injured knee to the contralateral normal knee while viewing them from the foot end of the examination table. (Reproduced with permission from the Norwegian Sports Medicine Association.)

KNEE

Varus or valgus stress test at 20°. This clinical test (Figure 12.5) is used to determine whether or not the patient has a collateral ligament injury. The knee is held at 20° flexion and loaded in a varus or valgus manner so that the collateral ligaments are stretched. The practitioner places his or her fingers along the joint space to feel whether it gaps open. Medial and fibular collateral ligament injuries are graded subjectively according to how large the opening in the joint space is, as follows: grade I, painful, but with no gapping; grade II, gapping, but with an endpoint present; and grade III, no endpoint to stress testing. The test may also be positive for physeal injuries in children and tibial plateau fractures in adults.

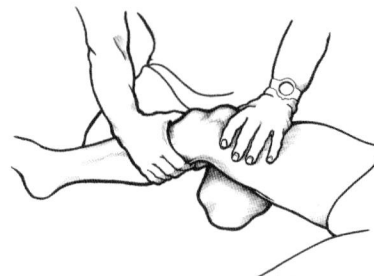

Sag test. The test (Figure 12.8) is used to evaluate the posterior cruciate ligament. The patient is placed in a supine position with the hips flexed to about 45° and the knees flexed to 90°. When a posterior cruciate ligament injury exists the tibia will sag backward compared to the healthy side.

Meniscus tear assessment (Figure 12.9). To test the medial meniscus, the practitioner holds one's fingers along the medial joint space while the tibia is externally rotated and slight valgus pressure is applied to the knee. The lateral meniscus is tested by applying pressure to the lateral joint space with simultaneous internal rotation and varus stress. The test is considered positive when a patient feels deep pain in the joint space. If a meniscus injury has occurred, a click can sometimes be palpated over the joint line as the knee is flexed. In addition, pain in the posterior aspect of the knee with maximal knee flexion or when the patient squats is commonly indicative of a meniscus tear.

Pivot shift test. This clinical test (Figure 12.10) is used to evaluate for a complete ACL tear. It is especially important for this test to have the patient completely relax to avoid a false negative test. With the patient lying on their back with the affected knee fully extended and tibia internally rotated, the tester stresses the knee with a coupled valgus and internal rotation force and flexes the knee. An appreciable clunk felt around 30° of knee flexion indicates that the subluxed joint has reduced and is indicative of a complete ACL tear.

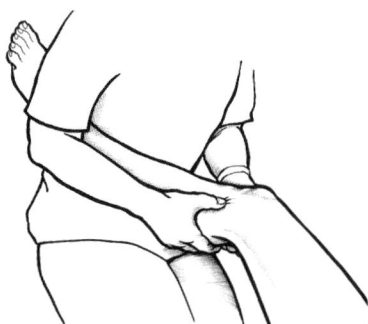

Figure 12.6 Lachman test. With the joint flexed to 30°, an anterior drawer movement is applied to the tibia in relation to the femur. (© Medical Illustrator Tommy Bolic, Sweden.)

Figure 12.7 Varus/valgus stress test. Hold the knee at 20° of flexion and load in varus or valgus, stretching the collateral ligaments. Place your fingers at the joint line to detect joint space opening. (© Medical Illustrator Tommy Bolic, Sweden.)

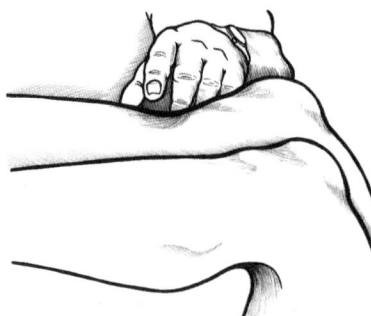

Figure 12.8 Sag test. In this position, the tibia will sag posteriorly compared to the uninjured side if a posterior cruciate ligament injury is present. (© Medical Illustrator Tommy Bolic, Sweden.)

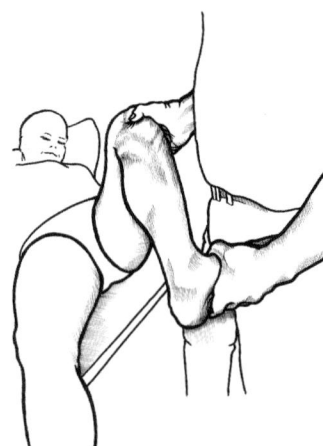

Figure 12.9 Meniscus tear assessment. Place one's finger over the joint line while the tibia is rotated and a varus/valgus stress is applied. A patient with a tear will feel pain deep within the joint. (© Medical Illustrator Tommy Bolic, Sweden.)

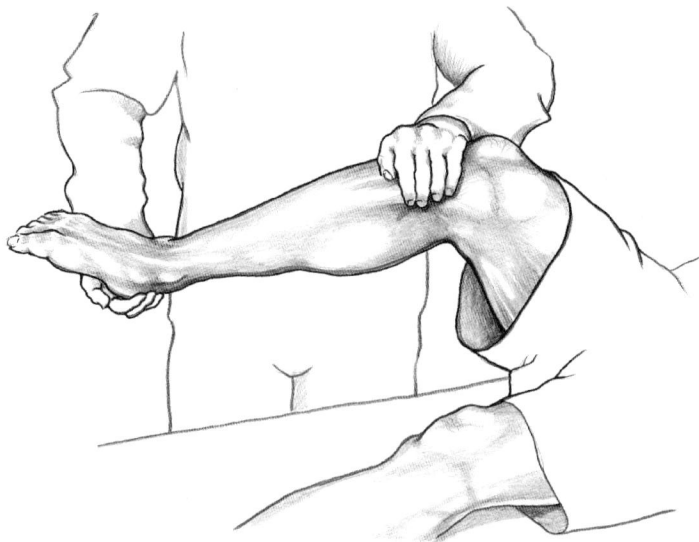

Posterolateral Lachman at 30°. The test (Figure 12.11) is used to evaluate whether an injury has occurred to the main structures in the posterolateral corner (i.e., the fibular collateral ligament, the popliteus tendon, and the popliteofibular ligament). The test is administered like a reversed Lachman test; with the knee flexed at about 30°, the tibia is pushed posteriorly in an externally rotated position.

Anteromedial drawer test. The test is used to evaluate for a combined superficial medial collateral ligament and posterior oblique ligament injury. With the knee flexed at 90° and the foot externally rotated to 15°, an anteromedial drawer force is applied. Increased anteromedial rotation of the tibia on the femur compared to the contralateral normal knee indicates a combined superficial medial collateral ligament and posterior oblique ligament injury.

Posterolateral drawer test. The test is used to evaluate for posterolateral corner injuries. With the knee flexed at 90° and the foot externally rotated to 15°, a posterolateral drawer force is applied to the knee. Increased posterolateral rotation compared to the contralateral normal knee indicates a probable injury to the popliteus tendon, poplitcofibular ligament, and fibular collateral ligament.

Posterior drawer test 90°. This clinical test (Figure 12.12) is used to evaluate the integrity of the posterior cruciate ligament. With the knee flexed at 90°, the tibia is pushed straight backward. If the posterior cruciate ligament is torn, the tibia will slip backward in relation to the femur. This test is utilized to assess the change in relationship between the proximal tibia to the distal femur.

External rotation recurvatum test. This clinical test (Figure 12.13) is also used to evaluate for a potential posterolateral ligament injury. With the patient supine, the great toe is lifted up from the surface while the thigh is immobilized. If a major injury to the posterolateral knee structures and other structures has occurred, the injured knee becomes hyperextended compared to the normal contralateral knee. Heel heights are the most accurate means to assess this clinical test. Most commonly this test is positive for a combined ACL and posterolateral knee structure injury.

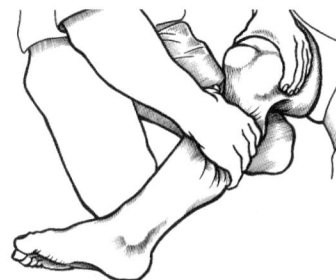

Figure 12.11 Posterolateral Lachman. "Reverse Lachman" where the tibia is pushed posteriorly in an externally rotated position. (© Medical Illustrator Tommy Bolic, Sweden.)

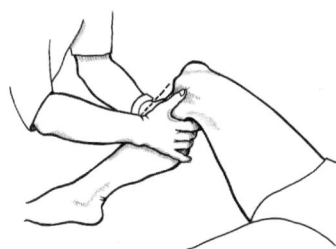

Figure 12.12 Posterior drawer test. With the knee flexed to 90°, the tibia is pushed straight backward and the step-off between the proximal anterior tibia and the distal aspect of the femoral condyles is observed. (© Medical Illustrator Tommy Bolic, Sweden.)

Dial test. This clinical test is primarily used to evaluate the integrity of the posterolateral corner and for a possible combined posterior cruciate ligament tear. With the patient lying supine, flex the knee off the edge of the examining table to 30° and then 90° while stabilizing the thigh. Externally rotate the foot and take note of the amount of external rotation experienced by the tibial tubercle compared to the contralateral normal side. An increase of more than 15° is a positive test. A positive test at 30° of flexion that is normal at 90° indicates a likely popliteus complex injury, while positive tests at both 30° and 90° of flexion suggests a combined injury to both the posterior cruciate ligament and posterolateral corner. This test can also be performed with the patient in the prone position. Beware that a person with a severe medial knee injury can also have a positive dial test.

Lateral patellar apprehension test. The test is used to evaluate the integrity of the patellar restraints and to check for patellar dislocation or subluxation. With the patient lying supine and their knee flexed at 30°, or fully extended, the tester applies pressure to the medial edge of the patella forcing it to move laterally. Pain and/or quadriceps contraction is suggestive of instability.

Medial/lateral patella restraint tests. This test is used to evaluate the stability of the patellofemoral joint. The patient should by lying supine with the knee and quadriceps relaxed. The patella is moved across its range of motion both medially and laterally. The amount of passive patella motion in a medial and lateral direction of the patella is measured against an imaginary midline of the patella in the resting position. This maneuver tests the static restraints of the medial and lateral extensor retinaculum complex. Any change from the patient's "normal" contralateral knee is suggestive of patellar retinacular injury. Most particularly, an increase in lateral patella translation represents laxity or incompetence of the medial patella femoral ligament and medial retinacular structures associated with lateral patella dislocation.

Straight leg raising against gravity. The test assess the integrity of the extensor mechanism, including quadriceps tendon, patella, and patella tendon. With the patient sitting at the edge of the examination table, passively extend their knee and then compared it to active extension. A "lag" sign represents the difference between passive and active extension of the knee. A lag signifies disruption and/or weakness of the extensor mechanism.

Supplemental Examinations

Routine radiographs should always be ordered for acute knee injuries, but an expert should decide if more specialized images or tests are necessary.

Radiographic examination. Fractures can usually be located with anteroposterior and lateral radiographs. A patellar tendon rupture will show increased height of the patella on lateral and anteroposterior radiographs. The practitioner should be aware that an ACL injury could cause an avulsion of the intercondylar eminence, especially in adolescent athletes. If a tibial plateau fracture is suspected, oblique radiographs should be ordered to properly view the plateau. Bilateral varus or valgus (Figure 12.14a) stress radiographs should be obtained to objectively determine the amount of increased joint line gapping if there is a concern about the integrity of the collateral ligaments. Kneeling posterior stress radiographs show the difference between posterior tibial translation in both knees and are useful to look for posterior cruciate ligament insufficiency (Figure 12.14b). Normal knees have between

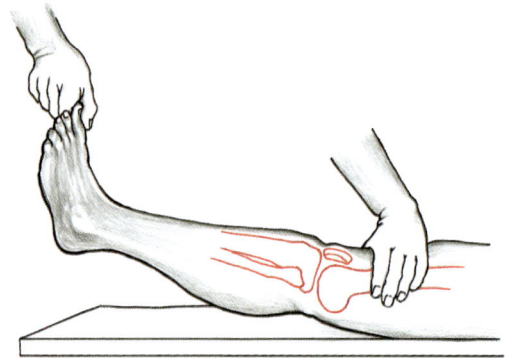

Figure 12.13 External rotation recurvatum test. With the patient in a supine position, lift the great toe off the surface while the distal thigh is stabilized. The patient's heel heights can be measured. (© Medical Illustrator Tommy Bolic, Sweden.)

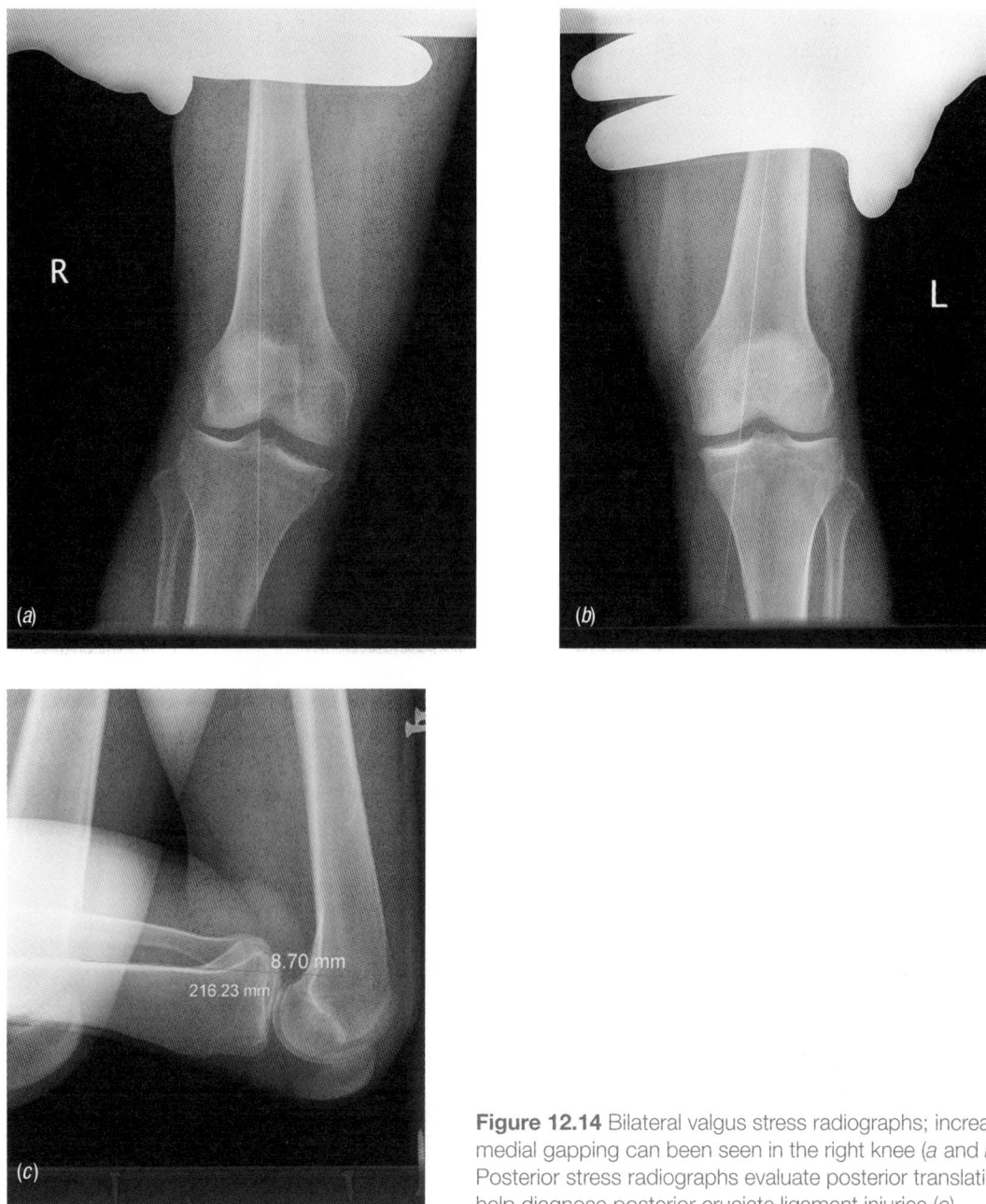

Figure 12.14 Bilateral valgus stress radiographs; increased medial gapping can been seen in the right knee (a and b). Posterior stress radiographs evaluate posterior translation and help diagnose posterior cruciate ligament injuries (c).

0–2 mm increased posterior translation, partial tears 2–7 mm, complete tears 8–11 mm, and combined injuries have greater than 12 mm increase. If a physeal (growth plate) fracture is suspected in a child or adolescent, bilateral radiographs should be ordered to compare the affected side to the healthy one. If the radiographs are negative, but palpation elicits pain at the growth zone, it is necessary to obtain varus or valgus stress radiographs.

Other examinations. MRI is an accurate method of demonstrating cruciate ligament, meniscus, and collateral ligament injuries. When a patient presents with locking in the knee, MRI can be useful to determine what structure is causing the joint to lock. Primary care physicians should refrain from ordering magnetic resonance images unless they feel that the images will provide or confirm a diagnosis within their realm to treat. Rather, they should refer the patient to an orthopedic surgeon or specialist who can insure the proper imaging tests are ordered to obtain an accurate diagnosis. Practitioners should be aware that MRI of the extremities does not routinely include the entire extensor apparatus. This can allow for quadriceps tendon ruptures to remain undetected in some cases. Tears in the extensor apparatus may be revealed by ultrasound, but the usefulness of this method is highly dependent on the skill of the operator.

Common Injuries

Medial or Fibular Collateral Ligament Injury

About 40% of all severe knee injuries involve the superficial medial collateral ligament; making it the most commonly injured knee structure. The mechanism of injury is commonly an opponent falling into the patient's slightly flexed knee, forcing it into valgus. These injuries are often isolated and are primarily limited to the origins (Figure 12.15) or the insertions of the medial knee structures. Fibular collateral ligament injuries are less common, but usually more complicated because the lateral side of the knee is made up of a series of ligaments and tendons that interact with one another to provide stability to the knee (Figure 12.16). Injuries here frequently involve the iliotibial band, fibular collateral ligament, biceps apparatus, popliteus apparatus, or lateral joint capsule, whereas a medial collateral injury usually involves only the superficial medial knee ligament. Posterolateral knee injuries are generally caused by external trauma directed at the medial side of the knee or by contact or noncontact hyperextension injuries. Ligament injuries are traditionally categorized into grades I, II, and III, based on the amount of opening in the joint space during stress tests when compared to the normal knee. Grade I injuries are painful, but with no gapping; grade II injuries have gapping, but with an endpoint present; and grade III injuries lack an endpoint with stress testing. Grades II and III are often combined injuries that may involve the cruciate ligaments and the menisci. A useful rule of thumb is that if a knee opens up on valgus or varus stress testing in full extension, the examiner should have a high index of suspicion for a collateral ligament injury.

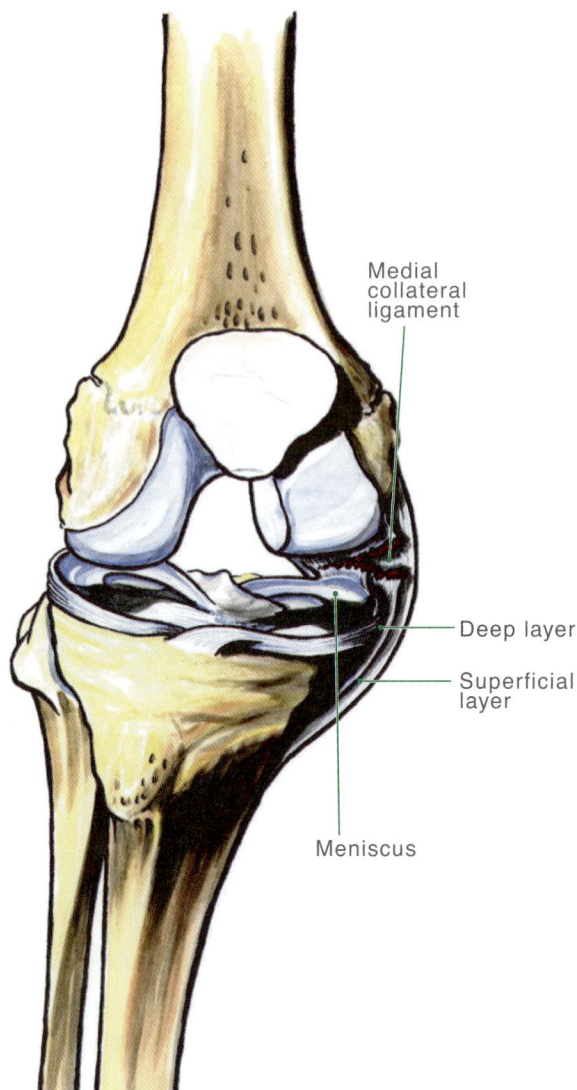

Figure 12.15 Medial ligament injury. If the knee is forced into valgus, the medial structures will be stretched and then torn. (© Medical Illustrator Tommy Bolic, Sweden.)

- Symptoms and signs: The patient has intense pain medially or laterally. The most common is a medial ligament injury. This does not usually cause swelling in the joint, but reduce flexion and extension are typical of the acute phase. Lateral/posterolateral knee injuries typically cause mild pain or swelling and may be overlooked if one does not include adequate clinical testing for posterolateral knee injuries during the examination. In children, physeal fractures often present with pain and symptoms similar to a collateral ligament injury and should not be overlooked.
- Diagnosis: The valgus stress test may be positive if the patient has sustained a medial knee injury. A positive varus stress test indicates a major posterolateral knee injury. Practitioners should compare the injured side with the healthy side first,

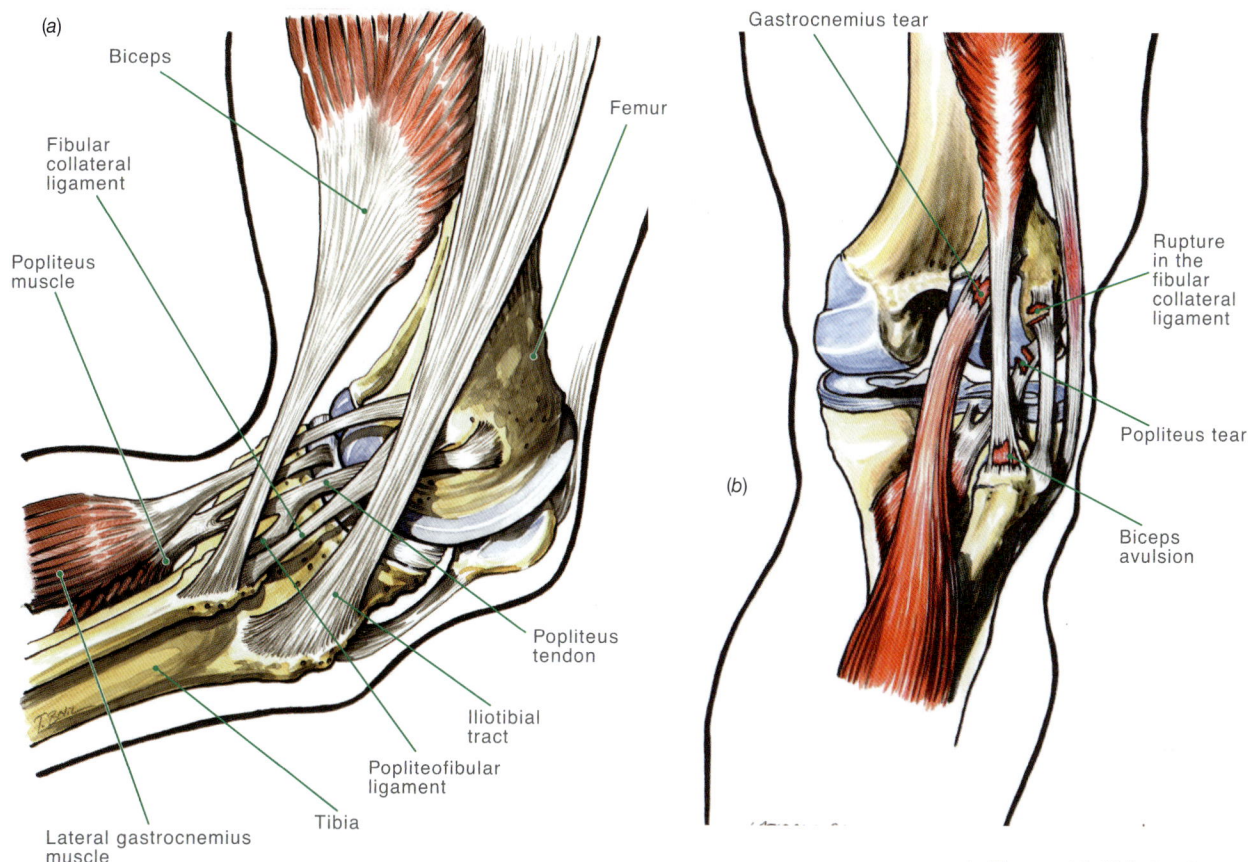

(a)
Biceps
Femur
Fibular collateral ligament
Popliteus muscle
Popliteus tendon
Iliotibial tract
Popliteofibular ligament
Tibia
Lateral gastrocnemius muscle

(b)
Gastrocnemius tear
Rupture in the fibular collateral ligament
Popliteus tear
Biceps avulsion

Figure 12.16 Lateral structures. The anatomy of the lateral side of the knee is more complicated than that of the medial side. Injuries on the lateral side are more typically complicated and require surgery more often than injuries on the medial side. Normal anatomy (a); common injuries (b). (© Medical Illustrator Tommy Bolic, Sweden.)

and then palpate the fibular collateral ligament. Inability to palpate the fibular collateral ligament indicates that the patient has a major injury that likely involves the popliteus tendon, the biceps femoris, and other structures on the lateral side. A complete tear of the fibular collateral ligament often causes less pain than other ligament injuries of the knee. The practitioner should always take routine radiographs to exclude a fracture of the fibular head or lateral capsule.

• Treatment by physician: Acute treatment of grade I injuries is administered according to the PRICE principle. Many patients benefit from special braces or immobilizers that contain ice water and apply compression. Following the PRICE principle, rehabilitation begins, emphasizing techniques to decrease swelling and restore strength, range of motion, and neuromuscular function. Grade II or III injuries on the medial side are treated for 4–6 weeks with a hinged knee brace, which allows for protected range of motion. An orthopedic surgeon experienced in complex knee injuries should evaluate grade II and grade III injuries on the lateral side, often with the assistance of MRI and varus stress radiographs. Grade III posterolateral knee injuries are normally treated via surgical intervention within the first 1–2 weeks following the injury. Practitioners should understand that major (grades II and III) medial and lateral injuries, combined with cruciate ligament injuries, will cause major knee instability if the central stabilizer (the ACL) is not reconstructed. The lateral side should be repaired or reconstructed concurrently during the ACL reconstruction. Collateral ligaments should never be surgically treated as the sole procedure if the ACL is also torn.

• Treatment by therapist: Exercises may begin as soon as pain allows, usually 1–2 days after surgery. The patient should avoid exercises that cause side-to-side stress. When swimming, patients should avoid the breaststroke and emphasize an up and down flutter kick.

- Prognosis: Grade I and II collateral ligament injuries often heal within 6–12 weeks. Recovery following a grade III tear depends significantly the accompanying injuries. Combined injuries usually require significantly longer time to heal compared isolated ones. With the exception of major injuries to the lateral ligaments, the athlete can usually return to normal sports activities without problems.

Anterior Cruciate Ligament Rupture

The reported annual incidence of ACL injuries is 5–10 injuries per 10,000 inhabitants; however, due to nonsurgical management of a high proportion of ACL injuries, the actual incidence is likely much higher. The ACL usually tears completely when it is injured (Figure 12.17), but because it consists of two functional bundles, cases occur in which only the posterolateral or the anteromedial bundle of the ligament is torn. Cruciate ligament injuries in children are rare, but they do occur and are occurring more often. In children, the ACL is particularly vulnerable to avulsions from the tibia. Of the patients with ACL injuries, about 75% sustain concurrent meniscal injuries, 80% have a bone contusion, and 10% have accompanying cartilaginous injuries that will require treatment. Still other patients will have accompanying injuries to the medial or fibular collateral ligaments. The most common injury mechanisms are shown in Figures 12.1–12.3.

- Symptoms and signs: ACL injuries usually cause rapid swelling (hemarthrosis within 12 hours) and immediate, sometimes intense pain. The patient often recalls that their knee gave way while attempting to bear weight on the leg immediately after the injury happened. A few hours after the injury occurs, it is often difficult to complete an adequate examination due to pain and swelling; however, a focused examination of the collaterals, a posterior sag or drawer test, and, most importantly, a Lachman's test are all that is necessary in this scenario. The usual tests can be administered as described after a few days (usually a week). The Lachman test is diagnostic of a torn ACL and is positive if the end point is soft. It may be unnecessary or even impossible to perform a pivot shift test during the acute phase. Avulsion injuries are more common than tears in children; in both cases, the child experiences acute swelling over the knee, significant pain, and limited mobility for stretching and bending.
- Diagnosis: Diagnosis is based on a positive Lachman test. The diagnosis is made clinically and is highly accurate when confirmed by a trained specialist (>90% accuracy in relation to arthroscopic findings). Significantly limited joint movement may be due to a bucket-handle meniscal tear or osteochondral injury. The practitioner should order MRI and radiographs to exclude a fracture or avulsion of the intercondylar eminence. Diagnostic arthroscopy is unnecessary for this injury as the diagnosis is made clinically.
- Treatment by physician: For acute injuries, the PRICE principle is recommended. The patient often needs crutches for ambulation, and analgesic medications to reduce swelling and pain. If a definite diagnosis is not possible during the acute phase, the primary-care physician should reexamine the patient after 5–7 days.

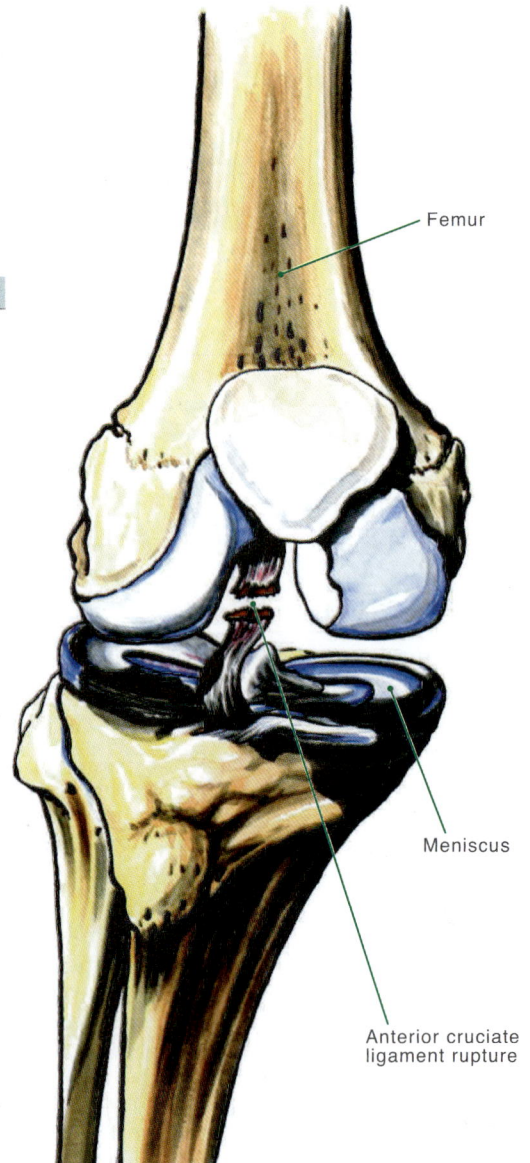

Figure 12.17 Anterior cruciate ligament (ACL) injury. ACL tears are usually total, and most are midsubstance ruptures that do not heal spontaneously. (© Medical Illustrator Tommy Bolic, Sweden.)

Femur

Meniscus

Anterior cruciate ligament rupture

Only patients with fractured or dislocated knees need to be admitted to the hospital emergently. Once diagnosed, a specialist should evaluate patients with ACL tears. The decision as to whether or not the ACL should be surgically reconstructed depends on the patient's requirements for future knee function. For patients with no associated injuries requiring treatment, one-third will manage well without the cruciate ligament, one-third will be required to significantly reduce their activity level to avoid surgery, and the remaining third will be so loose that they require surgery regardless. If a patient with an ACL tear requires surgery, the reconstruction should occur once the swelling has resolved and full active extension is present. This may take anywhere from 2 to 8 weeks. Other patient populations often undergo reassessment and rehabilitation for 6 months and are reevaluated for surgery if their quality of life is compromised due to the ligament deficiency or associated meniscal tears. Indications for surgery also depend on the extent of any additional injuries the patient may have sustained. Children with an ACL avulsion injury should undergo repair within the 2 weeks of the initial injury if possible. A midsubstance ACL tear usually requires reconstruction rather than repair. Due to the possibility of growth plate related problems, younger patients should be referred to a specialist. Braces can be used prophylactically for all twisting activities and will help prevent dislocations and further injury while the child or adolescent awaits surgery.

- Treatment by therapist: Physical therapy in which strength, movement, and neuromuscular function are emphasized is critical during the rehabilitation phase. The same type of program is used for conservative and surgically treated cruciate ligament injuries, but the progression is more rapid with conservative treatment. Rehabilitation is a long and difficult process for patients, and close adherence to the training program is important to successfully address all aspects of the rehabilitation. Patient follow-up should take place for 6 months, or longer if necessary.

- Prognosis: For high-level athletes, ACL tears make the patient feel as if the knee is unstable or giving way, and the risk of new meniscus and/or cartilage injuries is significantly increased without surgical reconstruction. After surgery, more than 80% of patients have a stable knee, and studies have reported that up to 90% of soccer players and about 60% of handball players return to their former level. Empirically, the majority of athletes perform better in their second season after returning to sport rather than the first. About 70% of conservatively managed patients have radiographic signs of arthrosis after 10 years. No similar follow-up of modern surgical treatment has been published. The athlete can choose surgery to prevent chronic instability in the joint but unfortunately, cannot be promised a reduced risk of arthrosis in the future. Follow-up studies of children who undergo surgery to repair cruciate ligament avulsions show excellent results with respect to stability and function.

Meniscus Injuries

The menisci act as the knees' shock absorbers and contribute to the normal stability of the joint. Meniscus injuries may be an isolated occurrence, or occur in combination with ligament injuries. Approximately 75% of patients with ACL injuries sustain a simultaneous meniscus injury. Damage to the medial meniscus increases loading on the cartilage in the medial joint compartment and the risk of arthrosis. In addition, patients who have their medial meniscus resected usually have increased laxity of their ACL or reconstruction graft. Nevertheless, a lateral meniscal injury is more serious than a medial one, because the lateral meniscus is of greater functional significance to joint loading. Therefore, this type of injury increases the risk of future early onset arthrosis. The risk of developing arthrosis depends on the location and

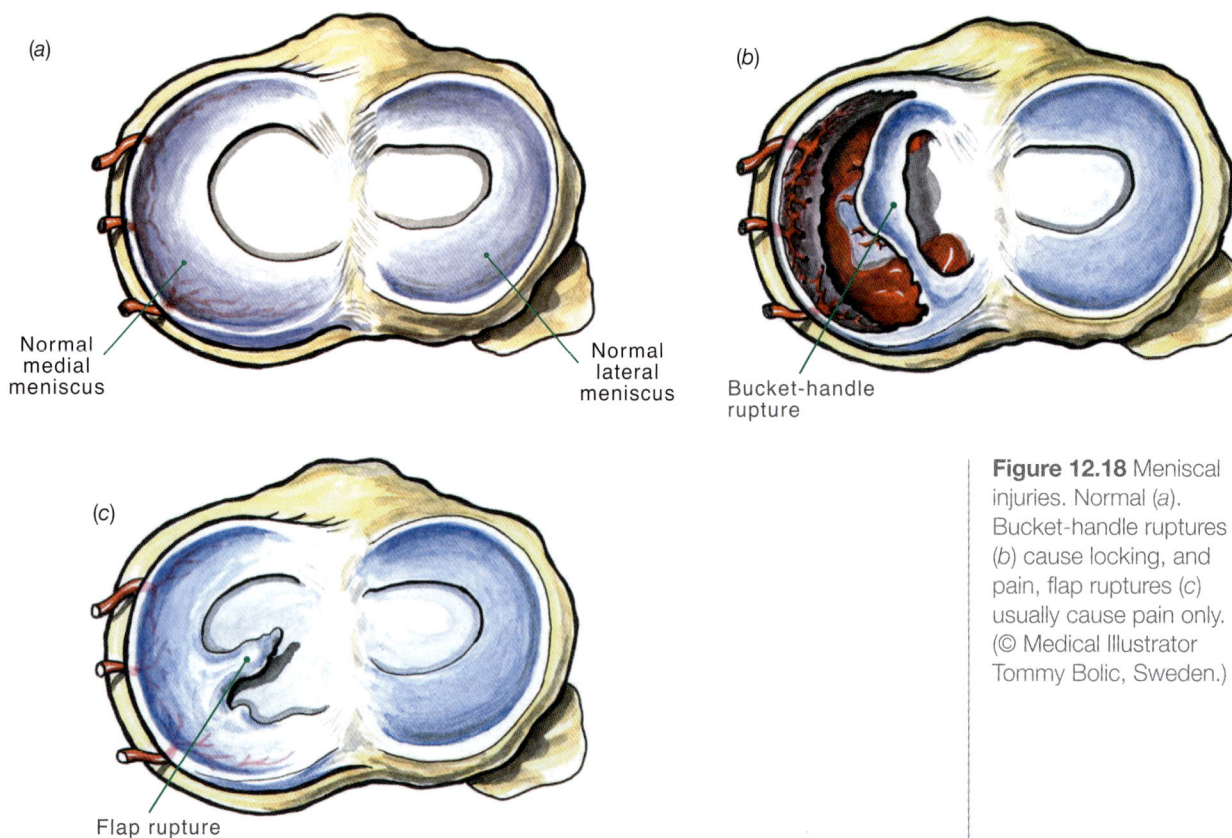

Figure 12.18 Meniscal injuries. Normal (a). Bucket-handle ruptures (b) cause locking, and pain, flap ruptures (c) usually cause pain only. (© Medical Illustrator Tommy Bolic, Sweden.)

amount of the meniscus that is injured. Figure 12.18 shows the most common types of injuries. The most important factor related to healing is the location of the injury. Peripherally located tears, in the so-called red zone (where there is a good blood supply), are amenable to repair. Centrally located tears, in the white zone (where there is no blood supply), usually must be shaved off and removed. Meniscus injuries in children are quite different from those in adults. Unlike adults, the majority of the meniscus of a child is circular, which provides better conditions for healing to occur. Enhanced healing increases the possibility of successful repair of a meniscus injury in a child, either by conservative measures or by surgery. This high probability of successful repair makes it is crucial to detect these injuries as early as possible. Children can sustain partial injuries and have meniscus cysts. Some children have what is known as a discoid meniscus, a large, oval-shaped meniscus that covers the entire surface of the tibia, which sustains unique types of tears.

- **Symptoms and signs:** Meniscus injuries that cause hemarthrosis are typically peripheral tears and are capable of being repaired due to adequate circulation in the outer parts of the meniscus. Unfortunately, peripheral injuries occur less often than central meniscus injuries, with radial and horizontal ruptures being the most commonly reported. These meniscal tears usually do not cause as much bleeding but do result in pain and eventually edema due to accompanying local synovitis. A peripheral meniscal tear (e.g., a bucket handle tear) may become unstable, which can cause locking in extension and is well suited to repair.
- **Diagnosis:** Diagnosis of a meniscal tear is based on pain in the joint space and in the posterior aspect of the knee with deep knee flexion. If hemarthrosis is present, joint range of motion is typically reduced. In contrast with a joint that is filled with blood, where decreased range of motion is caused by pain (pseudolocking),

a bucket-handle meniscal tear causes true locking and often demonstrates elastic resistance to extension. MRI is highly accurate in detecting meniscus injuries but is not always necessary to make the diagnosis.

- Treatment by physician: Arthroscopic repair of a peripheral meniscus tear should be performed within the first 2 weeks following the injury. If there is a minor tear, an arthroscopic partial resection is performed. Small partial tears (< 1 cm) that are associated with ACL injuries, and do not cross through the entire meniscus, may heal without surgery.
- Treatment by therapist: Physical therapy consists of general strength training and neuromuscular training after meniscus resection. The practitioner should be particularly aware of the potential for significant muscle atrophy in patients who had long-term knee pain prior to the injury being diagnosed. Rehabilitation continues until muscle strength and bulk are restored. Both the patient and the therapist should carefully monitor the knee for postoperative pain or swelling after a meniscus resection because this is may indicate the onset of osteoarthritis.
- Prognosis: The prognosis for meniscal tears is generally good. A sutured meniscal injury requires at least 4–6 months of rehabilitation before the athlete may return to sports activities in which the knee is subjected to torsional loading. The athlete may return to sports activities within 4 weeks of a minor resection. The long-term prognosis is unknown; however, a total resection of medial meniscus puts the patient at high risk for radiographic arthrosis within 2–10 years, whereas a partial resection appears to only moderately increase the risk of arthrosis during the same time. Lateral meniscus resections must be followed more closely as arthritis can develop in some athletes in less than a year. The prognosis of cartilage and meniscus injuries in children is also typically good, and they seldom cause symptoms into adulthood.

Dislocated Patella—*Dislocated Kneecap*

The most common cause of an acute knee hemarthrosis, other than a cruciate ligament or meniscus tear, is a lateral patellar dislocation (Figure 12.19). This injury can result from a direct blow, but is more commonly associated with noncontact twisting injuries involving external rotation of the tibia combined with a forceful quadriceps contraction. The patella dislocates laterally which disrupts the medial retinaculum. Spontaneous reduction frequently occurs when the patient instinctively attempts to straighten his or her leg. When the patella relocates, osteochondral fragmentation can occur as the medal patella facet abuts the lateral femoral condyle. These two areas, in particular, should be scrutinized for osteochondral damage.

- Symptoms and signs: While a patellar or quadriceps tendon rupture usually causes significant local swelling, a dislocated patella almost always causes a hemarthrosis. The patient will experience tenderness at the medial retinaculum.
- Diagnosis: Diagnosis is based on reduced range of motion, particularly with flexion, and pain along the medial patellar border. If an attempt is made to displace the patella laterally, the patient reacts by reporting pain and/or contracting their quadriceps muscle thus limiting patella excursion (positive lateral patellar apprehension test). In the acute setting, passive patella mobility is hard to judge secondary to pain. In the subacute or chronic setting, increased passive patella lateral translation is a necessary component to make the diagnosis of a lateral patella dislocation. The practitioner should always obtain radiographs since a dislocation may result in an avulsion or osteochondral fracture from the medial patella or lateral femoral condyle.
- Treatment by physician: The patella usually self reduces, which can be confirmed by anteroposterior radiographs. If the patella has not already

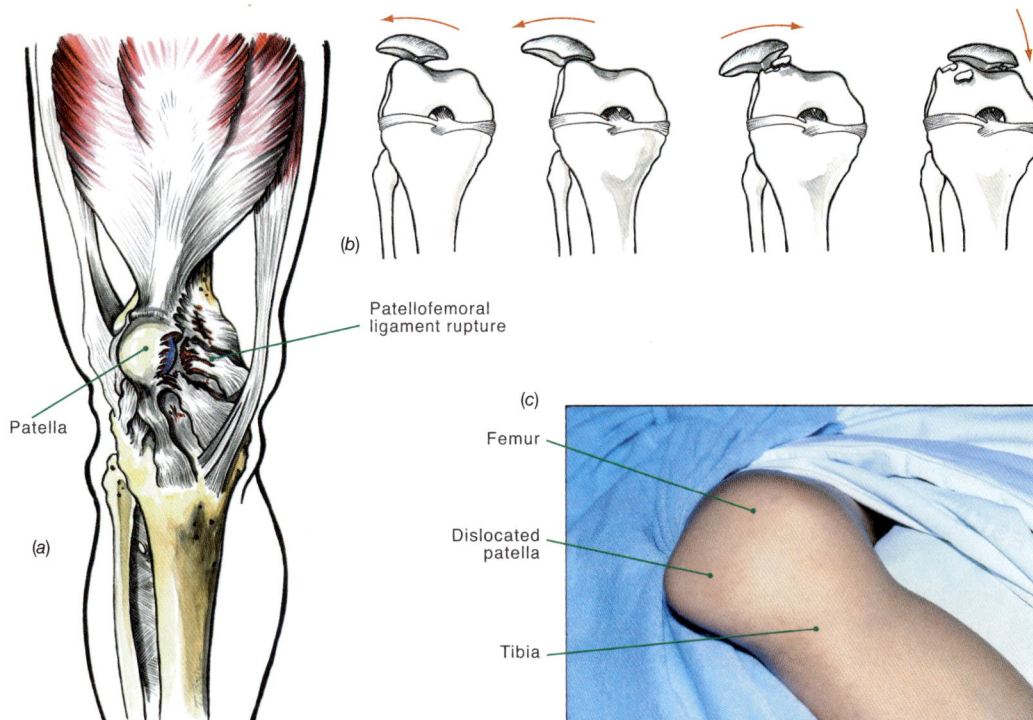

Figure 12.19 Patellar dislocation. The patella glides out laterally. The patellofemoral ligaments tear on the medial side, and severe bleeding occurs into the joint (a). Often a small fracture occurs at the femur when the patella dislocates (b). Typical clinical appearance (c). (© Medical Illustrator Tommy Bolic, Sweden.)

spontaneously reduced, a physician should immediately reduce it. This can typically be done under local anesthesia or conscious sedation by extending the knee while gently lifting the medial patella border. There is no consensus regarding *surgical treatment* for patella dislocations; however, most practitioners agree that patella dislocations associated with radiographic osteochondral fragmentation should undergo arthroscopy with debridement or fracture repair. Any tear in the medial retinaculum can be repaired at that same time. Nonsurgical treatments are directed at providing an environment where the patella does not dislocate and restoring joint motion and strength. While most physicians agree on the goals of such treatment, there is no consensus on the degree or length of knee immobilization. In the presence of a significant hemarthrosis, application of a compression dressing and immobilization in extension is appropriate until early motion and weight bearing are tolerated. The patient should increase weight bearing and independent knee motion as their knee pain and strength allow. Return to full activities should be based on functional strength rather than a specific time period from the original injury.

• Treatment by therapist: Initial physical therapy should be directed toward return of joint motion and reduction of swelling. The muscle groups targeted for strengthening are the core muscles and those that control limb rotation, in addition to the quadriceps muscles. Typically 6 weeks of monitored activities, which avoid pivoting and twisting activities of the knee, is recommended.

• Prognosis: Nonsurgical treatment of younger, active patients, with normal bony architecture of the patellofemoral joint is usually successful; however, in patients with significant patella alta and/or trochlea dysplasia, redislocation occurs in more than 50% of cases. Athletes typically return to sporting activities within 3–4 months.

Femoral Condyle/Tibial Plateau Fracture

Traffic accidents and falls are more likely to cause femoral condyle and tibial plateau fractures than sporting activities; however, tibial plateau fractures are relatively common in skiers, especially those over the age of 40. The same injury mechanisms leading to cruciate ligament and collateral ligament injuries may also cause fractures, most frequently in the tibial plateau (Figure 12.20) and less commonly in the femoral condyles or the patella. A tibial plateau fracture may cause a step-off in the joint surface and allow blood to enter the joint space from the bone marrow. If the articular step-off is more than 2–3 mm, the patient must undergo surgery to avoid subsequent development of arthrosis and instability in the joint. An acute knee effusion in an older skier should always be assessed to rule out a potential tibial plateau fracture.

- Symptoms and signs: The patient will have pain upon loading the knee and hemarthrosis will be present. Tibial plateau fractures must be ruled out when a patient has sustained a high-energy trauma, especially for elderly patients and patients with osteoporosis.
- Diagnosis: Radiographs will usually confirm the diagnosis, but occasionally depression of the tibial plateau can only be assessed on computerized tomography scanning or MRI due to bony overlap and/or mild joint space compression. Oblique view radiographs may also help determine the diagnosis. The practitioner should watch for epiphyseal injuries in children since they may be difficult to detect. For this reason, patients younger than 15 years should have radiographs of the healthy side taken for comparison.
- Treatment by physician: Patients who may have a fracture or who have a fracture verified by radiograph should be referred to an orthopedic surgeon for evaluation. Typically, these type of injuries need to be assessed to determine if they require surgery.
- Prognosis: The prognosis depends solely on the nature of the fracture, which may vary from major crushing of the tibia in ski jumpers to minimal depression fractures in recreational slalom skiers. A normal healing period for minor injuries is 6–12 weeks, but the athlete will be away from sports activities for a minimum of 3 months.

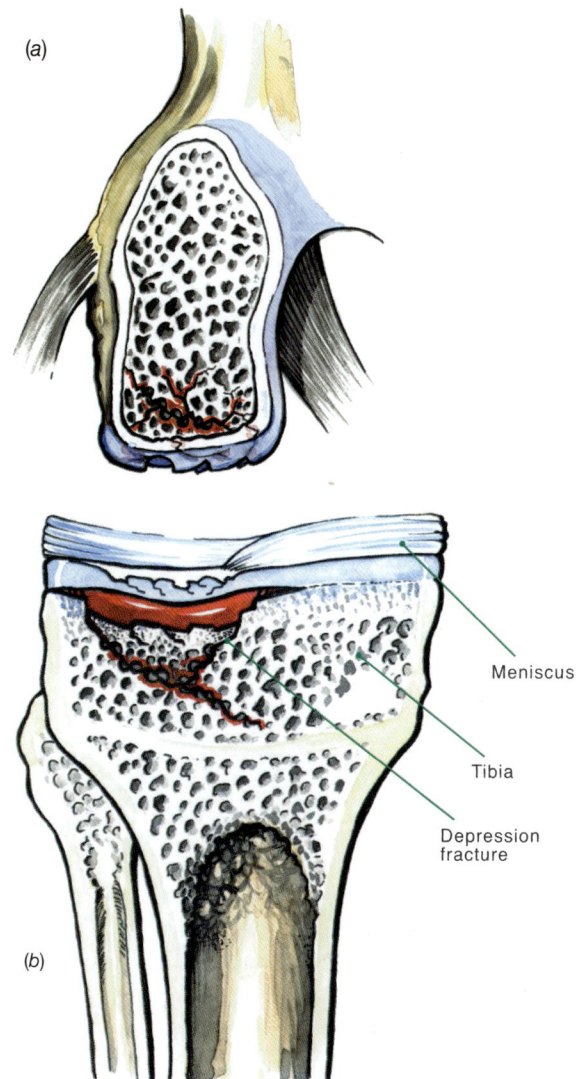

(a)

(b)

Meniscus

Tibia

Depression fracture

Figure 12.20 Femoral condyle fracture (a); tibial plateau fracture (b). (© Medical Illustrator Tommy Bolic, Sweden.)

Other Injuries

Posterior Cruciate Ligament Tears

Only one out of every ten cruciate ligament injuries involves the posterior cruciate ligament (Figure 12.21). Combined injuries occur in more than half of these cases. Approximately 50% of posterior cruciate ligament injuries are sports related injuries while the remainders are due to traffic accidents. The most common cause of posterior cruciate ligament tears is a direct blow to the upper portion of the tibia, such as can happen in a collision with a hockey sideboard or by an athlete falling directly

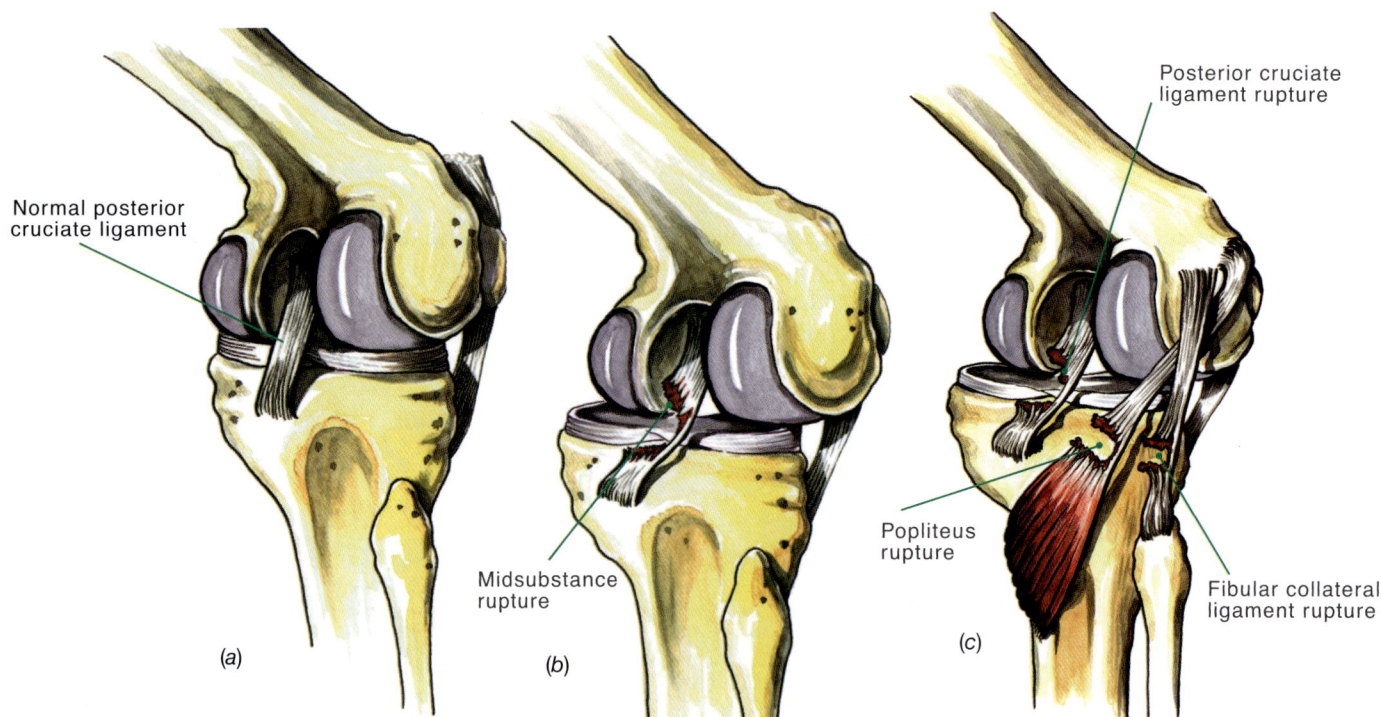

Figure 12.21 Posterior cruciate ligament injury. Normal (*a*). The injury may be isolated or (*b*) part of a combined, larger injury (*c*). (© Medical Illustrator Tommy Bolic, Sweden.)

on the tibia with the knee flexed, forcing the tibia posteriorly. A direct anterior blow will push the tibia backward in relation to the femur, causing damage to the posterior cruciate ligament. The blow is often not directed precisely anterior to the tibia, and there is a medial or lateral component to the force causing the posterior cruciate ligament to tear in combination with other structures, laterally or medially, respectively.

- **Symptoms and signs:** The patient often states that he or she sustained a direct blow to the front of their tibia, which can occur when an athlete dives into the goal area or into the sideboard in hockey. Generally, the patient experiences an acute onset of pain following the injury. Patients with posterior cruciate ligament injuries do not necessarily develop knee hemarthrosis with early onset swelling, but swelling eventually occurs in most patients.
- **Diagnosis:** The diagnosis is made clinically, based on a positive posterior drawer test. Patients frequently sustain combined injuries and must be carefully examined for such injuries. The patient should also undergo MRI if associated injuries are suspected following clinical examination.
- **Treatment by physician:** A patient with an isolated partial posterior cruciate ligament tear may be treated by active rehabilitation and does require referral to an orthopedic surgeon. Patients with a complete posterior cruciate ligament tears or combined ligament injuries, especially those with major posterolateral injuries or dislocated knees, are surgically treated, preferably within 2 weeks of the injury. As is the case for ACL tears, functional bracing has no documented positive effect on these injuries.
- **Treatment by therapist:** Patients often require several months of training, which focuses on increasing range of motion, decreasing edema and restoring quadriceps function. Training the quadriceps muscle after a posterior cruciate ligament injury is particularly important because it is a major dynamic stabilizer of the knee and may limit slipping of the femur in relation to the tibia. For the first 2 weeks

postoperatively knee flexion should be limited to 90° and range of motion exercises should be performed with the patient lying prone. After 2 weeks flexion can increase as tolerated and the patient should be put in a brace that protects the reconstructed ligament from posterior stress during normal range of motion.

- Prognosis: Isolated partial posterior tears seldom cause symptoms during sports activity; however, the patient may gradually experience instability as the scarred in posterior cruciate ligament tear stretches over time. This subset of patients will eventually require surgery.

Knee Dislocation *!*

Knee dislocations (Figure 12.22) are rare occurrence, but they are often accompanied by vascular and nerve injury, which makes early detection of these injuries extremely important. In sports activities, this injury can result from a major fall–for example, during ski jumping or when riding motorcycles–but dislocations also occur in football, basketball, soccer, and team handball. A dislocated knee is defined by a complete tear of at least three of the knee's four major ligaments– the medial and fibular collateral ligaments, and the anterior and posterior cruciate ligaments.

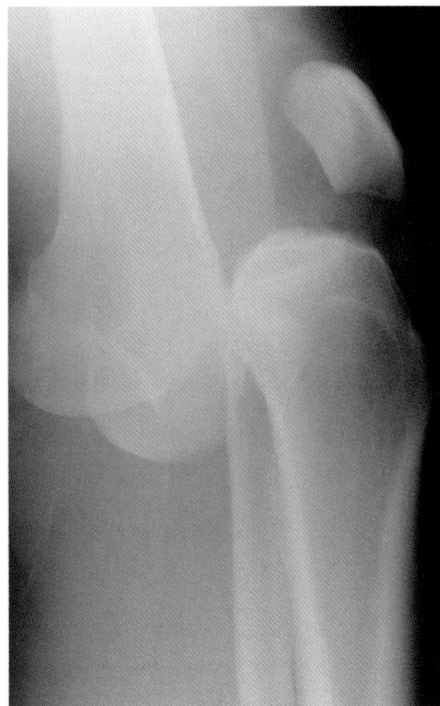

Figure 12.22 Knee dislocation. This injury is defined by a total tear in at least three of the four most important stabilizers in the knee, the medial and fibular collateral ligaments and the anterior and posterior cruciate ligaments.

- Symptoms and signs: Knee dislocation patients are usually in severe pain. Nearly one out of every three patients with a knee dislocation has signs of concomitant injury to the peroneal nerve. The practitioner should always check for a pulse at the dorsum of the foot: 10% or more of patients with a knee dislocation have an associated vascular injury. If the vessel is torn at the level of the knee, circulation must be restored within a few hours to avoid permanent damage or amputation. If more than 8 hours have elapsed, the amputation rate is nearly 90%.
- Diagnosis: Diagnosing a knee dislocation is based on the joint being unstable in at least three directions. There will be no doubt about the presence of a major injury. The Lachman test and posterior drawer test are positive, in addition to the varus or valgus test (or both) at 20° of knee flexion.
- Treatment by physician: In rare cases, reduction on site when the injury occurs may be difficult. If this situation, the physician must pull carefully along the extremity's longitudinal axis to reduce the tibia and the femur at the same time. If transport to a hospital is not readily available, the knee must be stabilized with an orthosis, cast or brace. Further orthopedic evaluation of this type of injury should take place immediately. At the hospital, the patient will undergo accurate neurological and vascular diagnostic tests followed by MRI to confirm the injury and rule out any fracture at the femur. If there is evidence of damage to the blood vessels, the patient will have immediate surgery to repair the vascular injury. If possible, a CT angiogram should be obtained to locate the area of the arterial injury, but this should not be done if a long delay is required for the test. In this case, injured ligaments will be attended to a few weeks later. If no vascular injury has occurred, a multiple ligament reconstruction can be performed within the first 2–3 weeks. The goal is to stabilize the patient for exercising and prevent reduced range of motion.
- Treatment by therapist: Recovery from a knee dislocation is a long-lasting and time-consuming process, often taking up to a year or more. Patients typically require mobilization of the knee joint as well as regular strength training and neuromuscular training.
- Prognosis: This is such a severe injury that few patients return to prior sports activities.

KNEE

Quadriceps/Patellar Tendon Rupture

Total rupture of the patella or quadriceps tendon is a rare occurrence. The injury mechanism is generally a fall on a flexed knee or sudden eccentric load in the presence of underlying degenerative change in the tendon. Patellar tendon tears and avulsions from the tibial tuberosity in children are often incorrectly diagnosed as Osgood–Schlatter disease. Instead of a torn patellar or quadriceps tendon, a child may have an injury known as a sleeve fracture. A sleeve fracture occurs when the patellar tendon, along with its insertion to the patella, tears off the patella like a glove. Medications, such as corticosteroids prescribed to rheumatoid patients, and anabolic steroids may contribute to weakening of the tendon.

- Symptoms and signs: The main symptom is an inability to actively extend the knee. If the patient's extensor apparatus is ruptured, he or she will be unable to keep the knee extended when the thigh is lifted off the table. Patients sometimes sustain only partial injuries that leave the extension mechanism intact. In children, avulsions of the tuberosity cause pain when the extensor apparatus is used, while sleeve fractures make it impossible for the child to keep the knee in an extended position.
- Diagnosis: Palpation of a complete tear will often reveal a gap above or below the patella. MRI or ultrasound examinations are not usually necessary, but they can be helpful in confirming the diagnosis.
- Treatment by physician: Extensor apparatus ruptures require surgery, ideally performed within 2 weeks. Infrapatella tendon ruptures require a longer time to heal before forceful knee extension is allowed. This prevents stretching of the tendon during the healing phase, which has been shown to cause patella alta. Grade I and II avulsions from the tibial tubercle in younger patients can be treated with immobilization for 4–5 weeks, whereas grade IV (total separation) must be evaluated for surgery. Sleeve fractures from the patella require surgical treatment.
- Prognosis: The prognosis is good, but athletes often have difficulty fully flexing the knee for the first year after injury.

Chondral and Osteochondral Injuries—*Cartilaginous Injury*

In up to 90% of major knee injuries, crushing of the subchondral bone occurs. This damages both the bone and the bone marrow under the cartilage (Figure 12.23), and eventually, the cartilage over the bone is also affected. Despite injury, the cartilage may look unremarkable to the naked eye. Approximately one out of every ten patients who is referred for arthroscopy has a cartilaginous injury, and about half of those would benefit from a surgery to resurface the cartilage. Osteochondritis dissecans (OCD) can often occur in patients with no previous history of knee trauma.

- Symptoms and signs: Patients provide a history of torsional trauma, which is often followed by activity-dependent swelling in the joint and periodic pain, sometimes with locking.
- Diagnosis: It is difficult to make a clinical diagnosis unless locking occurs. Therefore, arthroscopy is often used if the patient has recurring effusions or locking. Notch view radiographs are the most useful for revealing OCD, while MRI may reveal other cartilage disorders. The practitioner should be aware that smaller and less powerful MRI apparatus (<1.5 tesla magnets), designed for examining the extremities, are poorly suited to diagnosing cartilaginous injuries.

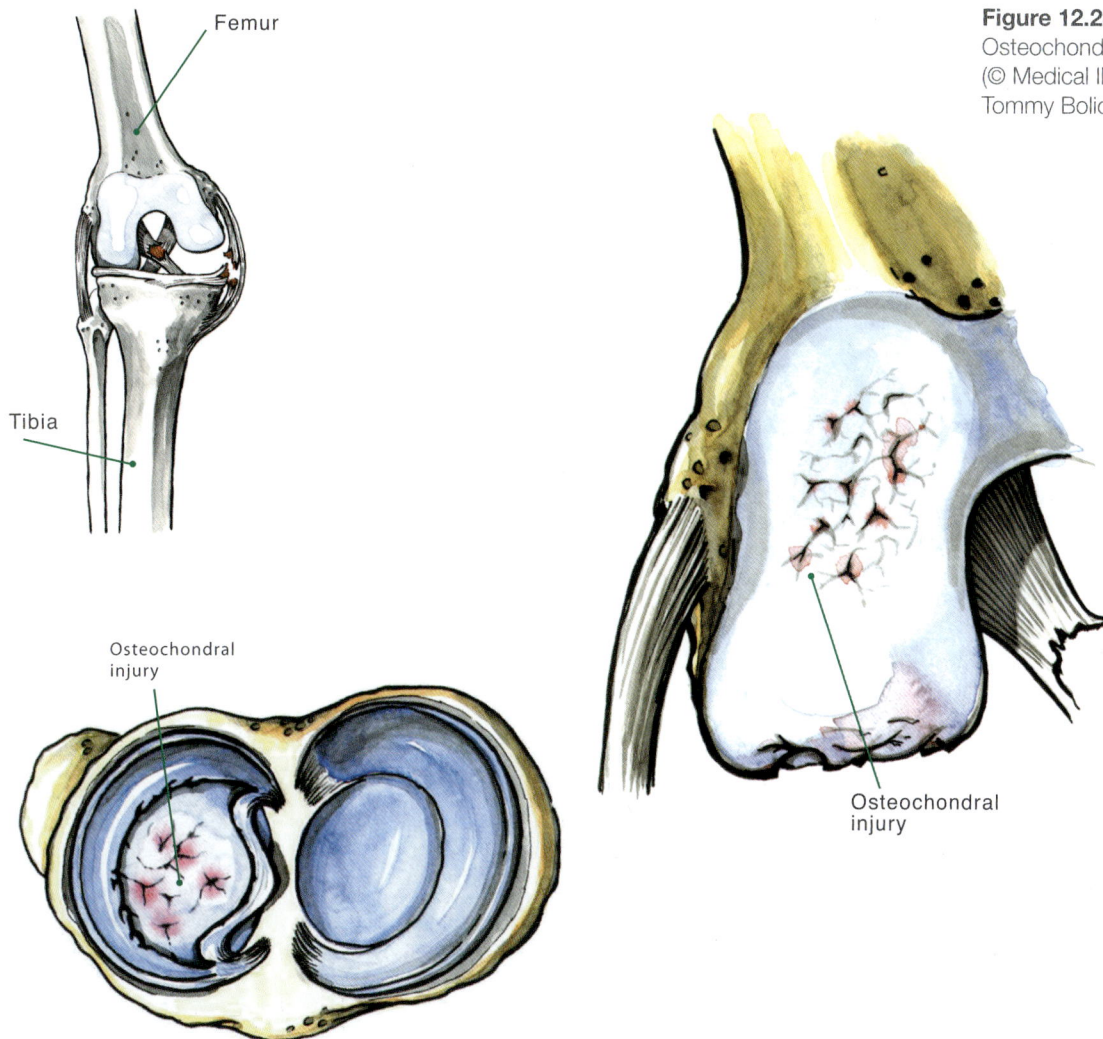

Figure 12.23
Osteochondral injuries.
(© Medical Illustrator
Tommy Bolic, Sweden.)

- **Treatment by physician:** Usually, a loose piece of cartilage will be removed via arthroscopy, but occasionally, it may be fixed with pins or screws. A number of possible treatments are available such as microfracture technique, mosaicplasty, cadaver allografts, and cartilage transplantation; however, the long-term results of these interventions are still not known.
- **Prognosis:** Prognosis is good in the short term. In the long term, lesions of more than 2 cm^2 increase the frequency of osteoarthritis and may significantly reduce knee function after 10 years.

Patellar Fracture—*Kneecap Fracture*

Patellar fractures occur as the result of direct trauma to the patella, such as a fall from a bicycle or a blow from a puck with inadequate knee padding. The most common patellar fractures seen in sports are transverse fractures, but longitudinal fractures also occur (Figure 12.24).

- **Symptoms and signs:** The patient experiences immediate strong pain and rapid swelling and is unable to stand upright. The fracture cleft can often be palpated.
- **Diagnosis:** Radiographs of the patella confirm the diagnosis.

- **Treatment by physician:** A nondisplaced patellar fracture that has an intact extensor mechanism may be treated nonoperatively via immobilization in a cast for 4–6 weeks. During that time, weight bearing is allowed on the cast. Once the patella is no longer tender to palpation and radiographic signs of healing are present, the cast can be replaced by a hinged brace and physical therapy aimed at strengthening and range of motion may begin. Displaced fractures or those with an interrupted extensor mechanism will require surgical repair using cannulated screws and steel wire. Restoration of articular congruity and the extensor mechanism continuity are critical with the goal of making the fracture stable for exercising without a step-off in the articular surface. Following surgery, a knee immobilizer is worn for protection until early union of the fracture can be seen on radiographs. Range of motion exercises are started in the postoperative period based upon the safe limits of motion determined by the surgeon. Fractures with stable internal fixation can start with early therapy and weight bearing as tolerated with flexion limited to the amount determined to be safe by the surgeon. With less stable fixation or in noncompliant patients, weight bearing is not allowed until 4–6 weeks after surgery.
- **Treatment by therapist:** Physical therapy focuses on flexibility training, which aims to increase range of motion and decrease swelling. Isometric strength training may begin after 2 weeks.
- **Prognosis:** Prognosis is good in the short term because patellar fractures usually heal within 6–8 weeks. Long-term problems include reduction of flexion, particularly from cartilage injuries where the symptoms usually do not appear until about 3–12 months after the initial injury, when the patient begins full loading of the knee. Cartilage injuries of the patella may limit stair climbing or other activities that require the knee to be loaded in flexion.

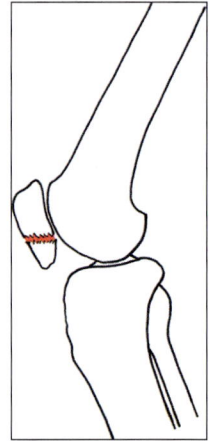

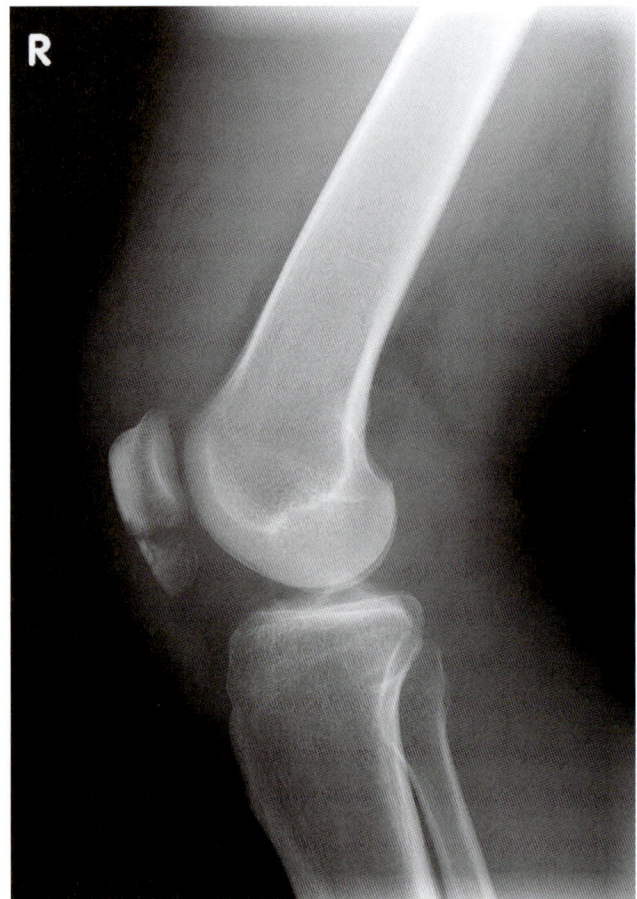

Figure 12.24 Lateral radiograph showing a transverse patellar fracture in the right knee. (© Medical Illustrator Tommy Bolic, Sweden.)

Knee Pain

Robert F. LaPrade[1,2], *Casey M. Pierce*[2], *Roald Bahr*[3], *Lars Engebretsen*[3], *Jill Cook*[4], *Elizabeth Arendt*[5], *and Nicholas Mohtadi*[6]

[1]*The Steadman Clinic, Vail, CO, USA*
[2]*Steadman Philippon Research Institute, Vail, CO, USA*
[3]*Norwegian School of Sport Sciences, Oslo, Norway*
[4]*Monash University, Frankston, VIC, Australia*
[5]*University of Minnesota, Minneapolis, MN, USA*
[6]*University of Calgary Sport Medicine Centre, Calgary, AB, Canada*

Definition

This chapter will discuss painful conditions in the area of the knee. In most cases, this pain develops gradually, without a history of trauma or acute injury. Occasionally, an overuse injury will develop as the result of a single hard or unfamiliar training session, but generally, pain gradually sets in over several days or weeks. Athletes may also have significant symptoms from a previous ligament injury if the knee has become unstable.

Differential Diagnoses

Table 12.2 provides an overview of the key differential diagnoses for knee pain. Meniscus injuries and overuse injuries, such as jumper's knee and patellofemoral pain syndrome (PFPS), are the most common causes of pain; however, recurring instability after a major knee injury often prevents athletes from returning to sports activities. Meniscus injuries are discussed in the previous chapter on acute injuries,

Most common	Less common	Must not be overlooked !
Meniscus injuries, p. 371	Osteochondral injuries, p. 378	Unstable osteochondritis dissecans
Patellofemoral pain syndrome, p. 384	Osteochondritis dissecans, p. 388	Posterior and combined instability, p. 387
Patellar tendinopathy, p. 385	Biceps tendinopathy, p. 389	Tumor
Quadriceps tendinopathy, p. 385	Popliteus tendinopathy, p. 389	Infection
Knee instability, p. 387	Iliotibial band friction syndrome, p. 390	
Post surgical scar tissue entrapment	Pes anserine or deep infrapatellar bursitis	
Bursitis, p. 391	Medial plica syndrome, p. 392	
	Osgood–Schlatter disease, p. 393	
	Sinding–Larsen–Johanson disease, p. 393	
	Knee osteoarthritis	

Table 12.2 Overview of the differential diagnoses of chronic knee pain. (Reproduced with permission from the Norwegian Sports Medicine Association.)

KNEE

but meniscus cysts caused by a chronic injury, usually in the lateral meniscus, and will be discussed here.

Diagnostic Thinking

The main concern when evaluating an athlete is to determine whether their chief problem is pain or instability. Most patients have anterior knee pain resulting from overuse rather than a specific trauma. Occasionally, pain develops following a single hard training session. For example, a patient with signs and symptoms of jumper's knee may experience sudden pain in connection with heavy weight training. In children and adolescents, usually the growth plates are the areas that are affected, but the physician should always order knee radiographs so that OCD is not overlooked. In addition, the diagnosis is usually based on the case history and the clinical examination. If pain persists despite a period of reduced training, the patient should be referred to a knee specialist for a more detailed evaluation. The case history of a patient with acute knee trauma may provide important information about the injury mechanism and can indicate the type of instability in an athlete in a twisting sport (such as soccer or handball) may have experienced.

Case History

A description of the pain and its location is central to the case history and diagnosis. Pain at the beginning of an activity that wears off after warming up but returns after the activity ceases indicates a tendinopathy, such as jumper's knee. Pain that worsens with warm-up and continues through the activity is more indicative of a structural injury, such as a meniscus tear.

Clinical Examinations

Inspection. First, the patient is examined while standing, which allows lower extremity alignment, valgus or varus alignment, and foot mechanics (e.g., flat foot or claw foot) to be evaluated. The quadriceps muscles should be inspected for signs of atrophy. The best way to assess this is with a tape measurer placed 15 cm proximal to the upper patellar pole; the measurement should then be compared to that of the healthy side. Next, the lower extremity is inspected while the patient is sitting down, and the position of the patella on the femoral condyles is noted (e.g., oblique, high, or low). Inspection will usually reveal whether or not the knee contains intra-articular fluid. Any bruising of the skin is also noted.

Palpation. Palpation of painful areas should provide an initial diagnosis for most patients. The patellar tendon, the patellar retinaculum, and the quadriceps tendon are palpated for pain and/or discontinuity. The examiner should push the patella distally while the knee is in extension to bring the origin of the patellar tendon closer to the surface, which allows for a more precise palpation. The quadriceps insertion to the patella should also be palpated, with special emphasis on the vastus medialis oblique muscle. The jumper's knee (patellar tendinopathy) test is administered by pushing the proximal origin of the patellar tendon in toward the distal patellar pole (Figure 12.33). If the patient experiences pain on palpation, the knee is flexed to 90° and the test is repeated. If there is less pain to palpation, the diagnosis of patellar tendinopathy is made. The joint space can be palpated, and a meniscus injury will usually cause pain there. In addition, the examiner should palpate the medial plica, pes anserine bursa, deep infrapatellar bursa, and posterior aspect of the knee (to look for a Baker's cyst). With the knee is full extension, palpation between the medial femoral epicondyle and medial patella should reveal the shelf formed by the medial plica. Pain with palpation of the plica indicates irritation, but should not be mistaken for irritation of the underlying synovium. The pes anserine bursa can be palpated just distal and approximately 3–4 cm medial to the tibial tubercle where the sartorius, semitendinosus, and gracilis tendons insert. Pain at this site indicates possible underlying bursitis. The deep infrapatellar bursa can be readily palpated on the distal 1–2 cm of the patellar tendon, slightly proximal to its insertion on the tibial tubercle. This is best accomplished with the knee in full extension and the quadriceps relaxed.

Mobility. Normal mobility in the knee joint is 0°–5° of hyperextension, and 135°–140° of flexion. Practitioners should be aware that individual patients can show variations in range of motion, so the injured knee should always be compared to the contralateral normal side to determine an individual patient's normal range of motion. If the patient has a chronic knee injury, both flexion and extension will often be reduced. This is often due to osteoarthritic changes, including osteophytes and a thicker and less elastic knee capsule. Normal mobility of the patella is relative to patellar size. If the patella is divided into four equal quadrants each representing 25% of the patellar width, normal range of motion is 1–3 quadrants of translation both medially laterally and inferior-superior in extension. Increased motion can indicate dislocation, while decreased motion can signal patellofemoral syndrome.

Neuromuscular function. The practitioner should palpate the pulses on the dorsum of the foot and behind the medial malleolus and compare them to the healthy side. Functional knee tests are used to detect lower limb dysfunctions: one-leg hop, triple jump, and stair hop tests. For the one-leg hop test, the patient stands on the uninvolved leg and jumps on to the same leg, as far as possible. The same procedure is repeated for the involved leg. For the triple jump test, the patient stands on the uninvolved leg, jumps twice onto the same leg, followed by a jump onto both legs. The same procedure is repeated for the involved leg. The jump distance for the uninvolved and involved leg for the one-leg hop and triple jump tests are recorded and compared.

Special tests. The stability of the knee joint is evaluated using the following special tests. These basic tests are critical in the initial evaluation of an acute knee injury and should be included in any practitioner's evaluation. The Lachman test at 30° (Figure 12.6), varus/valgus stress tests at 20° (Figure 12.7), sag test (Figure 12.8), pivot shift test (Figure 12.10), posterolateral Lachman test (Figure 12.11), posterior drawer test at 90° (Figure 12.12), and recurvatum test (Figure 12.13). The menisci are evaluated by the Meniscus tear assessment test (Figure 12.9). The jumper's knee test should be done with the knee in extension; the practitioner pushes the patella distally and palpates the origin of the patellar tendon from the lower patellar pole (Figure 12.26).

Supplemental Examinations

Routine anteroposterior and lateral radiographs are usually included in the initial evaluation of patients with knee pain. If indicated, a 45° axial radiograph should be included in the initial evaluation to examine the patellofemoral joint. Depending on the tentative diagnosis, a specialist should order additional examinations as necessary. Frontal images may be taken with the patient standing with their knees flexed to 45° in order to evaluate the height of the cartilage and the degree of radiographic osteoarthritis. If OCD is suspected, a tunnel image is also taken. Standing, long leg radiographs are used to measure varus or valgus knee alignment. To fully evaluate the patellofemoral joint, true lateral and anteroposterior radiographs taken at 20°–30° of flexion are necessary. MRI may be useful when diagnosing the causes of knee pain; however, radiographs are the gold standard for initial imaging evaluation.

MRI should be considered in situations where radiographs are negative and conservative treatment has not improved the patient's condition. Exceptions include elite athletes where an immediate diagnosis is required and patients who are a high surgical risk. Ultrasound, on the other hand, does not play much of a role in diagnosing the causes of knee pain. This is because ultrasound results are highly dependent on operator skill and not readily reproducible. Ultrasonography is typically useful only to determine the presence of joint effusion or cysts, and to guide a needle for aspiration or injection.

Common Injuries

Patellofemoral Pain Syndrome—*Anterior Knee Pain*

This is the most common cause of knee pain seen in the primary care setting and usually stems from overuse, but may also be caused by direct trauma to the patella, such as would be sustained during a fall. A number of other causes have also been suggested. Excessive knee valgus (increased Q angle) creates a tendency toward lateralization of the patella, which potentially increases loading of the medial patellofemoral ligaments, possibly resulting in pain (Figure 12.25). Pathological nerve endings that have been found in these structures may also account for pain. In addition, leg length discrepancies, hamstring muscle tightness, hip/leg muscle imbalance, insufficient foot pronation, and abnormal patella or trochlea morphologies can contribute to PFPS. Any one of these anatomic factors may be trivial as a single entity; however, in combination with other anatomic variables and associated with overtraining and overuse, they can lead to overuse injury centered on the kneecap. Most younger athletes have normal cartilage on the patella, and superficial changes on the articular surface of the patella do not cause pain. However, athletes with established cartilaginous injuries that extend down to the bone experience pain in this area. Some patients who have sustained a powerful, direct trauma to the patella show initial subchondral changes on MRI that may later produce changes in the cartilage and bone leading to increased pressure inside the patella. Thus, the cause of PFPS is multifactorial. Practitioners should remember that at least 30% of all 16-year olds have such symptoms, 90% of which will recover without treatment.

- Symptoms and signs: Patients with PFPS may have pain in various situations, as shown in Table 12.3.
- Diagnosis: If three of the symptoms listed in Table 12.3 are present, the patient qualifies for the diagnosis of PFPS. The diagnosis is clinical, and as a result, routine radiographs, computed tomography, and MRI typically provide no further information and are usually unnecessary.
- Treatment by physician: In most cases, the athlete will be referred to a therapist who emphasizes thigh and hip abduction strengthening and neuromuscular training. Patients are told to avoid the activities that cause pain and may have to stop physical training to allow for sufficient healing. Many patients benefit from the McConnell program with taping (Figure 12.38) to correct and support patella position during the training phase, but reports demonstrating efficacy of

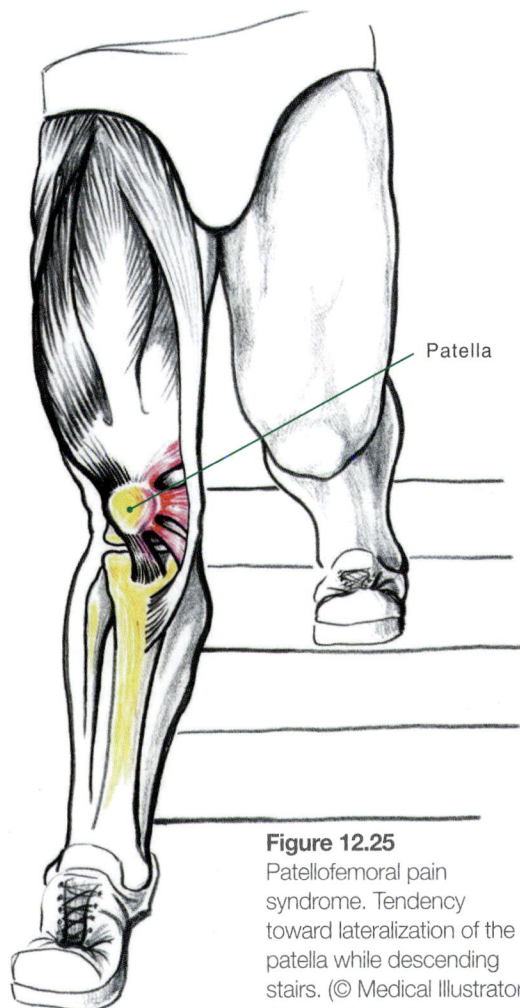

Patella

Figure 12.25
Patellofemoral pain syndrome. Tendency toward lateralization of the patella while descending stairs. (© Medical Illustrator Tommy Bolic, Sweden.)

Most common	Mechanism	Commentary
Pain when going downstairs	Eccentric use of the extensor apparatus causes pressure in the patellofemoral joint	Worst in patients with established osteoarthritis in the patellofemoral joint
Pain when squatting	Difficult to get down and unable to get up without assistance	
Pain when driving	Long-lasting pressure in the patellofemoral joint	
Pain when sitting for a long time (theater sign)	Long-lasting pressure in the patellofemoral joint	
Pain when braking	Developing strong force in the extensor apparatus	Most common in patients with irritation in the patellar tendon

Table 12.3 Overview of the typical symptoms of patellofemoral pain syndrome. (Reproduced with permission from the Norwegian Sports Medicine Association.)

the program are limited. The only indications for surgery are clearly documented findings of recurring patellar dislocations or subluxations or large symptomatic cartilage flaps from chondromalacia.

- **Treatment by therapist:** Therapy directed toward strengthening is the cornerstone for treating PFPS. Therapy is divided into two phases: the acute phase and the recovery phase. In the acute phase, the patient should rest the affected extremity and avoid activities that elicit pain. Nonsteroidal anti-inflammatory drugs and ice can help for symptom management during this process. Many patients will also benefit from taping or a brace to reduce pain. To take the stress off the joint and allow healing during exercise, patients can ride a stationary bike or run in a pool. During the recovery phase, patients will require guidance for therapy, in particular, strength training of the quadriceps and the gluteus medius. Strength is often so reduced in these muscles that several hundred quadriceps contractions will be required daily; therefore, patients require a home program in addition to supervised training. The hip abductors, hamstrings, iliotibial band, and core muscles should also be evaluated and conditioned as needed. Stretching of short muscles should also be included in the rehabilitation program, especially stretching of the lateral structures in the thigh. If present, excessive or insufficient foot pronation should also be addressed with proper shoes or a foot orthosis. Other tools such as orthotics, knee sleeves, and McConnell taping (Figure 12.38) can be used in combination with therapy techniques to treat PFPS.
- **Prognosis:** Prognosis is typically good as the majority of these patients report only mild or occasional symptoms at 5-year follow-up. 85% of patients have successful outcomes following therapy. Persistent symptoms should be evaluated to find specific causes for their pain. Continued abnormal tracking of the patella over the trochlea can lead to the development of arthritis and chronic pain, and surgical intervention may be necessary.

Patellar Tendinopathy—*Jumper's Knee*

Patellar tendinopathy (Figure 12.26) is a common sports-related diagnosis. The prevalence in volleyball players is around 40%, and the disorder is also common among top-level basketball (30–35%) and soccer players (10–15%). Pain is usually localized to the distal patellar pole but, in 10% of patients, the pain is localized to the quadriceps insertion to the patella. In some patients, pain begins after a single jump, lift, or landing; in others, it occurs after a hard training session or game; in still others, the onset is gradual. The cause of the disorder is unknown. In terms of histology, no signs of inflammation usually exist; instead, degenerative changes within the substance of the tendon are found. MRI and ultrasound examination can be normal in some patients with symptoms of jumper's knee.

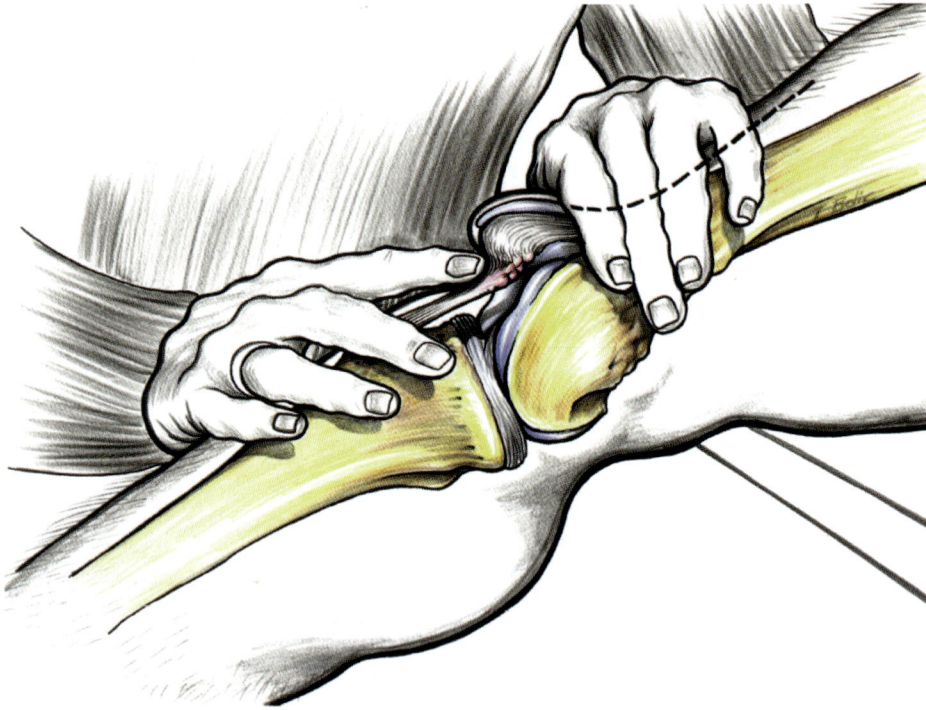

Figure 12.26 Patellar tendinopathy. The injury is usually located proximally in the deeper layer of the patellar tendon.
(© Medical Illustrator Tommy Bolic, Sweden.)

- **Symptoms and signs:** The patient describes activity-dependent pain, which is usually localized to the proximal portions of the patellar tendon and its origin from the inferior patellar pole. In some cases, the patient feels pain at the insertion of the quadriceps tendon on the superior patellar pole. Symptoms often progress with pain after exercise in the initial stages, then pain at the start of an activity, which subsides after warm-up but returns after exercise and, finally, pain both during and after activity. Patients often describe symptoms like those caused by PFPS—for example, pain when walking downstairs, driving a car, or sitting with a bent knee for an extended period of time (theater sign).
- **Diagnosis:** The diagnosis of "Jumper's knee" is made on the basis of distinct tenderness to palpation over the affected tendon insertion and activity-related pain in the same location. The diagnosis of patellar tendinopathy should be reserved for those with imaging findings corresponding to the painful area.
- **Treatment by physician:** Strength training that includes eccentric action, usually for a minimum of 12 weeks, should be the initial treatment for this group; however, patients who do not benefit from this training after 6 months may require surgery, which is probably best done as an arthroscopic procedure under ultrasound guidance. There is some evidence to suggest that ultrasound-guided sclerosing injections can improve symptoms substantially, but this rarely leads to complete resolution of symptoms. Evidence supporting the use of cortisone injections or other local therapy (such as electrotherapy or shock-wave therapy) typically shows initial improvements, but does not yield a lasting positive effect. Early clinical results for studies using platelet rich plasma to treat Jumper's knee have been encouraging, indicating that serial injections can potentially improve clinical outcomes; however further data is still needed to evaluate their long term efficacy. Nonsteroidal anti-inflammatory drugs often provide patients with temporary pain relief.
- **Treatment by therapist:** Eccentric strength training has a positive effect on some patients with this Jumper's knee. Eccentric training should be performed twice daily with three sets of 15 repetitions in each session. Each training

session takes about 5 minutes. The exercises can be done at home and should be performed on a 25°-declined board. Squats should go down to about 90° of knee flexion. The downward component (eccentric component) is on the affected leg, and the upward component on the asymptomatic leg. If both legs are injured, the patients should use their arms to maintain balance during the concentric phase. The eccentric component of each exercise should last for 2 seconds. The subjects should attempt these exercises despite mild to moderate pain with the movements but should stop or reduce load if the pain becomes disabling. Start the training without an external load and add load to a backpack in 5-kg increments as pain decreases. Heavy slow resistance training performed three times a week has also shown to be equally effective. This program includes three bilateral exercises (squat, leg press, and hack squat) with four sets of each exercise progressing from a 15 repetition maximum to a six repetition maximum during a minimum of 12 weeks. Patients should be instructed to spend 3 seconds completing each of the eccentric and concentric phases (i.e., 6 seconds per repetition). These programs are completed with the therapist closely monitoring the patient's entire exercise routine. Heavy slow resistance training performed three times a week has also been shown to be effective for this condition.

- Prognosis: Outcomes are typically good if conservative treatment is started early. When necessary, surgery yields positive outcomes in 60–70% of cases. Some patients are unable to return to sports activity at a high level, but the condition has not been shown to cause arthrosis or other chronic problems later in life.

Knee Instability

Most commonly, knee instability is caused by an untreated ACL tear. If an athlete continues to participate in his or her sport, the knee may be subjected to additional injuries (Figure 12.27). Combined instabilities or concurrent meniscal tears often make participation in twisting sports difficult if not impossible.

Figure 12.27 Injuries to the posterolateral corner. (© Medical Illustrator Tommy Bolic, Sweden.)

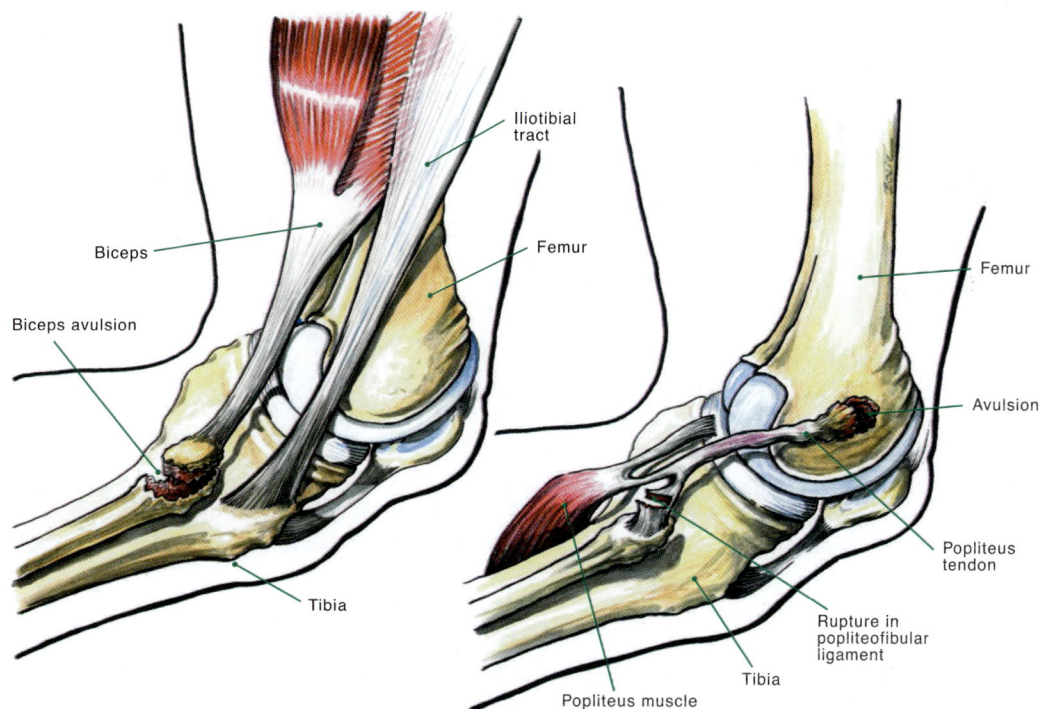

- Symptoms and signs: An accurate case history will almost always reveal a history of knee injury. Patients complain about joint instability more than they do about pain. The most bothersome symptom is usually constant subluxation caused by twisting movements. Subluxation eventually causes meniscal and cartilaginous injury with activity-dependent joint swelling as a clinical sign.
- Diagnosis: The diagnosis is made clinically with the help of stability tests. These are a positive Lachman and pivot shift test for ACL tears; a positive posterior drawer test at 90° flexion for posterior cruciate ligament tears; and a positive posterior Lachman at 30°, increased external rotation of the tibia at 30°, and a positive reversed pivot shift for posterolateral injuries. A positive external rotation recurvatum test also demonstrates a combined posterolateral corner injury and ACL tear. Routine radiographs are useful in evaluating the degree of osteoarthritis that has developed. Stress radiographs to evaluate posterior cruciate ligament tears or collateral ligament injuries are the gold standard in the diagnosis of chronic ligament injuries. MRI often does not help during the chronic phase with respect to evaluating instability.
- Treatment by physician: If an ACL injury has occurred, the athlete usually either has to stop participating in twisting sports or undergo surgery. Surgery is also indicated for combined instability, but even with surgery athletes will not always be able to return to their previous level of competition. Braces and other support devices do not help when participating in twisting sports, nor will functional training alone help athletes return to twisting sports if they have major instability.
- Treatment by therapist: Strength exercises and neuromuscular training will help to improve the patient's coordination, control, and daily life functioning.
- Prognosis: Athletes with major, combined instability will generally be unable to tolerate sports that require pivoting maneuvers.

Other Causes of Pain and Injuries

Osteochondritis Dissecans—*Separation of Cartilage and Bone Fragments*

OCD is a disorder in which the supply of blood to a piece of bone on the articular surface of the femur is reduced without a known trigger or previous trauma. This results in the eventual separation of the bone fragment from its insertion (Figure 12.28). Ultimately, the cartilage overlying the bone becomes unstable or comes completely loose, resulting in significant pain. Most patients are young, often less than 16 years of age. Older patients with OCD often recall having experienced mild symptoms for several years, indicating that the disorder had an early onset.

- Symptoms and signs: Patients with OCD often have no history of acute trauma in their case history, which is dissimilar to cartilaginous injuries in general.

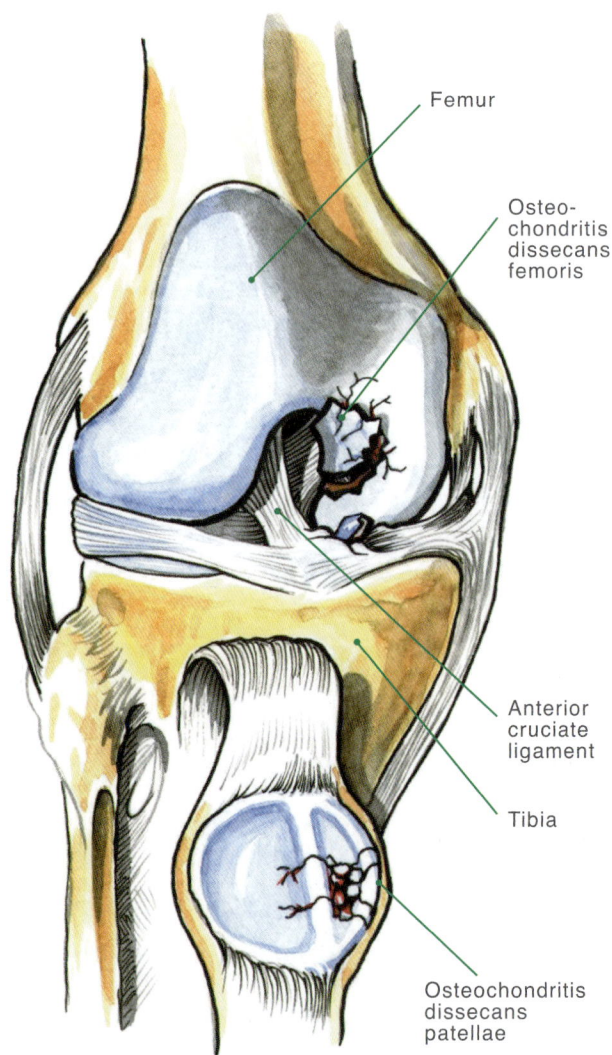

Figure 12.28
Osteochondritis dissecans. Loose bone fragments on the femoral condyle with overlying cartilage damage. The injury can also affect the patella. (© Medical Illustrator Tommy Bolic, Sweden.)

Symptoms though, are often the same as for traumatic cartilage injuries–pain with loading, locking of the joint, and load-dependent joint swelling.

- Diagnosis: The diagnosis is difficult to make based on clinical findings alone. Plain radiographs of the knee with tunnel views often produce the diagnosis. MRI is also useful, but high field strength MRI scans (> 1.5 tesla) are required to best demonstrate the articular cartilage lesions. To clarify whether the bone fragment is loose, magnetic resonance arthrography is best suited. Signal from contrast or joint fluid that has leaked in underneath the loose fragment is diagnostic for an unstable OCD lesion that requires surgical repair.
- Treatment by physician: This type of patient should be referred to an orthopedic surgeon. The preferred treatment for patients who are not fully grown is to avoid weight bearing, using crutches, and to work on maintaining range of motion for 6 weeks. An unloading brace for 6–s12 weeks has also been reported to help decrease symptoms and improve the lesion's chances of healing. Surgery is utilized as a last resort to either properly restore the blood supply or fix the fractured bone. Treatments often used for adults are arthroscopy with fixation of the bone and cartilage fragments, microfracture surgery, mosaicplasty, and cadaver allograft transplantation.
- Prognosis: The prognosis is excellent for children with OCD; more than 90% are left with no symptoms after 5 years. Unfortunately, the prognosis is not as good in adults, and the risk for early development of osteoarthritis is quite high. New methods of treating cartilage injuries appear promising in the short term; however, long-term results are not yet known.

Biceps Tendinopathy and Popliteus Tendinopathy

The thick, strong tendons surrounding the knee joint can become painful with overuse. This is particularly true of the two-headed biceps femoris and the popliteus tendon that is directly in front of the fibular collateral ligament (Figure 12.29). However, these are uncommon tendon problems compared to those affecting the quadriceps and patellar tendons.

- Symptoms and signs: If there is an overuse injury, the patient feels pain during flexion against resistance. Popliteus tendinopathy is usually found close to the origin of the popliteus tendon, about 18 mm in front of the origin of the fibular collateral ligament on the femur. In both cases, the patient will suffer from pain when running or participating in sports activities.
- Diagnosis: Diagnosis is clinical, by palpation and isometric testing of the biceps and popliteus muscles. Having the patient go for a long run, to provoke symptoms, is often useful before the physician begins the examination. A diagnostic block, with a small amount of local anesthetic, might also be helpful. A biceps femoris

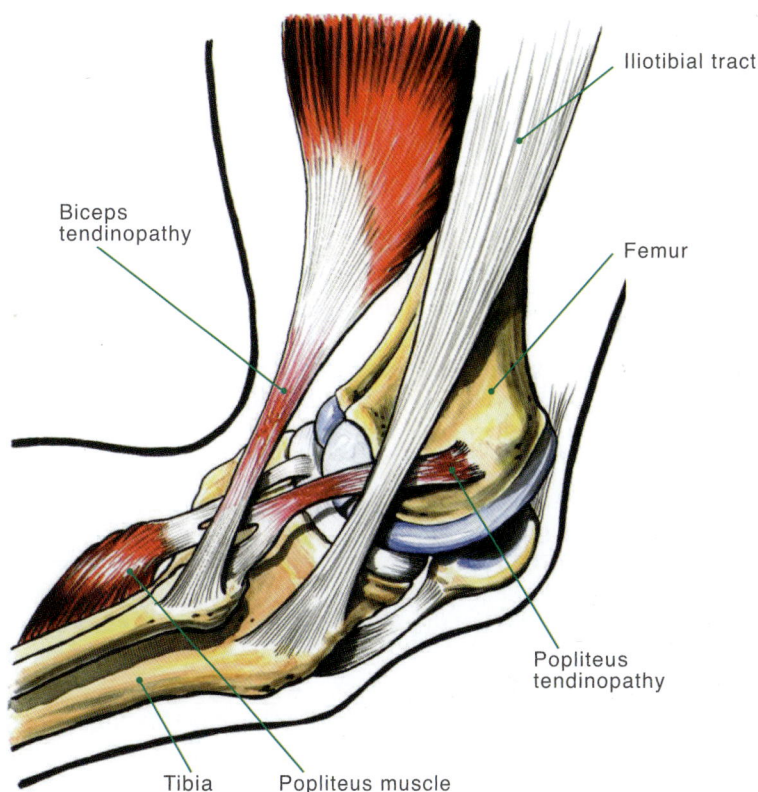

Iliotibial tract

Femur

Biceps tendinopathy

Popliteus tendinopathy

Tibia   Popliteus muscle

Figure 12.29 Biceps tendinopathy, popliteus tendinopathy. Other tendons in the area may also be affected, but these two are the most common. (© Medical Illustrator Tommy Bolic, Sweden.)

KNEE

injury is often caused by an acute avulsion at the insertion of the long and short biceps tendon on the fibula; therefore, early radiographs may be useful. A notch view radiograph can show osteophytes along the popliteal notch on the femur. MRI may reveal increased fluid content as a sign of active tendinopathy.

- Treatment by physician: If the radiographic examination is negative, a cortisone injection may be administered, but there are no studies in the literature to document a definite positive effect. Nonsteroidal anti-inflammatory drugs are a preferable alternative, possibly as a gel, during the early phase.
- Treatment by therapist: Adjusting training is important to alter the loading pattern of this patient group.
- Prognosis: With rest and treatment, the prognosis is good for biceps and popliteus tendinopathy.

Iliotibial Band Friction Syndrome—*Runner's Knee*

Tendinopathy of the iliotibial band (Figure 12.30) is known as runner's knee because it commonly affects long-distance runners. With overuse and monotonous running, the tendon of the iliotibial band becomes tender, and the athlete cannot tolerate running long distances. The distal portion of the tendon becomes irritated as it rubs against a layer of densely innervated fat tissue that covers the lateral femoral epicondyle. There is often a small bursa between the tendon and the bone, which may become inflamed as well.

- Symptoms and signs: The main symptom is activity-dependent pain located near the largest prominence of the lateral femoral condyle. There can be crepitation, but usually the patient only experiences distinct pain with palpation. The onset of pain varies, but most patients note onset after running 2–3 km or more. Additionally, patients often describe pain when climbing stairs or rising from a seated position.
- Diagnosis: Diagnosis is made clinically. The main finding on palpation is tenderness in the lateral lower thigh or upper knee. A diagnostic block with a small dose of lidocaine will confirm the diagnosis. Radiographs can be taken to help exclude other conditions.
- Treatment by physician: Alternative training, stretching of the iliotibial band and cortisone injections have a documented effect on this condition. Surgery is an option if the pain lasts longer than 6 months.
- Treatment by therapist: Stretching the iliotibial band (Figure 12.31a), as well as the gluteal and thigh muscles (Figure 11.31b and c), is generally helpful. Therapists should also direct training toward and provide advice about changing the patient's loading pattern and possibility changing the type running shoes.
- Prognosis: The prognosis for runner's knee is good with proper therapy and training.

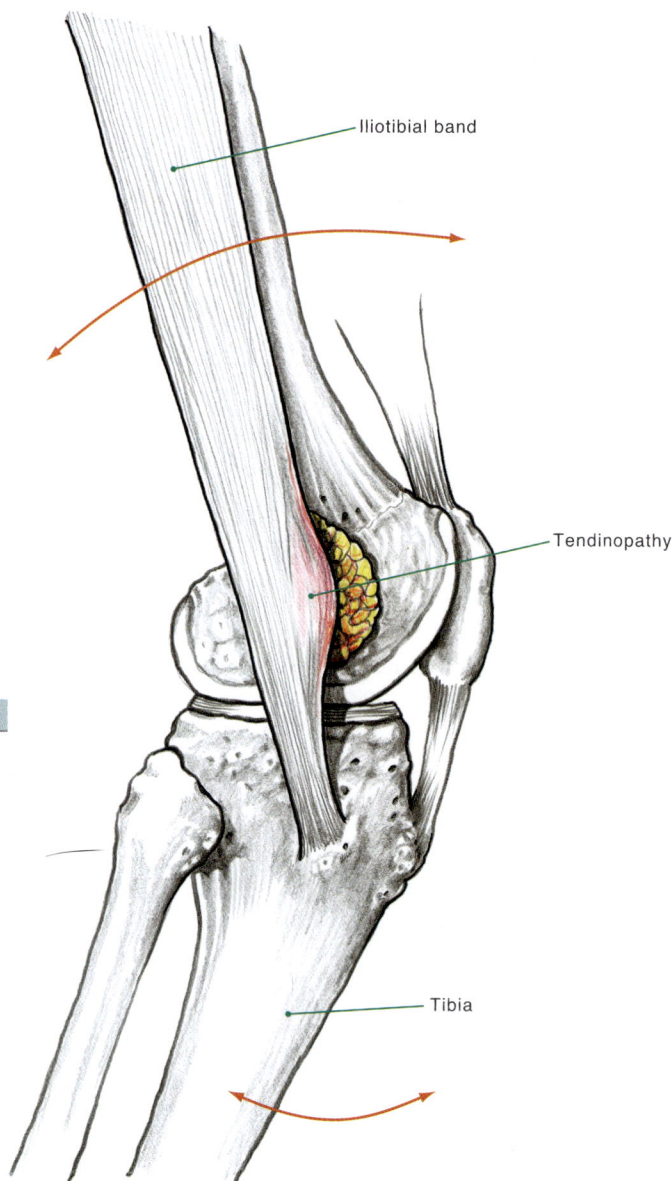

Figure 12.30 Runner's knee. The iliotibial band is affected where it glides back and forth over the lateral femoral Condyle. (© Medical Illustrator Tommy Bolic, Sweden.).

Labels: Iliotibial band, Tendinopathy, Tibia

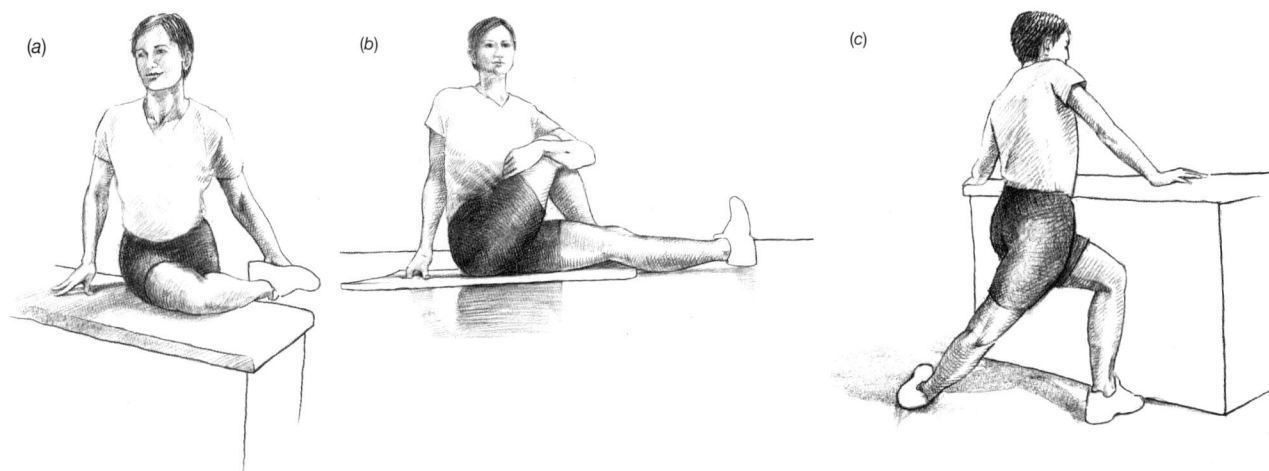

Figure 12.31 Stretching exercises to treat runner's knee, targeting the deep gluteal muscle (a), the gluteal muscle (b) and the iliotibial band (c). For each exercise, hold about 30 seconds, then release gently, and go a little farther in the path of motion. Repeat each stretch two or three times. (© Lill-Ann Prøis.)

Bursitis—*Bursa Inflammation*

Several bursae are found around the knee (Figure 12.32), all of which, in principle, can become inflamed. Inflammation is generally due to overuse of the surrounding tendinous structures but can also result from repeated trauma, for example, falling on the knee on the floor, or from bleeding in a bursa after a direct, powerful impact. Occasionally, as a result of scraped skin or a small wound over the bursa, patients can develop a bacterial infection in the bursa over the patella.

- Symptoms and signs: The prepatellar bursa is the one most commonly affected, often as a result of landing on or having an object strike the kneecap. Frequently, the bursa at the pes anserine or infrapatellar bursa becomes irritated, and in rare cases, the patient can develop bursitis at the biceps bursa where the fibular collateral ligament inserts on the fibula. The athlete has pain and swelling, and if infectious bursitis accompanies the injury, the skin is often red and warm to the touch and the patient can have a fever and general feeling of malaise.
- Diagnosis: The diagnosis is usually made clinically, based on palpating a local swollen or tender area corresponding to a specific bursa. MRI or ultrasound are usually not required, but sometimes are necessary to produce a definite diagnosis. The physician should be aware that MRI might demonstrate several bursae around the knee that may be completely normal. If infection is suspected (red, warm bursa) the bursa must be aspirated under sterile conditions. If the patient has aseptic bursitis, the contents are clear; however, if infected, the contents are cloudy, and the secretion should be sent for a bacterial culture with susceptibility testing and crystal analysis. In addition, the patient's rectal temperature should be taken and blood tests for C-reactive protein, white cell count and sedimentation rate should be ordered. If the patient has traumatic bursitis, the aspiration contents sometimes contain blood.
- Treatment by physician: If the patient has aseptic bursitis, it can be tapped and cortisone may be injected. If necessary, the bursa can be surgically removed to prevent recurrence. If the bursa is infected, antibiotics should be administered and adjusted as needed according to susceptibility testing. Surgical intervention is required only when needle aspiration fails to drain the bursa adequately,

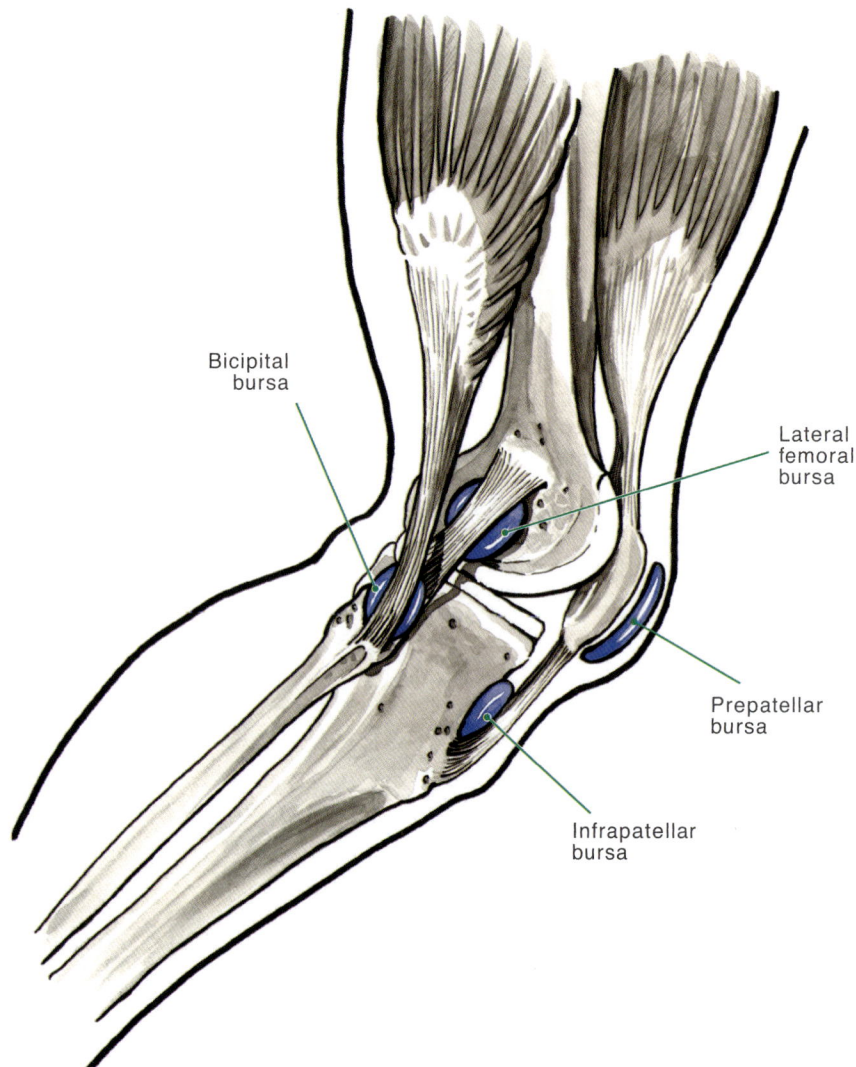

Figure 12.32 Bursae of the knee. The knee has several bursae, all of which are subject to inflammation. (© Medical Illustrator Tommy Bolic, Sweden.)

Bicipital bursa

Lateral femoral bursa

Prepatellar bursa

Infrapatellar bursa

the bursa site inaccessible to needle aspiration, or an abscess or sinus has formed.

• Prognosis: Prognosis is generally good for all types of bursitis. Most cases of bursitis typically resolve in 6–12 weeks with proper activity modification and physical therapy.

Medial Plica Syndrome—*Synovial Membrane Pain*

Patients with a thickened plica often have localized pain medial to their patella. The medial plica is a commonly occurring structure that extends from the suprapatellar fossa along the medial patellar edge and down toward the anteromedial recess (Figure 12.33). The plica may become enlarged, thickened, and irritated where it moves back and forth over the medial femoral condyle during flexion. Therefore, medial plica syndrome is often included in the differential diagnosis of patients with anteromedial knee pain. Symptoms appear when the membrane becomes thickened and appears inflamed under arthroscopy (Figure 12.33). Medial plica syndrome is reported to be a rare cause of knee pain among elite athletes.

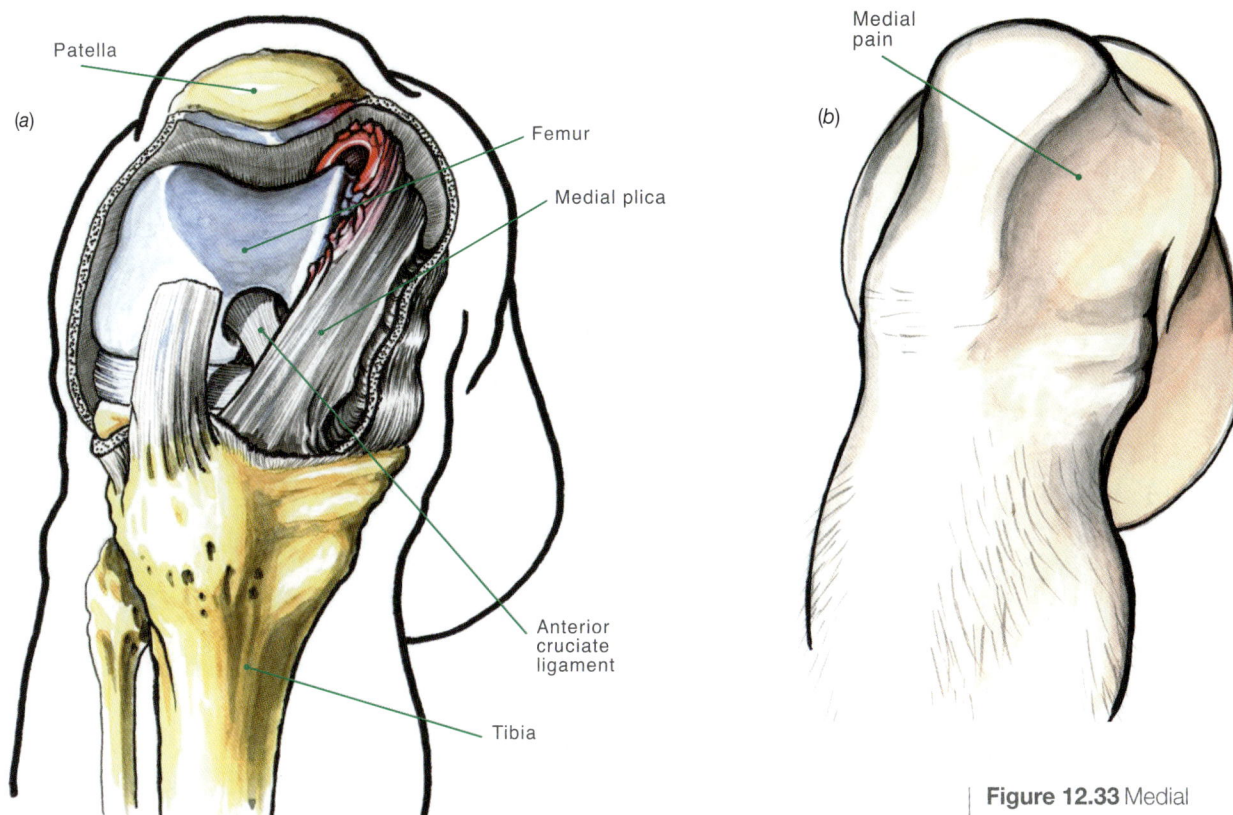

(a)

Patella

Femur

Medial plica

Anterior cruciate ligament

Tibia

(b)

Medial pain

Figure 12.33 Medial plica syndrome. The medial patellar plica in the knee is a common structure, but it can become enlarged and irritated (a) causing pain in deconditioned or post surgical patients. Typical maximal pain location (b). (© Medical Illustrator Tommy Bolic, Sweden.)

- Symptoms and signs: Activity-dependent anterior or medial knee pain. Palpation may reveal be a thickening along the medial patellar edge.
- Diagnosis: The diagnosis is made clinically. The structure is not easy to find using ultrasound but it is visible on MRI; however, the radiologist should be informed to specifically look for a plica. Arthroscopically, the plica looks like a thickened, reddish sail that spreads out over the medial femoral condyle.
- Treatment by physician: If other possibilities have been excluded, and all non-operative treatments fail, an arthroscopy can be done to remove the plica. Plica are often highly vascularized, so postoperative bleeding is a frequent occurrence, which prolongs rehabilitation times.
- Prognosis: Most athletes will be able to return to their sport, but the recovery time is typically about 3 months, sometimes more.

Osgood–Schlatter and Sinding–Larsen–Johansson — *Osgood–Schlatter Disease and Sinding–Larsen–Johansson Disease*

These diseases occur exclusively in older children and adolescents. They are caused by overuse of the patellar tendon, and occur either at its origin on the patella (Sinding–Larsen–Johansson) or its insertion to the tibial tuberosity (Osgood–Schlatter) (Figure 12.34). When growth zones of the distal patellar poles and the tibial tuberosity are overworked (usually as a result of jumping exercises in volleyball and basketball players or repeated long kicks or shots by soccer players), they can become irritated. The growth zone and the growth process will be disturbed, causing pain originating from the growth zones. Extra stress on the growth plate often results in a traction bump. Acute pain in the tibial tuberosity of a child is often misdiagnosed

KNEE

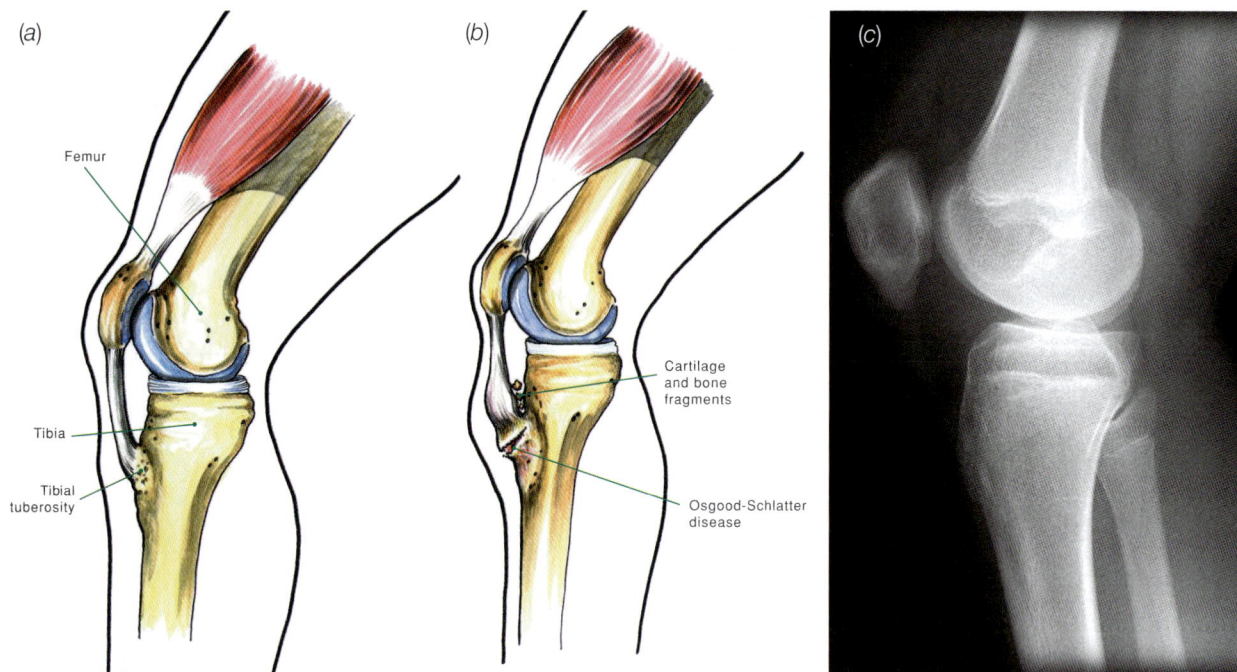

Figure 12.34 Osgood–Schlatter/Sinding–Larsen–Johansson disease: Normal (a). The tibial tuberosity often becomes large and tender in Osgood–Schlatter disease (b). The patella tendon is affected in Sinding–Larsen–Johansson disease (c). (© Medical Illustrator Tommy Bolic, Sweden.)

as Osgood–Schlatter disease, but instead it may be varying grades of avulsion of the patellar tendon from the tibial tuberosity.

- **Symptoms and signs:** The main symptom is pain with contraction of the extensor muscles. This is common in athletes in jumping and sprinting sports, such as track and field, soccer, volleyball, and basketball. The athlete, usually a younger male, is often in the middle of a growth spurt (12–18 years old). Swelling eventually occurs.
- **Diagnosis:** The diagnosis is clinical, but the physician should always take radiographs to exclude any tuberosity epiphysiolysis or tumors.
- **Treatment by physician:** Patients should refrain from placing heavy loads on the extensor apparatus for 6 weeks and work on quadriceps strengthening and hamstring stretching program. Most patients recover in that time, but a small percentage of these patients will have to refrain from jumping and sprinting sports for as long as 6 months. There is no relationship between Osgood–Schlatter disease and detachment of the tuberosity, so strict restrictions on the child's activities are unnecessary.
- **Prognosis:** Almost everyone recovers. At the latest, recovery occurs when the growth zones close, but there may be minor fragmentation of the tibial tuberosity in a small number of patients. This may cause symptoms when the patient is fully grown.

Rehabilitation of Knee Injuries

Robert F. LaPrade[1, 2], Casey M. Pierce[2], Roald Bahr[3], Lars Engebretsen[3], Jill Cook[4], Elizabeth Arendt[5], Nicholas Mohtadi[6], May Arna Risberg[3], and Grethe Myklebust[3]

[1]The Steadman Clinic, Vail, CO, USA
[2]Steadman Philippon Research Institute, Vail, CO, USA
[3]Norwegian School of Sport Sciences, Oslo, Norway
[4]Monash University, Frankston, VIC, Australia
[5]University of Minnesota, Minneapolis, MN, USA
[6]University of Calgary Sport Medicine Centre, Calgary, AB, Canada

Goals and Principles

The goals of acute knee injury rehabilitation are listed in Table 12.4.

When undergoing rehabilitation for knee injuries, healing of the injured ligament(s) without loss of mechanical stability is the main treatment goal. Whether there is an injury to the meniscus, ligament, cartilage, or cruciate ligament, the principles of rehabilitation are similar. The exercises used are basically the same for all types of injuries during the rehabilitation period; however, the progression may differ as to when the various exercises begin and when the resistance, number of repetitions, and speed are changed.

Following surgical intervention, the patient is usually sent home from the hospital with a rehabilitation routine that serves as a good starting point. Patients are then in the rehabilitation phase, and it is vital for the patient to begin active exercises. *Pain, swelling, and function* are used to guide the progression of rehabilitation. If exercise causes pain or swelling, thereby reducing function, the patient's routine needs to be modified to allow the knee to have a chance to recover. The patient should return to the level that was previously tolerated prior to the symptoms appearing.

	Goals	Measures
Acute phase	End swelling	PRICE principle with emphasis on good compression
Rehabilitation phase	End pain	Exercises, mobilization, stretching, ice
	Normal range of motion	
Training phase	Normal strength in the quadriceps and hamstring group compared with the healthy side	Strength training
	Normal sensory motor function: knee injuries may reduce neuromuscular function with a slow reaction to changes of position and new injuries caused by cutting and landing	Balance exercises, functional exercises, eventually controlled sport-specific training
	Reduce the risk of reinjury	Athlete should be fully recovered physically and mentally before resuming competitive activity

Table 12.4 Goals and measures for rehabilitation of acute knee injuries. (Reproduced with permission from the Norwegian Sports Medicine Association.)

KNEE

A commonly accepted recommendation is to change only one exercise at a time. This allows the therapist to accurately determine which type of exercise or movement or amount of loading that may be provoking the symptoms. Patients should be reminded to generously apply ice to the joint after exercising.

Rehabilitation typically begins with a higher number of repetitions (e.g., four series of 20–30 repetitions) and lighter loads, and should then gradually progress to heavier loads and fewer repetitions (e.g., three series of 12–15 repetitions). During the final phase of the rehabilitation period, the athlete's training should be aimed toward building maximum strength, depending on the type of activity the athlete will return to, which mean going down to three sets of 4–6 maximal repetitions for strengthening exercises (Figures 12.35 and 12.36). Collaboration with coaches regarding this type of training is important to insure that the training is both tailored to the patient's sport and managed with respect to what the knee can tolerate.

When retraining these patients, the therapist should focus on restoring neuromuscular function as well as rebuilding strength and range of motion. Starting neuromuscular exercises prior to strengthening exercises is usually a better tolerated program. Knee injuries change neuromuscular control, and retraining takes time. Therefore, it is important to motivate the patient to complete daily self-training exercises to restore normal neuromuscular function.

A high percentage of the most severe knee injuries cause a long-term absence from sports, and some athletes never return at all. This can be a traumatic experience for

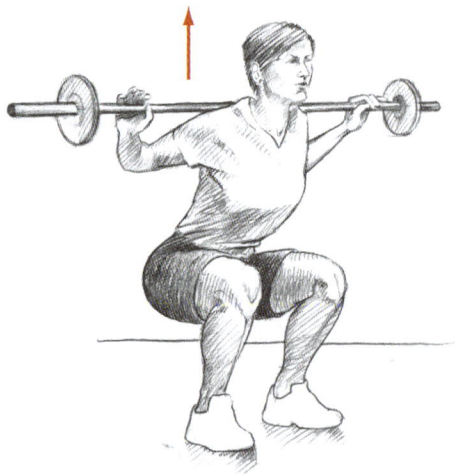

Figure 12.35 Squats with loading.

- Initially, use a bar to support your body weight, then use body weight, and eventually a load on your shoulders.
- Keep knees over toes.
- Keep hips level.
- Avoid getting your weight too far forward.
- Look up and straight ahead.
- Use a mirror to make yourself aware of knee position and weight placement during the start-up stage.

(Reproduced with permission from the Norwegian Sports Medicine Association.)

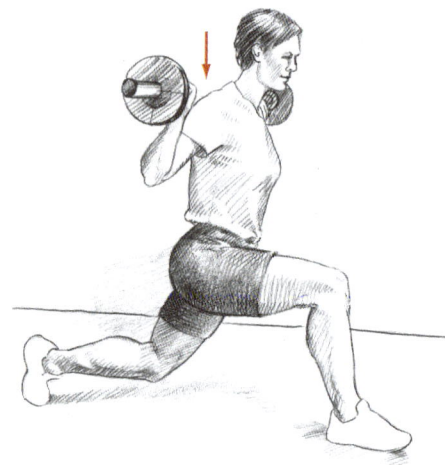

Figure 12.36 Lunges.

- Lower yourself a short distance at first, gradually longer and deeper (as shown in the figure).
- Keep knee over toes.
- Keep hips level.
- Do the same movement at an angle or straight out to the side.
- Use a mirror during the start-up stage.

(Reproduced with permission from the Norwegian Sports Medicine Association.)

the patient, and health care workers must be mindful and not discount the psychological aspects of dealing with a patient who has suffered a serious knee injury.

Return to Sport

Following surgical intervention, patients are provided with time frame when they can be expected return to full function. If the patient has an ACL injury, it is common to plan on 6–9 months of rehabilitation and recovery time before the athlete can return to sports that involve hard stops and sudden turns. After a meniscus resection, time off from athletic activities varies from 14 days to several months, depending on the amount of meniscus resected, which sport the patient plans on returning to and the amount of time elapsed before the intervention took place. The patient should wait a minimum of 6–8 weeks if he or she sustained a grade III medial ligament injury, because that is how long it takes the ligament to properly heal. These time frames are not absolute, and an athlete must not be sent back to contact or pivoting sports without being physically and mentally prepared to return. The patient's knee strength, balance, and function should be tested and compared to the contralateral healthy side before declaring the patient fully rehabilitated.

Strength test. Differences in muscle strength of the hamstring and quadriceps on the injured side as compared with the healthy side can be tested with the help of isokinetic testing equipment. Current recommendations require that the athlete's injured side be at least 90% of the strength on the healthy side before he or she returns to twisting sports. A quadriceps bench may be used for testing maximum strength as well as strength endurance. It should be pointed out that with major injuries and surgical treatment the normal contralateral side can also become weaker; therefore, baseline measurements of strength and function prior to injury serve as better comparators when available.

Functional tests. Before an athlete returns to sporting activities, leg function should be tested–for example, using timed running tests that include turns and dead stops or timed stair-jumping tests comparing the injured side to the healthy side. The athlete should be tested imitating, as closely as possible, the sport that he or she will return to. If it is possible to measure sport specific performance, these measures should be utilized in return-to-play decisions. These types of tests will reveal any lack of neuromuscular control. The patient should have nearly equal function on both sides prior to returning to normal competition. Utilizing such tests during the rehabilitation process will help to motivate the athlete to undertake additional training for strength and neuromuscular control on their own. If the patient is away from work or sport activity for a long time due to injury, it is also important for the athlete to mentally prepare to return to competition.

Preventing Reinjury

Athletes in twisting sports are at risk for reaggrevating a previously treated injury. Optimal rehabilitation can help to reduce the risk of a reinjury. This involves allowing adequate time for all structures to heal and reach the same strength, range of motion, and neuromuscular control as the healthy side. Including prevention exercises tailored for the special sport the athlete wants to return to is important to incorporate in the athlete's warm-up regime (12.37).

When patients sustain a major knee injury, they need to be carefully evaluated to determine to whether they can return to a twisting sport at all. The physician, the

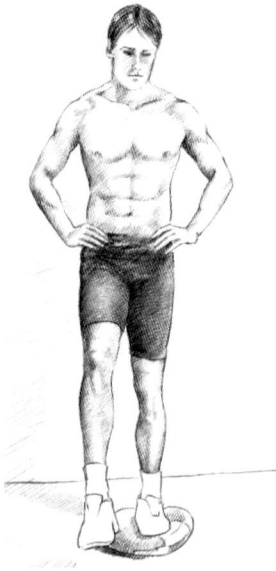

Figure 12.37 Neuromuscular training.

- Stand on one leg on a balance board or balance pad.
- Stand as still as possible for 15–20 seconds.
- Keep knees over toes.
- Stabilize your hip over the leg on which you are standing.
- Increase the degree of difficulty by using a ball or by closing your eyes.

(Reproduced with permission from the Norwegian Sports Medicine Association.)

therapist, and the athlete (and possibly his or her parents and trainer or coach), should discuss the problem with respect to the risk of reinjury and the long-term consequences of the injury.

Rehabilitation of Painful Conditions in the Knee

Two key aspects in the rehabilitation of patients with chronic knee pain are properly adjusting their training regimens and proper stretching. The examination should include assessment of the patient for possible foot or shoe problems. The practitioner should take a thorough case history with respect to the type and amount of physical training. The cause of overuse injuries can usually be understood if the amount and type of training are carefully reviewed. Symptoms are often triggered by an increase in the amount of training and/or change in the exercise conditions (e.g., temperature, surface, or shoe type).

The most common cause of chronic knee pain in recreational athletes is PFPS. Patients with this syndrome may benefit from bracing or McConnell tape, which is believed to change the position of the patella (Figure 12.38). This provides pain relief for many patients, enabling them to resume training nearly pain free. Electrostimulation to enhance muscle activation is used for patients having problem with activating the vastus medialis muscle. Impulses induce contractions of the vastus medialis oblique muscle. Electrostimulation can be used from several starting positions—lying, sitting, or standing—or it may be done during functional exercises, such as knee bends. This allows the patient to stop the vicious cycle of pain, reduced activity, poor muscle function, and atrophy (particularly in the vastus medialis or vastus medialis oblique) and to prevent further inactivity. When treating this type of patient, some pain during exercise is normal. When using a visual analog pain scale, where pain can be rated from 0 (no pain) to 10 (intolerable pain), it is common to accept pain up to 3 or even 5 on the scale during exercise and the period immediately afterward.

The muscles of patients who have had pain for a long time must be examined for possible painful points or trigger points and then treated.

In patients with "runner's knee," the patient needs to be examined thoroughly the reveal any weaknesses in core, hip, and lower extremity muscles. Their running technique should also be examined. Rehabilitation should include strength, neuromuscular, and endurance training. In addition, stretching of the lateral structures should be included until the patient can return to running without pain (Figure 12.31).

Training adjustments are necessary for patients with jumper's knee, so that the athlete can avoid exercises that push the extensor apparatus beyond the limits of pain. It should be emphasized that this disorder takes time to heal. An eccentric strength-training program using three sets of 15 repetitions twice daily for 12 weeks performing unilateral squats on a 25°-decline board. Recent literature also supports the use of heavy slow resistance training programs using four sets the exercises: squat, leg press, and hack squat, going from 15 repetition maximum to six repetition maximum during a 12 week program. In many cases, it is necessary for the practitioner to work together with the athlete's coach to adjust the amount of loading to which the athlete is subjected.

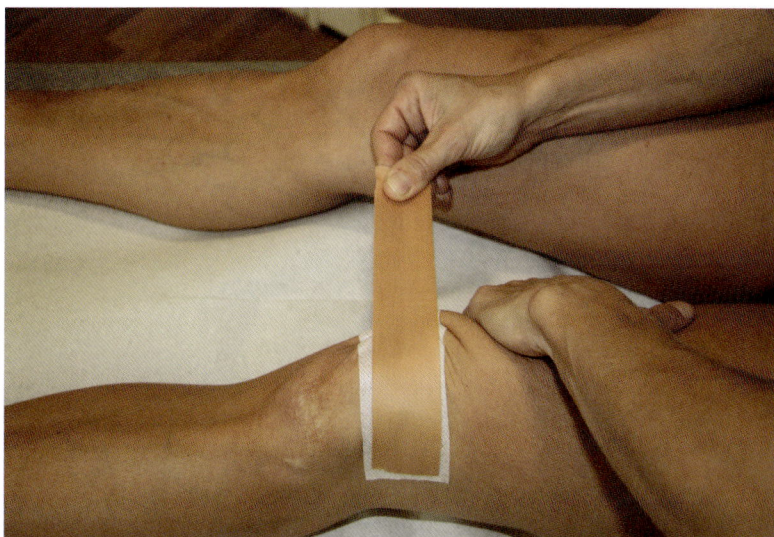

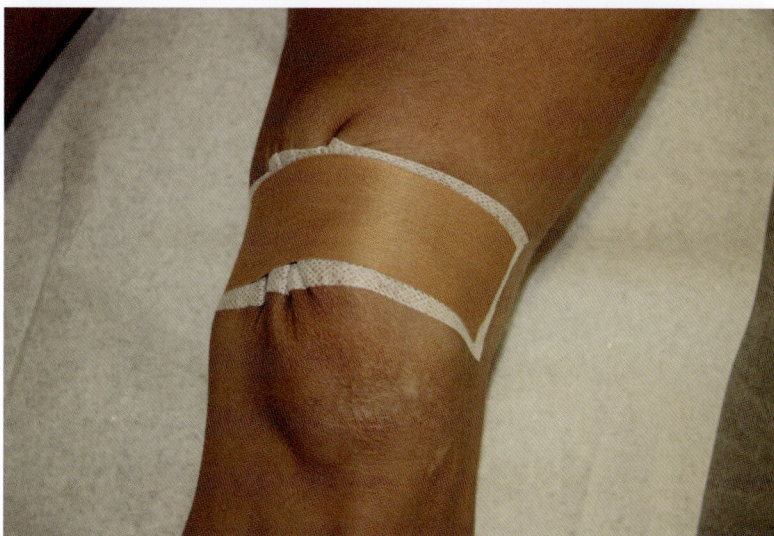

Figure 12.38 McConnell taping to relieve patellofemoral pain by changing the position of the patella, in this case more medially. (© Oslo Sports Trauma Research Center.)

Patients with chronic knee instability have shown to benefit significantly from a training program based on progressive strength and neuromuscular exercises. These exercises are similar to those used in the rehabilitation of acute knee injuries. Progression in load during strength exercises is needed to induce a strength improvement; this is usually tolerated well by these patients. Pain and swelling after exercise therapy are significant markers for a tailored exercise therapy program using the right progression for each patient. Quadriceps strength improvements are usually the hallmark for these patients. Neuromuscular exercises are used to normalize neuromuscular control using a progression of external stimuli and perturbations to improve dynamic stability. In addition to improve neuromuscular control, starting with balance exercises prior to strength training exercises have also shown to significantly improve quadriceps muscle strength.

Patients with a cartilage injury or a coexisting cartilaginous injury to the knee can expect mild pain when exercising; however, the pain should never exceed a value of 3 on a visual analog pain scale to 10. Swelling after exercise should also be used as a marker for the type and progression of exercises. These patients usually have a significant slower progression during the rehabilitation program as compared to chronic knee instability and, in particular, to knee ligament injuries. Patients with articular cartilage injury require a tailored exercise therapy program using individual adjusted weights and progression. Both clinical symptoms and cartilage health have shown to improve with an appropriately tailored exercise therapy program. However, some patients who sustain pain and swelling, therefore inability to undergo exercise progression, would need to be re-evaluated for other interventions by an orthopedic surgeon.

For all these chronic knee conditions patients should expect a minimum of 12 weeks in a rehabilitation program that includes at least three training sessions per week before they expect noticeable improvement. Before starting a rehabilitation program it is recommended to have the patient undergo clinical and functional tests to be able to monitor changes over time. Supervision by a physical therapist for the right progression of exercises is needed to achieve improvement in strength and neuromuscular control. Patient education should be part of the program for self-performance of the specific exercises and the progression of exercises.

13 Lower Leg

Acute Lower Leg Injuries

Jón Karlson[1], Håkan Alfredson[2], and C. Niek van Dijk[3]

[1]*Sahlgrenska University Hospital/Mölndal, Mölndal, Sweden*
[2]*University of Umeå, Sports Medicine Umeå Inc., Umeå, Sweden*
[3]*Academic Medical Center, Amsterdam, The Netherlands*

Occurrence

Acute lower leg injuries are relatively uncommon in athletes; however, chronic—in most cases due to overuse—injuries are a much bigger problem. Formerly, alpine skiers frequently sustained lower leg fractures (known as boot edge fractures), but because ski boots and bindings have changed, knee ligament injuries are more common now in adults. Still, tibia fractures remain a common problem among younger skiers. The mandatory use of leg padding in soccer may also have reduced the occurrence of lower leg fractures and muscle contusions.

Differential Diagnoses

Differential diagnoses for acute lower leg injuries are not very numerous (Table 13.1). Children, particularly adolescent boys who are growing rapidly (in height), may sustain avulsion fractures of the tibial tuberosity, and epiphysiolysis may occur in the proximal or distal tibia and fibula, even though this is not frequent and seldom related to sports. Tumors in the bone or soft tissues (usually sarcoma) may also cause acute symptoms if bleeding or a spontaneous fracture occurs. However, such tumors are infrequent, but should be forgotten or neglected as differential diagnosis.

Diagnostic Thinking

Diagnosis of acute lower leg injuries is usually made by means of a thorough case history and a clinical examination. The injury mechanisms are as a rule typical for the

Most common	Less common	Must not be overlooked !
Muscle rupture, p. 404	Acute compartment syndrome, p. 408	Epiphysiolysis, p. 411
Lower leg fracture, p. 405	Nerve contusion, p. 409	Peroneus tendons tendon rupture, p. 444
Fibular fracture, p. 406	Subperiosteal hematoma, p. 411	Tibialis posterior tendon rupture, p. 456
Achilles tendon rupture		
Tibial fracture		

Table 13.1 Overview of the differential diagnoses of acute lower leg injuries. (Reproduced with permission from the Norwegian Sports Medicine Association.)

The IOC Manual of Sports Injuries, First Edition. Edited by Roald Bahr.
©2012 International Olympic Committee. Published 2012 by John Wiley & Sons, Ltd.

most frequently occurring bone, muscle, and tendon injuries. Direct trauma, such as a kick in soccer, may cause muscle contusions and/or a fracture (usually the tibia). In case of a total rupture of the Achilles tendon, sometimes an audible snap will be heard. The athlete sometimes assumes he or she has been kicked from behind. Strong pain, best described as "pain out of proportion to the overall trauma," after a contusion injury or a lower leg fracture should always raise the suspicion of an acute compartment syndrome. This always needs immediate attention by the medical staff.

Case History

If the patient has an acute lower leg injury, the case history (including the injury mechanism) is in most cases a very good indicator of the correct diagnosis. Contusion injuries may cause a muscle contusion/bleeding and/or rupture, fracture, nerve contusion, or a periosteal injury, depending on the location of the contusion. A distention injury may on the other hand cause a muscle or tendon rupture or in some cases an avulsion fracture. Indirect trauma, such as bending of the lower leg over the edge of a slalom ski boot, may cause a lower leg fracture or a ligament injury, probably most often an anterior cruciate ligament (ACL) injury.

Clinical Examination

Inspection. A lower leg fracture, where the fracture ends are dislocated and perhaps even with skin perforation, is easy to diagnose by inspection. Major muscle ruptures and total ruptures of the Achilles tendon will initially be visible as a defect or indentation of the skin over the injury. The defect will shortly fill with effusion, blood, and edema, as the swelling increases. The magnitude of the injury is often directly related to the magnitude of the swelling. Later, discoloration of the skin will be visible, especially in case of intermuscular injury (where blood from the muscle belly spreads along the muscle fascia to the skin). If the patient has sustained a contusion of the anterior edge of the tibia with a periosteal injury, painful local swelling will usually develop rather quickly.

Palpation. If the patient has sustained a tibia and/or fibula fracture, without dislocation, the patient will upon palpation localize the pain to the site of the fracture, so called "direct pain." Minor swelling may be the only result of this type of injury. The patient will also indicate so called "indirect pain," where pressure applied to the tibia or fibula some distance away from the fracture will trigger pain corresponding to the site of the injury.

If the patient is examined immediately after a muscle rupture occurs, a tender defect can almost always be palpated in the muscle belly. However, this defect will quickly fill up with blood and edema, causing swelling. This makes the clinical diagnosis of a total muscle/tendon rupture less reliable the longer the time after the injury.

Achilles tendon ruptures are frequently missed, but it should in fact always be possible to definitely diagnose a total rupture of the Achilles tendon through a good clinical examination. A palpable "gap" in the tendon is almost always found, especially directly after the trauma. This gap is located 2–5 cm proximal to the insertion to the calcaneus.

The Calf squeeze test will always be positive if the patient has a total Achilles tendon rupture. This test is performed with the patient in the prone position with a slightly flexed knee joint, or kneeling with the affected leg on the examination table (and the affected leg outside the examination table) (Figure 13.1). Pressure applied from side-to-side to the calf musculature will cause reflexive plantar flexion of the ankle

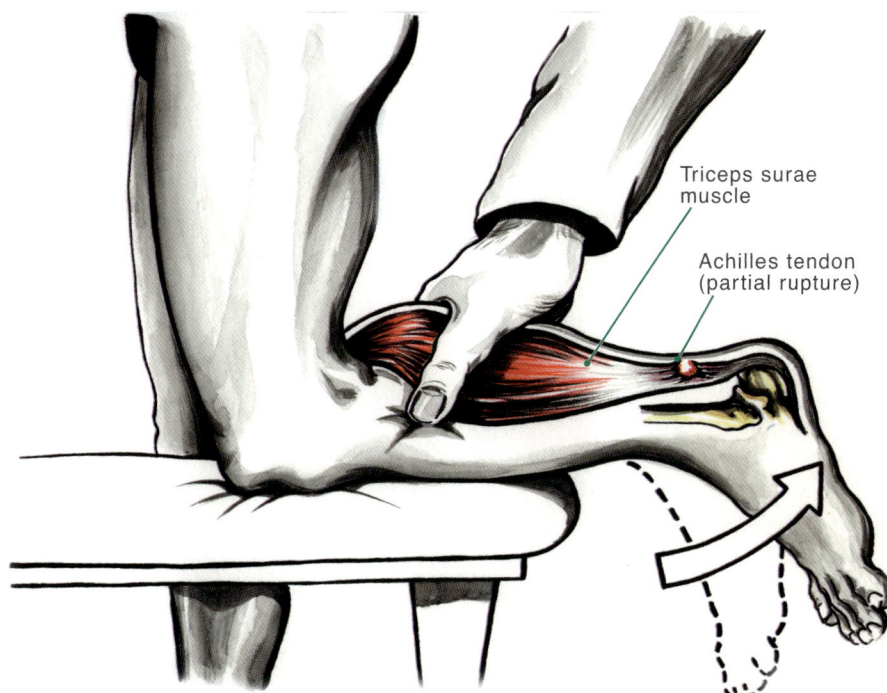

Figure 13.1 Calf squeeze test, which is used to demonstrate a total rupture in the Achilles tendon. If the tendon is torn, there is no reflex plantar flexion of the ankle joint when the calf muscles are abruptly compressed from side to side. (© Medical Illustrator Tommy Bolic, Sweden.)

Triceps surae muscle

Achilles tendon (partial rupture)

joint if the tendon is intact, but no movement will occur in case of a total rupture. The strength of active plantar flexion against resistance can also be tested. In case of Achilles tendon rupture, the plantar flexion strength is severely reduced or there is none at all.

Acute paratenonitis will cause the tendon to be tender and possibly somewhat thickened. Crepitation is typical and it can often be felt by applying pressure and palpating along the tendon, while the foot is being moved (like squeezing a wet sticky snowball).

Acute compartment syndrome causes the musculature to become painful, tense, and intensely tender to pressure. Passive movement of the ankle or toes always triggers significant pain in the affected musculature and is a strong "warning sign." Only late in the course the patient experiences a loss of sensitivity distally in the lower leg and in the foot. The medical staff must bear in mind that even with a full-blown acute compartment syndrome, the pulsations in the arteries on the dorsal side of the foot and behind the medial malleolus are normal.

Supplemental Examinations

Radiographic examination. An examination with plain radiographs in two planes (frontal and lateral) is necessary in order to clinically manifest fractures. Occasionally, a fracture in the fibula or tibia is only a thin fissure that may be difficult to detect on a radiograph. If a fracture is not revealed, but still strongly suspected, the patient should undergo a supplemental skeletal scintigraphic examination, or better still an magnetic resonance imaging (MRI) acutely. One or two days after the injury, scintigraphy will be positive, with strong uptake that corresponds to the fracture line. MRI will clearly demonstrate the fracture line, and it will give an even better image of edema formation in the surrounding cancellous bone. Therefore, if MRI is available, it should be the primary choice.

LOWER LEG

Pressure measurement. If the patient is suspected of having an acute compartment syndrome, he should be transferred immediately to a trauma hospital, where pressure in the affected compartment can be measured. Pressure is often increased in all four compartments of the lower leg if the patient has a fully developed compartment syndrome. A pressure of 45–50 mmHg is an indication for acute surgical intervention with division of the muscle fasciae of the compartments. In most cases 30 mmHg is the level that is defined as increased compartmental pressure.

Common Injuries

Muscle Rupture—*Muscle Injuries (Tennis Leg)*

Muscle injuries are often divided into contusion injuries and distention injuries (Figure 13.2). Contusion injuries are caused by direct impact or blow (such as a kick in soccer) to the lower leg. The musculature is crushed against the underlying bone, which may lead to deep muscle injury. Distention injuries are usually partial ruptures in the soleus or the gastrocnemius and most often affect the medial aspect of the gastrocnemius muscle. Athletes in sports in which jumping ability and speed are important factors (like tennis, badminton, squash, volleyball, basketball, handball, and soccer), as well as hurdlers and sprinters in track and field, are particularly vulnerable to such muscle ruptures. Tennis leg is a partial/subtotal rupture of the junction between the muscle and the distal tendon fibers of the medial gastrocnemius muscle (Figure 13.2).

- **Symptoms and signs:** The main symptom is pain that starts suddenly and corresponds to the location of the injury. The patient is unable to walk on his toes.
- **Diagnosis:** It may initially be possible to feel a small defect in the muscle belly, but shortly there is swelling due to bleeding and edema. Local tenderness is found on palpation at the rupture site. The muscle fasciae of the lower leg are thick, which makes the bleeding to remain inside the muscle belly. If the fascia tears, the skin will become discolored over and distal to the rupture in 2 or 3 days.
- **Treatment by physician:** Tennis leg may cause pain for several weeks, even though adequate initial treatment has been advocated. Surgery is practically never indicated. Caution is advised in using nonsteroidal anti-inflammatory drugs (NSAIDs) if major muscular bleeding has occurred, however. Paracetamol 1 g x 4 daily is recommended for pain.
- **Treatment by therapist:** Acute treatment using PRICE should be given for 2 days. On day 3, the patient should be reexamined, and the patient starts gradual rehabilitation with range of motion, as well as strength and flexibility exercises. In case of an intermuscular bleeding (with a rupture of the muscle fascia), discoloration of the skin can be seen.
- **Prognosis:** The athlete may return to sport activity once he achieves full painless flexibility equal on both sides and he has restored full strength in the muscle. In case of intermuscular bleeding, the duration is approximately 4–6 weeks, whereas

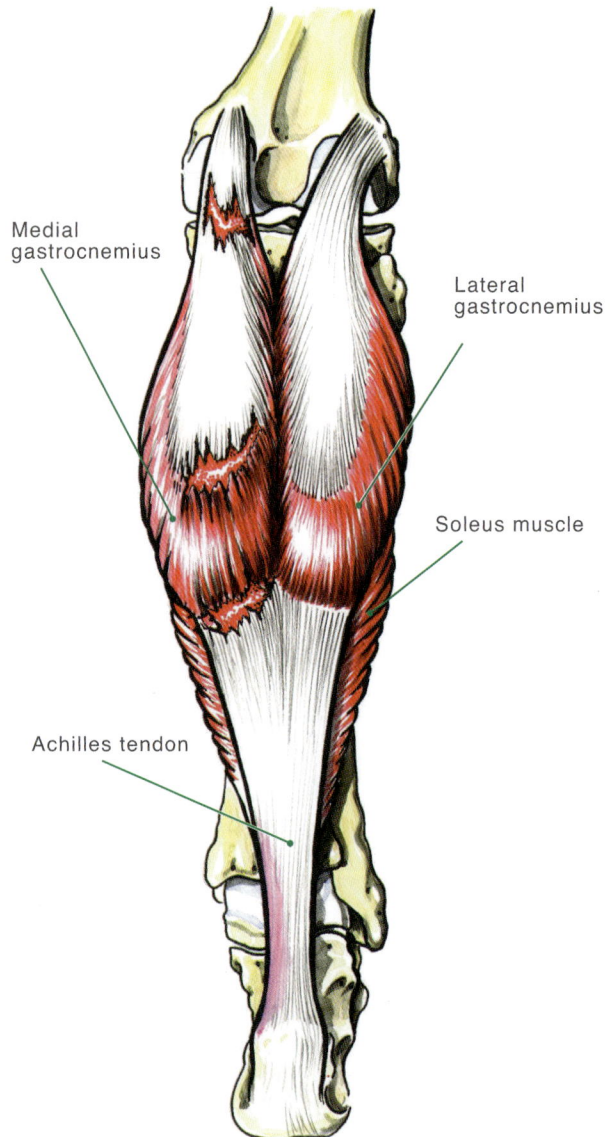

Figure 13.2 Muscle injuries of the lower leg. The muscle-tendon junction of the medial gastrocnemius head is the most typical location for such injuries (so-called tennis leg). However, the ruptures can occur at several locations in the muscle, usually at the muscle-tendon junction. (© Medical Illustrator Tommy Bolic, Sweden.)

Medial gastrocnemius

Lateral gastrocnemius

Soleus muscle

Achilles tendon

it may take as long as 8–12 weeks for a patient to fully recover from an intramuscular bleeding. If the injured area is allowed to heal with a permanent area of scar tissue that is insufficiently stretched, loading of the area may easily cause a relapse and a new rupture.

Lower Leg Fracture

Lower leg fractures are divided according to which bones are fractured; tibial fractures, fibular fractures or both (Figure 13.3). Such serious injuries occur most frequently in contact sports (e.g., soccer and ice hockey) and in high-energy sports (e.g., downhill skiing and motor sports). The injury mechanism may be a direct or indirect trauma, and the injury is correlated to either high- or low-energy activity. Direct trauma, such as a kick, usually causes a transverse fracture, whereas indirect twisting trauma causes an oblique or spiral fracture. Low-energy injuries are usually transverse, oblique, or spiral fractures, whereas high-energy trauma may cause complicated fractures with major or minor soft-tissue injuries. The physician should classify these injuries for treatment purposes and later on to evaluate the healing potential of the fracture.

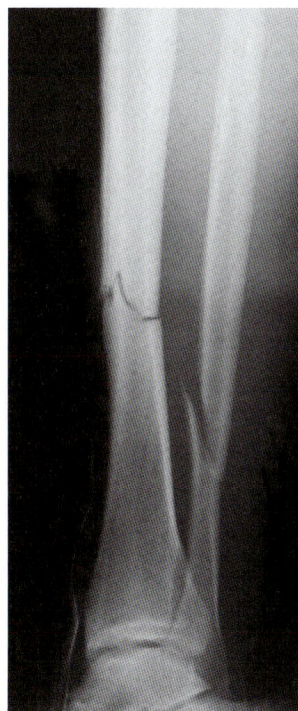

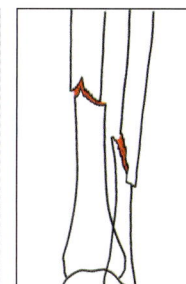

Figure 13.3 X ray of a lower-leg fracture with fracture lines through both the tibia and the fibula. (© Medical Illustrator Tommy Bolic, Sweden.)

- Symptoms and signs: Symptoms are strong pain with an acute onset, often dislocation of the fracture ends, and sometimes skin perforation. The fractured area may become swollen.
- Diagnosis: Clinical examination confirms the diagnosis if the fracture is unstable. Radiographs will usually confirm suspected fractures if they are simple fissures in the tibia or fibula. Sometimes supplemental skeletal scintigraphy or MRI will be necessary.
- Treatment by physician: Stable fractures are reduced, and a cast is applied; whereas unstable fractures, particularly open fractures, require surgical stabilization. Surgery may allow immediate knee and ankle joint mobility and some loading. If a lower leg fracture is treated with a cast, the cast must extend from the groin to the toes in order to achieve rotational stability. After 2–4 weeks the cast can be exchanged for a lower leg brace (walking boot). The patient can now start weight bearing with partial loading and range of motion training for the knee.
- Treatment by therapist: Initial on-site treatment consists of rough correction of the fracture dislocation and stabilization of the fracture as soon as possible (simple splinting, air-splints, pillows, or something similar), to avoid further soft-tissue damage and to reduce pain during transport. Any wounds are covered as sterile as possible. Immediately after the injury occurs, pain is often less intense, so rapid intervention may be possible without any type of pain-relieving medication.
- Prognosis: Tibia shaft fractures heal slowly, because of poor soft-tissue coverage and a poor blood supply to the anterior medial portion of the bone. It usually takes at least 8–12 weeks before healing is sufficient to allow the patient to gradually and carefully resume sport activity. There will be at least 6 months absence from contact sports and other sports that place a heavy strain on the lower leg after any tibia fracture, or even longer.

LOWER LEG

Fibular Fracture

This type of fracture is usually caused by direct trauma (such as a kick) or occurs in a patient with a sprained ankle who has a simultaneous syndesmosis injury. In the latter case, the fracture is usually located in the proximal part of the fibula (Figure 13.4).

Symptoms and signs: Strong pain with an acute onset after direct trauma to the fibula is the most common symptom. Proximal fibular fractures that occur in connection with ankle injuries are frequently overlooked. Significant tenderness on direct palpation is always present.

Diagnosis: Radiographs usually confirm the diagnosis of a fracture. Sometimes supplemental skeletal scintigraphy and/or MRI will be necessary.

Treatment: If major dislocation between the fracture ends has occurred, open reduction and osteosynthesis is necessary. An ankle fracture combined with an injury to the syndesmosis requires surgery of the fracture and stabilization of the syndesmotic ligaments.

Treatment by therapist: Simple fibular fractures without any major dislocation require only unloading, with crutches, until the patient is pain free. Because of good soft-tissue coverage and blood supply, these fractures usually heal well.

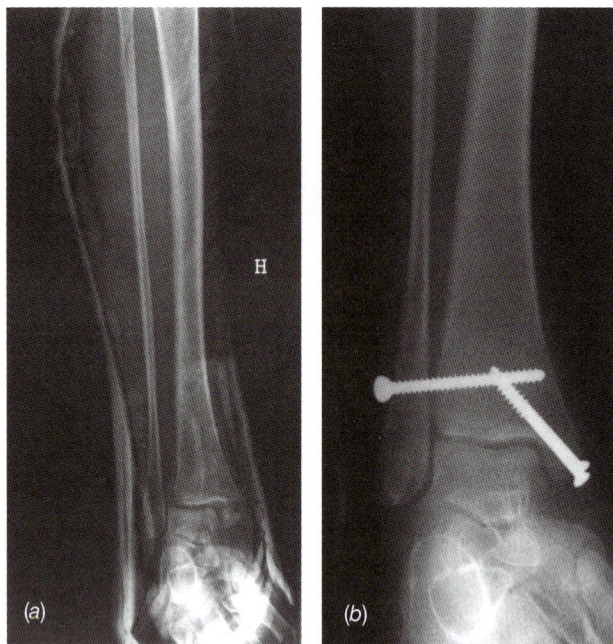

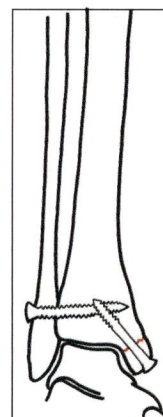

Figure 13.4 Syndesmosis injury. The X-ray demonstrates a proximal fibular fracture, syndesmosis rupture, and a fracture of the medial malleolus (*a*). The patient is first treated with a plaster cast. Thereafter screws through the fibula and into the tibia (to stabilize the syndesmosis), as well as screws stabilizing the fracture of the medial malleolus, are used to surgically treat the fracture (*b*). (© Medical Illustrator Tommy Bolic, Sweden.)

Achilles Tendon Rupture—*Tearing of the Heel Tendon*

The Achilles tendon is the thickest and strongest tendon in the human body. It plays a very important role in many sport activities and is particularly vulnerable to major loading from running and jumping. The Achilles tendon forms the common distal tendon of the gastrocnemius and the soleus muscles, that is, the triceps surae muscle (Figure 13.5). Athletes who sustain an Achilles tendon rupture most frequently are those who participate in sports characterized by rapid changes of direction and jumps (e.g., tennis, squash, badminton, and soccer) and runners and jumpers in track and field. However, sometimes not often a patient who sustains a tendon rupture has had a history of long-term pain localized to the tendon, but the rupture usually occurs without warning. Such ruptures may be caused by degenerative changes in the tendon (tendinosis), usually in the segment of the tendon with limited blood supply. This segment extends from 2 to 6 cm proximal to the insertion of the tendon to the heel bone.

Achilles tendon ruptures are divided into total and partial ruptures. However, partial ruptures are uncommon. Total ruptures usually occur in active recreational athletes (average age 40) who resume sport activity after having been away from it for some time. In these cases, degenerative changes may have weakened the tendon. To some extent, these changes in the tendon could have been prevented by regular physical

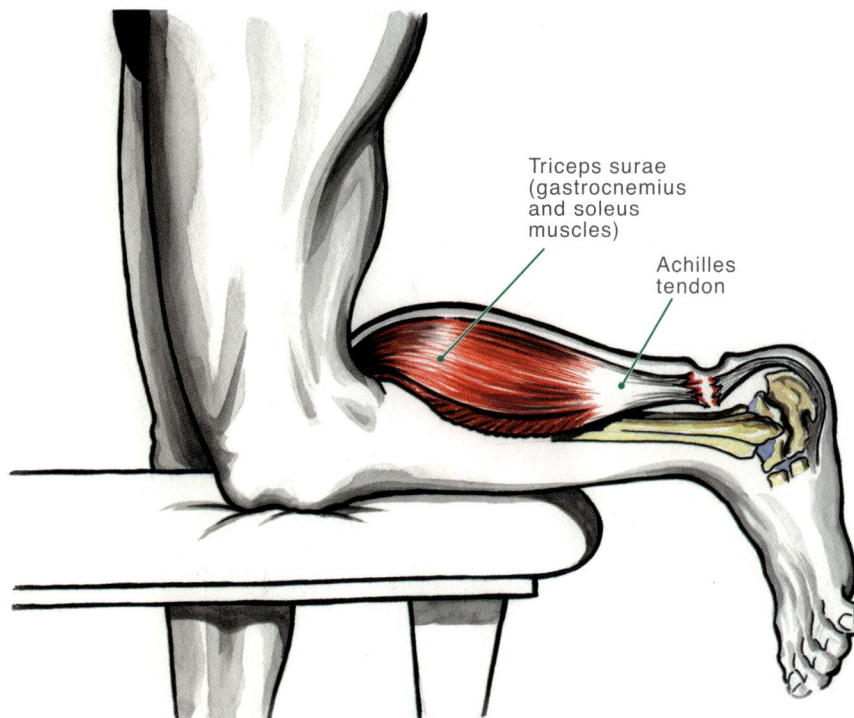

Triceps surae
(gastrocnemius
and soleus
muscles)

Achilles
tendon

Figure 13.5 Total Achilles tendon rupture. If the patient has a total rupture, the Calf squeeze test is positive, that is, there is no plantar flexion movement of the foot when the calf muscles are compressed from side to side. (© Medical Illustrator Tommy Bolic, Sweden.)

activity. In most cases, the injury mechanism is a strong contraction of the lower leg musculature, with simultaneous extension (eccentric loading) of the tendon. A typical mechanism is pushing off hard with the weight-bearing foot while the knee is extended (e.g., running uphill) or sudden unexpected dorsal extension of the ankle with reflexive contraction of the lower leg muscles (e.g., falling down into a hole, or missing the last step while walking downstairs).

- **Symptoms and signs:** The patient experiences acute, intense pain corresponding to the Achilles tendon, sometimes accompanied by an audible snap. The patient cannot walk on tiptoe, nor can he/she walk with a normal stride due to reduced power in plantar flexion.
- **Diagnosis:** During the clinical examination, the patient has significantly reduced (or no strength at all) plantar flexion strength. When the tendon is palpated, there is in most cases a "gap" in the tendon tissue, approximately 2–5 cm from the insertion to the calcaneus. If the injury is recent, the patient has pain corresponding to the site of the rupture. The defect eventually fills with blood and edema and the skin over the area becomes discolored. The Calf squeeze test is positive, that is, no plantar flexion movement upon quick compression of the calf muscles (Figure 13.5).
- **Supplemental examinations:** If the diagnosis is uncertain, ultrasonography and/or MRI may be useful.
- **Treatment by physician:** The most common treatment is direct suture of the Achilles tendon, with end-to-end suture. Nonsurgical treatment, with brace and gradual range of motion exercises, is indicated in patients with lower activity level. Postoperatively, the ankle is immobilized in a brace or cast for 2 weeks, where the foot is in moderate equinus position.
- **Treatment by therapist:** After 2 weeks the cast or brace is removed. Then the patient's ankle is mobilized in a range-of-motion walker (ROM-Walker) with free plantar flexion and gradually increasing dorsal flexion out from a zero position for the next 4 weeks. Beginning 6–8 weeks after surgery, the patient gradually increases the intensity of strength and flexibility training. This treatment plan usually

LOWER LEG

407

allows the athlete to return to full sport activity in approximately 4–6 months. Several studies have shown that early range of motion training and loading of a sutured tendon increases collagen formation, remodeling, and strength in the tendon. The risk of a rerupture after surgical treatment is approximately 3–4%, whereas the risk of rerupture after nonsurgical treatment is approximately 10% during the first 6 months (reruptures nearly always occur within the first 6 months). There is an increased risk of infection after surgical treatment.

Some authors have recommended nonsurgical treatment for total Achilles tendon ruptures. In such cases, patients are immobilized for 2 weeks and thereafter treated with brace for approximately 6 weeks, with gradually increasing range of motion. This treatment is usually not recommended for active athletes, due to somewhat higher risk of a rerupture, but taken as a whole the risk of complications is low and the functional outcome favorable.

Total Achilles tendon ruptures are sometimes missed and there is a risk of so-called doctor's delay to correct diagnosis. The patient who sustains this injury will complain of weak lower leg musculature, and he will not be able to maintain his normal stride. It is impossible for the patient to stand on tiptoe on the affected side, and plantar flexion strength is markedly reduced. These patients almost always require surgery to resect the scar tissue interposed in the rupture cleft, to mobilize the tendon, and to suture it end-to-end, in most cases with some kind of reinforcement, in most cases some kind of a fascia/tendon flap from the proximal part of the Achilles tendon for strength. Rehabilitation is similar to that used after the initial suturing; however, the progression is slower and more careful. The result with respect to strength and jumping ability is good in the majority of patients.

Other Injuries

Acute Compartment Syndrome

The lower leg's muscles are divided into four compartments (closed areas), surrounded by a relatively nonyielding muscle fascia. The four compartments are the anterior, lateral, deep posterior, and superficial posterior (Figure 13.6). Untreated acute compartment syndrome will always lead to an increased pressure inside one or more of the muscle compartments in the lower leg, resulting in more or less permanent muscle and nerve injury. This syndrome may occur in case of a fracture or muscle injury, or sometimes after acute overloading of the muscle groups, such as a long run on hard surfaces.

The mechanism behind the development of acute muscle compartment syndrome can be outlined as follows (Figure 13.6): increased interstitial pressure inside a compartment (e.g., resulting from bleeding or edema), reduced capillary circulation in the musculature, increased production of lactic acid, more edema (vicious cycle), increased venous stasis (i.e., compression of vessels that lead the blood out of the muscles), and further increase in pressure until all circulation in the affected musculature has ceased and the muscles first and thereafter the nerves in the affected compartment necrotize.

- Symptoms and signs: The major and most important symptom of acute compartment syndrome is strong pain, and it increases when the affected muscles are passively stretched. Muscle function is gradually reduced and ultimately lost after only few hours. Paresthesia (skin sensory disturbance) in the areas innervated by the affected nerves is a definite, but late, symptom.

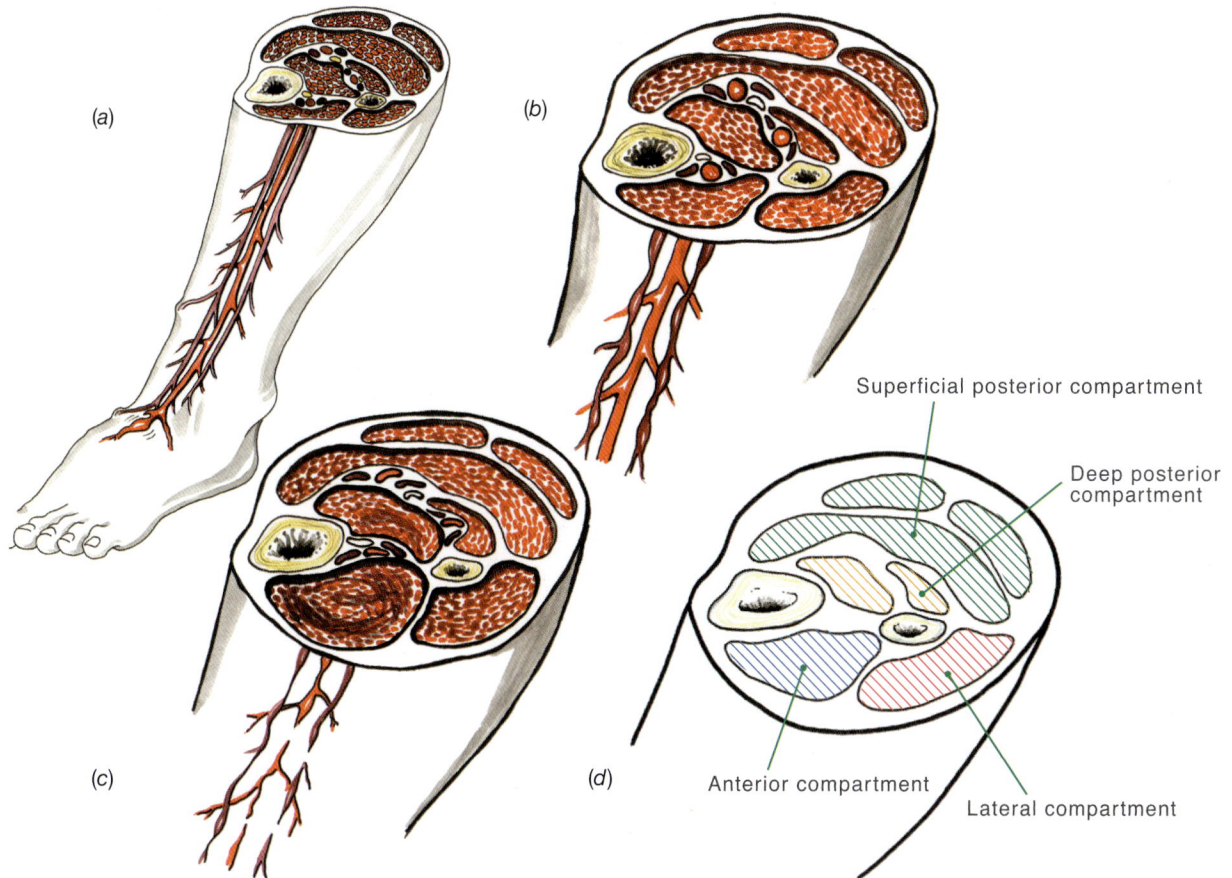

Figure 13.6 Development of acute compartment syndrome. The drawing shows normal circulation in the lower leg (a), venous stasis (b), and the last stage of compartment syndrome, where there is no circulation (c), The cross section shows the four compartments of the lower leg (d). (© Medical Illustrator Tommy Bolic, Sweden.)

- Diagnosis: The history of injury should arouse the suspicion of compartment syndrome. The lower leg musculature is swollen (even hard) and tender, and muscle/tendon function is increasingly diminished and finally totally absent. Paresthesias occur late in the course of treatment, although distal circulation in the foot and pulsations are normal.
- Treatment: The patient must be referred to a specialist for immediate medical surveillance and treatment. To measure the pressure in the affected compartment(s) can be an important, and equipment for this purpose should be available in all hospitals. If increased pressure is suspected on clinical examination, or if increased pressure is measured, that is, >30 mmHg, the patient must undergo surgery in order to open up all four compartments in the lower leg. This must happen without delay. If circulation is absent for longer than 4 or 5 hours, the damage will be irreversible.
- Prognosis: Prognosis is good with early and correct treatment. If the muscle is damaged (muscle necrosis) fibrosis, shortening, and contracture, as well as pain will occur.

Nerve Contusion

The common peroneal nerve (fibularis) is superficial and unprotected in the area where it passes directly behind t the fibular head (Figure 13.7). Direct trauma, such as a kick or a pressure injury over this area, may lead to total or partial paralysis of this nerve (peroneal paresis, so-called drop foot).

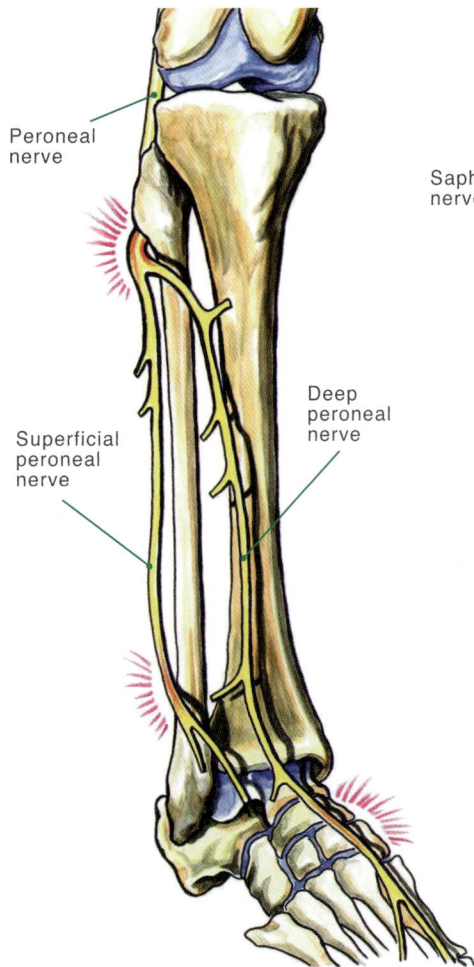

Figure 13.7 Peroneal nerve injury. This most often occurs just below the head of the fibula. Less common locations are just proximal to the lateral malleolus and on the wrist of the foot. (© Medical Illustrator Tommy Bolic, Sweden.)

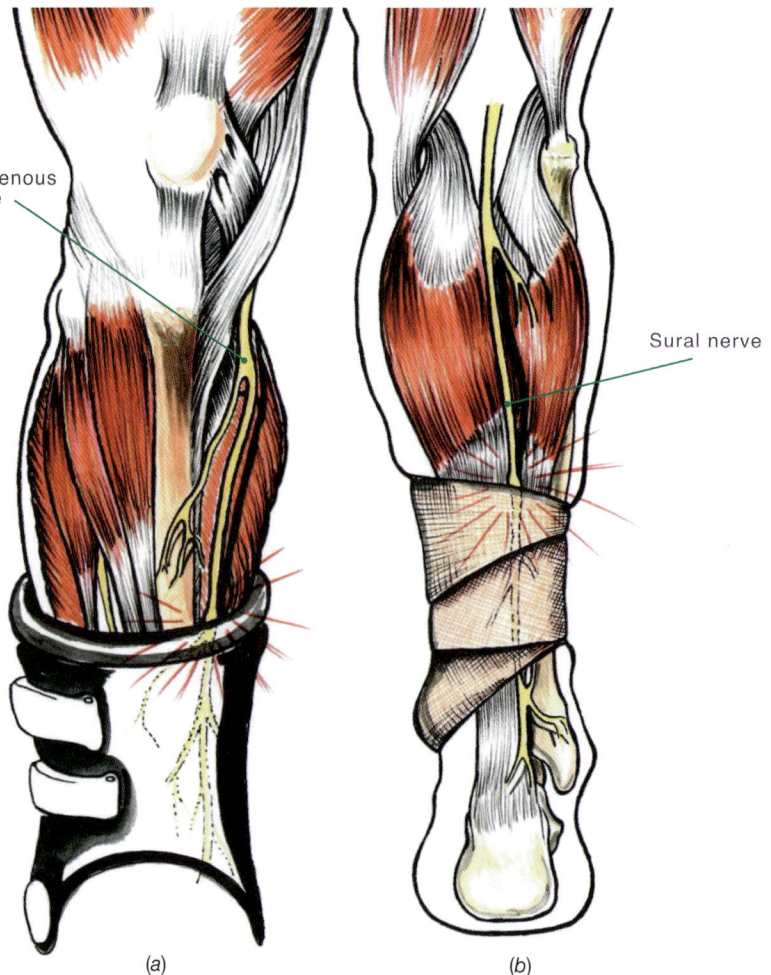

Figure 13.8 Saphenous nerve (a) and sural nerve (b) injuries. Entrapment of these nerves can be caused by a slalom boot or a firm elastic bandage. (© Medical Illustrator Tommy Bolic, Sweden.)

Other nerves in the lower leg that may be subjected to direct trauma or chronic irritation are the superficial distal cutaneous branch of the peroneal nerve, the sural nerve, and the saphenous nerve (Figure 13.8). A slalom ski boot that is strapped too tightly or a firm ankle tape may cause pressure injury to these nerves, sensory disturbance (paresthesia), and sometimes even pain in the skin area.

- Symptoms and signs: If peroneus nerve is injured at the fibular head, the patient will have weakened dorsal flexion and eversion in the ankle joint (drop foot), as well as paresthesia on the wrist of the foot and the ankle.
- Diagnosis: Diagnosis is to a large extent based on the case history and on clinical examinations. A supplemental neurophysiological examination will demonstrate whether the nerve damage is total or partial and also if regeneration has started.
- Treatment: If a contusion injury has occurred and the nerve is intact, function will gradually return without any type of treatment. If the nerve is torn, it must be surgically repaired.
- Prognosis: The athlete usually recovers completely after nerve contusion. It may take a few days to weeks or even longer time, depending on the injury mechanism. The prognosis after nerve suturing is not as good.

Subperiosteal Hematoma

Direct trauma, such as being kicked in the shin, may cause bleeding under the periosteum on the tibia. Subperiosteal hematoma is immediately painful, and the symptoms may last a long time (until the bleeding is resorbed). In some cases, part of the hematoma is converted to fibrous scar tissue, which may partially or even totally turn into bone.

- Treatment: Treatment is in accordance with the rest, ice, compression, and elevation (RICE) principle during the acute phase. Bleeding must be limited as much as possible using compression bandage. Later, a specially adapted plastic brace can be made to protect against similar new blows to the same area. However, the most important "treatment" is prophylaxis, such as wearing well-adjusted leg padding, for instance when playing soccer.

Epiphysiolysis—Slippage of the Growth Plate !

Epiphysiolysis (Figure 13.9) may occur both proximally and distally in the tibia and fibula, that is, close to the knee or ankle joints. In the proximal tibia, avulsions usually occur through the apophysis of the tibial tuberosity or the epiphysis just below the knee joint. These injuries mainly affect boys during the last stages of their pubertal growth spurt, when the musculature becomes stronger. Upon maximal contraction of the quadriceps (such as caused by jumps in basketball or volleyball), loading via the patellar tendon may become so great that the growth plate is injured.

Epiphyseal injuries of the proximal fibula as well as distally in the tibia and fibula (ankle joint injury) results from an injury mechanism similar to what would cause an ankle fracture (with or without a syndesmosis injury) in an adult.

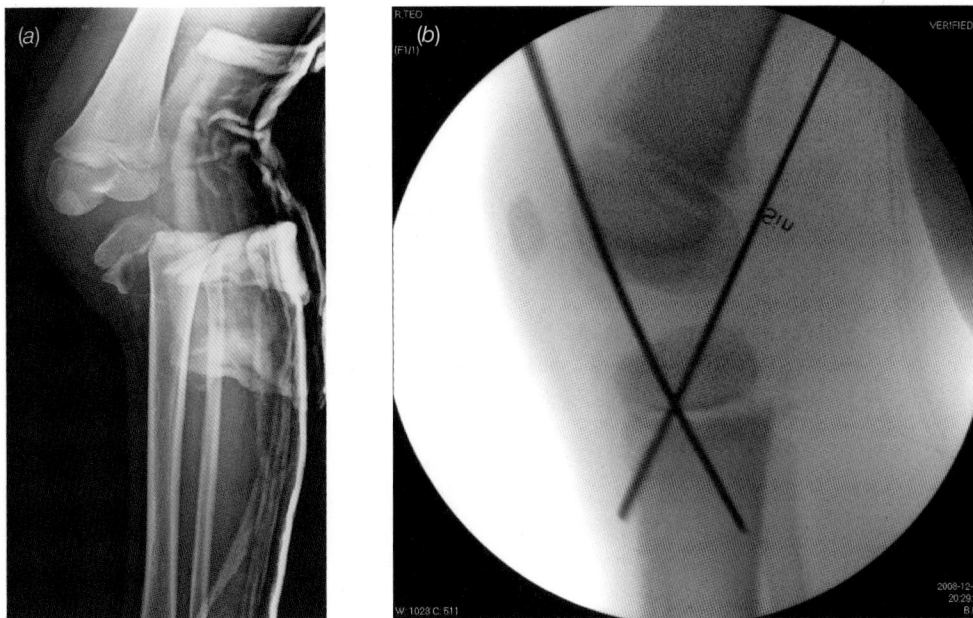

Figure 13.9 Epiphysiolysis of the proximal tibia is a serious injury in children and adolescents, as in this case (a), resulting from a biking accident. The injury was operated on with closed reduction and percutaneous fixation (b). (Reproduced with permission from the Norwegian Sports Medicine Association.)

LOWER LEG

- Symptoms and signs: The main symptoms are acute pain and sometimes dislocation similar to those caused by a fracture. As there is less bleeding compared with a fracture, less swelling usually occurs.
- Treatment: Proximal growth plate injuries are usually easy to reduce and to immobilize, for example using cast or a brace. In case of cast being used, a brace s should replace it after 2 or 3 weeks, after which the patient can start weight bearing to enhance healing. After 6 weeks, the athlete may start range of motion training and thereafter gradually increased strength training. Distal epiphysiolysis is treated according to the same principles; however, sometimes it requires exact surgical reduction and fixation, due to the risk of a growth zone injury in combination with a bone fracture. Syndesmosis injuries always require surgical stabilization.
- Prognosis: Prognosis is good provided exact reduction is achieved and thereafter adequate immobilization. In some cases, all or part of the epiphyseal plate may be so damaged that premature union of the epiphysis with the diaphysis (epiphysiodesis) occurs. This causes asymmetrical growth, which in turn may make corrective surgery necessary.

Chronic Lower Leg Pain

Jón Karlson[1], Håkan Alfredson[2], and C. Niek van Dijk[3]

[1]*Sahlgrenska University Hospital/Mölndal, Mölndal, Sweden*
[2]*University of Umeå, Sports Medicine Umeå Inc., Umeå, Sweden*
[3]*Academic Medical Center, Amsterdam, The Netherlands*

Occurrence

The lower leg is the most common location for chronic overuse disorders. These disorders are caused by external and internal factors and often by several factors in combination. The most common external cause is sometimes mentioned as "too much too soon"—that is, too rapid an increase in terms of the amount and intensity of training, running on hard (asphalt) or icy surfaces, poor training shoes, and training in cold climate. Malalignment is the most important internal cause, with the most common types being foot malalignment such as hyperpronation (longitudinal flatfoot), knee malalignment, such as varus (bow legged) or valgus (knock knees), increased anteversion of the femoral neck with toeing in, anisomelia (leg length discrepancy), and poorly rehabilitated musculature after previous injury and/or surgery. Athletes in all sports in which running is an important part of the activity may be affected by chronic overuse disorders in the lower leg.

Differential Diagnoses

The most common overuse disorders of the lower leg are medial tibia syndrome, stress fractures, Achilles tendinopathy, and chronic compartment syndrome (Table 13.2). In the same manner as for acute lower leg injuries, differential diagnoses for chronic overuse injuries are few. It is important not to miss bone and soft-tissue tumors. They can in many cases resemble the symptoms of overuse disorders. One such tumor is osteogenic sarcoma of the proximal tibia, which is most common in children. Osteoid osteoma, a benign bone tumor, is also often located in the lower extremities. Pain from osteoid osteoma often mimics pain caused by a stress fracture. Because some of these differential diagnoses are serious, the physician should always carefully evaluate patients who have long-term or noncharacteristic symptoms, especially with skeletal scintigraphy and/or MRI.

Most common	Less common	Must not be overlooked !
Medial tibia syndrome, p. 418	Peroneus tendinopathy, p. 422	Nerve contusion
Stress fracture, p. 419	Tibialis anterior tendinitis/paratenonitis, p. 422	Tumors
Achilles tendinopathy, p. 420	Chronic compartment syndrome, p. 423	Sciatica
	Retrocalcaneal bursitis, p. 424	Intermittent claudication
	Calcaneal apophysitis, p. 425	
	Retrocalcaneal bursitis and superficial bursitis, p. 425	
	Tibialis posterior tendinopathy, p. 456	

Table 13.2 Overview of the differential diagnoses of chronic lower leg injuries. (Reproduced with permission from the Norwegian Sports Medicine Association.)

LOWER LEG

Other relatively common differential diagnoses are sciatica with pain radiating to the lower leg, and intermittent claudication, caused by a poor blood supply to the lower leg musculature.

Diagnostic Thinking

It is as important to document the causes of chronic overuse injuries of the lower leg. In most cases, if the symptoms are treated and the causes are left untreated, the patient will eventually return to the doctor with the same symptoms. A thorough physical examination will often reveal one or more internal factors and the intensity of training is often only the triggering factor. If internal factors are minor, it usually takes a major change in the training "dose" to trigger overuse injuries, whereas the opposite is true of major congenital or acquired malalignment (Figure 13.10).

Case History

A thorough case history is important in order to determine what causes the patient's symptoms. The physician must document factors such as the amount and intensity

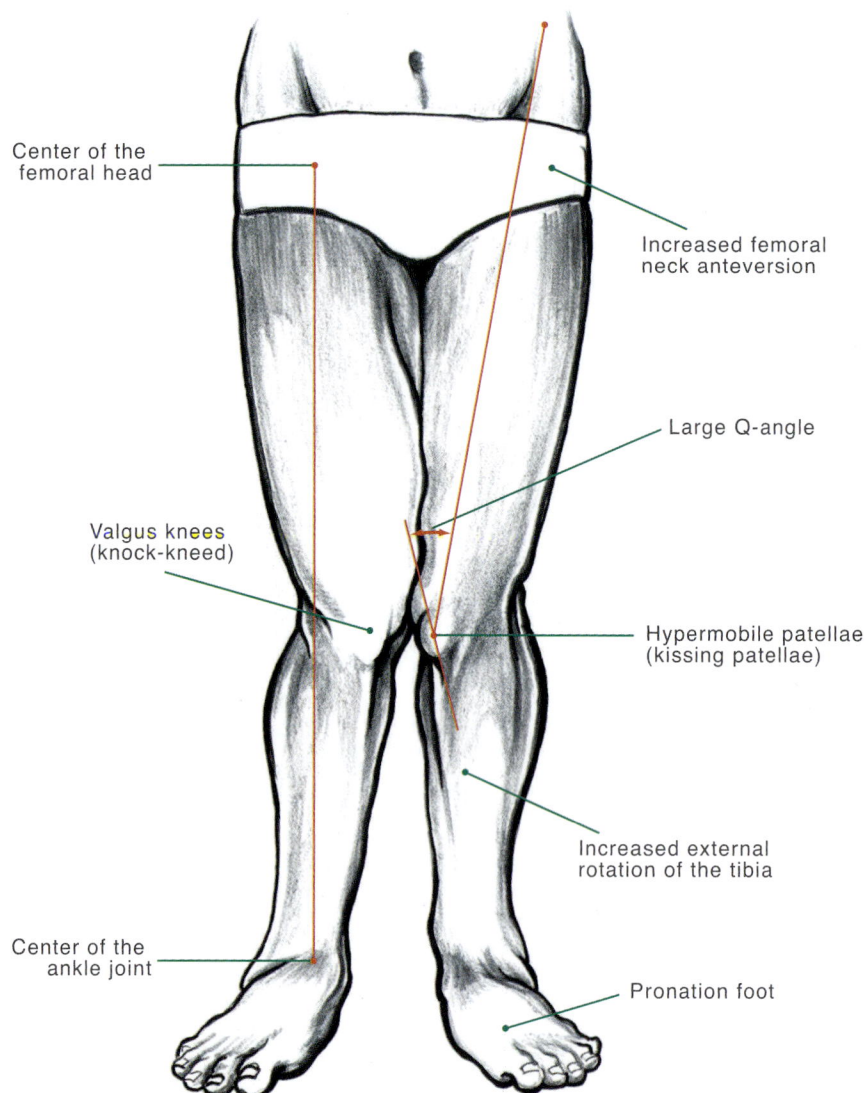

Figure 13.10 Malicious malalignment syndrome. This patient has increased anteversion of the hip, large Q-angle, increased external rotation in the tibia, and hyperpronation of the foot. When there is increased valgus positioning of the knee, the weight-bearing line is located lateral to the center of the knee joint. (© Medical Illustrator Tommy Bolic, Sweden.)

of training, increases in loading, the training surface, the footwear, and the timing of the symptoms in relation to these factors. It is also necessary to accurately document the exact location of the pain (Figure 13.11), whether it is local or diffuse, whether it started suddenly or gradually, whether it is continuous or only occurs during training, and whether it continues for a while after training is terminated. In addition, the physician should document whether the pain was initially a minor annoyance and gradually increased in connection with activity, or whether the pain remained unchanged during activity. In an athlete with medial tibia syndrome, the pain will start gradually during loading and will be localized to approximately the distal two thirds of the medial margin of the tibia. The pain often lasts for some time after weight bearing and will increase in intensity if the athlete does not reduce the amount of training. However, a stress fracture starts more suddenly, usually while running, and pain is localized to a smaller area. Pain also disappears quickly as a result of unloading and returns when the athlete attempts to run again.

Clinical Examination

Inspection. With the patient standing, the physician looks for scoliosis (curvature of the spine), anisomelia (one leg longer than the other), toeing in (as a sign of increased anteversion of the femoral neck), and varus or valgus malalignment of the knees (Figures 13.11 and 13.12), whether the patella (on both sides) are pointing straight forward or internally rotated (kissing patella), and whether there is hyperpronation of the feet (Figure 13.13). General posture should also be noted. It is often easy to uncover a moderate degree of pronation if the patient walks back and forth,

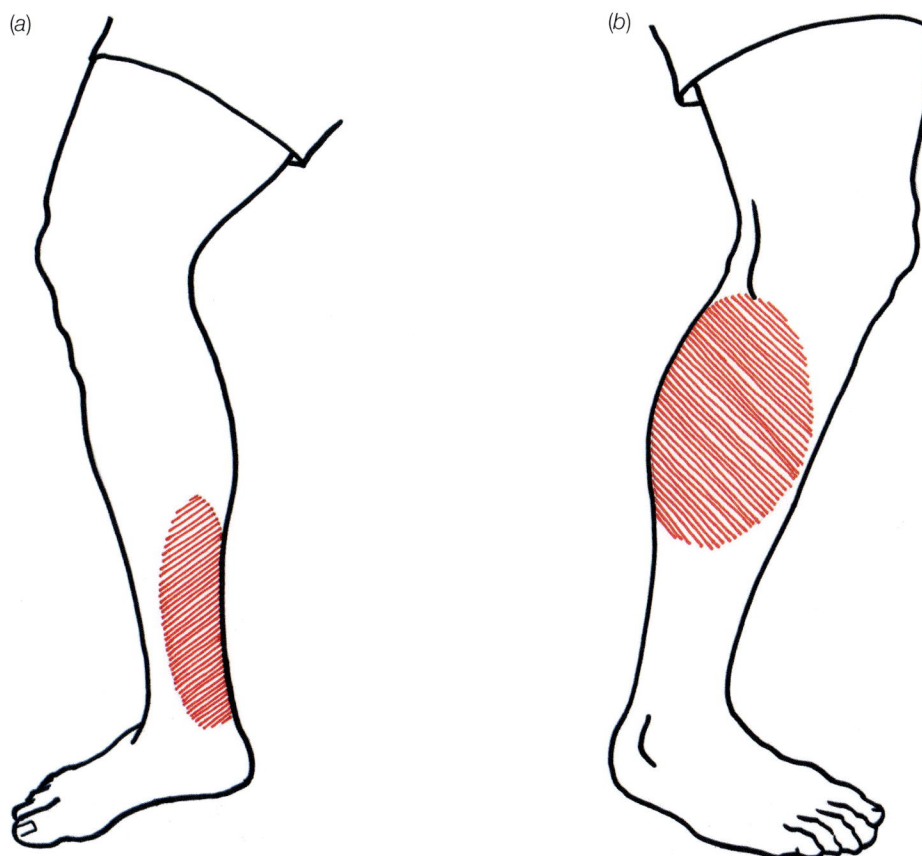

Figure 13.11 In athletes with medial tibia syndrome, the pain is usually located on the medial side of the leg (a), approximately 5–10 cm from the ankle joint. In patients with stress fracture, the pain is located more proximally in the leg (b). (© Medical Illustrator Tommy Bolic, Sweden.)

LOWER LEG

or walks or runs on a treadmill. The best method is to videotape the athlete on the treadmill from behind and thereafter watch the video in slow motion.

Functional testing. An athlete with a stress fracture of the lower leg usually shows a positive hop test. In case of a stress fracture, axial loading will trigger localized pain, in contrast to a more diffuse type in case of medial tibia syndrome. With the patient lying in a supine position, the physician looks for local swelling, or discoloration of the injured area.

Palpation. In a patient with medial tibia syndrome, palpation of the distal two-thirds of the medial margin of the tibia causes pain. The bony edge may feel irregular and sometimes bumpy. A stress fracture will cause local pain and possibly some swelling. In case of chronic compartment syndrome, the affected compartment is more tense than normal; the musculature is tender on palpation, especially directly after a training session. Chronic Achilles tendinopathy is often manifested by local thickening of the tendon and it may be tender to palpation (Figure 13.14). Retrocalcaneal bursitis is easy to detect by fluctuation, and pressure makes the bursa painful as well. Calcaneal apophysitis causes local pain and sometimes mild swelling at the insertion of the Achilles tendon to the calcaneus.

Supplemental Examinations

Radiographic examination. Radiographic examination of the entire lower leg in two planes is indicated in most chronic painful conditions of the lower leg. It is particularly useful for excluding possible serious differential diagnoses. If the patient has long-term chronic compartment syndrome, radiographic examination

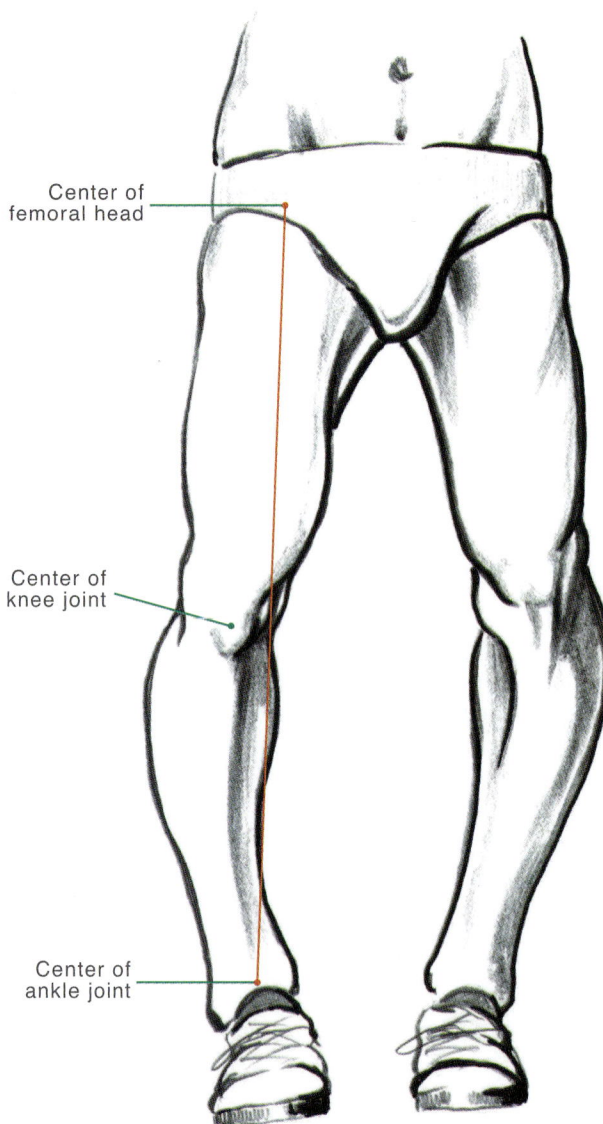

Center of femoral head

Center of knee joint

Center of ankle joint

Figure 13.12 Varus knees. If there is increased varus position of the knees, the weight-bearing line is located medial to the center of the knee joint. (© Medical Illustrator Tommy Bolic, Sweden.)

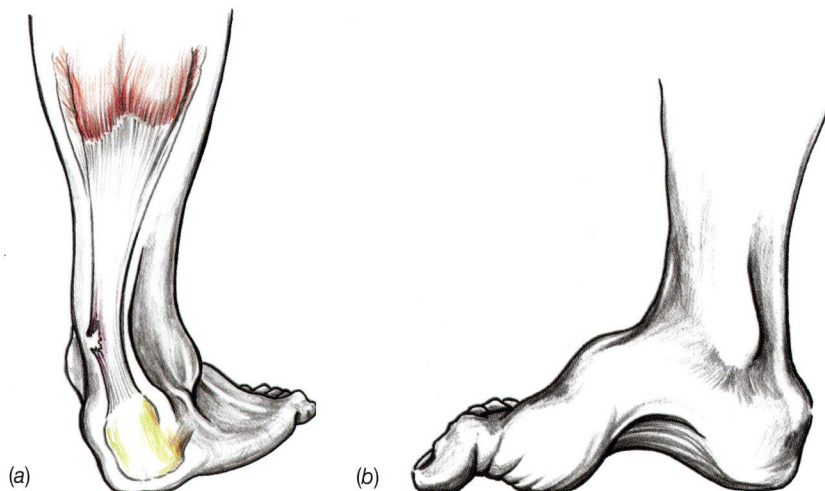

Figure 13.13 Pronation foot (flatfoot) (a) and cavus foot (claw foot) (b). Pronation foot may predispose to overuse injuries of the foot, ankle, lower leg, and knee. (© Medical Illustrator Tommy Bolic, Sweden.)

(a)

(b)

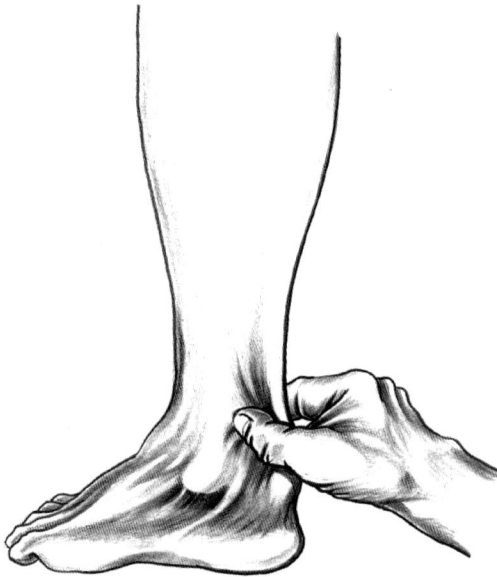

Figure 13.14 Palpation technique. Palpation of the Achilles tendon, approximately 2–6 cm from the insertion to bone triggers pain in the patient with Achilles tendinopathy. (© Medical Illustrator Tommy Bolic, Sweden.)

Figure 13.15 Stress fracture of the anterior cortex of the tibia. Sometimes stress fractures are difficult to see on x-rays. In most cases, there is thickening of the bone. This stress reaction happens before a stress fracture occurs. (© Medical Illustrator Tommy Bolic, Sweden.)

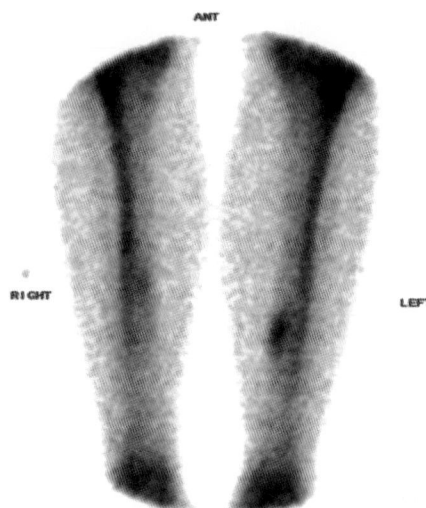

will often demonstrate a somewhat thickened and uneven medial cortex of the distal two-thirds of the tibia, whereas a stress fracture may be difficult to reveal. Stress fractures of the anterior margin of the tibia will appear as small rarefactions (mouse bites) in the cortical portion of the bone (Figure 13.15), but it is important to note that radiographs can only detect stress fractures in their later stages. If the patient has calcaneal apophysitis, the radiograph may show sclerosis and possibly fragmentation of the calcaneus at the insertion of the Achilles tendon.

Skeletal scintigraphy. Scintigraphy [or single-photon emission computed tomography (SPECT), if available] is an important examination in patients with chronic overuse injuries and is of particular diagnostic value in terms of stress fractures. One or 2 days after the symptoms begin, scintigraphy will show increased activity at the fracture site (Figure 13.16), while there is increased but more diffuse activity related to high loading of the skeletal substance, for instance, medial tibia syndrome.

Ultrasonographic examination. Scar changes in the musculature after partial or total ruptures as well as changes in the Achilles tendon from chronic tendinosis can be demonstrated using ultrasonography.

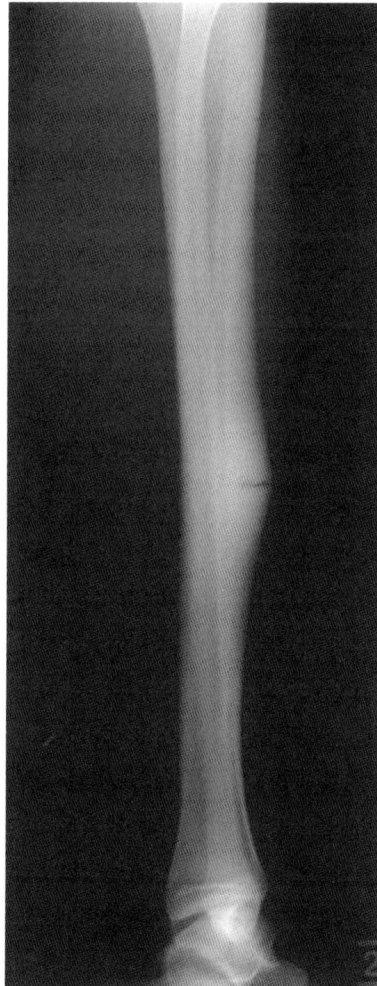

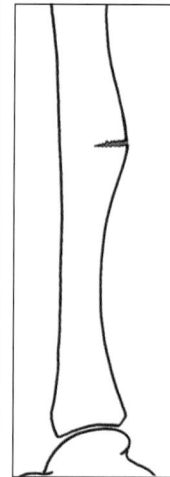

Figure 13.16 Skeletal scintigraphy. Stress fracture of the left tibia. (Reproduced with permission from the Norwegian Sports Medicine Association.)

LOWER LEG

417

MRI. MRI is used for the same purposes as ultrasound. In addition, MRI can also be used in the evaluation of tumors.

Pressure measurement. Several studies have shown that increased pressure can be measured in the anterior and lateral compartment of the lower leg when clinical symptoms indicate chronic compartment syndrome, especially after weight bearing. However, measurements of the deep and superficial posterior compartments have not produced similar results.

Common Injuries

Medial Tibia Syndrome— "Periostitis" of the Medial Margin of the Shin Bone

This is one of the most commonly occurring chronic overuse injuries in athletes. It occurs in all sports in which running and jumping constitute a major part of the activity. Muscular hypertrophy and stiffness related to intense training periods are assumed to be an important triggering factor of medial tibia syndrome, and the pain is associated with thickening of the fascia close to the periosteum at the medial margin of the tibia, particularly the distal two-thirds. Important predisposing factors are increased external rotation of the lower leg and hyperpronation. Both of these malalignments will cause the athlete to deviate his step onto the medial aspect of the foot (Figure 13.17), which increases medial load on the longitudinal arch of the foot

- Symptoms and signs: During and for a while after training the athlete experiences tenderness and sometimes pain along the medial tibial margin at the distal one-third of the lower leg. Pain gradually increases with the intensity of training and may become so incapacitating that the affected athlete will have to end his/her running and jumping exercises.
- Diagnosis: The diagnosis can be made based on history and a thorough clinical examination. Palpation findings are intense tenderness and sometimes swelling at the medial tibial margin. Most patients with this disorder have either externally rotated lower legs or hyperpronated feet. A poorly defined thickened medial cortex in the tibia will be visible on plain radiographs, and diffuse increased activity along large portions of the tibial margin (known as a stress reaction of the bone) will be visible by skeletal scintigraphy.
- Treatment by therapist: During the acute phase, the disorder is primarily treated with rest, alternative training, stretching of the lower leg musculature, and NSAIDs. At the same time, any malalignment should be

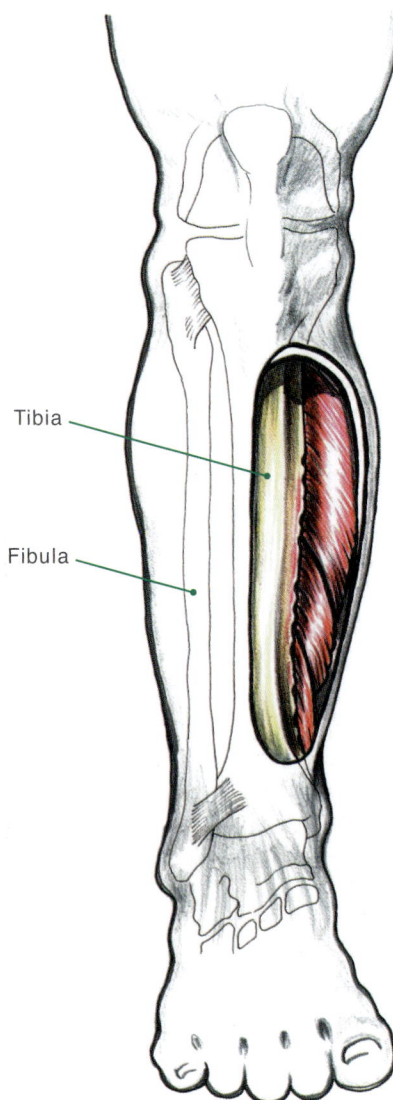

Tibia

Fibula

Figure 13.17 Medial tibia syndrome. Increased external rotation of the tibia and hyperpronation of the foot can result in increased loading on the insertion of the periosteum on the medial aspect of the tibia. This may also occur in athletes with normal alignment. (© Medical Illustrator Tommy Bolic, Sweden.)

corrected with specially fitted training shoes and/or insoles, and any training problems (e.g., intensity or surface) also need to be corrected. In case of hyperpronated feet, insoles should be used to correct valgus positioning of the heel and to provide good support under the longitudinal arch of the foot. It is often difficult to make the proper insole at the first attempt, and the orthopedic technician may need to make several adjustments. In some cases, the results of nonsurgical treatment are not satisfactory.

- Treatment by physician: Several studies have shown that the outcome is satisfactory in 80–90% of the patients who undergo surgical division of the superficial and deep posterior muscle compartments at the medial edge of the tibia. Therefore, this has become a routine intervention in many athletes with long-term disorders. The athlete can resume running training after 4–6 weeks.

- Prognosis: Prognosis is good if the external and internal triggering factors are corrected early. The athlete should plan to be away from high-level sport for approximately 6 months after surgical treatment.

Stress Fracture

Stress fractures of the tibia and fibula occur frequently in athletes, in which running and jumping constitute a major portion of their training and competitive activity. Several studies have shown that up to 50% of all stress fractures in the body occur in the lower leg. The fractures are primarily localized to the distal and proximal part of the tibia and the distal part of the fibula (Figure 13.18). Stress fractures typically occur between a few weeks and a few months after the athlete starts training; in athletes, who are active at a high level, they occur in connection with increased training intensity, usually when the athlete is preparing for a major competition. High loading on hard surface and insufficient shock absorption of the running shoes, combined with rapid increment of the training intensity, are the most important external factors. Malalignment may also be a contributing factor, but not to the same extent as in the development of medial tibia syndrome.

- Symptoms and signs: Significant pain of an acute onset from loading, usually during a long training session, is the primary and most important symptom. The pain is localized, and often disappears during rest. It returns as soon as the athlete attempts to start running again.

- Diagnosis: The history is the typical onset of pain and should raise the suspicion of a stress fracture. Examination includes tenderness and in some cases swelling over the fracture area and a positive hop test. Plain radiographs during the early phase are often negative, but callus may sometimes be demonstrated at the fracture site several weeks later. Skeletal scintigraphy must be performed to confirm the diagnosis, and this examination can be positive 1 or 2 days after the symptoms begin. MRI is, however, the most sensitive investigation during the early stages.

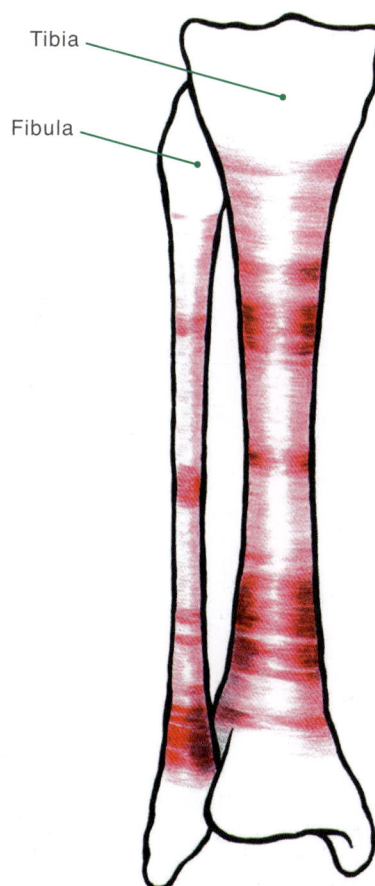

Tibia

Fibula

Figure 13.18 Location of stress fractures in the tibia and fibula. The color intensity shows where stress fractures usually occur. (© Medical Illustrator Tommy Bolic, Sweden.)

LOWER LEG

- Treatment by therapist: No weight bearing, using crutches for 6–8 weeks in terms of tibial fractures and 4 weeks in terms of fibular fractures is normally sufficient for healing, depending on the location of the fracture, especially in case of tibia stress fracture. During this period, it is important for the athlete to perform alternative training, that is, other activities that running, jumping, and direct loading of the affected lower extremity. Bicycling and running in water may be useful to maintain endurance, and strength training that does not include weight bearing is allowed. The physician should inform the patient of the necessity of adequate unloading; in order to avoid recurrence. During the unloading period, it is important to document why the patient has sustained a stress fracture and to correct both the training errors and malalignment.
- Treatment by physician: In rare cases, the stress fracture is located at the anterior cortex of the mid portion of the tibia. These fractures are known to be difficult to heal and may in some cases develop pseudoarthrosis, apparently because the blood supply in this part of the leg is poor. Even unloading for a long period does not lead to desired result. The patient remains pain free during normal daily activities; however, he has a recurrence of symptoms as soon as running training is resumed. Several different treatment methods have been suggested for these fractures. The most-used methods are surgical fixation of the anterior cortex with a plate and screws, medullary nailing of the tibia, excision of the fracture area, bone transplantation, or excision and drilling of the anterior cortex. Good results have been achieved by all these methods, but no large case series are reported. However, they involve surgical intervention, with the risk of complications that are related to any surgery. Therefore, in recent years, these fractures are sometimes treated with extracorporal shock wave therapy. However, the results are variable.
- Prognosis: Most stress fractures in the lower leg will heal if they are diagnosed early and adequately unloaded. Prophylaxis is the key to both primary fracture treatment and recurrences, including education of the patient in terms of proper footwear, avoiding too much training on hard surface, and to avoid to increase the intensity of training too rapidly. Sometimes an athlete (usually a thin, female athlete) will sustain several stress fractures at the same time. If this occurs, it is necessary to investigate the athlete for amenorrhea, anorexia related to the stress fractures.

Achilles Tendinopathy—*Chronic Painful Conditions in the Achilles Tendon*

Of the tendons in the lower leg, the Achilles tendon is the one that is most often affected by chronic changes. In such cases, degenerative changes (tendinosis) will occur in the tendon in the long term. Hyperpronation is one primary cause of chronic pain in the Achilles tendon. This condition will cause the foot to deviate into a valgus position after a heel strike, which in turn causes major loading of the medial fibers due to angulation of the Achilles tendon (Figure 13.19). This overloading may result in chronic irritation of the paratenon on the medial side of the tendon and in the tendon itself. External factors, such as running on a hard surface, cold climate, poor shock absorption of the footwear, and shoes with stiff soles, often contribute to the development of chronic Achilles tendinosis.

- Symptoms and signs: Pain is the major symptom. It can be divided into four stages. In stage 1, pain is felt only after activity and disappears after a period of rest. In stage 2, pain is felt during the activity, but does not limit the activity. In stage 3, pain is felt during the activity and is so intense that it prevents the athlete from participating in normal training. In stage 4, chronic pain is experienced, even while the patient is at rest. Morning stiffness and pain are typical early signs.

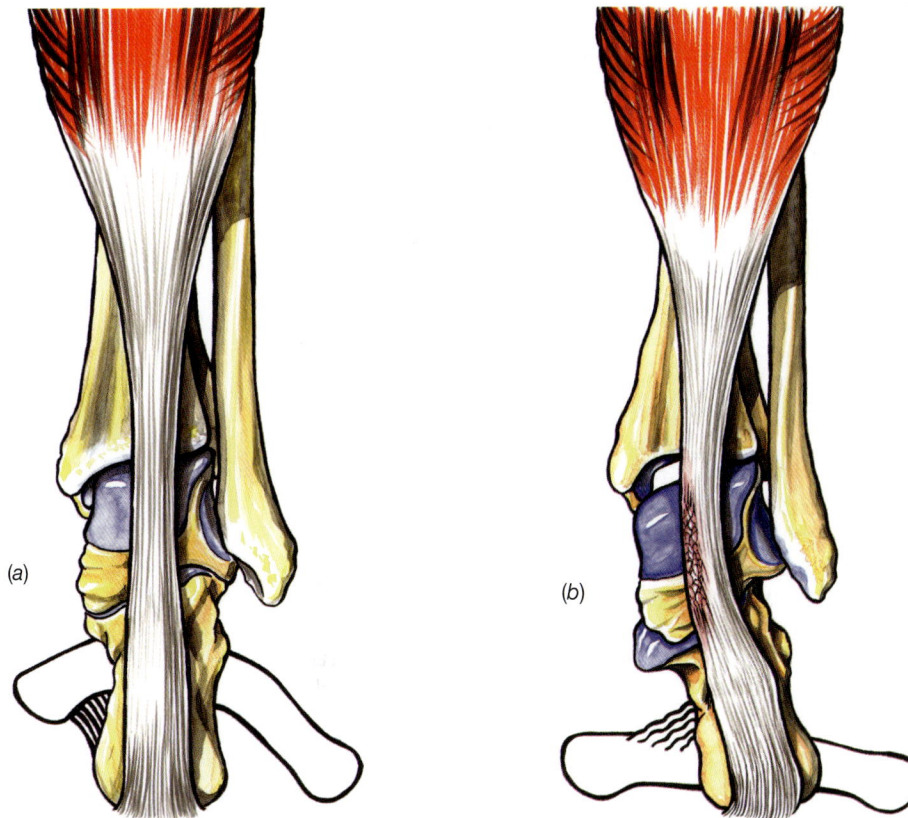

Figure 13.19 Achilles tendinosis—pronation foot. If the patient's foot position is normal (*a*) the Achilles tendon is straight, whereas a pronation foot (*b*) causes malalignment of the Achilles tendon with increased load on the medial part. (© Medical Illustrator Tommy Bolic, Sweden.)

- Diagnosis: Palpation findings are swelling and tenderness over the tendon. Both dorsal and plantar flexion movements of the ankle trigger pain. Thickening of the tendon is often present, approximately 2–6 cm proximal to the calcaneus. Ultrasonography and/or MRI will demonstrate thickened tendon, and in some cases degenerative tendon tissue.
- Treatment by physician: During the early-phase unloading, stretching the leg musculature, alternative training, and correction of the triggering factors (such as hyperpronation and training surface problems) can help. In some athletes injections using sclerosing agents and more recently platelet-rich plasma may give some improvement, but few are cured, and should not be considered until an eccentric training program has been completed for at least 3 months. Corticosteroid injections should neither be given into nor around the tendon. Nonsurgical treatment may not be successful in all patients. Surgical treatment, where the paratenon is divided and separated from the tendon, and in some cases degenerated tissue is removed from the tendon itself may produce satisfactory results, but the rehabilitation time is long, at least 6 months. Today, mini-invasive surgery, including arthroscopic methods, is being tested.
- Treatment by therapist: Patients with chronic Achilles tendinopathy have achieved good results after eccentric or eccentric-concentric strength training of the triceps surae muscle and the Achilles tendon itself. The athlete must do this training routine regularly, for 3–6 months, and with gradually increasing loads. After any surgical treatment, the retraining must be individualized according to the findings made during the surgery, but generally, athletes must gradually increase loading to a normal gait after 4–6 weeks. In order to avoid adhesion between the tendon and

LOWER LEG

421

the skin, mobility training in the ankle joint without loading is started as soon as pain allows. Beginning on the 6th postoperative week, the athlete can gradually increase strength training of the triceps muscle. Running training may begin, with caution in the beginning, when full range of motion and full strength is achieved, usually after about 3–4 months.

- Prognosis: Prognosis is usually good with proper treatment. Most patients become fully or partially asymptomatic and can resume their previous sports activity. However, rehabilitation after either nonsurgical or surgical treatment may take a long time. The need for surgical treatment is limited.

Other Injuries

Peroneus Tendinopathy—*Painful Conditions in the Peroneus Tendons*

Peroneal tendon problems are important differential diagnosis after ankle injury, especially partial longitudinal rupture that is always located behind the lateral malleolus (Figure 13.20). This injury is sometimes seen in patients with chronic recurrent ankle instability. This injury should especially be taken into consideration in athletes who do not recover well after ankle ligament injury.

- Symptoms and signs: There is moderate, but chronic swelling behind the lateral malleolus. There is always pain on palpation in the retromalleolar area.
- Diagnosis: Ultrasonography and/or MRI can be used to establish the diagnosis and to evaluate the extent of injury to the tendon. There is a longitudinal splitting of the tendon, in the majority of cases the peroneus brevis tendon is the one affected.
- Treatment by therapist: Rehabilitation with range of motion, balance training, and muscle strengthening. In case of moderate to major tendon damage, physical therapy is often not successful, but surgical treatment is needed.
- Treatment by physician: In many cases surgical treatment is needed. The tendon is explored, the degenerated tendon tissue removed and the tendon reconstructed. In case of concomitant ankle laxity, the ligaments (anterior talofibular and calcaneofibular) are reconstructed at the same time. Postoperative the ankle is immobilized for 6 weeks, before rehabilitation is started. Full weight bearing is allowed.
- Prognosis: The prognosis after surgical treatment is good; the majority recovers well and athletes are able to return to their previous activity level after approximately 3–4 months.

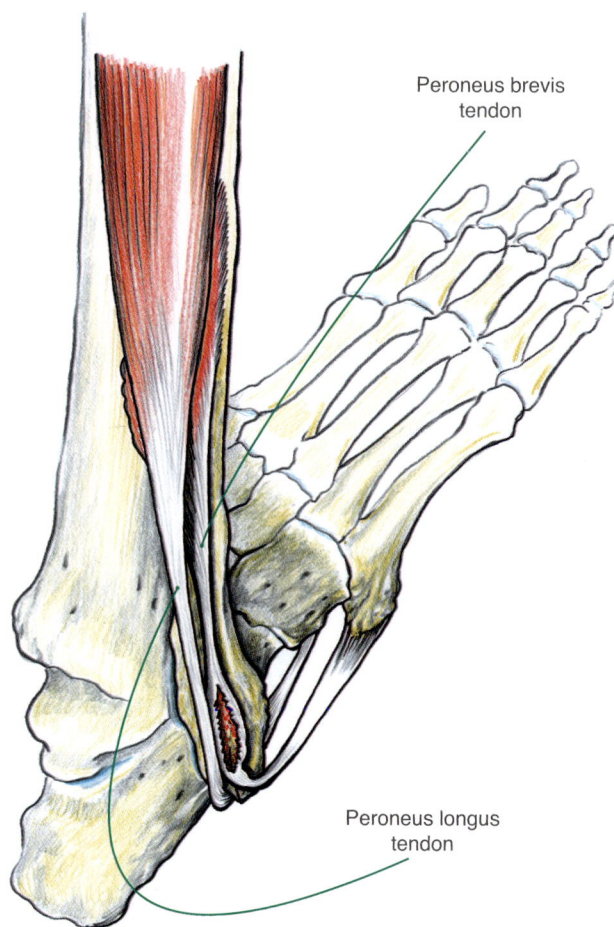

Peroneus brevis tendon

Peroneus longus tendon

Figure 13.20 Longitudinal partial rupture of the peroneus brevis tendon behind the lateral malleolus. This injury sometimes happens in athletes with recurrent ankle instability. (© Medical Illustrator Tommy Bolic, Sweden.)

Tibialis Anterior Tendinitis/Paratenonitis—*Acute Tendon/Tendon Sheath Inflammation*

Acute, inflammatory reactions are sometimes seen around the ankle, mainly in the tibialis anterior tendon sheath. In most cases, it is triggered directly by "too much too soon," that is, the patient has increased the amount and intensity of loading too rapidly. External factors, such as running on a hard surface, cold climate, poor footwear, and internal factors (such as foot malalignment, particularly hyperpronation), are important contributing factors. If these factors are not corrected at the same time as the training errors are corrected, there is a great likelihood that the athlete will experience a recurrence of the symptoms even if the initial treatment is successful.

- Symptoms and signs: Patients experience pain of acute onset, caused by movement of the ankle joint, and pain localized over the affected tendon.
- Diagnosis: Diagnosis is established based on local swelling, tenderness, and possibly crepitation when the tendon is palpated.
- Treatment by physician: Physicians should identify any triggering factors and correct them as necessary. NSAIDs are often useful.
- Treatment by therapist: Recommended treatment is unloading until asymptomatic. The athlete should start alternative training during the initial period, that is, should engage in activities that do not cause pain in the affected area.
- Prognosis: Prognosis is usually good, if unloading and other treatment are started early. The symptoms will usually disappear in 1 or 2 weeks. However, the condition can easily become chronic if the athlete continues excessive loading despite the pain.

Chronic Compartment Syndrome—*Chronic Increased Compartmental Pressure*

Chronic compartment syndrome of the lower leg is a relatively rare disorder that primarily affects the anterior, and less often the deep posterior muscle compartment, and very rarely the lateral and superficial posterior compartments. The disorder is most common in athletes who are engaged in running and jumping exercises such as team handball and football, but also in athletes who engage in strength sports, like weight lifting. Chronic compartment syndrome is usually caused by rapidly increasing muscle volume in connection with intense training. Muscle volume will increase during exercise, because of the increased blood volume and the retention of fluid, which leads to increased pressure in the compartment, reduces capillary circulation, and eventually causes ischemic pain. When loading stops, the pressure decreases, the blood supply normalizes, and pain disappears.

- Symptoms and signs: Patients experiences pain from loading starting gradually. The pain usually rapidly disappears at rest. The disorder may become so intense that the athlete has problems with dorsal flexion of the ankle and may have paresthesia (numbness), particularly in the area innervated by the peroneus nerve. The pain is always localized to the affected compartment.
- Diagnosis: Diagnosis is based on tender, tight musculature, particularly after provocation (running). The diagnosis is confirmed by pressure measurements of the affected compartment after loading. Pressure in a muscle compartment of the lower leg is normally between 10 and 15 mmHg, both at rest and during activity, whereas loading may increase the pressure to over 30 mmHg, when a chronic compartment syndrome is present by definition.
- Treatment by therapist: During the early stages, the recommended treatment is unloading and stretching of the lower leg musculature, alternative training, and short period of rest. It is especially important for the athlete to avoid running on hard surface and to wear well-adjusted footwear with good shock absorption and necessary correction of any malalignment. The athlete should avoid loading that provokes the symptoms for up to 3 months and then gradually resume training.
- Treatment by physician: If the disorder is chronic, it may be necessary to surgically unload the affected muscle compartment. To avoid scar formation and adhesions in the area where the surgery was performed, the patient must begin mobility training and light strength training of the lower leg musculature as soon after surgery as possible.

LOWER LEG

• **Prognosis:** Prognosis after surgical treatment is good. The athlete can in most cases return to full training activity 6–8 weeks after surgical treatment.

Retrocalcaneal Bursitis

A bursa is normally found in the area between the calcaneus and the Achilles tendon (Figure 13.21). It may become inflamed because of chronic irritation, such as from direct pressure from tight shoes, or indirectly via chronic tendinopathy of the distal portion of the tendon.

• **Symptoms and signs:** Patients experience pain, and often swelling, particularly on the lateral side. Pressure from shoes may cause significant discomfort.
• **Diagnosis:** Pain, swelling, and possibly fluctuation when the bursa is palpated will help to establish the diagnosis. Ultrasonography and MRI show an increased amount of fluid in the bursa.
• **Treatment by therapist:** The primary treatment is to avoid pressure on the tendon insertion. This may be achieved by shoe modification or by using a piece of foam rubber and placing it over the painful area.
• **Treatment by physician:** If the symptoms continue, corticosteroid injection into the bursa may be effective. The physician should avoid injecting cortisone into the tendon insertion because this may increase the risk of tendon rupture. If non-surgical treatment is not successful, surgical treatment may become necessary. Arthroscopic extirpation is recommended.

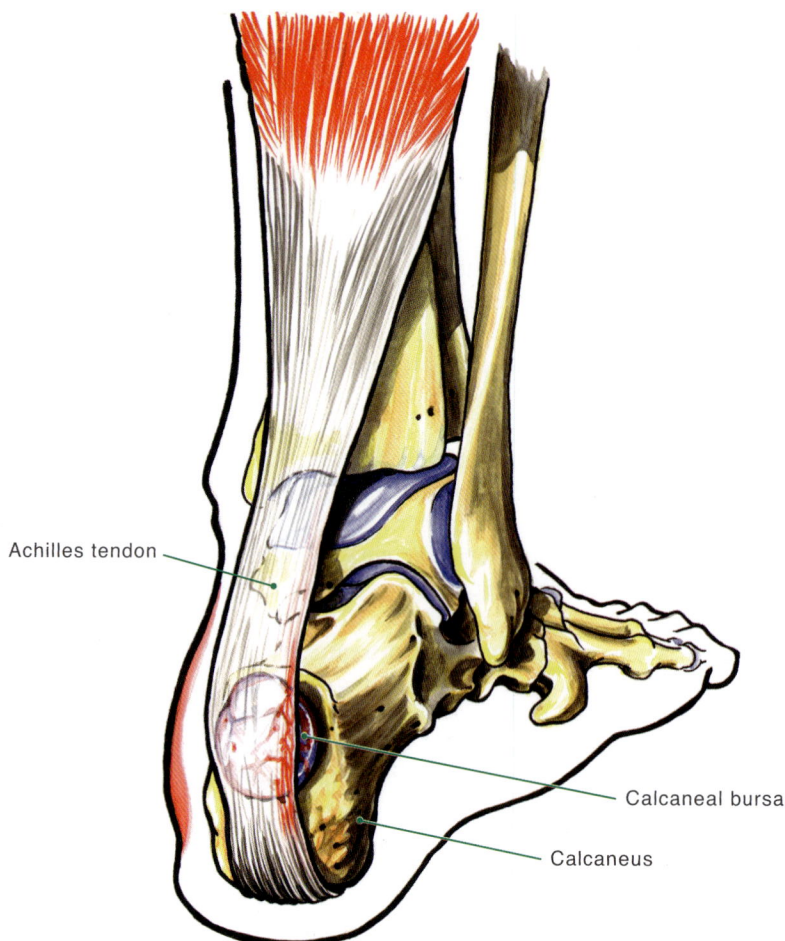

Achilles tendon

Calcaneal bursa

Calcaneus

Figure 13.21
Retrocalcaneal bursitis. The retrocalcaneal bursa is located beneath the Achilles tendon pointing toward the distal insertion on the calcaneus. Bursitis is often accompanied by a bony spur on the calcaneus. (© Medical Illustrator Tommy Bolic, Sweden.)

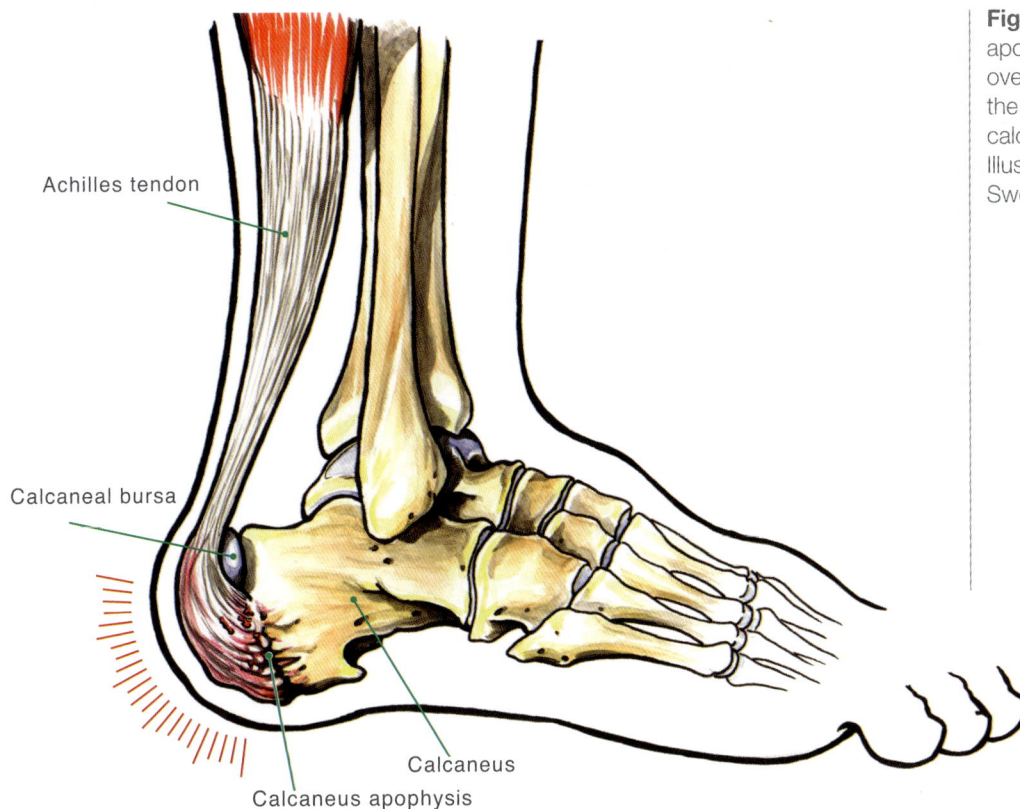

Figure 13.22 Calcaneal apophysitis. This is an overuse injury that affects the growth plate of the calcaneus. (© Medical Illustrator Tommy Bolic, Sweden.)

Achilles tendon

Calcaneal bursa

Calcaneus

Calcaneus apophysis

Calcaneal Apophysitis (Morbus Sever)

This condition occurs in active adolescents (primarily between the ages of 10 and 15 years), during the pubertal growth spurt when the child's height increases rapidly and muscle strength develops somewhat more slowly. It is caused by overloading of the tendon insertion to the calcaneus and of the growth plate (apophysis) in this area, in combination with fragmentation and possibly sclerosis of the bone nucleus (Figure 13.22).

- Symptoms and signs: Pain is localized to the posterior portion of the calcaneus during and after exercise. The area often feels stiff, and the child may limp.
- Diagnosis: Diagnosis is established based on tenderness on palpation and possibly mild swelling over the tendon insertion. Radiographs may show fragmentation and sclerosis of the posterior portion of the calcaneus.
- Treatment: The physician should inform the patient and the patient's parents that the disorder will resolve spontaneously when the patient is between 16 and 18 years old. The athlete's activity is limited only by pain.

Retrocalcaneal bursitis and superficial bursitis—*Bony Prominence at the Achilles Tendon Insertion*

Long-term chronic irritation around the insertion of the Achilles tendon, such as bursitis, will cause a periosteal reaction with bone formation in the area between the tendon and the heel bone (Figure 13.23), most often with overgrowth in the lateral direction. Pressure in this area, for instance, related to tight shoes will make the disorder worse, eventually causing significant pseudoexostosis (bone spur) (Figure 13.24), often combined with an inflamed subcutaneous bursa.

- **Symptoms and signs:** The patient experiences pain over a protruding bump, which is beneath and lateral to the tendon insertion.
- **Diagnosis:** Diagnosis is made by clinical examination. Radiographs are helpful to show the bony outgrowth.
- **Treatment:** If the patient must unload because of symptoms, alternative training (not running training) and corrective insoles are recommended. The athlete's activity is limited only by pain. If the symptoms are long lasting with significant bony outgrowth, surgical treatment may become necessary (arthroscopic treatment is recommended).

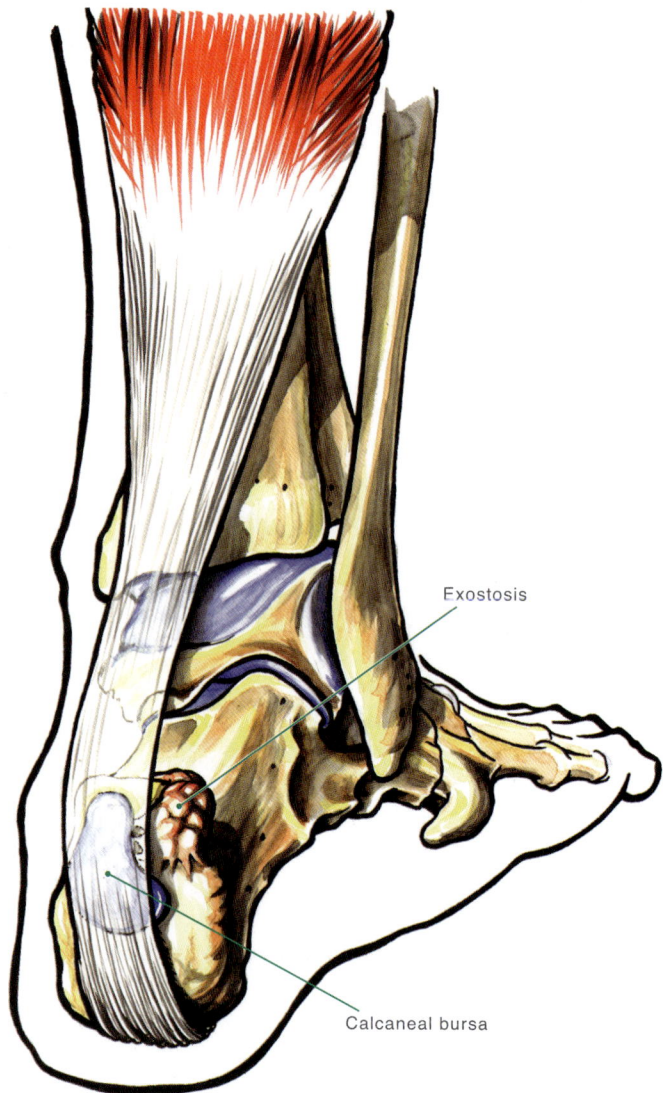

Exostosis

Calcaneal bursa

Figure 13.23 Posterosuperior calcaneal exostosis. The pseudoexostosis of the calcaneus is visible on the lateral side of the Achilles tendon. (© Medical Illustrator Tommy Bolic, Sweden.)

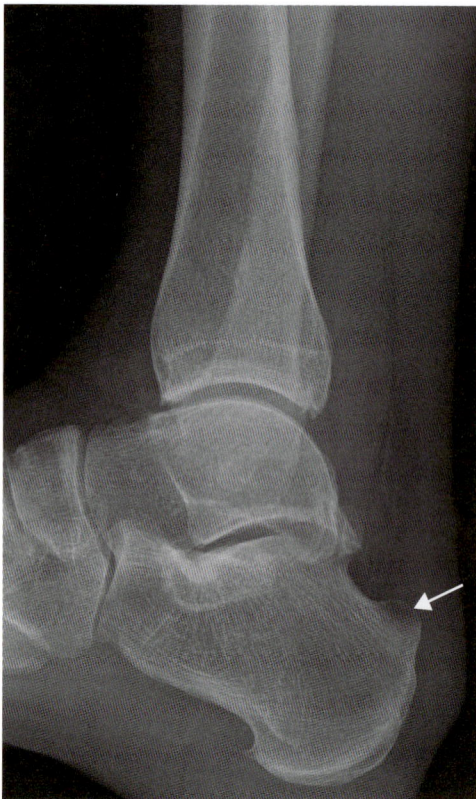

Figure 13.24 Radiograph showing the typical bone spur formation often seen in athletes with retrocalcaneal bursitis.

Rehabilitation of Lower Leg Injuries

Roland Thomée

Sahlgrenska University Hospital, Göteborg, Sweden

Acute Lower Leg Injuries: Goals and Principles

Table 13.3 lists the goals for rehabilitation of acute lower leg injuries.

During the acute phase, which usually last for 1–3 days after an acute injury, tape, bandage, or an orthosis may be used to provide protection and some compression. The rehabilitation should start as soon as possible with general exercises for the rest of the body. The physiotherapist can help the injured athlete with a rehab program with knee extension, knee flexion, leg press, hip muscle exercises, core exercises on a balance ball, and shoulder/arm exercises (Figure 13.25). Often can cardiovascular training start early with bicycling on an ergometer and as soon as tolerated on a cross trainer or a rowing machine. As soon as allowed and tolerated, exercises for the lower leg, ankle, and foot should be started. The main goal is to aid in the healing process. With low loading exercises there will be an increase in blood circulation, which aids the removal of waste products and provides nutrients for the injured tissue. Also the low load (compression, tension, and torsion) provides important stimuli for the ongoing repair phase (Figure 13.26).

Many injuries of the lower leg are treated with an orthotic device instead of a cast, allowing some range of motion and some loading of the injury. One example is a total Achilles tendon rupture, where a brace will help maintain mobility in the ankle joint while allowing some loading of the injured tendon.

Lower Leg Pain: Goals and Principles

The principles of rehabilitation for lower leg pain from an overuse injury are mostly the same as for an acute injury. However, the rehabilitation involves identifying the causes of the injury, usually to be found among external and internal factors. This helps the patient to avoid sustaining the same injury again. Overuse of the lower leg usually involves intense running and/or jumping with high forces from eccentric loading in the stretch shortening cycle of the muscle tendon complex. Running

	Goals	Measures
Acute phase	Reduce swelling	PRICE principle with emphasis on good compression
Rehabilitation phase	Normal mobility and able to train with normal function	Exercises for increased circulation and improved range of motion, strength and function
Training phase	Normal strength and sensory motor function Reduce the risk of reinjury	Sport-specific strength training and sensory motor training

Table 13.3 Goals and measures for rehabilitation of acute lower leg injuries. (Reproduced with permission from the Norwegian Sports Medicine Association.)

LOWER LEG

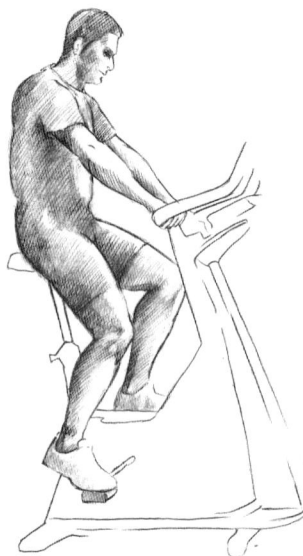

Figure 13.25 Bicycling (1–30 minutes, several times daily) for foot and ankle range of motion and for general conditioning. (Reproduced with permission from the Norwegian Sports Medicine Association.)

and jumping also involves high compression, tension, and torsion forces on skeletal structures. Therefore, it is important during rehabilitation to gradually improve the overall capacity of the lower leg structures to tolerate these high forces. The physiotherapist can design an individual rehab program with the adequate exercises and gradual increase in intensity. It is clear that the rehabilitation for many lower leg injuries takes a long time, that is, 6–12 months, sometimes longer.

The most important part of the rehabilitation program after a lower leg injury is a gradually increasing strength, running, and jumping program. A gradually increasing toe raise protocol for improved muscle strength and muscle endurance of the lower leg is presented in Figures 13.27 and 13.28. The physiotherapist can, when necessary, provide further specific strengthening exercises for the lower leg. When the speed of movement is increased the high forces of the stretch shortening cycle becomes more prominent. Therefore, the running and jumping programs should, with caution, be gradually increased and in close cooperation between the athlete and

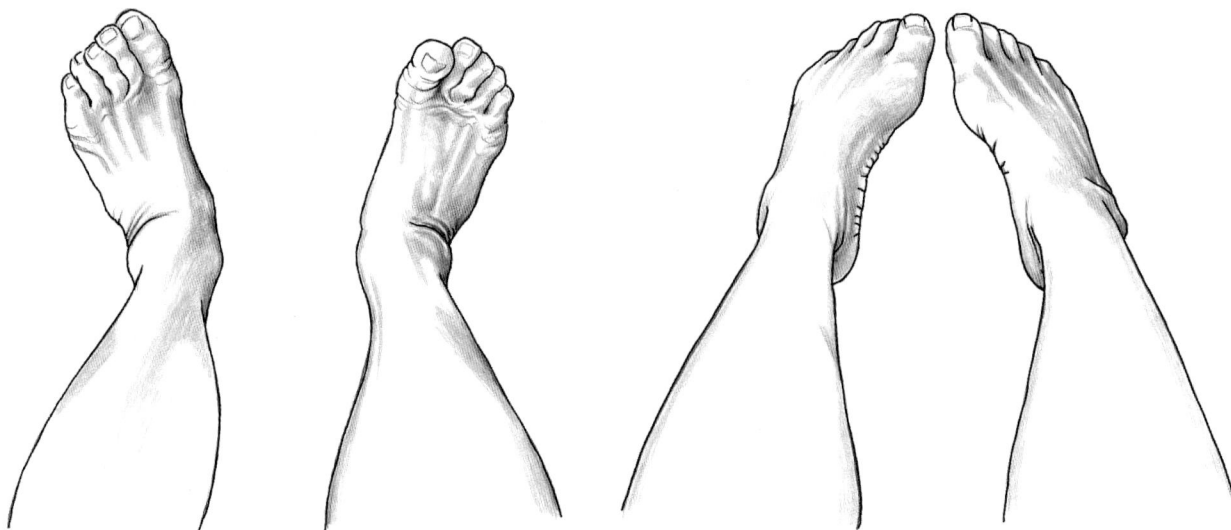

Figure 13.26 Ankle dorsi-/plantarflexion for increased circulation in the lower leg and for foot and ankle range of motion. Four sets of 20 repetitions of each exercise several times per day. (Reproduced with permission from the Norwegian Sports Medicine Association.)

the physiotherapist. When needed, the physiotherapist can also add specific range of motion exercises as well as specific exercises to improve neuromuscular control, for example, balance and coordination.

Preventing Reinjury

A training phase that is sufficiently long, correcting external and internal causes of injury, reaching sufficient criteria for muscle function and a gradual return to sport are keys to prevent reinjury.

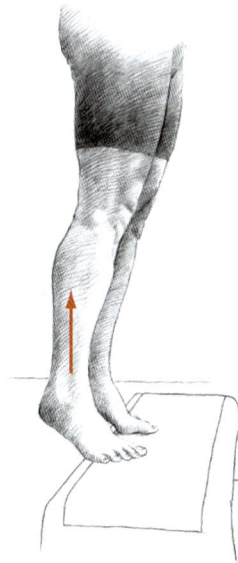

Figure 13.27 Toe raises on an edge on two feet and on one foot. Four sets of 5–30 repetitions with increasing external load 3–5 days per week. Gradually increase range, tempo, and emphasis on the eccentric phase. (Reproduced with permission from the Norwegian Sports Medicine Association.)

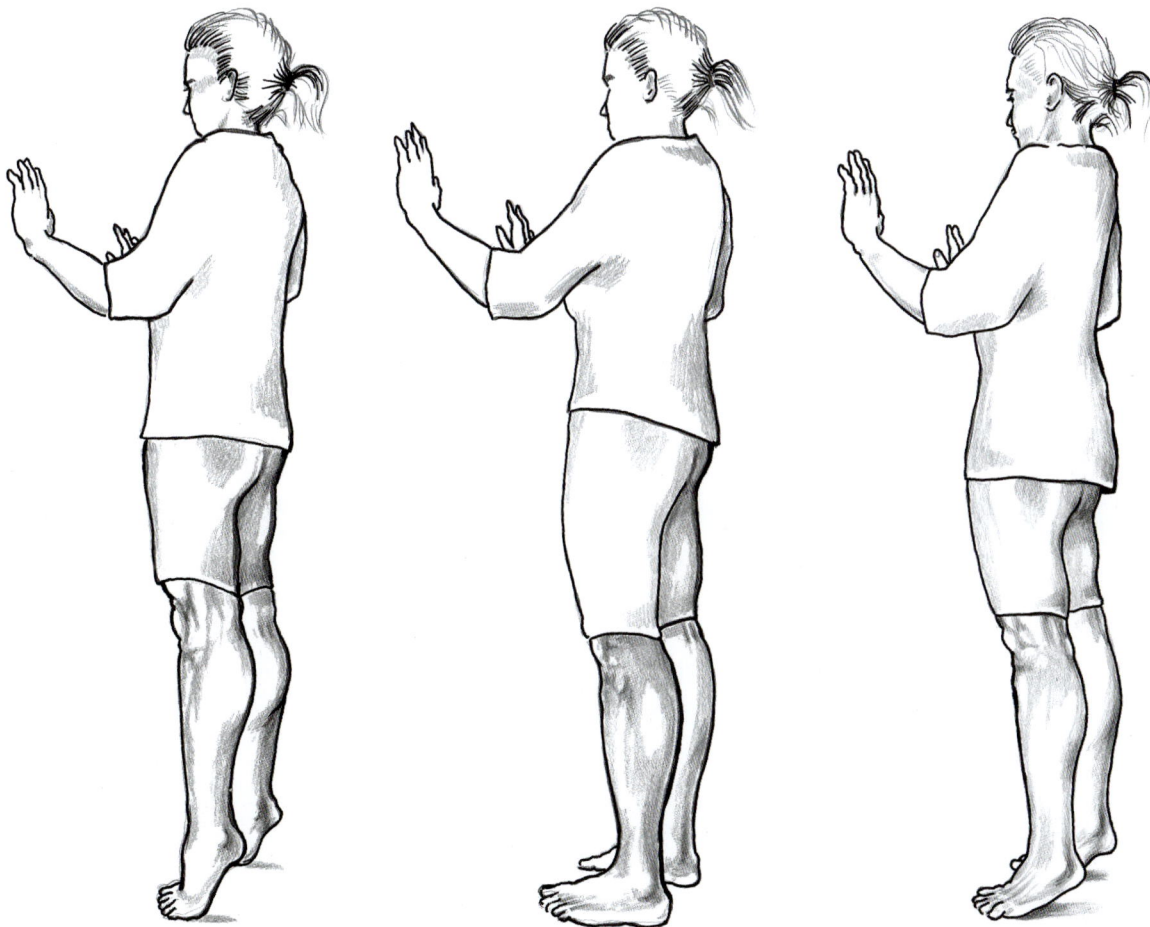

Figure 13.28 Rebounding fast toe raises—involving the stretch-shortening cycle. Performed like skipping rope without leaving the floor. Start up on toes, fall down and, before the heel touches the floor, rebound backup mainly utilizing the elastic properties of the Achilles tendon and calf muscle, 2–4 sets of 20–100 repetitions 2–4 days per week. (© Medical Illustrator Tommy Bolic, Sweden.)

14 Ankle

Acute Ankle Injuries

Roald Bahr[1], Ned Amendola[2], C. Niek van Dijk[3], Jón Karlson[4],
Umile Giuseppe Longo[5], and Gino M.M.J. Kerkhoffs[3]

[1]*Norwegian School of Sport Sciences, Oslo, Norway*
[2]*University of Iowa, Iowa City, IA, USA*
[3]*Academic Medical Center, Amsterdam, The Netherlands*
[4]*Sahlgrenska University Hospital/Mölndal, Mölndal, Sweden*
[5]*University Campus Bio-Medico, Rome, Italy*

Occurrence

Acute ankle injuries constitute approximately 10% of all acute injuries that are treated by physicians. It is estimated that one ankle injury occurs per 10,000 inhabitants every day. Ligament injuries of the ankle are the most common injury in sport, accounting for about one-fifth of all sport injuries. In some sports, especially team sports like football, basketball, volleyball, and team handball, ankle injuries total up to half of all acute injuries. This is also true of some individual sports, in which landing after a jump or running on an uneven surface (such as in orienteering) are risk elements.

Differential Diagnoses

Table 14.1 provides an overview of the differential diagnoses of acute ankle injuries. Young, active patients whose inversion trauma occurred when the patient ran, jumped, or fell, usually sustain lateral ligament injuries. Children can sustain

Most common	Less common	Must not be overlooked ❗
Lateral ligament injuries, p. 435	Achilles tendon rupture, p. 406	Syndesmosis injury, p. 440
	Medial ligament injuries, p. 436	Epiphyseal plate injuries (children)
	Base of the fifth metatarsal, p. 437	Tarsal coalitions
	Lateral malleolus fractures, p. 439	
	Medial malleolus fractures, p. 439	
	Ankle dislocation, p. 443	
	Talar fracture, p. 443	
	Peroneal tendon dislocation/rupture, p. 444	
	Tibialis posterior tendon rupture, p. 456	
	Calcaneal fracture, p. 464	

Table 14.1 Overview of the differential diagnoses of acute ankle injuries. (Reproduced with permission from the Norwegian Sports Medicine Association.)

epiphyseal plate injuries as a result of this type of trauma, whereas older patients commonly sustain a fracture of the lateral malleolus or, less commonly, at the base of the fifth metatarsal. Syndesmosis injuries are rare, but can occur alone or, much more commonly, in combination with other ligament injuries or ankle fractures. In addition, underlying tarsal coalition may present as recurrent ankle sprains.

Diagnostic Thinking

Most ankle injuries should be treated at the primary-care level. Usually, the main problem is to distinguish between lateral ligament injury and a fracture of the lateral malleolus. Fractures at the base of the fifth metatarsal and syndesmosis injuries are commonly overlooked during the initial examination. This is also true for the very rare tendon injuries. A precise clinical examination is necessary to determine whether the patient should be referred for a radiographic examination to exclude a fracture. If the patient needs radiographs, they should be taken without delay. If surgery is needed for an ankle fracture, it should take place within 8–12 hours before swelling is pronounced.

Thus, the goal of the clinical examination during the acute stage is to determine whether the patient has sustained a lateral ligament injury or some other injury that may require immobilization or acute surgical treatment. If the most important differential diagnoses can be excluded by means of the clinical examination, additional examinations are usually unnecessary during the acute stage.

Case History

A precise description of the injury mechanism is the key to establishing the correct diagnosis, particularly in terms of suspecting less common injuries.

Inversion trauma (Figure 14.1), which causes approximately 85% of all ankle injuries, usually damages the lateral ligaments in younger patients. Three anatomically and functionally separate units—the anterior talofibular, the calcaneofibular, and the posterior talofibular ligaments—provide the ligament support on the lateral side. Normally, the anterior talofibular ligament is torn first (about two-thirds of

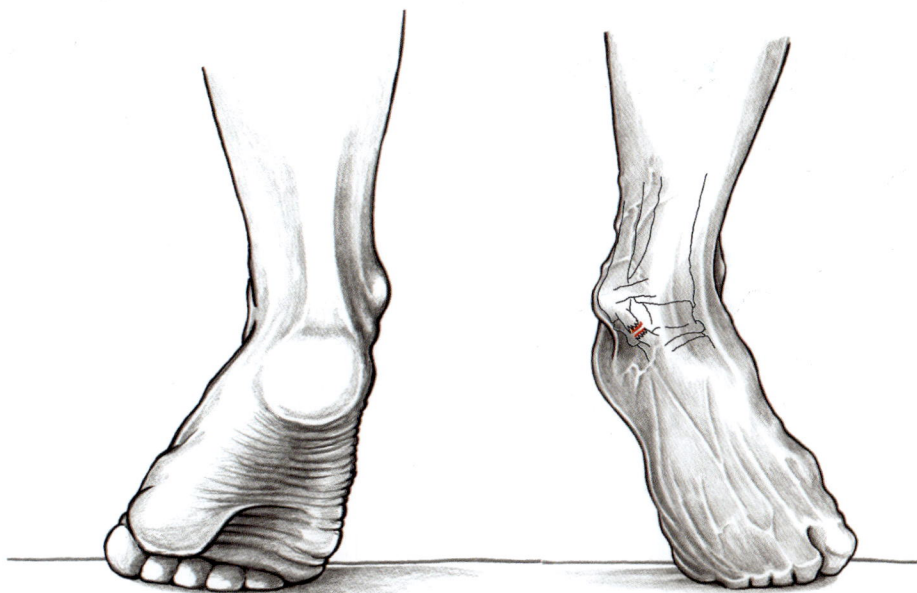

Figure 14.1 Inversion trauma. This is the most common injury mechanism for sprained ankles. Injuries occur when the ankle is internally rotated and supinated when the athlete lands in plantar flexion (equinus position). The most common injury is an anterior talofibular ligament rupture (as shown). (© Medical Illustrator Tommy Bolic, Sweden.)

ANKLE

431

all injuries are isolated ruptures of the anterior talofibular ligament), then in approximately one-third of all injuries the calcaneofibular ligament is also torn, and only in rare cases (about 1%) are all three of the lateral ligaments torn. The proportion of patients with combined ruptures (i.e., ruptures of both the anterior talofibular and the calcaneofibular ligaments) is higher among patients who have been injured before. The proportion of combined injuries is probably lower if patients are seen at the primary care level (e.g., by the team doctor or a general practitioner) than in the hospital setting. Be aware that, in conjunction with ligamentous injury, medial or lateral talar dome chondral injuries or bony contusions may occur.

Young patients seldom sustain fractures as a result of moderate trauma, such as inversion trauma, for instance, during running. If the forces are greater (e.g., that caused by a jump from a height of 2 m or more), a fracture should be suspected, usually in combination with a syndesmosis injury. However, moderate inversion trauma commonly causes fractures in middle-aged or older patients–either of the lateral malleolus or at the base of the fifth metatarsal. Avulsion fractures of the fifth metatarsal occur because the most important active stabilizer against inversion trauma, the peroneal muscles (especially the peroneus brevis muscle) are activated to control the foot so the athlete can make a flatfooted landing, thus preventing a ligament injury.

Eversion trauma usually causes an injury to the deltoid ligament (a continuous ligamentous unit that runs along the entire medial malleolus). This ligament is in two layers, one deep and one more superficial). Medial ligament injuries occur with or without simultaneous syndesmosis injuries and fractures of the lateral malleolus. Isolated ligament injuries on the medial side are rare, totaling approximately 1–2% of the ligament injuries in the ankle. There are probably several reasons for this, including a movement pattern in which a natural landing occurs with the foot in plantar flexion and slight supination. Other important factors, however, may be that the deltoid ligament has greater rupture strength than the lateral ligaments and the bony anatomy on the medial side of the ankle compared with the more unstable lateral side. For that reason, eversion injuries usually cause fractures or syndesmosis injuries, in addition to the medial ligament injury. In rare cases, eversion injuries may also result in isolated syndesmosis injury or even peroneal tendon dislocation.

Strict external rotation trauma may cause an isolated anterior syndesmosis injury. If the ankle is locked in plantar or dorsal flexion, strong external rotation of the ankle may cause the tibia and the fibula to be pressed apart so that the anterior syndesmosis tears. This may occur, for example, if the ankle is locked in a downhill ski boot, jumping boot, or ice hockey skate (Figure 14.2).

If an athlete lands flatfooted after jumping from a great height (usually more than 2 m), a calcaneus fracture or some other less common fracture should be suspected.

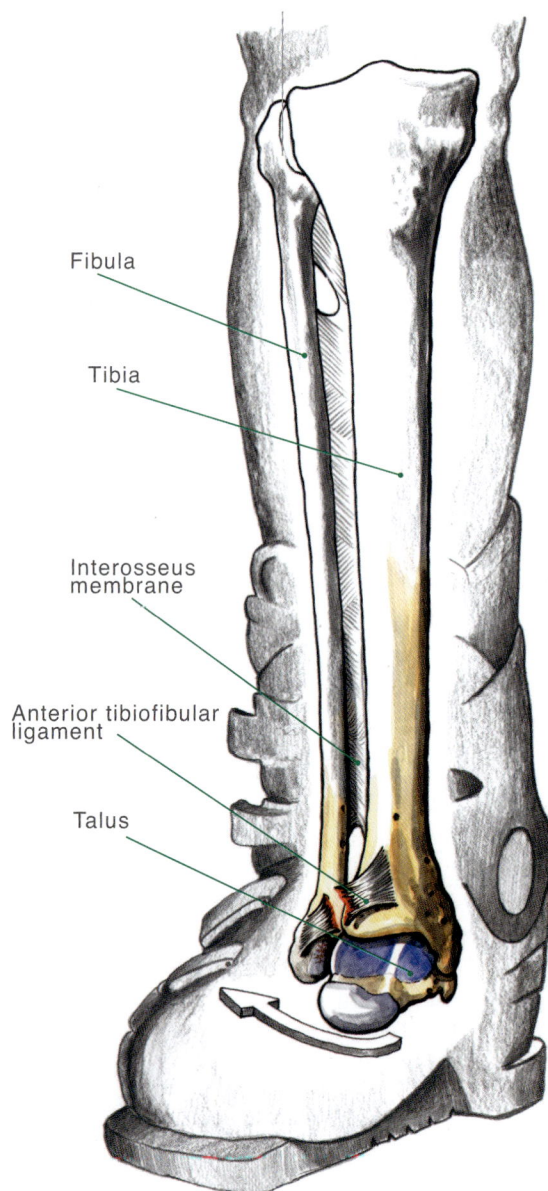

Fibula

Tibia

Interosseus membrane

Anterior tibiofibular ligament

Talus

Figure 14.2 External rotation injury with a syndesmosis rupture. If the foot is locked in plantar flexion in a downhill ski boot or ice hockey skate, an isolated rupture in the anterior syndesmosis (the anterior talofibular ligament) may occur. (© Medical Illustrator Tommy Bolic, Sweden.)

Clinical Examination

Inspection. A lateral ligament injury usually causes swelling in front of and below the lateral malleolus. This may happen quickly (sometimes within 5–10 minutes, if untreated) and may be pronounced. However, athletes, in particular, are likely to have received such good acute treatment (with compression) that there is minimal or no swelling when the patient is being examined. If the examiner is unaware of this, an injury may be overlooked or underestimated. Cold treatment may provide such good pain relief that palpation tenderness is significantly reduced, as well. However, cold treatment alone will not affect the swelling to any major extent.

Palpation. Thorough palpation is the most important examination. The physician should bear in mind that the anterior talofibular ligament attachment is located anterior to and proximal to the tip of the fibula. According to the Ottawa rules, emphasis is placed on palpation of the following four structures: the lateral malleolus, the medial malleolus, the base of the fifth metatarsal, and the navicular bone (as shown in Figure 14.3). The sensitivity to clinically significant fractures is 100%, but the specificity is as low as 59%. Hence, it is necessary to order radiographs only if there is a positive palpation finding or the patient is unable to bear weight on the injured leg.

Neuromuscular function. It is seldom possible to evaluate neuromuscular function completely during the acute stage, because pain inhibition is often significant. Nevertheless, it is usually possible to check that peroneal tendon function is intact, to palpate the course of the tendon, and to determine whether to suspect an injured retinaculum or a rupture of the brevis tendon's insertion at the fifth metatarsal. Longitudinal rupture (splitting) of the peroneal tendons (in the majority of cases to the peroneus brevis tendon) may also occur. Also, if patients are seen on subsequent days after injury, they may also complain of soreness in the peroneal muscles. Most likely, this occurs in patients who were able to contract their peroneal muscles in an attempt to protect themselves against injury; a maximal eccentric contraction may have caused a partial muscle rupture.

Sensory motor function. Sensory function cannot be evaluated during the acute stage, but should be monitored repeatedly during the rehabilitation stage, especially before the athlete returns to competitive sport. Function can be evaluated by means of a simple test (see page 448).

Figure 14.3 Ottawa rules. Palpate along the mid-margin of the fibula and tibia, the base of the fifth metatarsal, and over the navicular bone. If the patient does not have tenderness to palpation in these areas and can bear weight on his leg, radiographs are not necessary during the acute stage. (© Medical Illustrator Tommy Bolic, Sweden.)

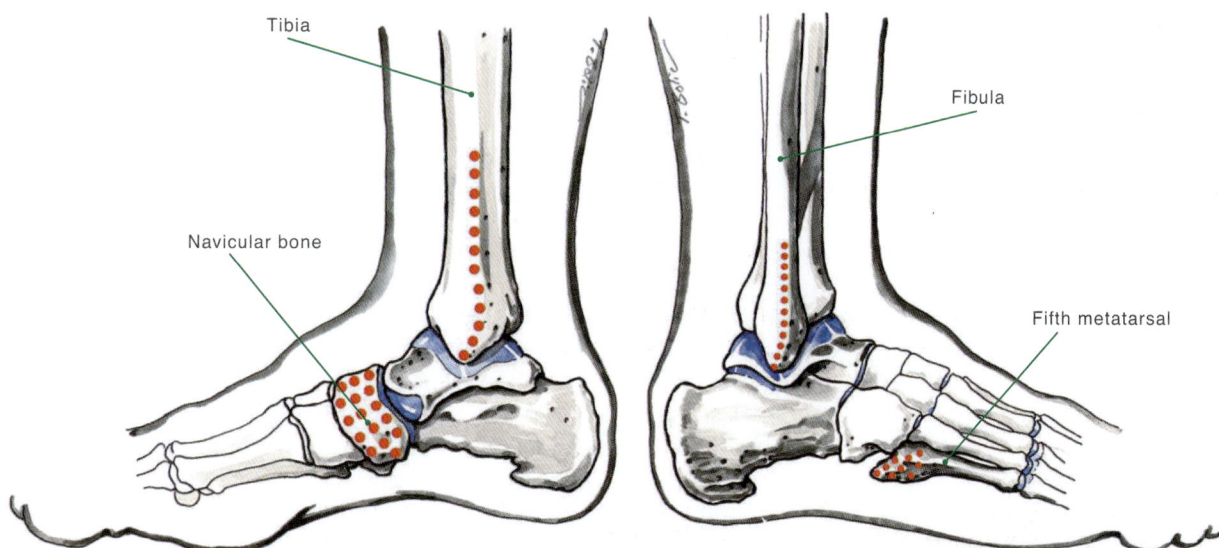

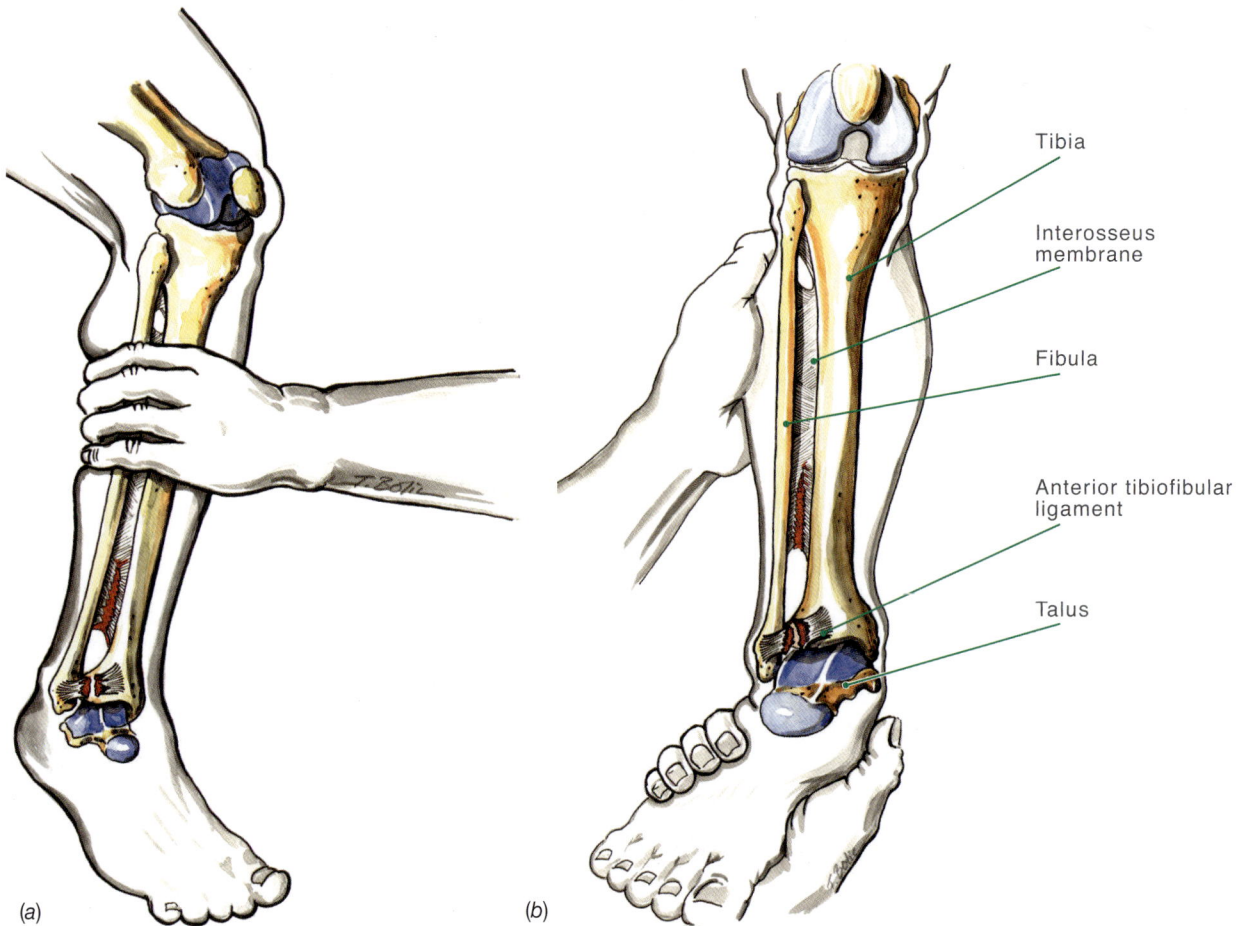

Figure 14.4 Testing the syndesmosis. The squeeze test (*a*) is done by compression of the fibula and tibia at the middle of the lower leg, whereas the external rotation test (*b*) is performed by rotating the foot externally with the ankle in neutral position (90°). The tests are evaluated as positive if they cause pain in the syndesmosis area. They usually do not result in any significant pain if only a lateral ligament injury has occurred. (© Medical Illustrator Tommy Bolic, Sweden.)

Syndesmosis tests. One "specific" syndesmosis test is called the squeeze test (Figure 14.4). It consists of compression of the lower leg and thereby squeezing the fibula and the tibia together. If this causes pain distally in the syndesmosis area, an injury should be suspected. If the test is positive, the patient also needs to be evaluated for alternative diagnoses, such as fibula or tibia fractures, compartment syndrome, or contusion of the lower leg musculature. An alternative test is the external rotation test (Figure 14.4). This test is done in the same manner as that for the injury mechanism previously described for downhill skiers. Pain in the syndesmosis area caused by external rotation in neutral flexion may indicate an injury to the anterior syndesmosis. The external rotation stress test can be performed in the standing position, fixating the foot on the ground while asking the patient to externally rotate on the planted foot, reproducing the pain. In addition, a syndesmosis injury usually causes pain when the ankle is in forced dorsal flexion. Combined with the palpation findings, these tests at least give some indication of whether or not the patient has a syndesmosis injury. To establish correct diagnosis of syndesmosis injury is often difficult and the injury is often missed, which may lead to serious consequences.

Stress tests. Two stress tests—the anterior drawer test and the talar tilt test (see page 448)—are used to evaluate the integrity of the lateral ligaments and the laxity of the ankle ligaments. The principle behind these tests is that it should be possible to grade lateral ligament injuries. However, in practice, this may be difficult to accomplish, especially during the acute stage. In addition, the choice of treatment is not dependent on an accurate grading of the ligament injury; therefore, there is no need to emphasize stress tests during the acute phase.

Supplemental Examinations

Radiographic examination. Unless the clinical examination has caused the suspicion of a fracture (see Ottawa rules) or of a syndesmosis injury, there is no reason to routinely take radiographs of patients with acute ankle injuries. If radiographs are taken, a standard ankle series should include frontal, lateral, and a mortise view (which shows the talus projected in the ankle mortise). The physician should look for malleolar fractures and syndesmosis injuries in particular. Syndesmosis injuries may cause lateral displacement of the talus and/or increased mortise width (medial joint space widening) (Figure 14.12). Sometimes eggshell-shaped avulsion fractures from the tip of the fibula (avulsion of the anterior talofibular and/or the calcaneofibular ligament bony insertion) are visible.

Other radiographs may be indicated in special cases:

- Oblique images may help if a malleolar fracture is suspected and the standard ankle series is difficult to evaluate.
- If a fracture at the base of the fifth metatarsal is suspected, frontal and lateral images of the fifth metatarsal should be ordered.
- An examination using fluoroscopy may be useful in evaluating syndesmosis injuries, but should be ordered by an orthopedic surgeon.

Common Injuries

Lateral Ligament Injuries

Injuries to the lateral ankle ligaments are usually classified according to the number of injured ligaments (Figure 14.5). Grade I is defined as a partial rupture of the

Figure 14.5 Lateral ligament injury. Partial ruptures of the anterior talofibular ligament (grade I) may occur (*a*), but total ruptures are much more common (grade II, *b*), and sometimes occur in combination with a total rupture of the calcaneofibular ligament (grade III, *c*). (© Medical Illustrator Tommy Bolic, Sweden.)

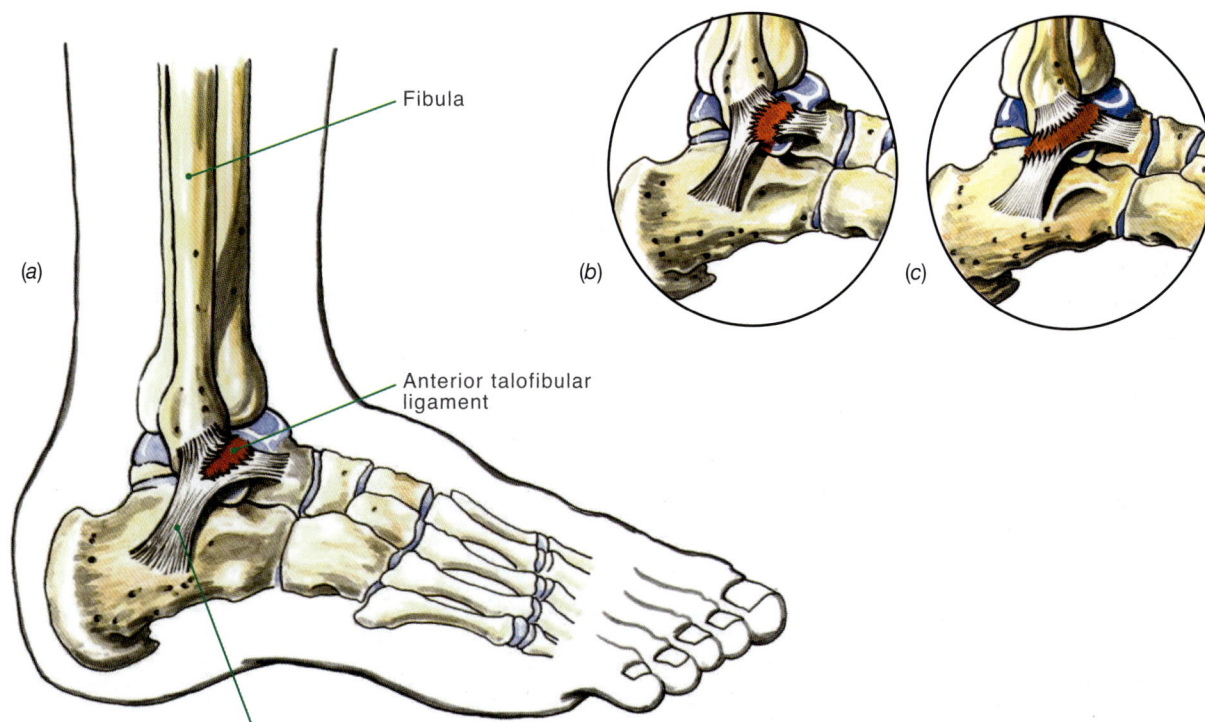

(*a*)   Fibula

Anterior talofibular ligament

(*b*)   (*c*)

anterior talofibular and/or the calcaneofibular ligaments; grade II, as a total rupture of the anterior talofibular ligament, but with an intact calcaneofibular ligament; and grade III is a total rupture of the anterior talofibular and calcaneofibular ligaments. Partial ruptures are uncommon, that is, the ligament injury is almost always a complete rupture. This means that the patient almost always has a grade II or grade III injury.

Early functional treatment is always indicated for grade I and II injuries, whereas immobilization in a cast, surgical treatment, and functional treatment have all been used for grade III injuries. However, functional treatment of grade III injuries restores stability nearly equal to that achieved by other methods, and it provides full mobility and full function earlier than the other treatment alternatives, with less risk of complication. Therefore, most physicians prefer functional treatment for all lateral ligament injuries. This implies that it is not necessary to distinguish between grades I, II, and III injuries by means of stress tests or diagnostic imaging (including stress radiographs) during the acute stage.

- Symptoms and signs: Patients experience swelling and tenderness in front of and below the lateral malleolus. Findings are usually localized directly over the ligaments if examined immediately after the injury occurs. However, many patients do not seek medical attention until 1 or 2 days after the injury occurs, and then they often have significant swelling and subcutaneous bleeding over the lateral side of the ankle. In such cases, it may be difficult to distinguish between a ligament injury and a fracture.
- Diagnosis: The diagnosis is made clinically, but radiographs with a standard ankle series are indicated to exclude fractures or syndesmosis injuries, in accordance with the Ottawa rules or positive syndesmosis tests. The anterior drawer test and the talar tilt test (see page 448) are of minor value during the acute stage.
- Treatment by physician: During the acute stage (i.e., the first 24–48 hours) the goal is to limit bleeding, and this is most effectively achieved through intensive PRICE treatment, including nonweight bearing with crutches. Compression is crucial. Treatment with nonsteroidal anti-inflammatory drugs (NSAIDs) provides good pain relief and enables more rapid mobilization of the patient. This treatment should be continued for 4–5 days, provided that there are no contraindications. This therapy has a. Weight bearing, preferably without crutches, should be started after 24–48 hours, Instead of cast immobilization, brace mobilization is recommended.
- Treatment by therapist: The patient should be referred to a therapist as soon as possible, for detailed instructions of rehabilitation exercises (see page 459) and possibly for taping or fitting a brace. No effects of ultrasound, electrotherapy, electricity, laser, or the like have been documented.
- Prognosis: The prognosis is good. The ligament usually heals in 6–12 weeks; however, full function can be achieved much earlier with good treatment during the acute stage. However, 10–20% of the patients have persisting problems after an acute ankle injury, either recurrent instability and/or pain (see page 449–452). Therefore, the patient should be told to contact a physician in case of late symptoms.

Other Injuries

Medial Ligament Injuries

Eversion injuries may cause a rupture, usually partial, of the deltoid ligament (Figure 14.6). Medial ligament injuries are also seen in combination with malleolar fractures or syndesmosis injuries.

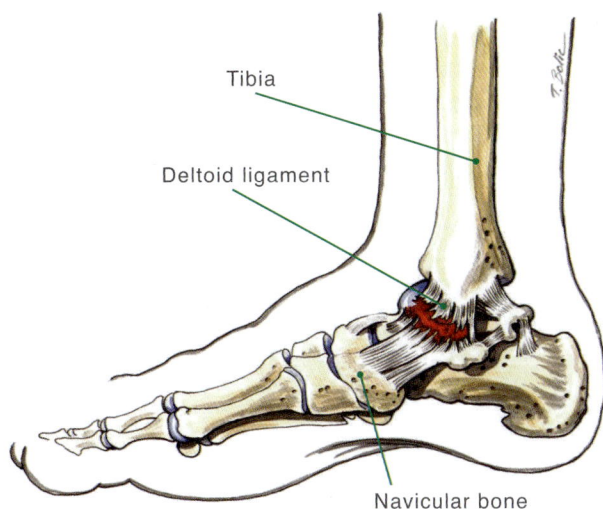

Figure 14.6 Medial ligament injury. Far less common than lateral injuries, medial injuries should be suspected after an eversion trauma. (© Medical Illustrator Tommy Bolic, Sweden.)

- Symptoms and signs: The main findings are tenderness to palpation and swelling below the medial malleolus. If a total rupture of the deltoid ligament occurs, a defect can be palpated in the ligament. However, this is very rare as an isolated injury.
- Diagnosis: The diagnosis is established clinically, but radiographs with a standard ankle series are indicated to exclude fractures or syndesmosis injuries in patients with positive palpation findings (in accordance with the Ottawa rules) or if the syndesmosis test is positive.
- Treatment: PRICE treatment, brace, and functional treatment are all used for isolated medial ligament injuries in the same manner as that for lateral ligament injuries. A medial arch support can also provide some pain relief.
- Prognosis: Prognosis is good, but the progression is generally slower than for lateral ligament injuries. Whereas, for instance, a soccer player can return to play after 7–10 days after lateral ligament injuries, it takes 4–6 weeks after a significant medial injury.

Fracture at the Base of the Fifth Metatarsal

Inversion injuries may cause a fracture at the base of the fifth metatarsal. These fractures are caused by strong traction from the lateral bands of the plantar fascia or the peroneus brevis tendon on a weight-bearing inverted foot. There are three types of fractures in the area: avulsion fractures (most common), oblique fractures through the diaphyseal-metaphyseal junction (true Jones fractures), and a fracture through the diaphysis (Figures 14.7 and 14.8). The former two are acute fractures, whereas a diaphysis fracture is usually a stress fracture (see page 472).

- Symptoms and signs: The main finding that makes it easy to distinguish between this injury and lateral ligament injuries is the distinct tenderness over the base of the fifth metatarsal (Figure 14.3). It is palpated as a marked prominence along the

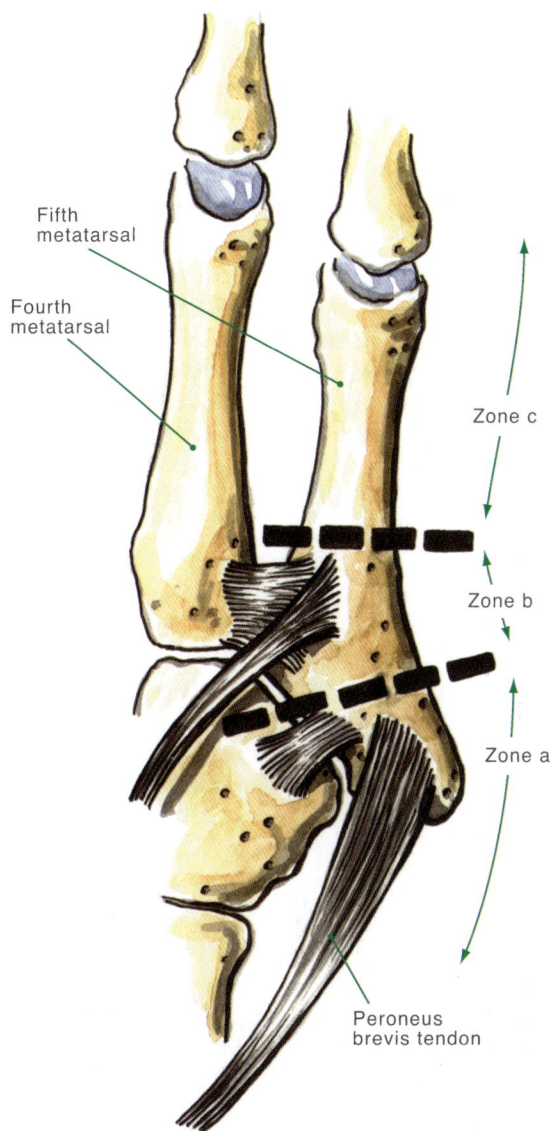

Figure 14.7 Classification of fractures of the fifth metatarsal. Acute fractures are usually avulsion fractures (zone *a*) or oblique fractures through the diaphyseal-metaphyseal junction (so-called Jones fractures, zone *b*). The third type of fracture, the diaphysis fracture (zone *c*), occurs primarily as a stress fracture. It is important to distinguish between different fracture types because they have different prognosis for healing, and therefore differing treatments. (© Medical Illustrator Tommy Bolic, Sweden.)

ANKLE

lateral edge of the foot. Swelling eventually occurs but is often minimal on the day of the injury.

- Diagnosis: The diagnosis is established with radiographs of the fifth metatarsal (lateral and frontal views to reveal displacement or angulation and, if necessary, oblique views to look for periosteal reaction). *On a routine ankle series of radiographs, the base of the 5th metatarsal should be included on the lateral view.* The images must be carefully examined to distinguish between avulsion fractures (Figures 14.7 and 14.8) and oblique fractures through the diaphyseal-metaphyseal junction (true Jones fractures) (Figure 14.7). In addition, stress fractures often present with acute pain. These fractures usually have evidence of increased repetitive stress with cortical thickening prior to fracture, and a history of some pain in the area for some time before the fracture occurs.
- Treatment: Avulsion fractures without significant dislocation will usually heal with nonsurgical treatment. Immobilization is necessary only as long as needed to reduce pain and in most cases immobilization is not needed at all. Generally, the patient may weight bear without pain after 1 or 2 weeks, followed by mobilization and rehabilitation as soon as pain allows. True Jones fractures go through a zone with a poorer blood supply, and late healing or nonunion are likely to occur. Jones fractures without displacement may be treated by immobilization in a cast for 4–6 weeks without weight bearing. Jones fracture with displacement should be operated on with intermedullary compression screw fixation. Surgical fixation may also be indicated for an athlete who wants to return to sport early, even if there is no dislocation. Stress fractures should always be evaluated for surgical fixation.
- Prognosis: Prognosis is good in avulsion fractures, and function is usually normal in 4–6 weeks after nonsurgical treatment. The result after surgical treatment of Jones fracture is good, and the healing time is usually 10–12 weeks.

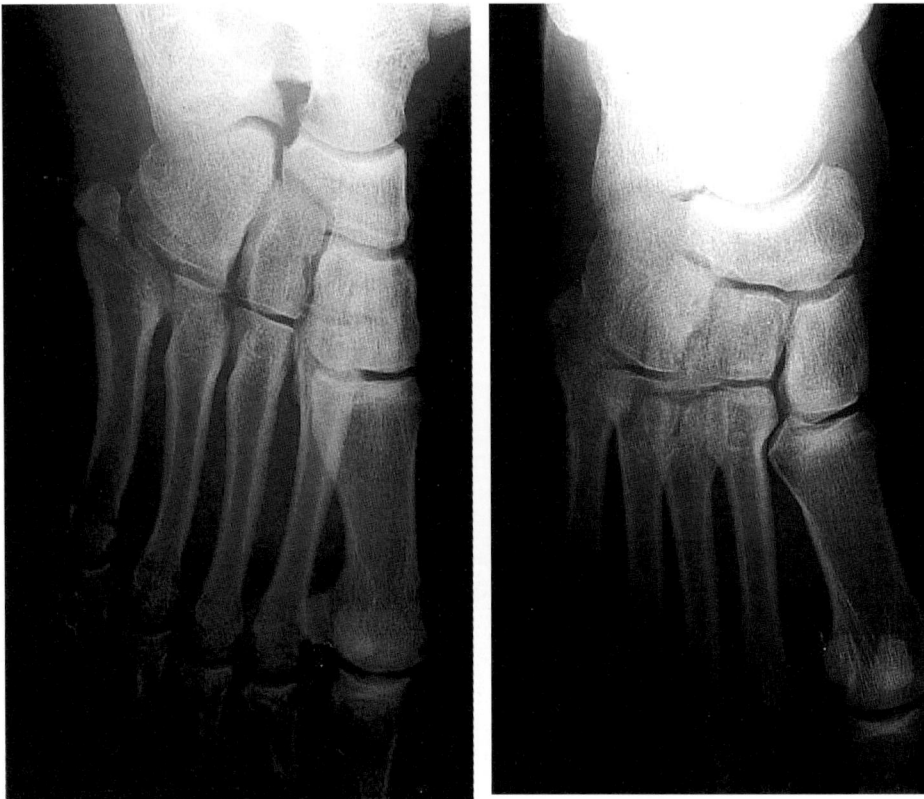

Figure 14.8 Avulsion fracture through the base of the fifth metatarsal. (© Medical Illustrator Tommy Bolic, Sweden.)

Malleolar Fractures

Isolated fractures of the lateral malleolus are the most common, but with higher energy trauma these fractures often occur in combination with medial malleolar fractures (bimalleolar fractures) or fractures of the posterior malleolus (trimalleolar fractures). Fractures are usually also accompanied by ligament injuries and/or syndesmosis injuries. Ankle fractures can be classified according to the location of the fracture line through the lateral malleolus (AO classification, Figure 14.9).

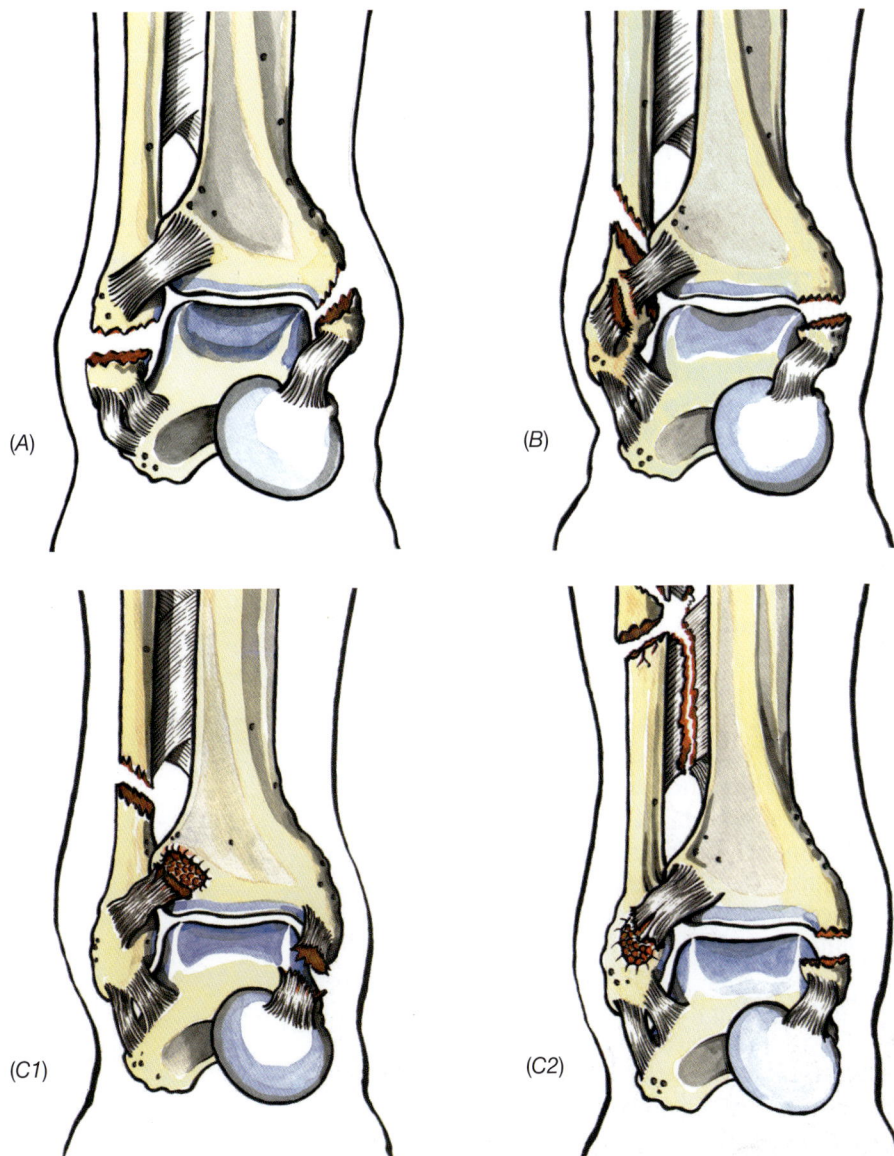

Type	Syndesmosis rupture (%)	Dominant force
A	0	Supination
B	50	External rotation
C1	100	Pronation
C2	100	Pronation

Figure 14.9 Classification of ankle fractures (AO classification). The classification system is based on the location of the fracture line through the lateral malleolus. (© Medical Illustrator Tommy Bolic, Sweden.)

ANKLE

- Symptoms and signs: Symptoms are significant swelling, positive Ottawa sign, and obvious dislocation. To reduce the risk of skin damage dislocated ankle fractures must be reduced and stabilized without delay–even before radiographs are taken.
- Diagnosis: The diagnosis is established with a standard radiographic ankle series. Oblique views may be helpful if standard images are difficult to interpret. Skin color should be checked, as should capillary filling distally and the pulsations on the dorsum of the foot and the posterior tibial artery. Distal skin sensitivity should also be checked.
- Treatment principles: The main goal of treatment is to maintain (for fractures that are not dislocated) or restore (for dislocated fractures) the normal relationship between the articular surfaces on the talus on the one side and the tibia and fibula on the other. Dislocation as little as 1–2 mm can change the loading pattern of the ankle joint and increase the risk of osteoarthritis. An important factor is to evaluate whether the fracture line through the lateral malleolus is below, in, or above the syndesmosis. Ankle fractures in children may damage the growth zones in the distal fibula and tibia. This may cause growth disturbance that eventually results in asymmetry in the ankle, angulation, and/or leg shortening.
- Treatment of type A fractures (Figure 14.9): Small avulsion fractures from the tip of the lateral malleolus are treated in the same manner as ligament injuries, with early mobilization and functional treatment. Lateral malleolar fractures below the syndesmosis are stable if the medial malleolus is intact and there is no ligament rupture of the deltoid ligament. These fractures may also be treated functionally using a brace and weight bearing is allowed as soon as pain and swelling allow.
- Treatment of type B fractures (Figures 14.9 and 14.10): Lateral malleolar fractures at the syndesmosis level without significant dislocation are treated with a walking cast (or lower leg brace, e.g., Walker Boot) for 4–6 weeks. Weight bearing is allowed as soon as pain and swelling allow it. If the dislocation is more than 2 mm and the talus is displaced laterally, the fracture is unstable, especially if combined with a simultaneous medial injury (either a rupture of the deltoid ligament or a fracture of the medial malleolus). Surgery is recommended.
- Treatment of type C fractures (Figure 14.9): These fractures are characterized by a high fibula fracture, a syndesmosis rupture, and a rupture of the interosseous membrane. The fracture is unstable, and surgical treatment should be undertaken as soon as possible, preferably within 8 hours. The fracture should be reduced and stabilized before the patient is transported to the hospital. This can usually be achieved easily by grasping the heel, pulling it in the longitudinal direction, and the tibia is then carefully pushed posteriorly, if necessary. Apply a U-cast (or similar immobilization) before the patient is transported to the hospital.
- Treatment of epiphysiolysis fractures in children: Often no changes in the epiphyseal line are visible in undisplaced (type 1) injuries. The diagnosis is clinical if the patient has distinct palpation tenderness over the epiphyseal line, especially on posterior palpation pressure. It may be helpful to compare radiographs of both ankles. Growth plate injuries without any visible dislocation should be treated with a short walking cast for 3–4 weeks. However, if dislocation is present, the patient should be operated on, without any delay.

Syndesmosis Injury—*Injury to the Ligament between the Tibia and the Fibula* !

A partial or total rupture of the anterior syndesmosis (anterior inferior tibiofibular ligament) (Figure 14.11) usually occurs in combination with medial ligament injuries and/or malleolar fractures. Type A fractures of the lateral malleolus (Figure 14.9) rarely involve syndesmosis injuries, type B involve syndesmosis

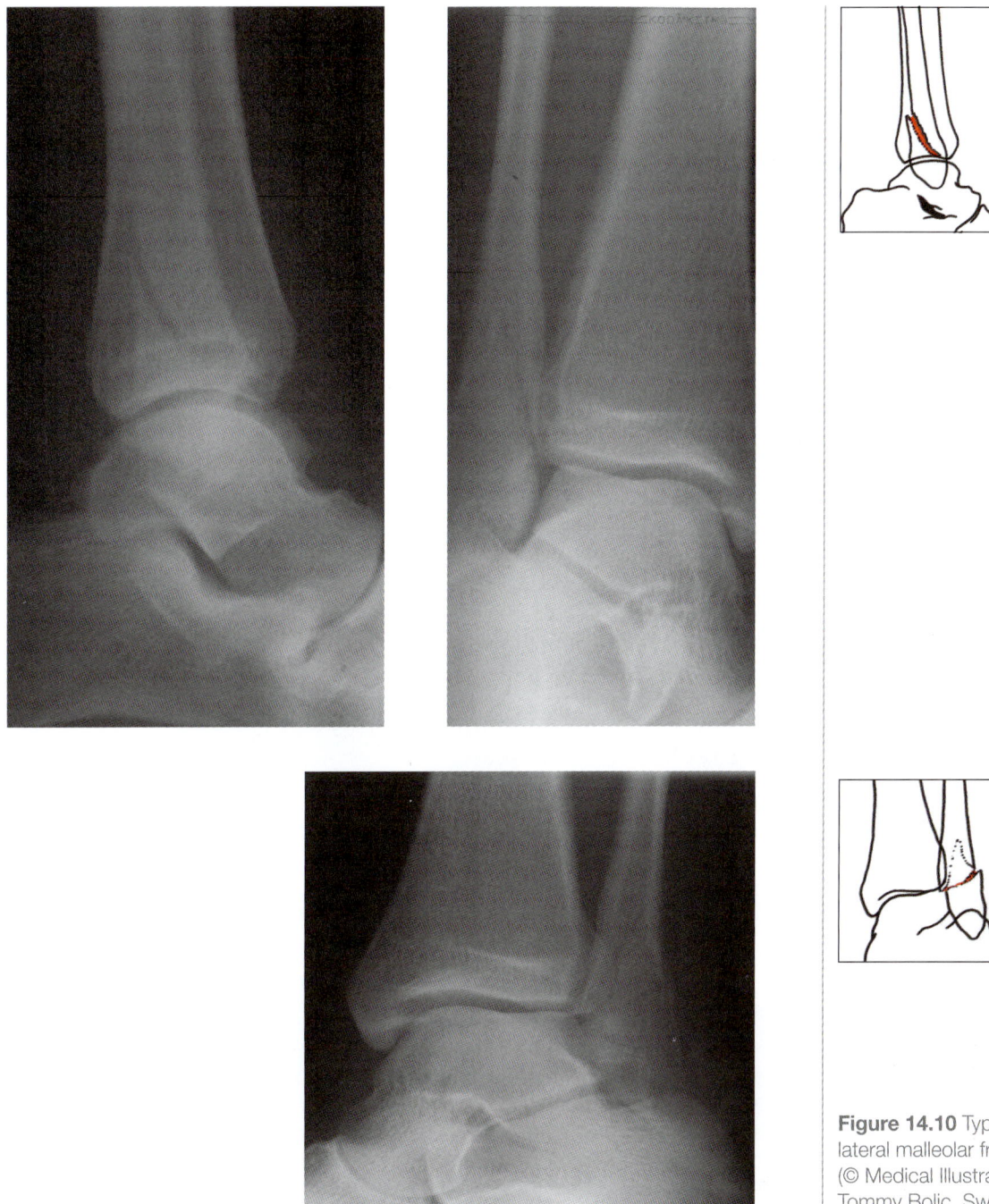

Figure 14.10 Type A lateral malleolar fracture. (© Medical Illustrator Tommy Bolic, Sweden.)

injuries in 50% of the cases, and type C almost always involve syndesmosis injuries. Isolated syndesmosis ruptures may also result from strict external rotation trauma— for example, in a downhill ski boot (Figure 14.2).

- **Symptoms and signs:** Patients experience swelling, often moderate, and maximum palpation tenderness over the syndesmosis just proximal to the joint space. Positive squeeze test, positive external rotation test, and pain from forced dorsal flexion all indicate syndesmosis injuries. Patients who are suspected of having a syndesmosis injury must be carefully examined for this type of injury and for other

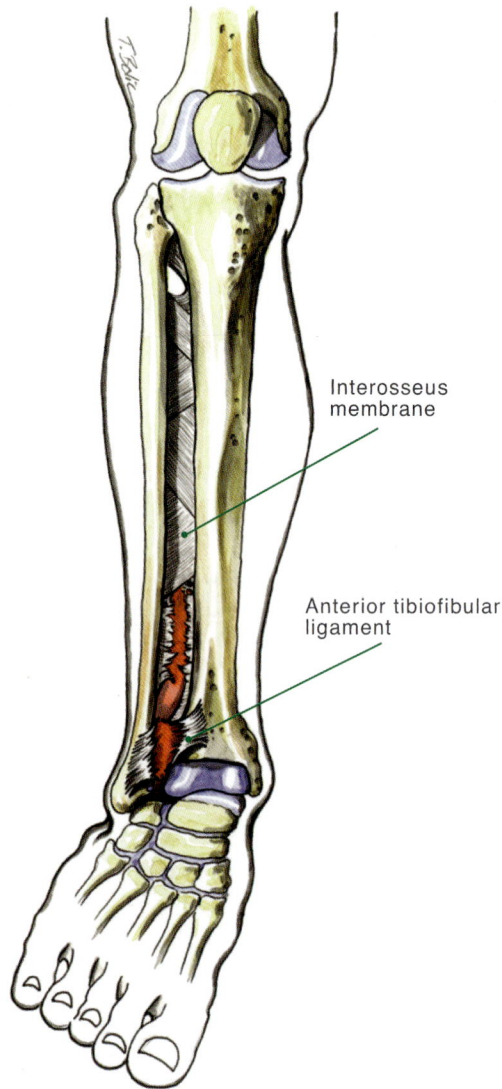

Figure 14.11 Syndesmosis rupture. Often overlooked, particularly when isolated and occurring as a result of pure external rotational trauma inside a hockey skate or downhill ski boot. (© Medical Illustrator Tommy Bolic, Sweden.)

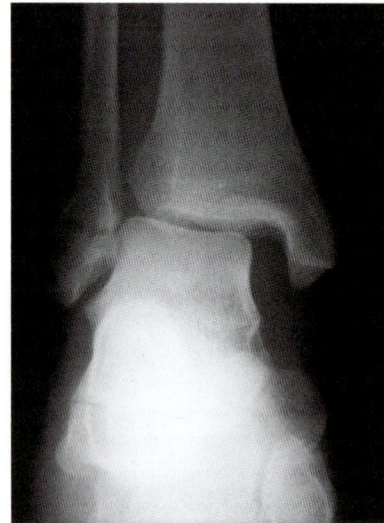

Figure 14.12 Syndesmosis rupture. A radiograph of a total syndesmosis injury demonstrates widening of the ankle mortise, resulting in increased space between the fibula and the talus.

ligament injuries or fractures of the ankle. The proximal fibula should be examined for possible fracture.

- Diagnosis: The diagnosis is made clinically, but radiographs of the ankle are necessary. In such cases, radiographs should ideally include the entire fibula. If the patient has a total syndesmosis rupture, widening of the ankle mortise (Figure 14.12) will be visible on the radiographs. Magnetic resonance imaging (MRI) may be necessary as a supplementary investigation.
- Treatment by physician: The treatment is the same PRICE principle as for lateral ligament injuries. Partial ruptures are treated functionally, and a period of immobilization (often 2 weeks or longer) in a walking cast may be necessary until the patient can weight-bear again. The patient should be mobilized, and rehabilitation should start as soon as pain allows. Total ruptures with diastasis are surgically treated with stabilization using syndesmosis screws, sometimes also suturing of the ligament, and

a cast/brace for 6 weeks. Partial weight bearing, within the limits of pain, is allowed after 3–4 weeks. Untreated total syndesmosis ruptures may lead to osteoarthritis of the ankle.

- Treatment by therapist: The training program should emphasize range of motion training, strength exercises, and neuromuscular function. This is particularly true if the patient underwent surgical treatment and subsequent immobilization.
- Prognosis: If the patient has a partial syndesmosis rupture, the rehabilitation period for accompanying ligament injuries or fractures often becomes protracted. If the patient has an isolated total syndesmosis injury, it will usually take 4–6 months before he can return to competitive activity. Ossification of the ligament (synostosis) may occur in rare cases. This is characterized by increasing stiffness and pain when kicking 3–12 months after the injury.

Ankle Dislocation

A dislocated ankle is a rare injury (Figure 14.13), caused by landing at high speed, falling from height, and landing with the ankle in an inverted or everted position, or external trauma to the weight-bearing foot.

- Symptoms and signs: The patient may experience significant swelling, obvious deformity, complete dysfunction, and pain. To reduce the risk of skin damage that may complicate further treatment, dislocated ankles should be reduced and stabilized immediately, before the patient is transferred to the hospital.
- Diagnosis: The diagnosis is based on the obvious dislocation, but it may be difficult to distinguish it from a dislocated ankle fracture (bi- or trimalleolar). The practitioner should check skin color, distal capillary filling, and arterial pulsations. Distal sensitivity should also be checked.
- Treatment by physician: The dislocation is reduced by grasping the heel and forefoot and pulling in the longitudinal direction. A cast should be applied before the patient is transported to the hospital. The patient is as a rule treated by surgery.

Talar Fractures

A talar fracture is a rare injury but may result from a fall from a height, strong plantar flexion, or inversion or eversion injuries. It is also seen in athletes as a stress fracture. The fracture is either located in the talar body or the neck of the talus (Figure 14.14). Snowboard ankle is a rare type of fracture through the lateral process of the talus. This type of fracture constitutes approximately 3% of the ankle injuries sustained by snowboarders. Major portions of the talus are intra-articular and the talus does not have any muscle insertions. Therefore, the bone has a poor blood supply and the healing period is often long, sometimes with a risk of avascular necrosis.

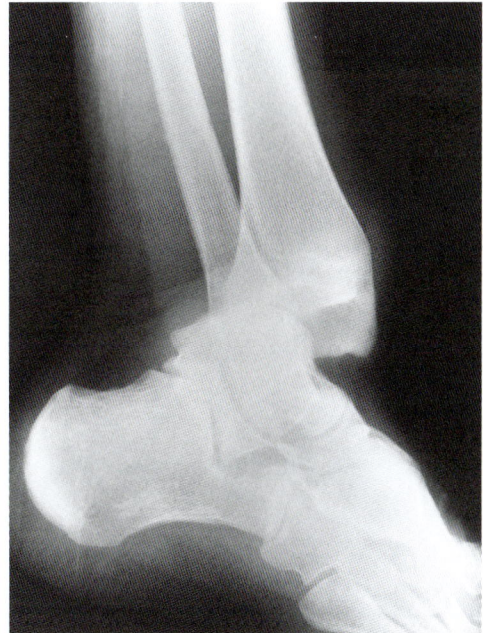

Figure 14.13 Dislocated ankle.

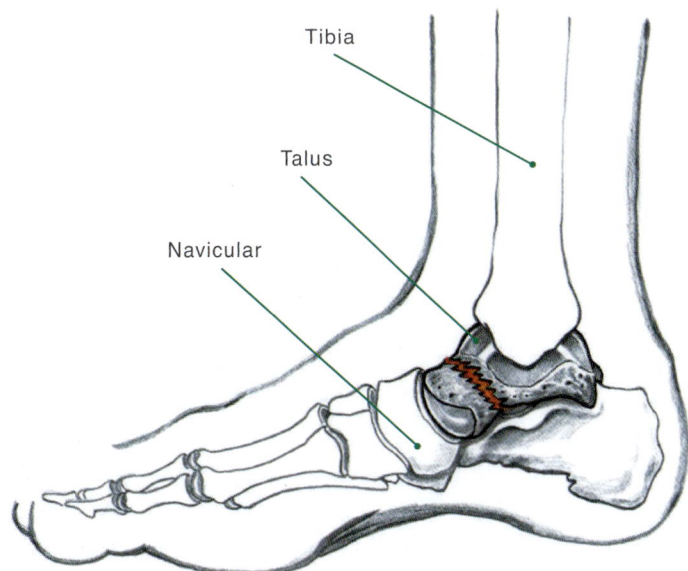

Figure 14.14 Talar fractures. Typical location, talus fracture through the neck of the talus, but other fracture types may occur. (© Medical Illustrator Tommy Bolic, Sweden.)

Tibia

Talus

Navicular

ANKLE

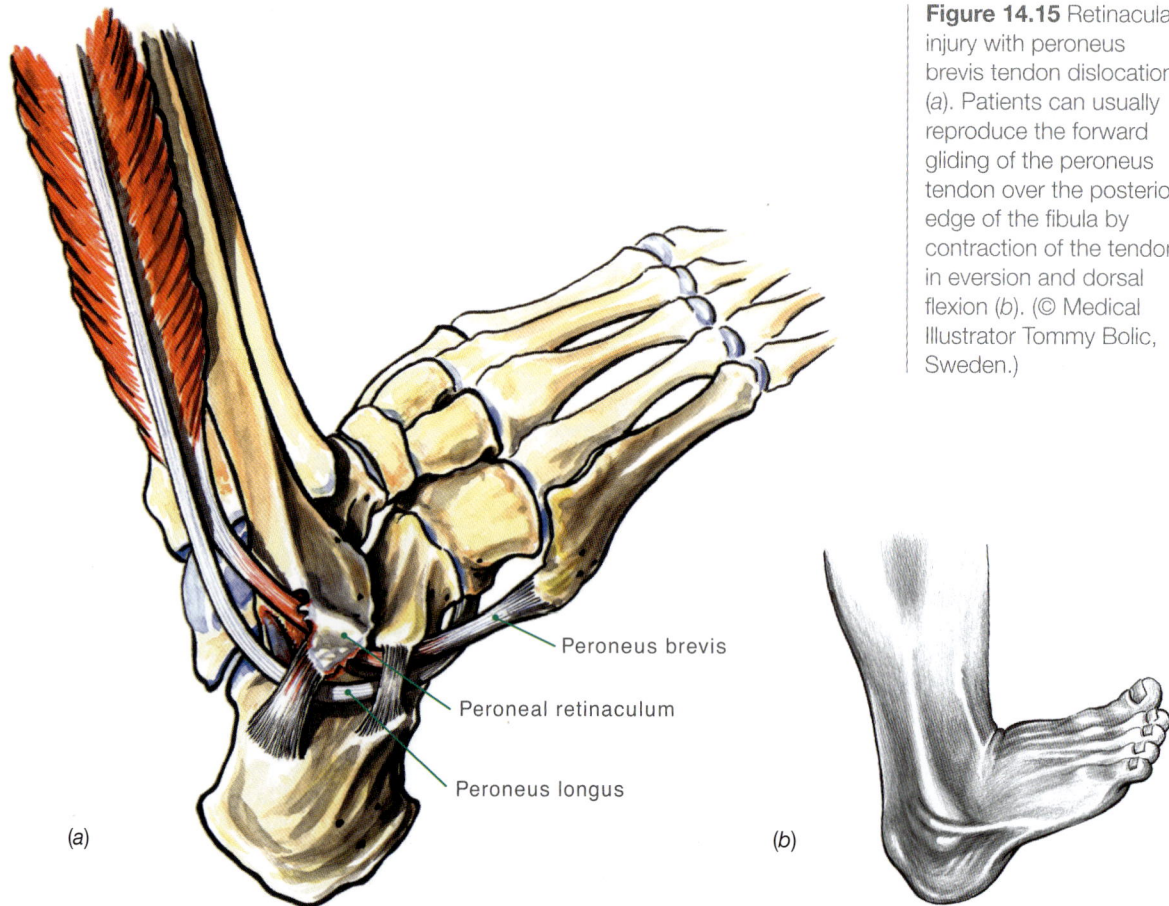

Figure 14.15 Retinacular injury with peroneus brevis tendon dislocation (*a*). Patients can usually reproduce the forward gliding of the peroneus tendon over the posterior edge of the fibula by contraction of the tendon in eversion and dorsal flexion (*b*). (© Medical Illustrator Tommy Bolic, Sweden.)

Peroneus brevis

Peroneal retinaculum

Peroneus longus

(*a*)   (*b*)

- Symptoms and signs: Symptoms are swelling and tenderness deep inside the ankle joint or in front of the anterior joint space, as well as pain from weight bearing.
- Diagnosis: The diagnosis is usually established with a standard ankle series, but a computerized tomography (CT) scan may be indicated, to document the fracture in more detail. Snowboard ankle is rarely visible on a standard radiograph, so the patient should undergo a CT scan if there is continuous lateral pain after an acute ankle injury, particularly in a snowboarder.
- Treatment by physician: The patient is in most cases treated by surgery.

Dislocation/Rupture of the Peroneal Tendons

The peroneal tendons may be injured in the area behind the lateral malleolus, particularly from contraction of the peroneus muscles with the foot in plantar flexion and eversion. This may result in longitudinal rupture of the tendon (in almost all cases the peroneus brevis tendon) in this area or in tearing of the peroneal retinaculum, so that the tendon is dislocated anteriorly on the lateral malleolus, particularly in dorsal flexion (Figure 14.15). Partial ruptures of the distal portion of the peroneus brevis tendon close to the insertion on the base of the fifth metatarsal bone also occur with inversion trauma, but this is rare.

- Symptoms and signs: The athlete often states that she heard a crack or felt something snapping behind the lateral malleolus. The patient can often reproduce this snapping during the examination if the peroneal tendons are dislocated. The easiest way to do this is to have the patient contract the peroneal musculature with the foot in eversion and dorsal flexion against resistance. The entire tendon can be seen and palpated over the lateral malleolus. Some patients have a congenital or permanent subluxation/dislocation where the gliding cannot be reproduced. In case of a partial rupture, the tendon is usually tender and thickened in the affected area. Partial rupture is an important differential diagnosis in athletes who do not recover well after lateral ligament injury.

- Diagnosis: The diagnosis is based on symptoms and on the clinical examination, but a standard radiograph of the ankle is indicated. In 15–50% of the patients, an avulsion fracture of the posterior edge of the lateral malleolus is visible. This type of avulsion fracture is pathognomonic for the diagnosis. Subluxation makes the diagnosis more difficult, and usually leads to delay of correct diagnosis and treatment.
- Treatment by physician: In most cases, the treatment is surgical, either to stabilize the peroneal tendons with retinacular plasty (or some similar method), or in case of longitudinal rupture, reconstruction of the tendon, and stabilization. In some patients, ligament reconstruction is needed as well, as concomitant injury of the lateral ligaments and partial peroneal rupture is more frequent than previously thought.

ANKLE

Pain in the Ankle Region

Roald Bahr[1], Ned Amendola[2], C. Niek van Dijk[3], Jón Karlsson[4],
Umile Giuseppe Longo[5], and Gino M.M.J. Kerkhoffs[3]

[1]*Norwegian School of Sport Sciences, Oslo, Norway*
[2]*University of Iowa, Iowa City, IA, USA*
[3]*Academic Medical Center, Amsterdam, The Netherlands*
[4]*Sahlgrenska University Hospital/Mölndal, Mölndal, Sweden*
[5]*University Campus Bio-Medico, Rome, Italy*

Definition

Painful conditions of the ankle are discussed in this section. Sometimes, overuse injuries occur after a single hard training session or training under unusual conditions, but generally the pain starts gradually over days or weeks. This section also describes disorders that may occur in the previously sprained ankle, often with gradually increasing pain.

Differential Diagnoses

Table 14.2 provides an overview of the most relevant differential diagnoses of ankle injuries. Pains in the heel region, in the middle of the foot, and in the forefoot are discussed in chapter 15. The most common cause of ankle pain is a previous or recurrent ankle sprain(s). Ankle sprains can result in osteochondral injuries, chronic synovitis, and/or recurrent instability. The symptoms may have persisted after an acute injury or may present long after the injury occurred. The patient does not always make the connection between the pain and previous ankle sprains. Another injury that is often overlooked is stress fractures. Less common causes of ankle pain, which are also often related to previous ankle sprains are sinus tarsi syndrome, syndesmosis injuries, anterior and/or posterior impingement (often simultaneous), ruptures of the tibialis posterior tendon (infrequent in young people, for instance, athletes), an injury to the peroneal or

Most common	Less common	Must not be overlooked !
Symptoms after previous ankle injuries:	Sinus tarsi syndrome, p. 452	Complex regional pain syndrome, p. 457
Osteochondral injuries, p. 449	Anterior impingement, p. 452	
Stiffness	Posterior impingement, p. 454	
Synovitis in the ankle joint, p. 451	Stress fractures, p. 455	
Chronic ankle instability, p. 451	Tibialis posterior syndrome, p. 456	
	Nerve entrapment, p. 456	
	Osteoarthrosis, p. 457	
	Peroneus tendinopathy/tendon rupture	

Table 14.2 Overview of the differential diagnoses of ankle pain. (Reproduced with permission from the Norwegian Sports Medicine Association.)

the tibialis anterior tendons, and reflex sympathetic dystrophy (very uncommon in athletes). Other painful conditions are rare, although some may be typical for certain sports.

Diagnostic Thinking

If the pain appears to be related to a previous ankle injury (which may have occurred some time ago), a primary goal of the examination is to distinguish between osteochondral fractures or chronic instability. For athletes who load the ankle in extreme positions, such as soccer players, ballet dancers, and gymnasts, anterior or posterior impingement disorders are frequent and should be suspected. Athletes with repeated high-intensity loading of the foot must always be evaluated for possible stress fractures. The initial evaluation of patients with ankle injuries should take place at the primary-care level, but a number of conditions require further evaluation by a specialist.

Case History

Patients must be thoroughly examined with respect to previous ankle injuries. Patients with ankle trauma are usually primarily affected by pain (e.g., from osteochondral fractures, chronic synovitis, and sinus tarsi syndrome) or a sensation of functional instability. In other patients, the case history usually indicates overuse, particularly from running (e.g., stress fractures), ballet, gymnastics, or soccer (e.g., anterior or posterior impingement). Localization of pain, instability problems, and accompanying symptoms should be documented.

Clinical Examination

Inspection. Malalignment is a predisposing factor to overuse injuries in the ankle, for instance, stress fractures. The patient should be examined during standing and walking, the arch of the foot should be evaluated, and an increased tendency for pronation and varus/valgus positioning should be assessed. A tibialis posterior injury is indicated if the patient has visible asymmetry with increased valgus of the hind foot and a positive "too many toes" sign (Figure 14.23). The practitioner should also evaluate function by having the patient balance, jump, and run.

Palpation. All relevant structures—the lateral malleolus, the medial malleolus, the navicular bone, the tarsal sinus, the course of the peroneal tendons, and the tibialis posterior tendon—should be palpated carefully. The ankle and subtalar joint lines should also be palpated. It may be necessary to have the patient run something similar in order to provoke symptoms before the examination. A positive Tinel sign and radiating pain provoked by lightly tapping over the posterior tibial nerve indicates tarsal tunnel syndrome. However, it should be born in mind that tarsal tunnel syndrome is rare and it is very difficult to correctly establish a diagnosis. Sometimes entrapment of one of the calcaneal branches of the posterior tibialis nerve (Baxter's nerve) may be suspected.

Movement. Active and passive movement of the ankle should always be carefully examined. Pain upon forced plantar or dorsal flexion may indicate posterior (ballet ankle) or anterior (soccer ankle) impingement. Pain at maximum inversion or eversion may indicate an osteochondral injury. Normal range of motion in the ankle joint is 15°–20° dorsal flexion, 30°–50° plantar flexion, 15°–30° pronation, and 45°–60° supination. The best way to evaluate movement is by comparing the injured ankle with the uninjured one.

ANKLE

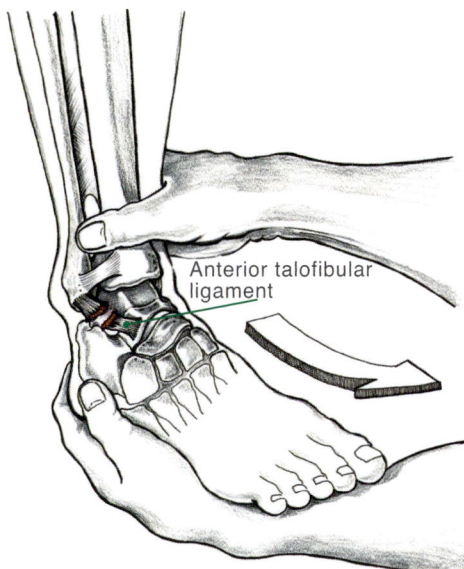

Figure 14.16 Anterior drawer test. The anterior drawer test is performed by holding the calcaneus with the foot resting on the forearm in slight plantar flexion, bringing the foot forward in relation to the tibia. The knee should be flexed in order to relax the gastrocnemius muscle. The movement takes place around an imaginary axis located in the intact deltoid ligament. (© Medical Illustrator Tommy Bolic, Sweden.)

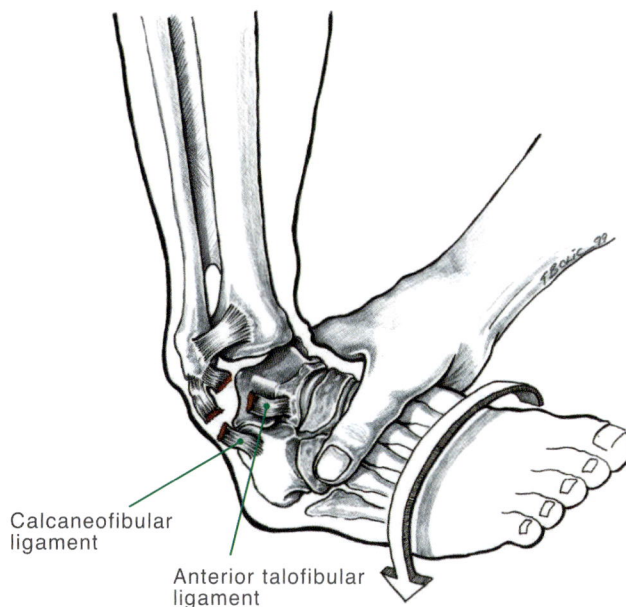

Figure 14.17 Talar tilt test. The talar tilt test is performed by supinating the foot while holding the calcaneus, with the foot in a slight equinus position. (© Medical Illustrator Tommy Bolic, Sweden.)

Stress tests. The integrity of the ligaments and the laxity of the ankle can be evaluated with the help of two stress tests: the anterior drawer test and the talar tilt test. If the patient has a ruptured anterior talofibular ligament, anterior translation will be increased during the anterior drawer test (Figure 14.16). If the calcaneofibular ligament is also torn, increased supination during the talar tilt test will also be present (Figure 14.17). The physician should always compare laxity tests with the uninjured side.

Neuromuscular function. The physician should evaluate the peroneal and tibialis anterior/posterior tendons and should palpate the course of the tendons. Neuromuscular function is extremely important to the functional stability of the ankle and is often impaired after a previous ankle injury. Function can be evaluated by means of a simple balance test where the patient stands on one leg with his arms crossed over his chest while he is looking straight ahead (Figure 14.18, Solec test; basic position). Normally, the patient should be able to accomplish this using only his ankle to correct balance. If the patient is forced to use his hips, knees, or upper body to correct balance, or if he loses his balance, the

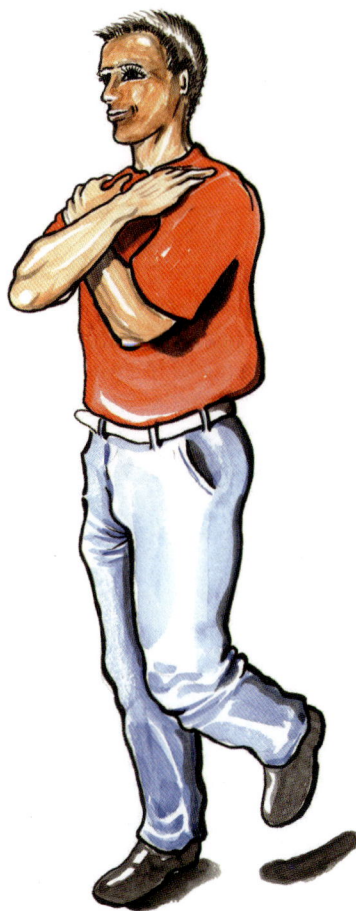

Figure 14.18 Balance test. The patient stands on one leg with the other knee slightly flexed. He crosses his arms over the chest and looks at a point straight ahead. If he can balance for 1 minute with his eyes open, he closes his eyes and balances for another 15 seconds. (© Medical Illustrator Tommy Bolic, Sweden.)

Evaluation	Quantitative (time)	Qualitative (movement pattern)
Above normal	Stands on one leg for 1 minute	Uses only the ankle to correct balance the entire time, then manages to stand with his eyes closed for 15 s without losing his balance
Normal	Stands on one leg for 1 minute	Manages >45 s using only the ankle to correct balance
Slightly abnormal	Stands on one leg for 1 minute	Has to correct balance with the knees, hips and upper body once in a while; otherwise makes corrections using the ankle
Abnormal	Stands on one leg for 1 minute, but sometimes uses the other leg for support	Unable to correct balance with the ankle alone; has to use the knees, hips, and upper body the entire time
Severely abnormal	Manages to stand on one leg, but only for short periods	

Table 14.3 Classification of sensory motor function in the ankle joint. (Reproduced with permission from the Norwegian Sports Medicine Association.)

test is positive and indicates a neuromuscular functional problem (Table 14.3). The physician should always evaluate the functional stability by comparing it with the opposite side as well.

Supplemental Examinations

If the patient is suspected of having a tendon injury, diagnostic imaging is usually indicated. Plain radiographs of the ankle joint, which often demonstrate calcification or accessory bones, are indicated if anterior or posterior impingement is suspected. However, routine radiographs have low sensitivity to show suspected osteochondral fractures or stress fractures. Skeletal scintigraphy or MRI is required to exclude this type of injury. CT scan is often the best examination when a stress fracture is suspected.

Common Injuries

Osteochondral Injuries

Osteochondral fractures and chondral injuries are common after ankle sprains, particularly when the injury is caused by landing from a jump or by high-speed running. Inversion trauma causes the talus to tilt in the ankle mortise, inflicting a compression injury of the upper medial corner of the talus (Figure 14.19). Correspondingly, cartilage or bone on the articular surfaces of the tibia and fibula may be injured. The injury may vary from minor (compression of the bone) to major (a separated piece of bone, leading to a loose body in the ankle joint). A traumatic osteochondral injury may cause osteochondritis dissecans (OCD), but this also often occurs without known trauma. Osteochondral defects of the ankle account for approximately 4% of the total number of osteochondral defects. These occur most frequently in 20- to 30-year-old men. Defects can be found on the medial and lateral sides of the talar dome, and occasionally are located centrally.

- Symptoms and signs: Generally, the injury is not recognized when the initial trauma occurs, but eventually the patient seeks medical assistance due to persisting or recurrent pain. In addition, there may be stiffness and/or locking. The ankle is not always tender to palpation.
- Locking and catching are symptoms of a displaced fragment. In most patients who have a nondisplaced lesion after supination trauma, in the acute phase the symptoms cannot be distinguished from the soft tissue damage. Chronic lesions classically present as deep lateral or medial ankle pain associated with weight bearing.

ANKLE

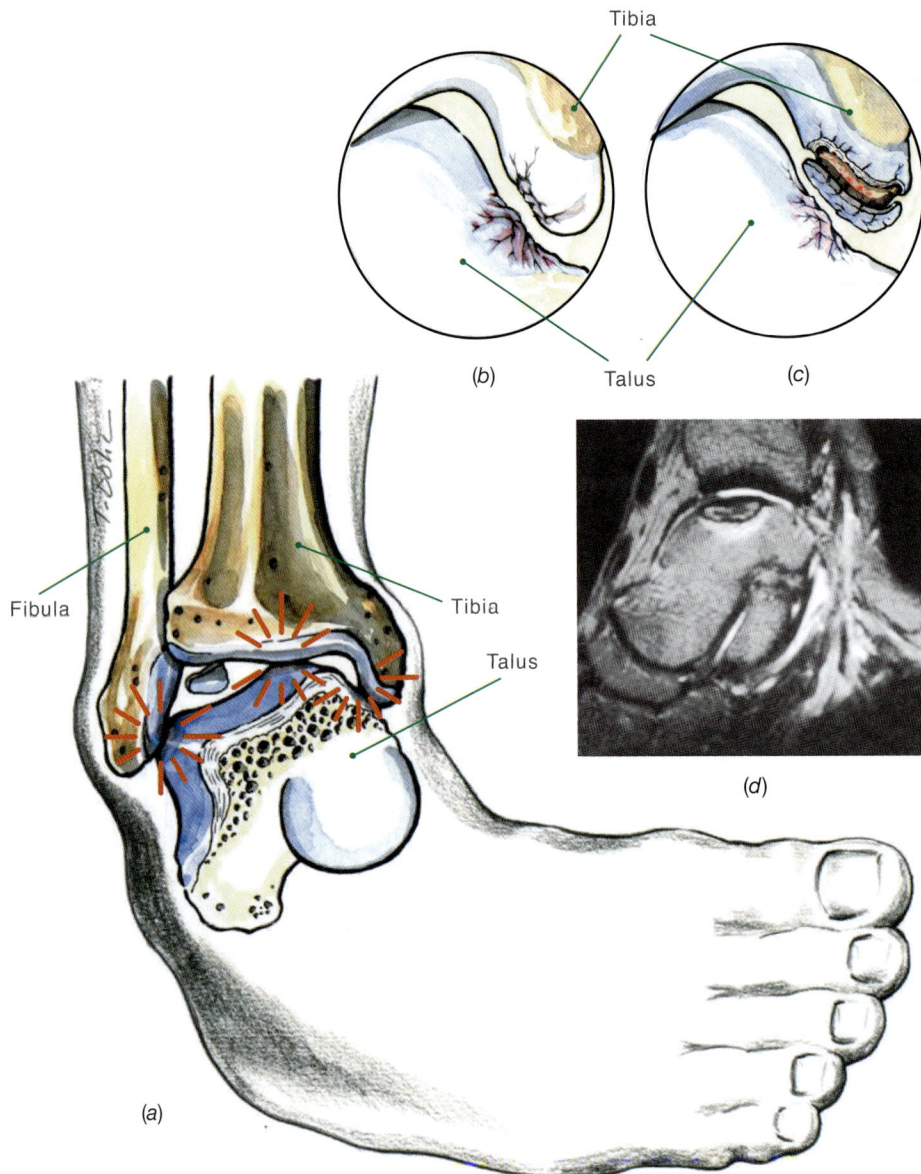

Tibia

(b)   Talus   (c)

Fibula

Tibia

Talus

(d)

(a)

Reactive swelling and stiffness can be present, but absence of swelling, locking, or catching does not rule out an osteochondral defect. Recognizable pain on palpation is typically not present in these patients. Some patients have reduced range of motion.

• Diagnosis: After careful history taking and physical examination of the ankle, routine radiographs of the ankle are taken, consisting of weight-bearing anteroposterior, mortise, and lateral views of both ankles. The radiographs may show an area of detached bone surrounded by radiolucency. Initially, the damage may be too small to be visualized on routine radiography. By repeating the imaging studies in a later stage, the abnormality sometimes becomes apparent. A heel-rise view with the ankle in a plantar-flexed position may reveal a posteromedial or posterolateral defect. MRI is often used for detection of these lesions. CT is useful for better defining the exact size and location of the lesion and, therefore, more valuable for preoperative planning. The diagnosis is established by CT or MRI. Scintigraphy with focally increased uptake also indicates osteochondral damage. CT or MRI makes it possible to distinguish between subchondral fractures (grade I), chondral fractures without detachment (grade II), chondral fractures with detachment but without dislocation (grade III), and chondral fractures with dislocation (grade IV).

- Treatment: Fractures without dislocation (grades I and II) are immobilized using a lower leg cast or brace for 6–8 weeks without weight bearing, whereas dislocated fractures (grades III and IV) require surgery, either to remove or reattach the osteochondral fragment. This is often accomplished using arthroscopic techniques. After treatment, a graded rehabilitation program is necessary before the athlete can return to sport.
- Prognosis: The younger the patient, the less the damage, the better is the prognosis. Approximately 70–90% of patients with grades III or IV injuries regain normal ankle function; however, several of them after surgical treatment and prolonged rehabilitation period.

Synovitis in the Ankle Joint

Intra-articular bleeding is often present after a ligament injury occurs. This blood is usually absorbed quickly, but in a few cases it contributes to persisting synovitis. Later in the course, the anterolateral corner of the joint capsule of some patients becomes more voluminous, sometimes producing a meniscoid lesion that bulges into the joint (and may cause impingement and pain). Usually, patients with anterior osteophytic impingement have accompanying soft-tissue changes (synovitis or scar tissue).

- Symptoms and signs: Pain from weight bearing may be localized both laterally, medially, anteriorly, and posteriorly. Palpation tenderness corresponds to the localization of pain.
- Diagnosis: MRI and arthroscopy may be indicated, especially if anterior impingement is suspected.
- Treatment: The treatment is primarily NSAIDs and a short period of rest. A corticosteroid injection may be necessary. If instability is present, the patient should use a stabilizing brace until symptoms subside. Patients, who do not respond to nonsurgical treatment within 4–6 weeks, should be evaluated with MRI and considered for arthroscopic removal of meniscoid lesions. Before surgical treatment is decided on, the exact diagnosis must be established.

Chronic Ankle Instability

After an ankle is sprained, some patients experience recurrent instability problems from repeated inversion trauma, and they may have the feeling that the ankle will give way in some situations. It may be correlated with functional instability or laxity, that is, elongation of the ligaments or a combination of both. Impaired neuromuscular function and peroneal muscle strength are related to functional instability.

- Symptoms and signs: The patient reports repeated ankle sprains (usually minor sprains) or a feeling of the ankle giving way. Some patients report pain as well.
- Diagnosis: Positive anterior drawer and talar tilt tests indicate ligament laxity. The balance test is used to evaluate neuromuscular function. Reduced neuromuscular function may cause functional instability, even without signs of ligament laxity.
- Treatment by physician: The patient should use tape or brace during the period of rehabilitation, completing a program that includes balance and peroneal strength exercises. If there is ligament laxity and the rehabilitation program is not successful with persisting functional instability, surgical stabilization, that is, ligament reconstruction should be considered.

ANKLE

451

• Treatment by therapist: The patient gradually progresses in balance exercises in which he stands on the floor to exercise using balance mats and wobble boards daily for at least 10 weeks. During this period the patient should be instructed in self-training and how to evaluate the progress.

• Self-treatment: The patient should use tape or a brace in at-risk situations and should complete a self-training program in collaboration with a therapist.

• Prognosis: Most patients with instability problems benefit from balance exercises. Surgical stabilization with ligament reconstruction (there are more than 60 different methods described in the literature) produces good outcome in most cases. Athletes can be expected to return to sports activity approximately 12 weeks after surgical stabilization.

Other Injuries

Sinus Tarsi Syndrome

Sinus tarsi syndrome is a description of painful conditions localized to the tarsal sinus, usually on the lateral side (Figure 14.20). It occurs in patients who have previously injured their ankle, with damage to the subtalar joint or ligaments, or as an overuse injury caused by subtle subtalar laxity or subtalar overpronation.

• Symptoms and signs: The patient usually experiences continuous symptoms after what was considered a moderate inversion trauma. Pain is localized on the lateral side around the sinus tarsi in front of the lateral malleolus. Pain is often most pronounced in the morning and is reduced after warm-up. Pain provoked by running on grass or another soft irregular surface is typical.

• Diagnosis: Tenderness to palpation over the tarsal sinus. Pain can often be provoked both in full supination and in full pronation. The diagnosis is confirmed if the patient is pain free after an injection of local anesthesia into the tarsal sinus.

• Treatment by physician: Corrective shoe insoles should be used if the patient has an increased tendency toward pronation to stabilize the subtalar joint and provide heel control. An injection of a corticosteroid often brings rapid improvement, but underlying causes such as joint injury, impingement, or laxity should be examined for.

• Self-treatment: The patient can treat herself by unloading, applying ice, corrective training, and wearing different shoes that fit well with a stable heel counter.

Anterior Impingement—*Soccer Ankle*

This pain syndrome is called "soccer ankle" because it is usually seen in soccer players, but it also occurs in athletes in other sports. Anterior impingement of the ankle joint may cause chronic pain, and it may reduce function. One cause is repeated, strong plantar flexion from kicking the ball, causing a rift in the joint capsule anteriorly (Figure 14.21). Another cause may be strong dorsal flexion, resulting in contusion of the

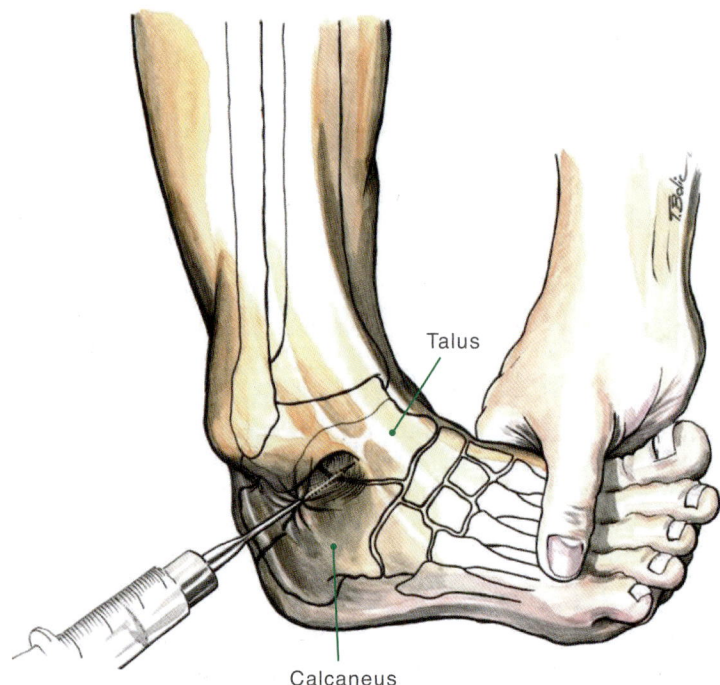

Figure 14.20 Sinus tarsi syndrome. The corticosteroid injection is given from the lateral side into the tarsal sinus, a finger's width in front and a finger's width below the tip of the lateral malleolus. The tip of the needle should be aimed toward the tip of the medial malleolus and must enter into the open soft-tissue sport in the sinus tarsi. In most cases fluoroscopy is recommended. (© Medical Illustrator Tommy Bolic, Sweden.)

Talus

Calcaneus

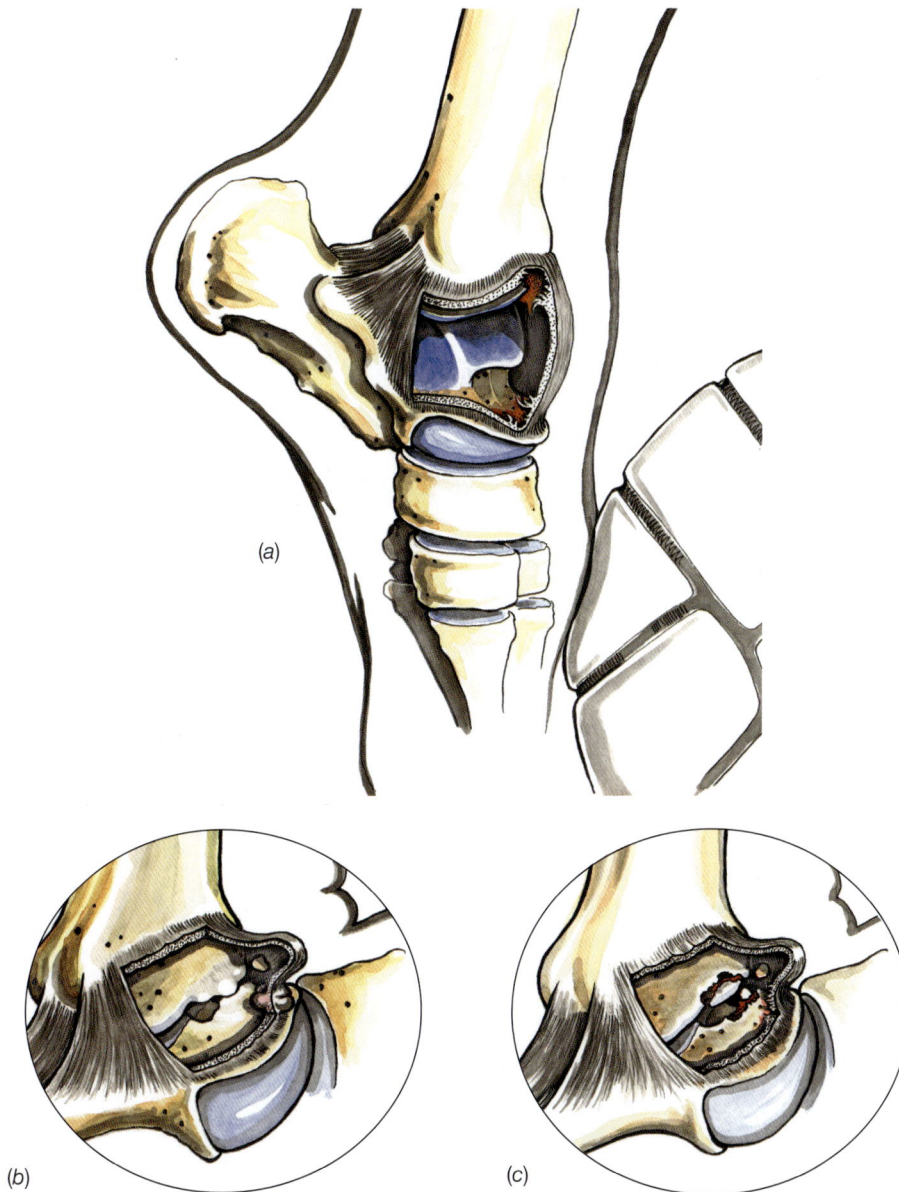

Figure 14.21 Soccer ankle. Possible injury mechanism with anterior impingement. The injury may be the result of anterior osteophyte formation related to bone or capsular injury because of hyperextension in plantar flexion when kicking a ball (*a*), or the result of contusion injuries in forced dorsal flexion (*b*, *c*). (© Medical Illustrator Tommy Bolic, Sweden.)

anterior tibia and the talus against each other. This causes osteophytes to develop on the anterior edge of the tibia and later the talus. Underlying ankle instability will also cause osteophytes to form as a means of stabilizing the joint. The osteophytes will increase the anterior impingement and cause pain. In some cases, osteophyte formation can be seen anteriorly on the tibia, causing a depression (divot sign) on the talus (instead of osteophyte formation there).

- Symptoms and signs: Pain is activity dependent and is usually triggered in maximal dorsiflexion, generally in connection with starting and stopping movements. In subacute cases, the pain may begin after forced dorsal flexion. The area is not necessarily tender to anterior palpation. Ankle ligament laxity after a previous injury may contribute to increased impingement.
- Diagnosis: Pain may be reproduced by using a starting movement where the ankle is loaded in forced dorsiflexion. The osteophytes can be palpated with dorsiplantar

ANKLE

453

flexion and are tender on the anteromedial joint line. Radiographs usually demonstrate osteophytes over the neck of the talus or at the anterior margin of the tibia on a lateral view or oblique (approximately 30° of external rotation will give a better view of the anterior tibial osteophyte).

- Treatment by therapist: In cases in which instability contributes to the symptoms of impingement, an ankle tape or brace may help. Emphasizing good muscle strength and control will also help in reducing symptoms.
- Treatment by physician: In subacute cases, NSAIDs may be indicated, and if this is not helpful, an injection of corticosteroids may be attempted. When radiographs show more prominent osteophytes, arthroscopic removal of the osteophytes and surrounding synovitis should be considered.
- Self-treatment: The patient can treat himself by applying ice, changing the loading pattern, and resting. Ankle taping, in order to avoid extremes of dorsiflexion is often helpful, at least in the short term.
- Prognosis: The prognosis is good, even in cases that require surgery. Most soccer players are back at full function after 4–6 weeks after arthroscopic treatment.

Posterior Impingement—*Ballet Ankle*

Posterior impingement is caused by impingement between the posterior part of the talus and the tibia. The condition is usually called "ballet ankle" because it is common among ballet dancers. Forced plantar flexion (demi-pointe and pointe positions) (Figure 14.22) causes pain. The condition is also common in gymnasts and soccer players (after kicks with the ankle extended). In patients with these types of symptoms, osteophytes usually develop posteriorly on the talus, or a prominent posterior process is present. The bone may become detached, creating a loose body. In some cases an os trigonum is present (Figure 14.22). All of these conditions may irritate the flexor halluces longus tendon, as part of the impingement process. An os trigonum (a bone that is not attached to the tibia) is found normally in approximately 10% of the population; however, not all have symptoms. In sports in which forced plantar flexion is frequent, an os trigonum may cause impingement.

- Symptoms and signs: The primary symptom is pain from forced plantar flexion. The patient usually experiences posterolateral tenderness in the area behind the peroneal tendons. Palpation of the flexor hallucis tendon through a range of motion on the posteromedial side of the ankle is important.
- Diagnosis: Pain can be reproduced with the ankle weight bearing during forced plantar flexion. Plain radiographs (preferably of both ankles for comparison) may show osteophytes at the posterior tubercle of the talus or an os trigonum. However, large osteophytes with few symptoms, and pronounced symptoms without any major osteophytes, can also be seen. Inflammation of or around the flexor hallucis longus tendon may cause similar symptoms, and the conditions may occur simultaneously. MRI may be useful to clearly diagnose structures involved. The injection of a small amount (0.5–1.0 mL) of local anesthetics can help to confirm the diagnosis. This should be done using fluoroscopy or ultrasound guidance. Crepitations and triggering of the flexor hallucis longus should also be born in mind as differential diagnosis.
- Treatment by physician: In subacute cases, anti-inflammatory medication (NSAID) may be indicated, and if this does not work, a corticosteroid injection may be attempted, preferably under fluoroscopy guidance. If neither therapy is effective, arthroscopic removal of an os trigonum, loose body or osteophytes should be considered.

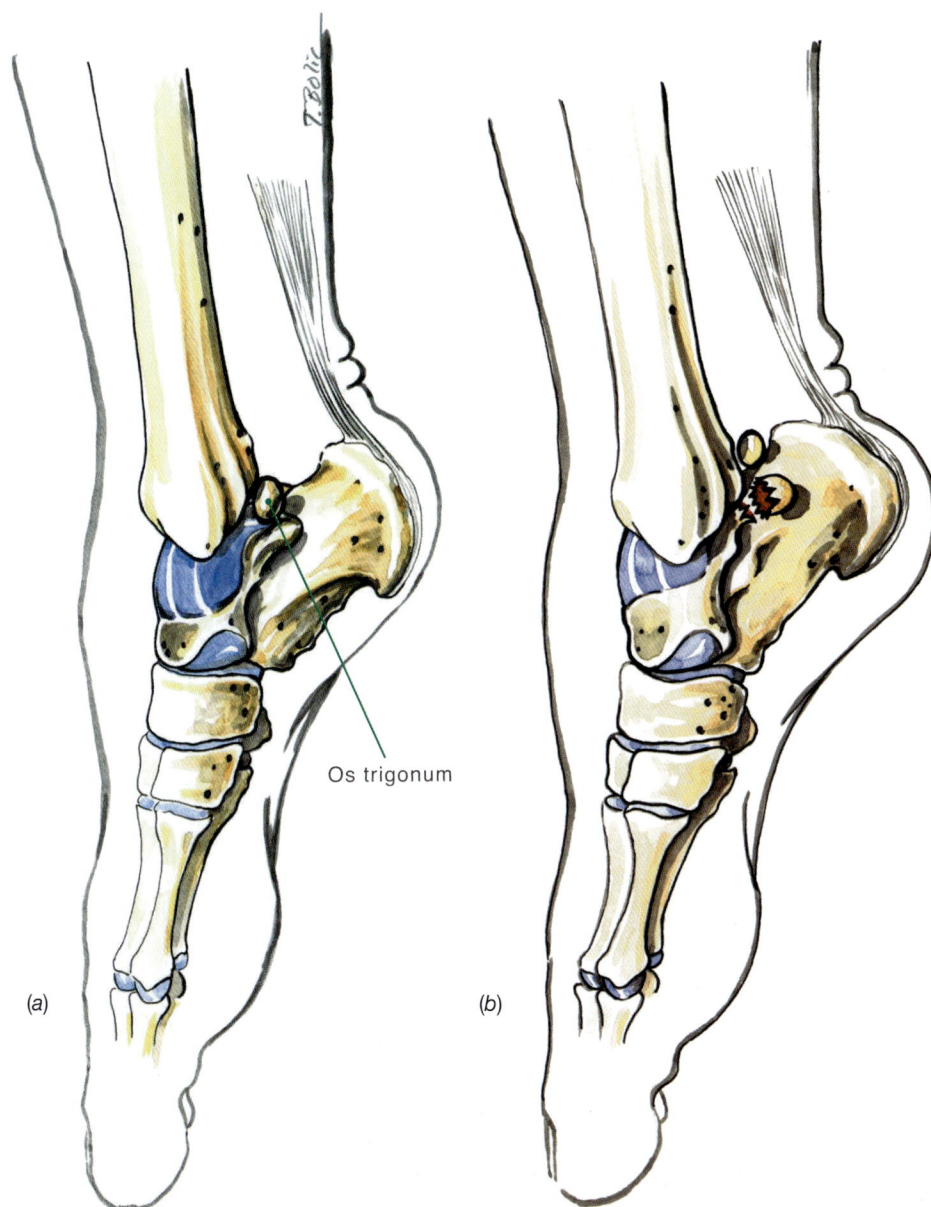

(a)

Os trigonum

(b)

Figure 14.22 Ballet ankle. In forced plantar flexion, such as the pointe and demi pointe positions in ballet, the posterior tubercle or an os trigonum (*a*) is impinged against the posterior aspect of the tibia (causing pain). Pain may also be caused by the formation of osteophytes come loose (*b*) and flexor hallucis longus irritation may occur from impingement or low lying muscle belly impinging in the tendon tunnel. (© Medical Illustrator Tommy Bolic, Sweden.)

- Self-treatment: The patient can treat herself by applying ice, changing the loading pattern, and a short period of rest.
- Prognosis: The prognosis is good, even in cases that require surgery; however, rehabilitation may require more than 6 months.

Stress Fractures

Stress fractures may occur in most bones of the foot and ankle, for instance, the talus and navicular bones. However, stress fractures of the calcaneus are less frequent. Navicular stress fractures are more common than talar fractures and mainly occur in athletes in flexibility and sprinting sports. Stress fractures of the fifth metatarsal are discussed on page 472.

- Symptoms and signs: *A high index of suspicion is required.* Symptoms are exercise-related pain in the affected area, sometimes diffuse, and usually radiating

ANKLE

455

to the forefoot. There is almost always palpation tenderness in the affected area. The navicular bone is palpated by localizing the talonavicular joint first (by moving the forefoot in supination and pronation) and then by palpating the "N-point" (the proximal dorsal portion of the navicular bone). Malalignment, such as overpronation (which presumably predisposes the athlete to the injury), is often found. Reduced ankle dorsiflexion flexibility may predispose to increase talonavicular stress.

- Diagnosis: The primary examination for a suspected stress fracture is scintigraphy or MRI, due to the poor sensitivity of plain radiographs. A positive scintigraphic examination is usually followed by an MRI or a CT, to distinguish between a stress reaction (negative CT) and a stress fracture (positive CT/MRI). CT evaluation for bone healing in navicular fractures is ideal.
- Treatment: Stress reactions are treated by nonweight bearing combined with immobilization. Patients with stress fractures should be referred to an orthopedic surgeon for evaluation. Both the navicular and the talus have poorly vascularized zones, where delayed healing or nonunion may occur. Surgery may be indicated in some patients. Normally, the lower leg is immobilized in a cast or brace for at least 8 weeks without weight bearing, after which activity can be gradually increased within the limits of pain. To avoid delayed healing, weight bearing should not be allowed during the immobilization period. Malalignment should be corrected with shoe insoles.

Tibialis Posterior Syndrome—*Rupture of the Tibialis Posterior Tendon*

Young athletes very rarely sustain ruptures of the tibialis posterior tendon (Figure 14.23), but such injuries may occur in older athletes in the area behind the medial malleolus. Painful conditions are also common in the tendon close to the insertion. The tendon has a broad insertion surface that includes the navicular bone, all three cuneiform bones, and the second, third, and fourth metatarsals. In rare cases, ruptures may also occur in connection with ankle sprains, usually behind the medial malleolus.

- Symptoms and signs: When the rupture is subtotal or there is synovitis of the tendon sheath, the main symptom is continuous activity-related pain along the course of the tendon, either behind the medial malleolus or near the insertion. In more advanced cases, tenderness will be present at the rupture. The patient may be unable to stand on her toes, the hind foot has a valgus position and the "too many toes" sign is positive (acute flat footedness) (Figure 14.23). Generally, the patient will state that he had long-lasting pain and throbbing in the area. However, many patients will not seek medical assistance in the acute situation. In fact, the patient delay is in many cases over 12 months. These patients often present with fixed hind foot valgus position and increased pronation of the forefoot, which in most cases is very difficult to treat.
- Diagnosis: The best way to establish the diagnosis is thorough clinical examination, but an MRI, and ultrasonography may also be useful.
- Treatment: If a rupture of the tibialis posterior tendon is suspected, surgical treatment is often needed.

Nerve Entrapment—*Tarsal Tunnel Syndrome*

Nerve entrapment may cause local injury to a nerve or inflammation due to a direct injury or compression from surrounding structures. The primary symptom is almost always pain and later dysesthesia (e.g., numbness, pricking, or a burning sensation). Pain is usually limited if a sensory nerve is involved, and it is more diffuse when the motor nerves are affected. In the ankle area, the posterior tibial nerve is affected most often, where it passes behind the medial malleolus and behind the tibialis posterior tendon. This is the tarsal tunnel syndrome. Entrapment of other nerves (such as the deep peroneal nerve or the superficial peroneal nerve) is less common. Also, the sensory nerves on the medial aspect of the heel may be inflicted (Baxter's nerve). Entrapment disorders must be carefully evaluated in case of pain and dysesthesia; patients should be referred for electrophysiological or nerve conduction velocity examinations.

Osteoarthritis

Osteoarthritis in the ankle joint primarily affects elderly patients who have sustained ankle fractures previously. The main symptoms are pain and stiffness. The diagnosis is established using plain radiographs.

Complex Regional Pain Syndrome !

Complex regional pain syndrome, or reflex dystrophy, may occur after ankle injuries (both fractures and ligament injuries), but is not frequent. After a few weeks or months of initial improvement, symptoms increase. The symptoms consist of increasing pain, swelling, and the skin feels warm or cold. Local sweating and changes in skin color or temperature may occur. Early diagnosis is the key to successful treatment, because the prognosis depends on how soon treatment is started. Radiographs may eventually show demineralization. Patients with reflex dystrophy that do not respond rapidly to conventional pain therapy should be referred to a pain clinic for evaluation.

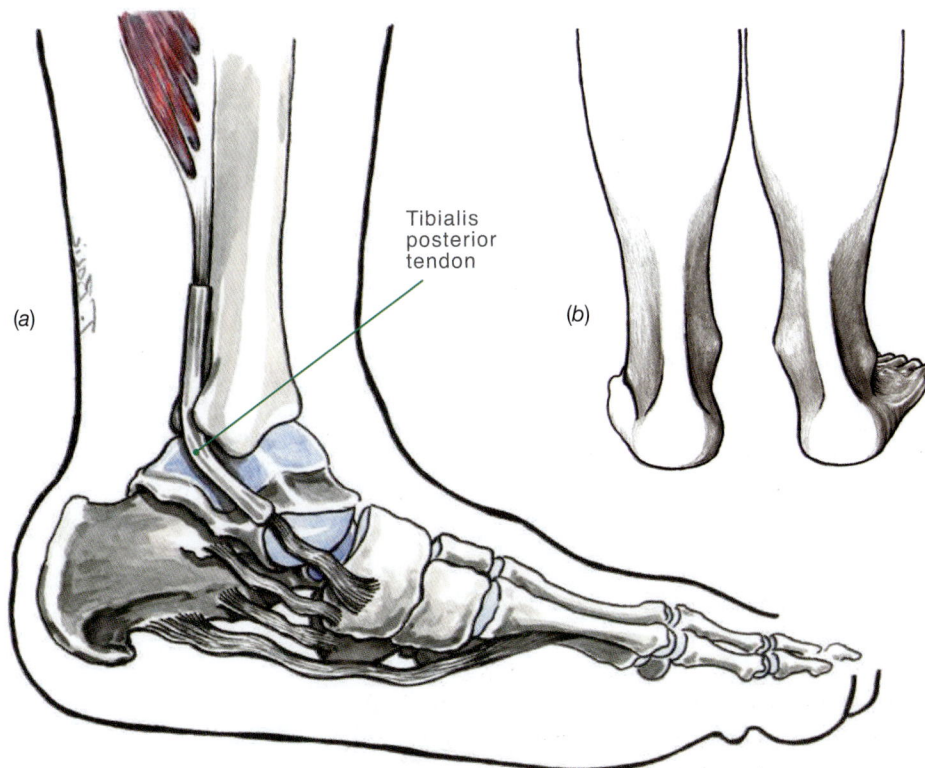

(a)

Tibialis posterior tendon

(b)

Figure 14.23 Tibialis posterior tendon rupture (a). If a rupture occurs, it will look like the patient has acutely acquired flatfoot. Inspection from behind reveals asymmetry where several toes are visible on the affected side ("too many toes" sign) (b). In addition, the patient may have difficulties standing stand on her toes on the affected side. (© Medical Illustrator Tommy Bolic, Sweden.)

ANKLE

Rehabilitation of Ankle Injuries

Roald Bahr

Norwegian School of Sport Sciences, Oslo, Norway

Acute Ankle Injuries: Rehabilitation Goals and Principles

Table 14.4 lists the goals for rehabilitation of acute ankle injuries.

Warm-up may be passive at first, including warm baths, but it should be active as soon as possible—for example, with the use of a cycle ergometer (Figure 14.24). Mobilization of the ankle and the joints of the foot may be necessary in rare cases. This can be both active and passive.

The exercise program reflects the goals listed in Table 14.4 below and uses mobility exercises, strength exercises, functional exercises, and specific exercises to improve neuromuscular function with a gradual progression towards more challenging exercises.

Tape, elastic bandages, or a brace are used to provide compression during the acute stage. During the rehabilitation stage, tape or a brace is used to provide compression and for support, so that training for normal function can begin more quickly. During the training stage, tape or a brace is primarily used to prevent reinjury, particularly if the athlete trains on an uneven surface or in other situations that may involve a risk of reinjury.

Ankle Pain and/or Instability: Goals and Principles

The rehabilitation of patients with chronic ankle pain generally involves focusing on neuromuscular function. The most common cause of ankle pain is a previously sprained ankle that resulted in osteochondral injury and instability. The instability

	Goals	Measures
Acute stage	Reduce swelling	The PRICE principle with emphasis on compression
Rehabilitation stage	Normal and pain free range of motion so that the patient can train with normal function	Exercises
Training stage	Normal neuromuscular function; a consequence of ankle injuries may be reduced neuromuscular function with a slow reaction to changes in position	Exercises
	Healing of the injured ligament(s) without the loss of mechanical stability or tensile strength	
	Reduce the risk of reinjury	

Table 14.4 Goals and measures for rehabilitation of acute ankle injuries. (Reproduced with permission from the Norwegian Sports Medicine Association.)

may be because of increased laxity (i.e., the ligaments are permanently lengthened), or functional (i.e., no mechanical instability is present, but neuromuscular function in the ankle is impaired). In almost all cases, a 10-week neuromuscular training program that includes balance exercises will be attempted before the patient is evaluated for possible surgical treatment (Figure 14.25). The patient should do 10 minutes of balance training 5 days a week for at least 10 weeks–the 10-5-10 rule.

Preventing Reinjury

Because sprained ankles are the most common injuries in sport, prevention is key. This is particularly true for athletes with previous ankle injuries, for whom the risk of reinjury is 4–10 times greater than for athletes without previous injuries. The risk of reinjury is particularly high during the first 6–12 months after a previous injury in athletes who have not completed an adequate neuromuscular training program.

The following measures have had good results:

Neuromuscular training. Balance training on a wobble board should be done according to the 10-5-10 rule. The 10-week program may seem excessive, but experience shows that it can easily be completed if the athlete does the daily exercises while doing another activity, such as watching TV. Studies of athletes with instability problems after ankle injuries show that

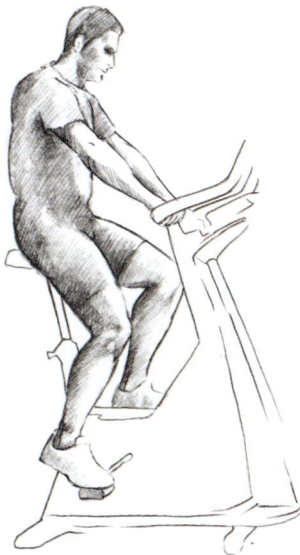

Figure 14.24 Bicycling to remove swelling and increase range of motion
- Use mild resistance.
- Use high frequency and low load.
- Start with your heel on the pedal, then move the loading forward to use your ankle more actively.
- The key is primarily to use the ankle joint to pedal.
(Reproduced with permission from the Norwegian Sports Medicine Association.)

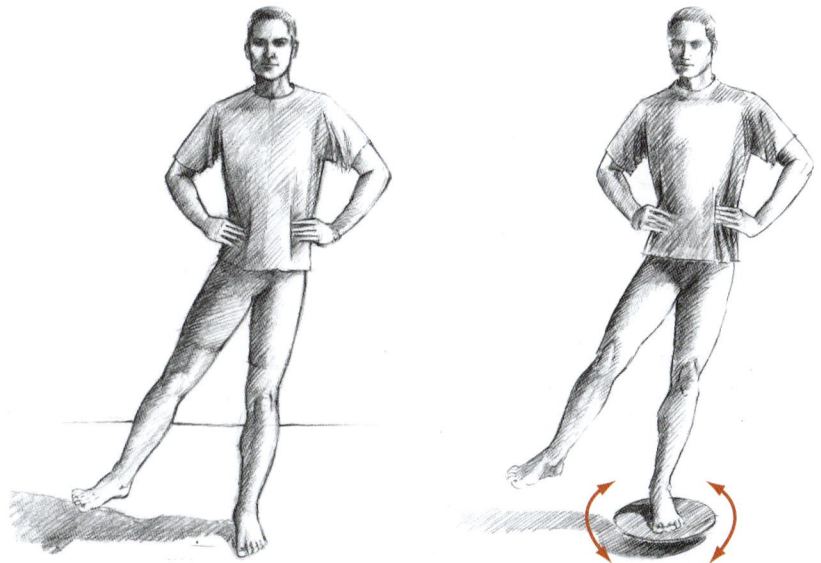

Figure 14.25 Neuromuscular function: standing balance exercises
- Be precise about your starting position; keep your knee over your foot and control your hip.
- Increase difficulty by closing your eyes or by adding distractions, such as a ball or other movements.
- Increase difficulty by switching from a soft to a hard surface.
(Reproduced with permission from the Norwegian Sports Medicine Association.)

ANKLE

- sensory motor function is reduced in patients with instability, including increased reaction time in the peroneal musculature to a sudden inversion stress.
- sensory motor function may be normalized with 10 weeks of training on a balance board.
- training on a balance board reduces the risk of a new injury to the same level as that of ankles that were not previously injured.

Taping or bracing. Athletes who do not achieve complete rehabilitation through neuromuscular training should use tape or a brace during at-risk activities until rehabilitation is completed. Tests have shown that taping or using an orthotic device prevents new injuries in athletes with previous ankle injuries. Recent studies show that the use of a brace does not reduce performance with respect to flexibility or speed. If an athlete uses taping or a brace, he needs to be well informed about the importance of continuing to use support until full function is achieved.

15 Foot

Acute Foot Injuries

Ned Amendola[1], Tom Clanton[2], and Andrew Franklyn-Miller[3]

[1]*University of Iowa, Iowa City, IA, USA*
[2]*The Steadman Clinic, Vail, CO, USA*
[3]*Aspetar, Qatar Orthopaedic and Sports Medicine Hospital, Doha, Qatar*

Occurrence

The foot serves a complex purpose for athletes. It absorbs impact from the ground, carries body weight, and converts energy from the thigh and lower leg into effective motion for running, jumping, lateral movement, acceleration, and braking. These movements involve major loading, and a number of factors may cause foot injuries. Therefore, foot injuries occur most commonly in athletes in sports that involve considerable walking, running, jumping, cutting, and other loading of the feet (Table 15.1). In a study of more than 16,000 athletes, 15% of the injuries were localized to the feet. Informing athletes and trainers about simple prophylactic measures, such as training conditions, choice of footwear, and the appropriate use of insoles, may prevent many foot disorders.

Differential Diagnoses

Contusions (injuries caused by impact) and sprains (twisting) are the most common of all acute foot injuries. Direct trauma, such as a kick or having the upper side of the foot stomped on by cleats, is common in soccer, whereas orienteering runners usually sprain the ankle because of an uneven surface. More violent high-energy injury mechanisms may cause a fracture or a dislocation in various locations in the foot. The foot contains 26 bones that are bound together by 30 different joints, and all these bones and joints are vulnerable to injuries. Fractures are most common in

Most common	Less common	Must not be overlooked ❗
Fifth metatarsal fracture, p. 437	Dislocations, p. 464	Gout
Talus fracture, p. 443	Metatarsophalangeal joint injury (turf toe), p. 465	
Metatarsal fracture, p. 463	Toe joints	
Phalanx fracture, p. 463	Tarsometatarsal joints (Lisfranc joint)	
Calcaneal fracture, p. 464	Talonavicular and calcaneocuboid joints (Chopart joint)	
Contusions and sprains, p. 465	Subtalar joint	
Blisters, p. 466		

Table 15.1 Overview of the differential diagnoses of acute foot injuries. (Reproduced with permission from the Norwegian Sports Medicine Association.)

the toes and metatarsals, less common in the calcaneus and talus, and rare in the other tarsal bones (navicular, cuboid, and the three cuneiform bones). Dislocations are most common in the toe joints, less common in the tarsometatarsal joints (Lisfranc joints), and rare in the other foot joints. Turf toe refers to a spectrum of injury, mild sprain to a complete rupture, of the plantar plate of the great toe. Foot blisters are common and may be very annoying until the affected area is unloaded. Gout may cause acute severe pain, usually localized to the area around the great toe metatarsophalangeal (MTP) joint, with warm, erythematous skin, and swelling. In athletes, this may be misinterpreted as an acute injury.

Diagnostic Thinking

A good case history is essential if the patient has an acute injury. Depending on the force of the trauma, it may be possible to determine whether the patient has a fracture or just a contusion or sprain. If the patient has a mild soft-tissue injury or a sprained joint, it is often possible for the patient to bear weight on the foot; however, if the foot is fractured or dislocated, pain makes weight bearing almost impossible. A thorough clinical examination that includes inspection, palpation, and manual testing the structures in the foot will also provide good information about how severe the injury is and whether supplemental examinations, such as routine X-rays, computed tomography (CT), ultrasound, or MRI are necessary. Generally, the patient is referred for X-rays anytime there is deformity, inability to weight bear, or suspicion for a fracture.

Clinical Examination

Inspection. If the patient has an acute injury, the practitioner should look for malalignment, discoloration of the skin, and swelling, as well as wounds. Dislocated toe joints are easily diagnosed by inspection. In such cases, the differential diagnosis is a significantly displaced fracture.

Palpation. This is the most important part of the examination, to localize the site of injury. Thorough palpation of bones, joints, ligaments, and tendons, of the foot provides important information about what is injured, and it can often be used to determine whether dislocation or a fracture has occurred. If a metatarsal fracture has occurred, pressure or pulling in the bone's longitudinal direction via the corresponding toe triggers pain (indirect tenderness). If a Lisfranc injury is suspected, abduction stress of the foot will exhibit significant pain. The ability to correlate an area of tenderness to palpation with a corresponding knowledge of the underlying anatomical structures is crucial to musculoskeletal diagnosis.

Movement. The various joints in the foot are tested for the ability to move and to determine whether movement triggers pain. The best way to determine whether foot movement is normal or not is to compare it with the opposite, healthy side.

Supplemental Examinations

Radiographic examination. X-rays must be taken for acute injuries if there is the slightest suspicion of a fracture. Comparison X-rays should be taken for suspicion of MTP plantar plate ruptures and Lisfranc joint injury. In addition, stress radiographs of the tarsometatarsal joint may be of value if the plain X-rays do not show any abnormality but significant injury is suspected.

CT. If fractures or dislocations in the midfoot or tarsus have occurred, CT is often indicated. A CT scan can provide very good supplemental information to routine

X-rays, particularly if three-dimensional reconstruction is planned. A CT scan is done routinely if surgical treatment of complicated foot injuries is planned.

MRI. MRI imaging is indicated to assess soft-tissue injuries, plantar plate injuries, and Lisfranc sprains without any displacement.

Common Injuries

Fractures in Phalanges and Metatarsals—*Toe and Midfoot Bone Fractures*

Metatarsals and phalanges are often fractured in athletes and in nonathletes. The injury is usually caused by direct trauma to the back of the foot or to the toes or by strong torsional trauma. Fractures resulting from direct trauma are usually transverse but may be comminuted, whereas fractures resulting from indirect trauma are oblique or spiral (Figure 15.1). Intra-articular fractures occur most often in the MTP joint of the big toe.

- Symptoms and signs: Symptoms are pain (particularly from loading), swelling, possibly discoloration of the skin or skin perforation, and malalignment.
- Diagnosis: Palpation causes significant pain that corresponds to the fracture. Indirect tenderness is typical of metatarsal fractures. The diagnosis is confirmed by X-rays.
- Treatment: Fractures in the metatarsals and phalanges that are not displaced or are only slightly displaced, are treated by unloading, until the patient is pain free, and possibly by short-term (3–4 weeks) treatment in a cast or walking boot, if the patient has much pain. Wearing stiff-soled shoes provides sufficient pain relief for most patients. Displaced fractures, particularly intra-articular ones, must be surgically reduced and fixed. It may be somewhat difficult for avulsion fractures at the base of the fifth metatarsal to heal, because the lateral band of the plantar aponeurosis puts tension on the end of the bone. Therefore, open reduction and fixation with a screw often becomes necessary.
- Prognosis: Simple fractures in the metatarsals and phalanges heal quickly, and the athlete can usually return to a complete training routine in 4–6 weeks. If surgery is necessary, the patient can count on a somewhat longer rehabilitation period.

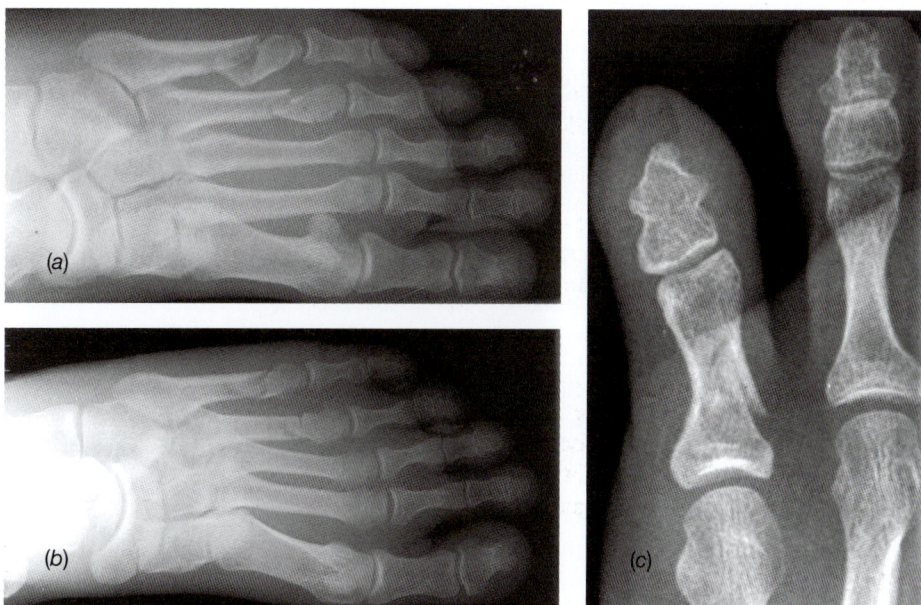

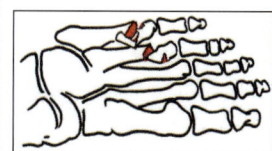

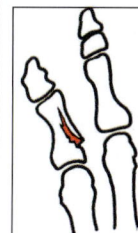

Figure 15.1 Fractures. Oblique fractures through the distal portions of the fourth and fifth metatarsals (*a* and *b*). Fractures of the proximal phalanx of the little toe (*c*). (© Medical Illustrator Tommy Bolic, Sweden.)

Calcaneal Fractures—*Heel Bone Fractures*

The cause of a calcaneal fracture (Figure 15.2) is usually a jump or a fall from a height, with the patient landing on his heels. The resulting injury is often bilateral. Parachute jumpers frequently sustain calcaneal fractures, and the force of the trauma affects how severe the injury is. Slight force (low-energy trauma) usually results in a simple fracture without significant malalignment, which can be treated conservatively. High-energy trauma causes crushing of the calcaneus. The angle the heel bone forms with the rest of the foot (tuber-joint angle) becomes straighter, causing the foot to be flat, and the subtalar articular surface on the heel bone is more or less pressed out of place.

- Symptoms and signs: Pain and tenderness is localized to the calcaneus, particularly when loading is attempted or when the heel is compressed from side-to-side. Slight swelling occurs during the early phase. Deformation of the foot with flatfoot, a dislocated Achilles tendon insertion, and a widened heel are visible even before swelling and discoloration of the skin begin. Ankle joint movement is often normal while subtalar joint motion of inversion and eversion is usually painful.
- Diagnosis: Diagnosis is based on X-rays of the heel in two planes. To demonstrate the injury before surgical treatment, CT is often used to reconstruct the calcaneus in three dimensions.
- Treatment: Fractures without malalignment are treated with a cast or walking boot for 4 weeks, and the patient is allowed to bear weight as soon as it can be done pain free. Fractures with malalignment should be treated surgically, to restore normal anatomy.
- Prognosis: Fractures that are not displaced heal without sequelae, and the patient regains normal foot function. In case of major crushing of the calcaneus, particularly depression of the subtalar articular surface, the outcome is primarily determined by the extent of the articular damage though this may be improved by how well the bone is surgically reconstructed. A good portion of these patients end up with a somewhat flatter and wider foot, and many patients eventually develop post-traumatic arthritis in the subtalar joint.

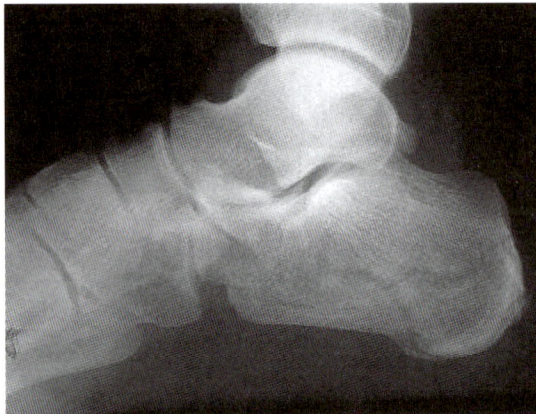

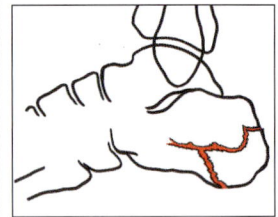

Figure 15.2
Nondisplaced Y-fracture in the calcaneus.
(© Medical Illustrator Tommy Bolic, Sweden.)

Dislocations

Dislocations in the foot are relatively common in the toes and in the tarsometatarsal joint (Lisfranc joint). They are less common in the talonavicular and calcaneocuboid joints (collectively called the Chopart joint) but may be seen between the talus and the calcaneus (the subtalar joint).

- Symptoms and signs: Pain, malalignment, and swelling are the primary symptoms.
- Diagnosis: Diagnosis is based on clinical examination, with frontal and lateral X-rays, usually supplemented with oblique images. CT may provide a good image of a dislocated bone for three-dimensional reconstruction of the tarsus. The dislocation

is often combined with a fracture in these areas. MRI and/or stress X-rays may be of value with undisplaced sprains when significant injury is suspected.

- Treatment: If the dislocation is unstable, the treatment is exact anatomical reduction and fixation with pins, screws, or plates. Early mobilization is important in preventing joint stiffness. If stress X-rays are stable, more aggressive weight-bearing treatment may be instituted in the nonoperative setting.
- Prognosis: Prognosis is good if exact reduction is achieved and the patient is mobilized early. If subluxation persists, the patient often has chronic pain from loading and post-traumatic arthritis will develop in the affected joints.

Contusions and Sprains—*Injuries Caused by Impact and Torsion*

Contusions and sprains often affect soft tissues and joints in the foot. Most of the time, if no dislocation has occurred, the articular capsules and ligaments will heal without lasting symptoms.

- Symptoms and signs: Pain, swelling, and discoloration of the skin over the injured area are the primary symptoms.
- Diagnosis: Case history and clinical examination are usually sufficient to make the diagnosis. In doubtful cases, the patient must be given X-rays to exclude a fracture.
- Treatment: PRICE (rest, ice, compression, and elevation) and nonsteroidal anti-inflammatory drugs (NSAIDs) are used during the acute phase. To avoid stiffening of the foot, the athlete must begin weight-bearing and mobility training as soon as pain allows. Sometimes taping provides good pain relief.
- Prognosis: Prognosis is good. If a contusion has occurred, the athlete is usually able to return to full activity after a few days, whereas painful sprains in the tight articular capsules of the foot may take 4–6 weeks to heal.

Metatarsophalangeal Joint Injuries—*Turf toe*

This injury most commonly occurs with a forced hyperdorsiflexion of the great toe, either with a landing from a jump or load on the back of the leg and ankle while getting tackled, that is, in football (Figure 15.3). This was originally described on turf because of the traction between the shoe and the foot. Preexisting hallux rigidus may predispose to this injury. The injury can be classified into a hyperextension injury, a hyperflexion injury, or a dislocation. Hyperplantarflexion injuries to the MTP joint of the great toe (and the lesser toes) are not uncommon in professional beach volleyball players, and have therefore been referred to as "sand toe".

- Symptoms and signs: Patients with a turf (and sand) toe injury usually present with a history of an injury or multiple injuries to the great toe with resultant activity-related pain, ecchymosis, redness and swelling around the MTP joint. Associated abnormal findings may include deformities such as hammering, subluxation, varus, valgus, or hypermobility. Push-off, forward drive, running, and jumping are compromised.
- Diagnosis: Suspicion of this injury is important. Standing AP X-rays of both feet to determine the position of the sesamoids is necessary. Live fluoroscopic examination may help delineate the lack of distal sesamoid excursion with toe extension, or dorsiflexion. Lateral X-rays taken with the toe in flexion and extension can also confirm whether or not the sesamoids move with the base of the proximal phalanx or not. MRI can help assess the extent of soft-tissue injury defining tears in the plantar plate, metatarso-sesamoid ligament, and/or the intersesamoid ligament as well as associated osseous or cartilage injury.

FOOT

465

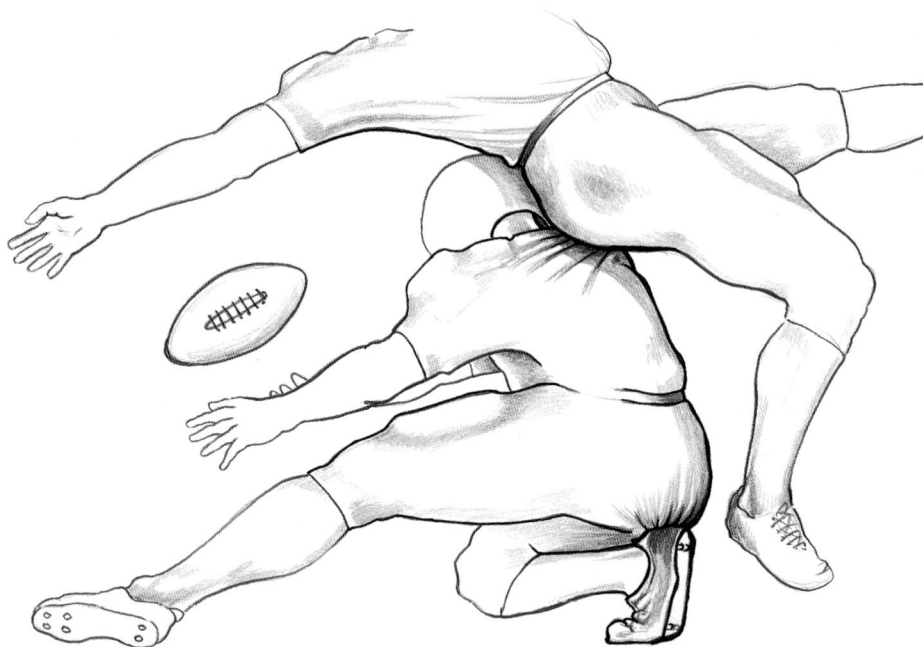

Figure 15.3 Typical injury mechanism for turf toe. (© Medical Illustrator Tommy Bolic, Sweden.)

- Treatment: For mild to moderate injuries with no displacement of the sesamoids, symptomatic treatments are usually sufficient, including use of footwear with a stiff insole, taping, NSAIDs, and continuation in athletic events according to pain. More severe injuries may require immobilization until healing or consideration for surgical repair when there is sesamoid displacement. Patients who experience sand toe injuries should be treated conservatively, with taping, anti-inflammatory medications, shoe wear modification, ice, and rest.
- Prognosis: Good with milder sprains without any sesamoid displacement or migration. With sesamoid fracture or displacement, surgical repair to reduce and repair the plantar plate will yield better outcomes than nonoperative treatment.

Blisters

Blisters are harmless but sometimes extremely painful and disabling injuries that affect all types of athletes, particularly those for whom running and cutting is a major part of their sport, such as in basketball and tennis. Blisters are usually caused by new shoes or by switching to an unfamiliar surface, such as from outdoor to indoor training.

- Symptoms and signs: The patient experiences gradually increasing pain above the area that is subjected to friction, usually over the calcaneus or ball of the big toe. The skin turns red and a blister develops. At first the blister contains a clear fluid (edema), but it may become bloody. Puncturing a blister creates an open wound and should be performed with sterile technique, if it is necessary. A blister can become an ulceration if friction and irritation continue, but the most critical concern is infection.
- Diagnosis: Diagnosis is made on the basis of case history and inspection.
- Treatment: Prophylactic treatment is undoubtedly the best type. If friction is likely, the skin over the affected area is treated with ointments or salicylic acid ointment or is protected with special bandages (e.g., Compeed, Second Skin, or a similar product). These choices may also be effective when symptoms first appear. Clean,

dry, soft socks also provide good protection. When injury first occurs and a blister forms, aspiration of fluid using sterile technique with a sterilized needle to empty the blister without damaging the skin above it is reasonable. If sterile conditions cannot be employed, then it is best to leave the skin intact. Regardless, the layer of skin above the blister should not be removed. It makes a good bandage and protects the wounded subcutis while new skin forms. The dead skin can be cut off after a few days. Use of moleskin and felt or other similar materials to form an off-loading buttress around the blister can also be effective in an athlete who must continue with competition or potentially stressful activities. When an open wound forms, no loading is allowed, and it must be kept as clean as possible, to avoid infection, until it heals. Treat serious infections with a soft-soap bath, systemic antibiotics, and daily changes of sterile bandages.

Chronic Foot Pain

Ned Amendola[1], Tom Clanton[2], and Andrew Franklyn-Miller[3]

[1]*University of Iowa, Iowa City, IA, USA*
[2]*The Steadman Clinic, Vail, CO, USA*
[3]*Aspetar, Qatar Orthopaedic and Sports Medicine Hospital, Doha, Qatar*

Occurrence

Running, jumping, and lateral movements cause major loading of the foot, which transfers these movements up through the ankle, lower leg, knee, thigh, hips, pelvis, and finally into the spinal column. Loading of the foot by running on a flat surface has been measured at about three times body weight, and jumping and running downhill increase this loading up to nine times body weight. The foot hits the ground 480–1200 times per kilometer when running, so that, with time, significant loading must be absorbed by the foot and transferred elsewhere. The ability of the foot to tolerate this loading depends on normal anatomy with normal foot biomechanics and an appropriate combination of stiffness and elasticity. A foot that deviates significantly from normal will have a lower tolerance limit for triggering chronic overuse injuries. Although this type of injury is caused by anatomical deviation (malalignment), it is triggered by weight bearing. Variation from a typical foot alignment is relatively common, even among athletes, but it is important to recognize that different individuals tolerate biomechanical and anatomical variations to greater or lesser degrees, and this can often change over time. A foot that was originally typical, with good height on both the longitudinal and the transverse arches, may gradually become a pronated foot. A runner who formerly never had problems with overuse disorders may suddenly trigger an injury, such as Achilles pain, stress fractures in the tarsus, or plantar fasciitis, during an intense training period or when recovering from another injury for which he may be compensating.

Differential Diagnoses

The most common chronic painful conditions in the foot are caused by stress fractures and plantar fasciitis (Table 15.2). Chronic irritation of the soft parts around a sesamoid bone (sesamoiditis), injuries to the joint capsule of the MTP joint of

Most common	Less common	Must not be overlooked ❗
Stress fractures, p. 472	Calcaneal apophysitis, p. 425	Sinus tarsi syndrome, p. 452
Plantar fasciitis, p. 473	Sesamoiditis, p. 475	Tarsal tunnel syndrome, p. 456
	Hallux rigidus, p. 476	Osteoarthritis, p. 457
	Hallux valgus, p. 476	Morton syndrome, p. 478
	Metatarsalgia, p. 477	Cuboid syndrome, p. 480
		Heel pain
		Inflammatory joint disease

Table 15.2 Overview of the differential diagnoses of chronic foot pain. (Reproduced with permission from the Norwegian Sports Medicine Association.)

the big toe, and irritation of the periosteum and soft parts around the heads of the second to the fourth metatarsals (metatarsalgia or synovitis) also occur frequently. A Morton's neuroma may occur in athletes causing pain can mimic metatarsalgia or synovitis. Cuboid syndrome is rare, and produces pain at the lateral hindfoot. Injuries caused by an impact to the heel pad that irritates the underlying periosteum are common in sport and in some cases may be difficult to treat. Rheumatic disorders may affect the joints in the feet initially, and gout causes typical pain, rubor, and swelling over the MTP joint of the big toe and to a lesser degree, other joints of the foot. Sciatica may cause pain that radiates into the foot and a reduced blood supply due to arteriosclerosis, particularly in diabetics can produce ischemic pain in the foot.

Diagnostic Thinking

Chronic overuse disorders may be difficult to diagnose. There are certainly multifactoral reasons for overuse injuries including extrinsic factors such as training load, volume, preexisting conditioning and training surface alongside intrinsic factors such as small muscle development of the foot or indeed musculature of the shank. Older evidence is available to suggest that traditional morphological descriptions of the foot as varus or valgus at the calcaneus and or pes planus or cavus can predispose to overuse injury but more recent work casts doubt on this. The two goals of the examination are to make the diagnosis and to identify any anatomical or biomechanical predisposing factors. The patient must be examined while sitting, standing, walking, and maybe even while running on a treadmill, to determine whether there are significant biomechanical issues contributing to the patient's chronic pain. A video taken while the patient is running, which can be watched in slow motion, may be useful. Minor axial deviation can be discovered and possibly corrected with simple aids such as insoles or custom orthoses. Therefore, the goal of treatment of chronic overuse disorders is to change the athlete's loading pattern by correcting training problems improve muscular control and support axial deviation. Another common problem can be vitamin D deficiency or other nutritional issues, particularly in the female athlete.

Case History

If the patient has a chronic overuse disorder, a more detailed case history is necessary to determine whether the injury was caused by internal or external factors or by a combination. Information about when and where the foot symptoms originated with respect to loading and rest is key in making the proper diagnosis. For example, an acute stress fracture in the metatarsal can occur during loading in the form of localized pain, whereas the symptoms of midfoot plantar fasciitis develop more gradually and are diffusely localized under the foot. A detailed training history should map surface, volume, and intensity changes along with a careful history of running shoe changes and interventions to date.

Clinical Examination

It is necessary to be familiar with the normal movements of a running foot during the gait cycle (Figure 15.4). Of course there is much development in the running technique as part of rehabilitation and so initially this text refers to a traditional rear foot strike. The first stage is heel strike, when the heel makes contact with the ground partly supinated, with the lateral calcaneus striking the ground. The next stage is mid-stance when the foot, with the heel planted on the ground, pronates until the sole of the foot touches the ground. Then the heel goes from a supinated to a more neutral position, and the shank or lower leg rotates inwardly. The third stage

FOOT

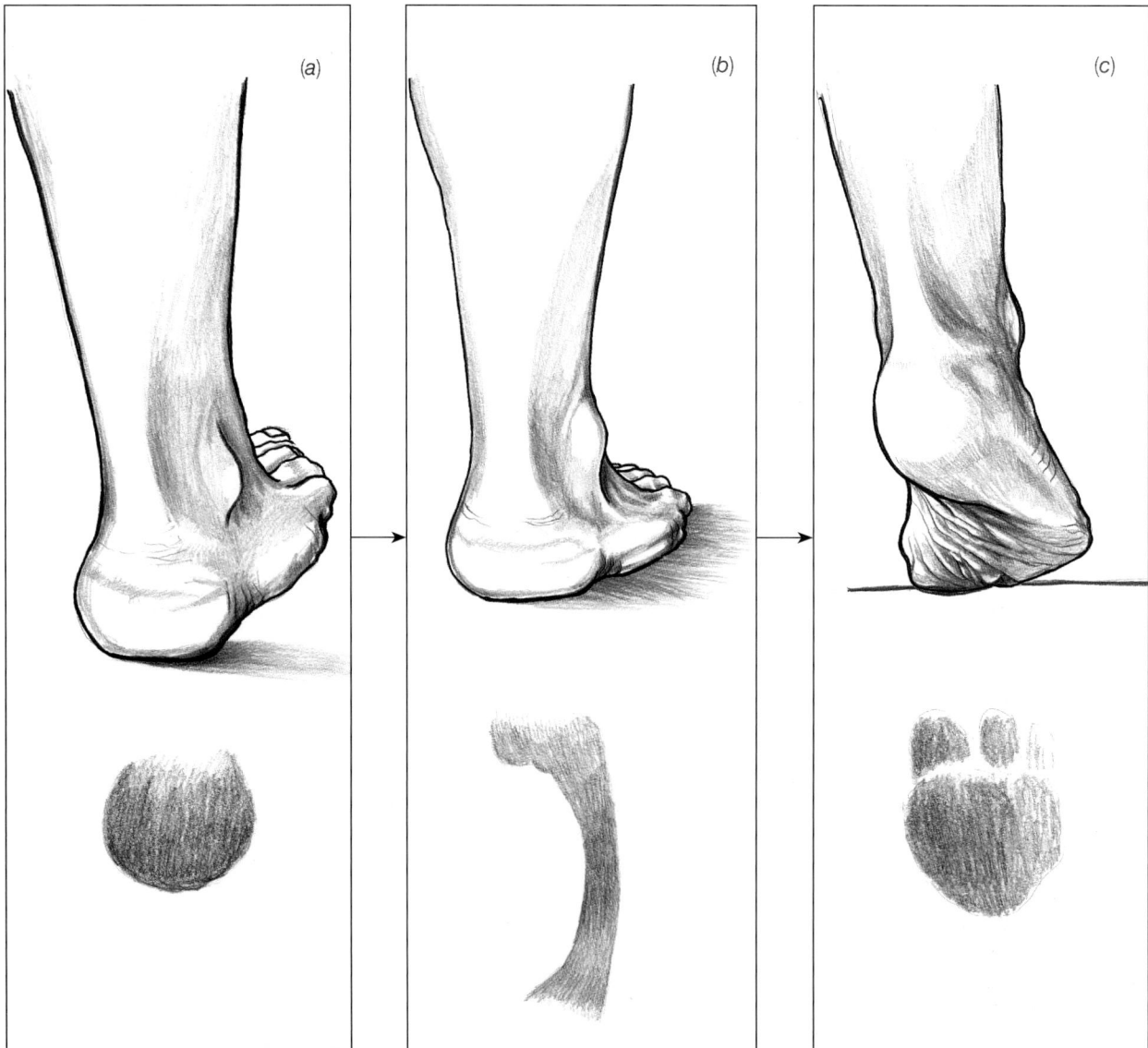

Figure 15.4 Foot motion during gait cycle: heel strike (a), mid-stance (b) and toe off (c). (© Medical Illustrator Tommy Bolic, Sweden.)

is the toe-off stage. The forefoot is pressed against the ground, the heel is lifted up, and the foot is supinated. This "locks" the tarsus, and the foot becomes stiff, providing a good toe-off. The fourth stage is the swing stage, where the foot prepares for heel strike again. Currently many runners do not conform to this model and use a "midfoot" or forefoot running style negating the heel strike and subsequent settling pronation that may either be palliative or indeed predictive of future overuse injuries—only time will tell.

Inspection. An athlete with a foot overuse injury must be carefully examined when sitting, walking, standing, and lying down. The entire lower extremity, the pelvis, and the back must be systematically examined. The physician must look for scoliosis, anisomelia (leg length discrepancy), toeing in, varus and valgus positioning of the knees, malrotation of the lower legs, tight Achilles tendons, and, last but not least, foot malalignment, particularly cavus foot and the over-pronated foot (Figure 15.5). All these conditions may be important contributing factors to chronic injuries. Well-worn jogging shoes should always be examined and will often indirectly reveal foot malalignment that may be difficult to see during a clinical examination. The well-worn shoes can also be an etiological factor due to uneven wear or excessive usage since maximum life expectancy in most running shoes is 650–800 km. It is also important to examine any foot orthoses in use and to the extent of their use in each shoe type.

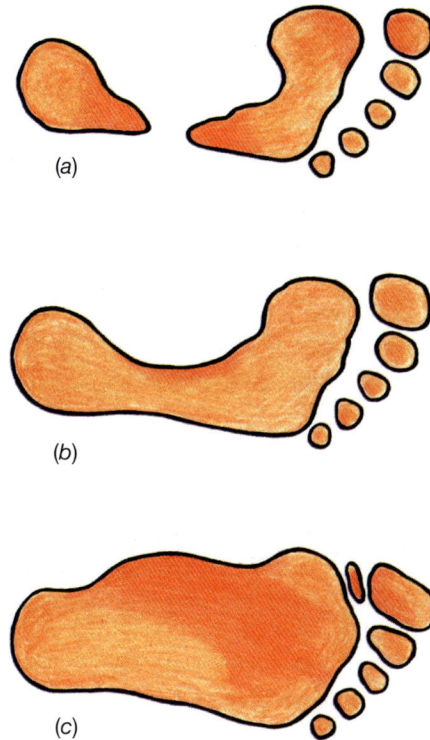

Figure 15.5 Footprints. Cavus foot (clawfoot, pes cavus) (a), normal foot (b), and overpronated foot (flatfoot, pes planus) (c). (© Medical Illustrator Tommy Bolic, Sweden.)

Palpation. If the patient has a stress fracture in the metatarsal, pain may be triggered by direct palpation over the area of the fracture and by indirect pressure in the bone's longitudinal axis. But equally pain may not be detected on palpation. Circulation in the foot is examined by palpating the pulse in the dorsal artery of the foot and in the posterior tibial artery (Figure 15.6). Capillary refill time can indicate the microcirculation and can be assessed by pressing on the pulp of the big toe to ensure refill is less than 5 s. Cutaneous sensation may be tested both by light and sharp touch alongside proprioception that is important to examine as an early sign of diabetic peripheral neuropathy. It may be assessed by sensation of distal interphalangeal joint movement.

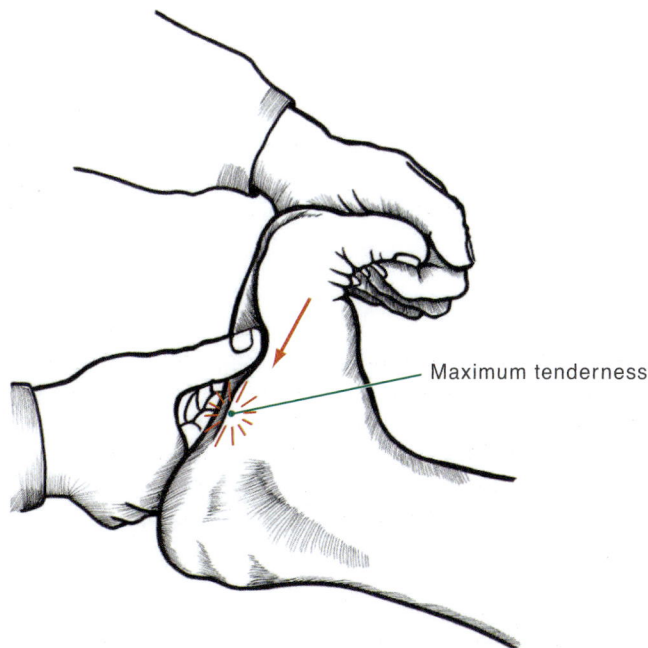

Maximum tenderness

Figure 15.6 Palpation of the plantar fascia if the patient has plantar fasciitis. In insertional disease, the most tender point is usually at the insertion of the plantar fascia to the calcaneus but can extend down the medial border. The toes are dorsally flexed to tense the plantar fascia. (© Medical Illustrator Tommy Bolic, Sweden.)

Supplemental Examinations

Radiographic examination. Standard X-rays on two planes are often indicated if the patient has a long-term, painful condition of the foot, and an oblique view may also be necessary. X-rays are useful in demonstrating any axial deviation but mainly serve to exclude other pathology. Stress fractures result in either callus formation or the development of a nonunion. Rheumatologic conditions can result in erosive changes in the periarticular areas. Gout can also cause erosive changes on both sides of a joint as can the rare condition of pigmented villonodular synovitis. Bone spurs, or exostoses, are frequently seen on X-rays of athletes and are often asymptomatic. The traction spur seen on the plantar heel has often been associated with plantar fasciitis but is actually a traction spur that occurs with calcification of the flexor digitorum brevis muscle that originates from this area of the calcaneus.

Ultrasound. Ultrasound examination can also reveal plantar fascia degeneration or inflammation, suggest cortical disruption of the metatarsals and identify a Morton neuroma.

Scintigraphy. Scintigraphy is a sensitive test for diagnosing a stress fracture. X-rays may take 10–21 days to demonstrate a stress fracture. It is particularly difficult to demonstrate stress fractures in the tarsus with X-rays, even if the disorder is long-term, although skeletal scintigraphy is positive after 1 or 2 days. MRI seems to have supplanted the use of scintigraphy and has become the gold standard.

MRI. MRI has become an increasingly valuable tool for diagnosing problems within the foot. Newer high-resolution scanners, better software, and more focused fields of view have enabled visualization of more subtle pathology, such as plantar plate tears, Morton's neuromas, partial tears of the plantar fascia, and subtle ligament injuries within the foot. An MRI can also demonstrate a stress fracture with great sensitivity and specificity and without radiation exposure shortly after onset of symptoms.

CT. CT may be indicated for evaluating stress fractures that do not become asymptomatic after adequate unloading. In such cases, CT will demonstrate the development of a nonunion or demonstrate an incomplete stress fracture that may not be evident as is frequently the case for the tarsal navicular.

Common Injuries

Stress Fractures

Foot stress fractures are relatively common in athletes who engage primarily in running and jumping sports. Several studies have shown that up to 25% of all stress fractures in the body are localized to the tarsus, particularly to the navicular bone. Both overpronation and cavus foot increase loading of the navicular bone, predisposing this bone to stress fractures. Stress fractures in the foot are almost always directly triggered when the patient increases the amount or intensity of training too quickly, in addition to exercising on a hard surface and wearing footwear with poor shock absorption. Other bones in the foot that are particularly vulnerable to stress fractures are the metatarsals (fatigue fractures) and the sesamoid bones under the head of the first metatarsal.

• Symptoms and signs: Patients feel pain that may gradually become increasingly painful but sharp on direct contact during a training session. The pain disappears at rest but rapidly returns during loading.

- Diagnosis: A case history with acute, localized pain from loading should generate the suspicion of a stress fracture. Examination findings are tenderness and possibly mild swelling above the fracture. The hop test is positive when the patient has localized pain. An X-ray may demonstrate a fissure in the shaft of the metatarsals, at the base of the fifth metatarsal, and through the affected sesamoid bone, but it is usually negative for a tarsal fracture. An MRI of the affected bone will confirm subcortical bone oedema and this would also result in a positive bone scan (Tc-99) (Figure 15.7).

- Treatment: The recommended treatment is not bearing weight, with crutches, for 4–8 weeks, depending on the location of the fracture. In the metatarsals, a brief period without weight bearing is often sufficient, whereas fractures in the tarsus and particularly in the navicular bone take longer to heal, due to increased compressive loading forces and reduced blood supply. Alternative exercises, such as bicycling, running in water, and strength training are important during the nonweight-bearing period. Active training with loading must be resumed gradually and carefully, preferably under the guidance of a physical therapist. The predisposing etiology such as training volume, poor mechanics or footwear must be addressed otherwise, the injury often recurs. Female athlete triad signs must be examined to exclude osteopenia secondary to anorexia and menstrual cessation as a predisposing factor. It is difficult to heal stress fractures at the base of the fifth metatarsal and in the sesamoid bone under the head of the first metatarsal using conservative treatment because of the pull of the lateral band of the plantar aponeurosis and the flexor hallucis brevis muscle, respectively. Therefore, these fractures are often treated surgically, with reduction and screw osteosynthesis of the fifth metatarsal and extirpation of one (the smallest) fragment in the sesamoid bone versus a complete sesamoidectomy in some circumstances. In some cases, a nonunion may be present in other bones as well, particularly in the navicular bone. A CT examination can demonstrate this, and if it does, treatment is surgical fixation of the two fragments to each other with screws.

- Prognosis: Stress fractures in the foot generally heal easily if the patient begins an adequate level of not bearing weight early. Once healing occurs, it is important to correct biomechanical abnormalities through physical therapy, use of orthoses, and better design of training programs and consideration of other factors such as shoes and surfaces. Vitamin D deficiency and nutritional issues should also be addressed if present.

Plantar fasciitis — *Tendinosis in the Tendon Capsule on the Sole of the Foot*

The most common cause of heel pain in athletes is plantar fasciitis. It is a chronic painful condition at the origin of the plantar aponeurosis on the calcaneus (Figure 15.8). Plantar fasciitis is caused by chronic traction in the plantar aponeurosis or at the common origin, often with microruptures within this tissue. It does not share the same etiology as tendinopathy with a more defined inflammatory stage and origin area, often with microruptures in the tendinous tissue. Long-term disorders can be associated a heel spur (calcification at the insertion of the calcaneus) to form, which can be demonstrated by plain X-ray. Cavus foot, overpronation, and over-training on hard surfaces are the most common predisposing factors.

- Symptoms and signs: Patients experience pain from weight bearing that is localized under the plantar heel that is particularly bothersome in the morning on arising from bed. In mild cases, pain occurs only at the start-up of training and abates after a warm-up period while in more severe cases the pain can be present throughout the day.

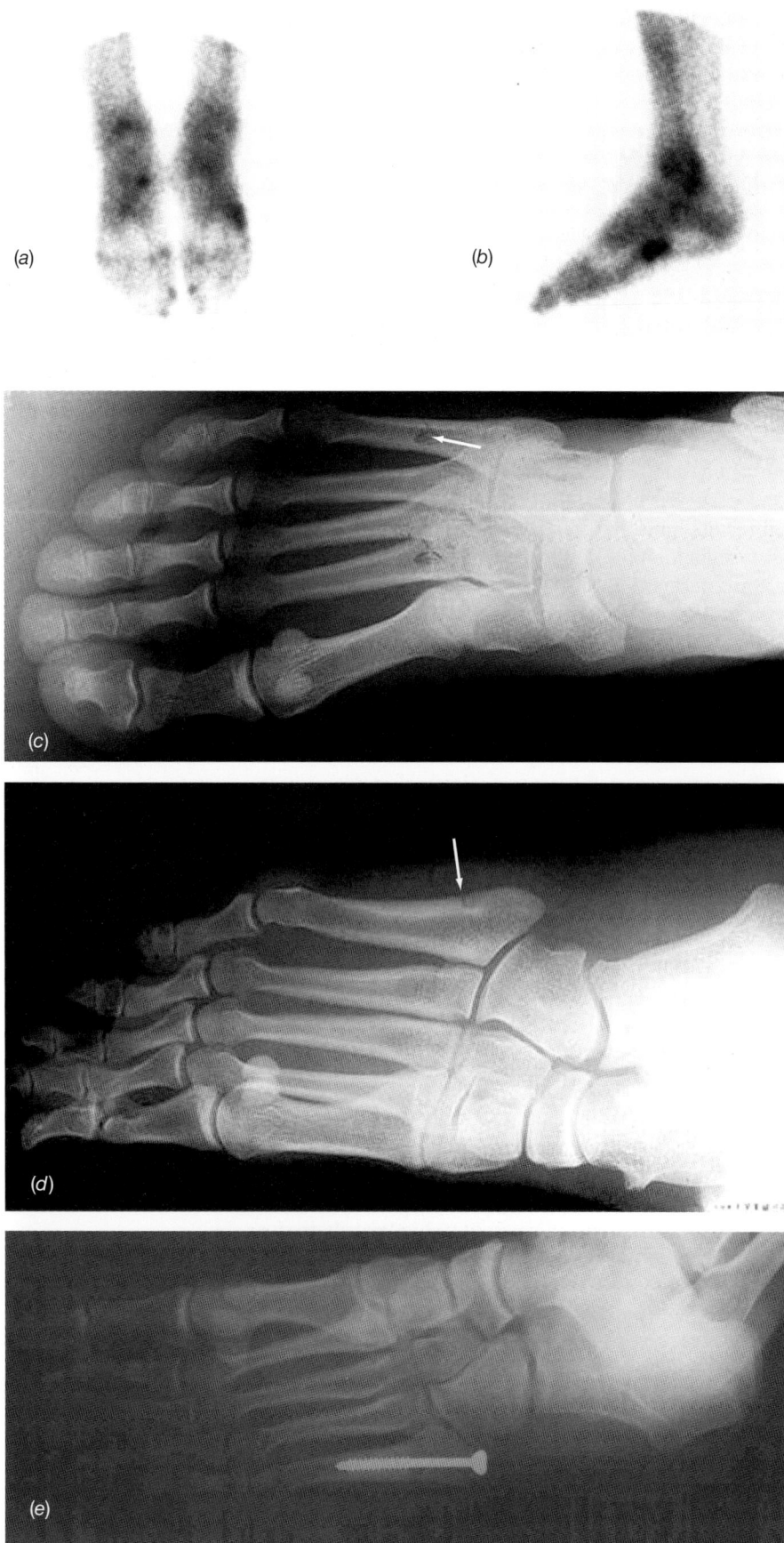

Figure 15.7 Stress fracture at the base of the fifth metatarsal. Skeletal scintigraphy demonstrates strong contrast uptake at the base of the fifth metatarsal (*a* and *b*). The X-ray view demonstrates a fracture line through the base of the fifth metatarsal (*c* and *d*). The X-ray view demonstrates the status after surgical fixation of the fracture using a compression screw in the bone marrow canal of the fifth metatarsal (*e*). (Reproduced with permission from the Norwegian Sports Medicine Association.)

- Diagnosis: A diagnosis is based on the case history, with gradually developing symptoms being typical. During palpation, the patient indicates pain corresponding to the fascia's insertion on the plantar medial heel bone most commonly.
- Treatment: Recommended treatments are modifying weight bearing activity, alternative exercises, NSAIDs, heel buildup, and possibly fitting special insoles with cutouts for the painful area. Stretching of the plantar fascia and the lower leg musculature are essential. Friction massage may be helpful. An injection of cortisone around the insertion of the fascia may be attempted once, but it should not be repeated if the desired effect is not achieved. If the injection is made wholly or partially into the fascia, it will very likely rupture. Good results have been achieved by using a night brace for 1 or 2 months (to stretch the plantar fascia), particularly for patients who have a great deal of morning pain. Correction of the external and internal factors that trigger the disorder is crucial for preventing a recurrence. In some cases, conservative treatment does not produce satisfactory results. In such cases, other treatments that can be effective include low intensity or high-intensity shockwave treatment or injection of platelet rich plasma. If this is ineffective, the patient may be offered surgery to separate the plantar fascia from the insertion on the calcaneus. It is not necessary to remove calcaneal spurs.
- Prognosis: This is a self-limiting problem that does improve with time and conservative treatment. The outcome of surgical treatment is not predictable; most patients become asymptomatic quickly and may resume their training routines within 4–6 weeks. It is possible for overpronation to occur following release of the plantar fascia, and it may be necessary to treat this with custom orthoses.

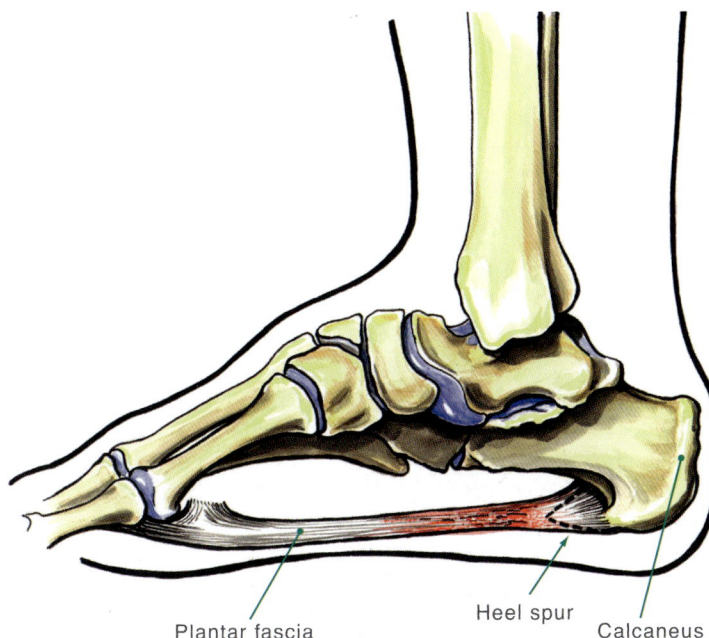

Figure 15.8 Plantar fasciitis. The figure shows the area for maximum tendinosis changes and pain in red and where heel spurs (calcification of the flexor digitorum brevis) may occur. (© Medical Illustrator Tommy Bolic, Sweden.)

Labels on figure: Plantar fascia, Heel spur, Calcaneus

Less Common Injuries

Sesamoiditis—*Inflammation Around the Sesamoid Bone*

The sesamoid bones under the head of the first metatarsal are surrounded by tendinous tissue, except for the articular surface against the metatarsal, where the sesamoid bone is covered with cartilage. The sesamoid bones are subjected to major loading, both from the longitudinal loading from pull by the flexor hallucis brevis tendon and by direct shock absorption from the ground. Overuse may trigger an inflammatory reaction (sesamoiditis) in the soft parts around the sesamoid bone. "Toe runners," athletes who only load the forefoot when running, are particularly vulnerable to this disorder.

- Symptoms and signs: Pain under the MTP joint of the big toe from weight bearing is the primary symptom.
- Diagnosis: Diagnosis is based on local tenderness and possibly mild swelling over the affected sesamoid bone. X-rays often do not show signs of a stress fracture, scintigraphy may demonstrate increased contrast enhancement but is usually unnecessary, whereas MRI is most likely to show the anatomy and the edema from stress.

FOOT

• Treatment: Recommended treatments are unloading, NSAIDs, reduction in training intensity, and perhaps, alteration in running technique. Footwear with good shock absorption, possibly with extra insoles and a cutout or relief pad for the painful area, is often the best therapy. Cases that are resistant to treatment for a long time may require surgical removal of the sesamoid bone.

Hallux Rigidus—*Beginning Degeneration in the Metatarsophalangeal Joint of the Big Toe*

Localized trauma or repeated minor hyperextension injuries (turf toe syndrome) or plantar flexion trauma (sand toe syndrome) to the MTP joint of the big toe may cause damage to the articular cartilage within the joint or inflammation in the joint capsule. This can result in a painful joint with loss of mobility, especially in dorsiflexion. Much training on artificial turf with rapid deceleration and dorsal shortening of the joint is a primary triggering cause. In athletes who play beach volleyball, the triggering cause is repeated plantar flexion trauma to the joint. Oftentimes, there is no clear etiology but the first MTP joint develops a degenerative process that is characterized by loss of the joint space and dorsal osteophyte formation on the first metatarsal head.

• Symptoms and signs: Patients experience pain around the MTP joint of the big toe from running and cross-country skiing. This pain is caused by the movement that involves dorsiflexion of the joint or by running and jumping on a soft surface, like sand.
• Diagnosis: The diagnosis is made on the basis of tenderness, particularly on the dorsal side of the MTP joint, and possibly swelling there. Often a protruding cartilaginous edge can be palpated near the joint and medially. Dorsiflexion is reduced and painful. An X-ray may demonstrate osteophytes, or joint space narrowing particularly close to the edge of the articular surface of the metatarsal.
• Treatment: The recommended treatments are PRICE and NSAIDs for the short term. Taping the joint to limit dorsiflexion should be attempted, and the patient may wear stiff-soled shoes with a slight rocker bottom. A cortisone injection may be given to relieve an acute exacerbation in symptoms but should not be used repeatedly. For long-term disorders with manifest osteophytes, surgery to remove cartilage and new bone formation (cheilectomy) is an option.
• Prognosis: Prognosis is good if degeneration of the cartilage in the joint is not extensive. If the degeneration is extensive, the patient will have lasting symptoms, and arthrodesis of the big toe's MTP joint may be necessary.

Hallux Valgus—*Abnormal Lateral Angling of the Big Toe*

Hallux valgus is excessive lateral displacement of the big toe (Figure 15.9). The condition is most common in older women but may even occur in teenage girls. The cause is one or more anatomical displacements in the foot, and the disorder occurs most often as part of the deformity with transverse flatfoot. In small children the axis goes through the first metatarsal and the big toe together, whereas at the end of the growth period the normal valgus position of the big toe is between 15° and 20°. This valgus position seems to be partially caused by wearing shoes, because the condition almost never occurs in people who do not wear shoes. If the valgus position exceeds the upper normal limit of 20°, pulling on the MTP joint, especially by flexor and extensor tendons, will further strengthen the big toe's tendency to go into a valgus position. The head of the first metatarsal will be pressed medially, and pressure from the shoe will cause chronic irritation of the bursa on the medial side of the metatarsal head. Eventually, an exostosis will form in this area, which will worsen the pressure. Lateral migration of the big toe will cause the toes closest to it to assume a position that resembles hammertoe.

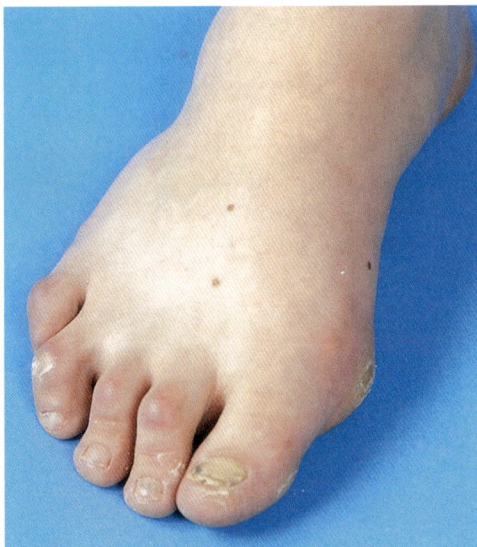

Figure 15.9 Hallux valgus. The patient is flatfooted and has significant valgus alignment of the first metatarsal. Pressure points are visible over the head of the first metatarsal medially and dorsally on the other toes. The patient also has nail fungus on the big toe. (Reproduced with permission from the Norwegian Sports Medicine Association.)

- Symptoms and signs: Pain gradually increases above a bump that develops on the medial side of the head of the first metatarsal. Pain also occurs from wearing tight shoes. The skin over the bump becomes red, irritated, and tender. The patient may also have pain in the second and third toes, because of increasing malalignment and pressure.
- Diagnosis: Clinical examination shows the typical bump with red and tender skin above it, a broadened forefoot, valgus positioning of the big toe, and possibly hammertoe positioning of the second and third toes. If movement in the big toe's MTP joint triggers pain, it may indicate that osteoarthritis is developing in the joint. X-rays of the foot are always indicated when evaluating the patient for surgical treatment.
- Treatment: For moderate malalignment and only a few symptoms, treatment is conservative. Initially treatment can be symptomatic and corrective with a transverse pad, which rests against the middle (second to fourth) metatarsal bones behind the heads of the metatarsals to lift them up from the sole of the shoe. In addition, the patient should wear footwear that is wide enough and high enough for the toes. Narrow and pointed shoes will worsen the symptoms. If the symptoms and the malalignment are extensive, the patient should be offered surgical treatment for definitive correction This is accomplished by removing the exostoses in combination with either corrective osteotomy of the first metatarsal or with a soft, plastic orthosis on the tendon and joint capsules to align the toe. Postoperatively, the patient has to wear a redressing cast for 6 weeks, after which free mobilization is allowed.
- Prognosis: Surgical treatment produces definitive results, but some patients have a recurrence of the malalignment and symptoms after a while. If cartilage in the big toe's MTP joint is damaged, primary arthrodesis must be performed in the joint.

Metatarsalgia—*Pain Under the Heads of the Second to Fourth Metatarsal Bones*

Metatarsalgia occurs frequently in overweight patients with transverse flatfoot where the heads of the second to the fourth metatarsals are deeper than normal. This results in slight hammertoe positioning of the corresponding toes, and the heads of the metatarsals are subject to greater loading than normal. Eventually, the periosteum and soft parts around the heads of these metatarsals become irritated.

- Symptoms and signs: Pain from weight bearing is the primary symptom.
- Diagnosis: Diagnosis is based on palpation tenderness over the heads of the metatarsals in the plantar area. Most patients have manifest transverse flatfoot, possibly combined with beginning hallux valgus malalignment.
- Treatment: Recommended treatment is unloading for a short period, concomitant with fitting of insoles that elevate the transverse arch of the foot.
- Prognosis: Prognosis is good with early correction of the transverse arch.

Morton Syndrome (Interdigital Neuroma)—*Ganglion Between the Two Metatarsals* !

The interdigital nerves become pinched where they pass the heads of the metatarsals, either due to direct injury or secondary to compressive footwear, repetitive load or other intrinsic factors. The nerve between the third and fourth toes is the most vulnerable to injuries. Pressure causes irritation of the nerve, and a neuroma eventually forms. This causes the pressure to increase and symptoms to worsen (Figure 15.10).

- **Symptoms and signs:** Pain in the forefoot upon walking and running may become very disabling.
- **Diagnosis:** Diagnosis is made on the basis of pain from pressure on the space between the metatarsals directly proximal to the heads of the metatarsals. Pain radiates out into the affected toes, and sensitivity may be reduced in the area where

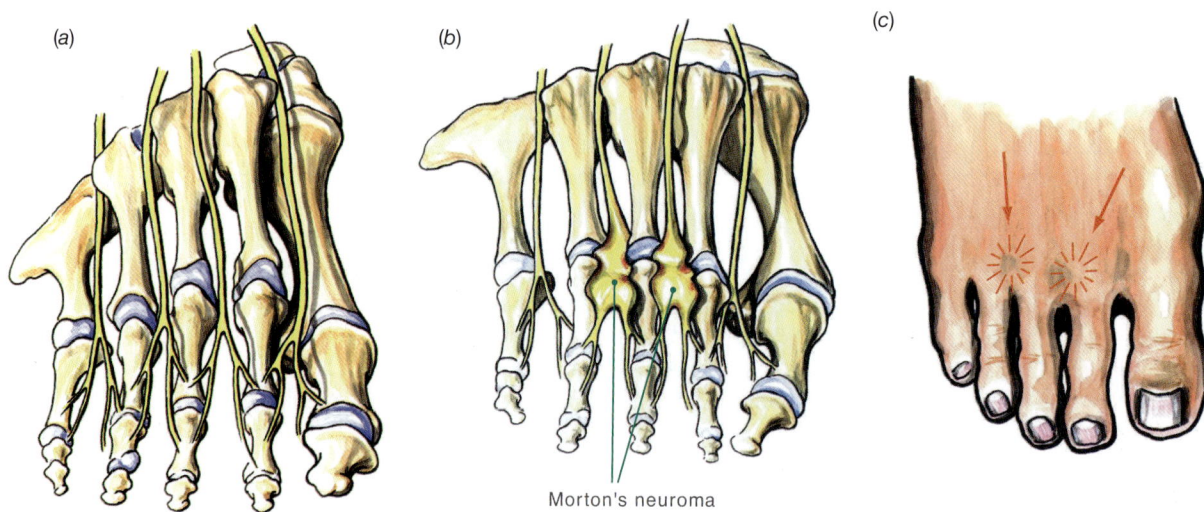

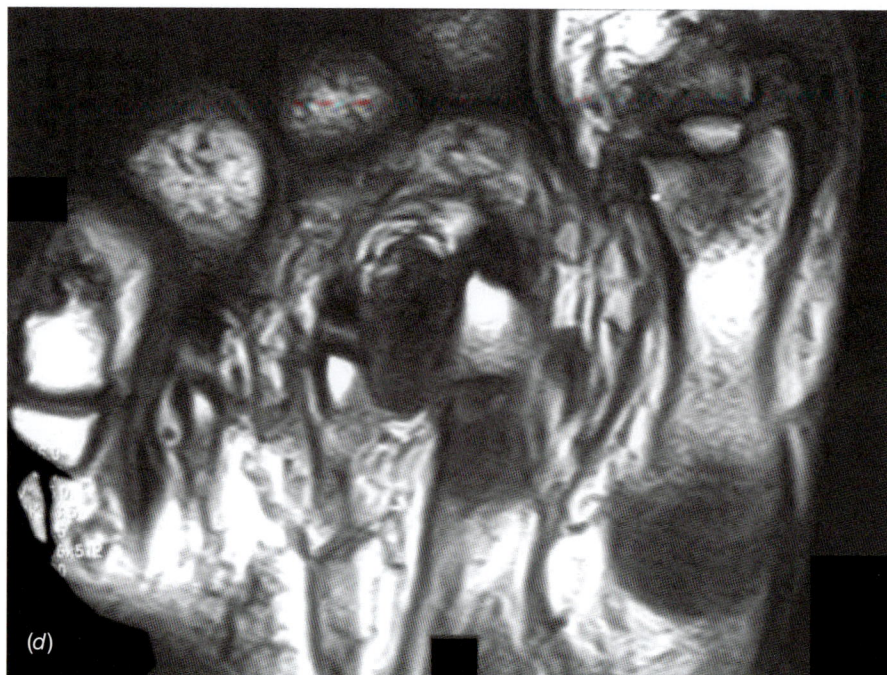

(a)

(b)

Morton's neuroma

(c)

(d)

Figure 15.10 Morton neuroma. Normal toe nervs (*a*). Morton neuroma (nerve tumors) between the heads of the second and third metatarsals, and between the third and fourth metatarsals (*b*). Areas for maximum tenderness with pressure from the dorsal and plantar side in the space between the metatarsal heads (*c*). MRI demonstrates a large neuroma between the second and third metatarsals (*d*). (© Medical Illustrator Tommy Bolic, Sweden.)

the nerves of the toes innervate. Pressing the forefoot together from side to side or dorsally flexing the toes hard will often provoke pain. An MRI will show possible thickening of the nerve (Figure 15.11).

- Treatment: Correction of forefoot arch with a metatarsal bar can provide symptomatic relief with insoles and the use of wide shoes often relieves symptoms. Longer term relief can be found with a corticosteroid injection with local anesthetic to settle the symptoms but if recurrent surgical excision of the neuroma is the most common method. Postoperatively, the patient should unload for 2 weeks, after which loading is gradually increased and the training routine is resumed at around 6 weeks.

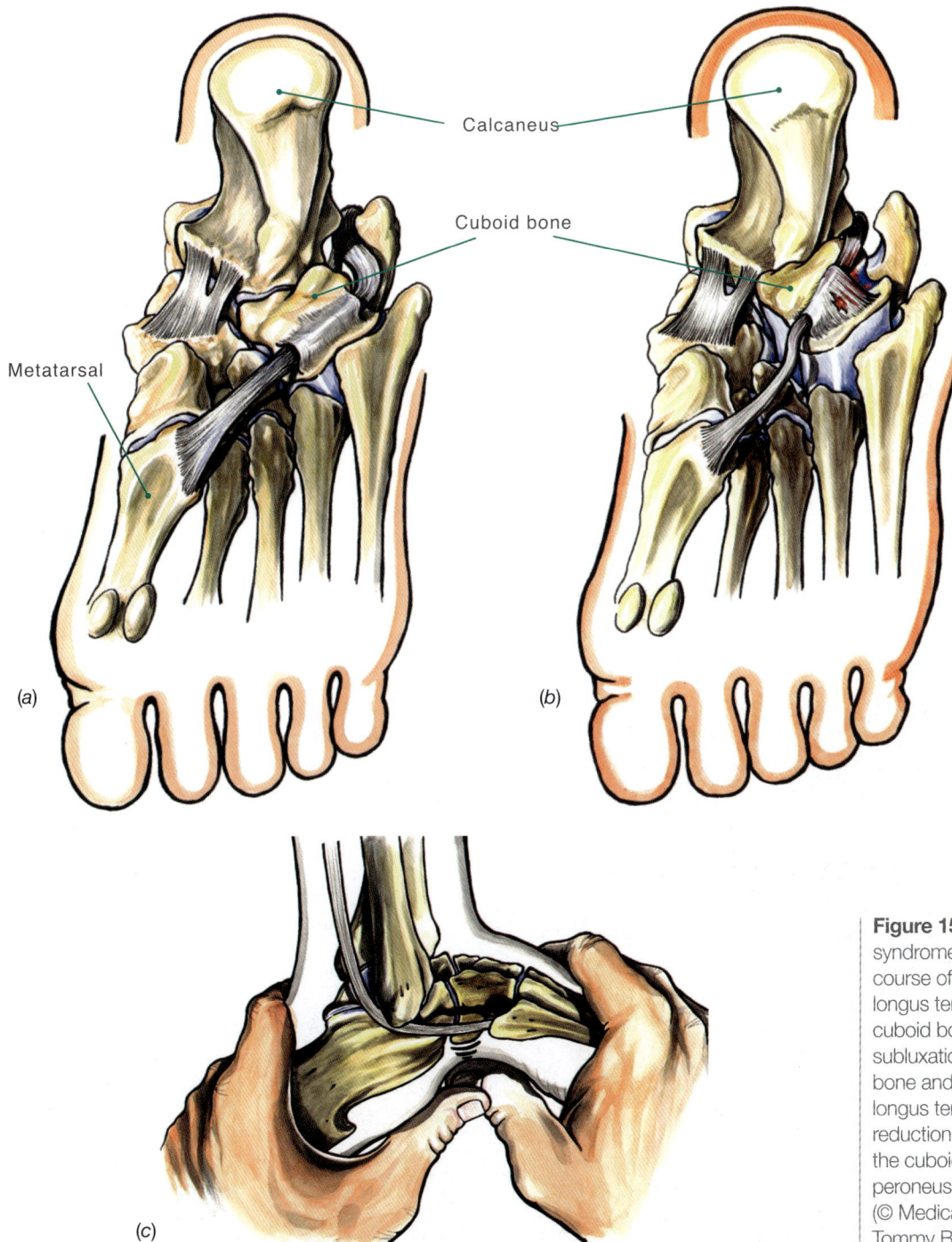

Calcaneus

Cuboid bone

Metatarsal

(a)

(b)

(c)

Figure 15.11 Cuboid syndrome. Normal course of the peroneus longus tendon under the cuboid bone (a). Plantar subluxation of the cuboid bone and the peroneus longus tendon (b). The reduction maneuver for the cuboid bone and the peroneus longus tendon (c). (© Medical Illustrator Tommy Bolic, Sweden.)

FOOT

• Prognosis: Surgical treatment may have a surprisingly positive effect on patients with long-term symptoms. Usually, the pain disappears completely, but some patients experience slight discomfort for a few weeks after the intervention.

Cuboid Syndrome—*Subluxation of Cuboid Bone* ❗

The peroneus longus tendon attaches to the base of the first metatarsal hooking under the arch of the lateral border of the foot (Figure 15.11). The tendon is normally located in a small groove on the underside of the cuboid bone. Although difficult to clinically demonstrate it is believed significant distance running training may cause the lateral border foot pain radiating along the peroneus tendon. Cuboid syndrome refers to an apparent plantar subluxation of the cuboid bone. Long-term loading would cause the cuboid bone to glide slightly downward. This in turn may allow the tendon to slide out of its groove, forcing the cuboid out of position.

• Symptoms and signs: Pain is localized to the lateral side of the foot under and slightly behind the lateral malleolus. Loading increases pain.
• Diagnosis: Diagnosis is based on palpation tenderness over the peroneus tendon that inserts under the heel bone. Tenderness in the middle underside of the foot, which corresponds to the underside of the cuboid bone, is also present.
• Treatment: Offloading and muscle retraining of the peroneal muscles often allows a reduction in symptoms and may be attributable to peroneal tendon inflammation. Some specialists advocate bony manipulation of the cuboid but this would suggest intra-articular ligament injury that is unlikely to respond to manipulation and sural nerve entrapment should be excluded. The authors believe careful examination of the foot is likely to reveal a more identifiable cause of the pain generating structure but a local anesthetic injection to the calcaneocuboid joint can help isolate this in dancers.

Heel Pain—*Injury to the Heel Fat Pad* ❗

An acute strong injury caused by impact or repeated impact to the heel (such as much running on a hard surface) may cause bleeding in the fat pad under the heel

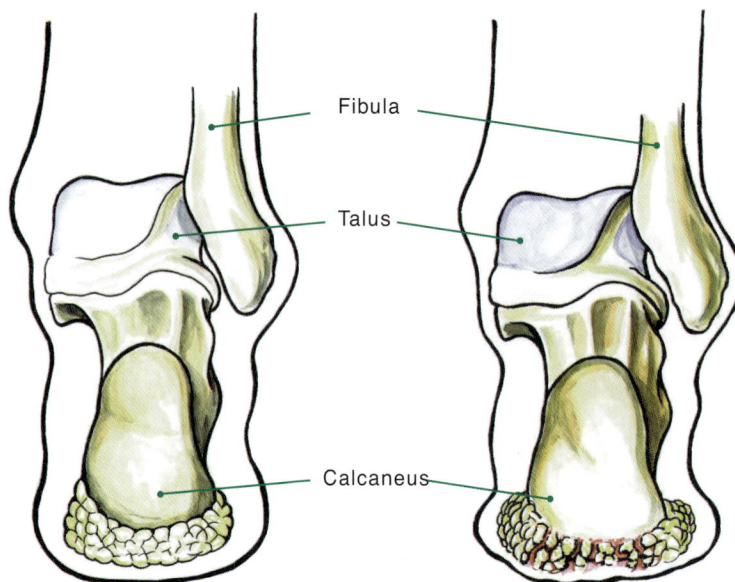

Figure 15.12 Injury of the heel pad. Normal heel pad with intact connective tissue septae and fatty tissue held in place in small cavities (*a*). If the fibrous septae are destroyed, the fat of the heel pad will be squeezed laterally and medially (*b*). (© Medical Illustrator Tommy Bolic, Sweden.)

Fibula

Talus

Calcaneus

and crushing of the connective tissue septae that hold the fatty tissue in place. This reduces the heel pad's shock-absorbing properties and eventually irritates the periosteum on the calcaneus. Long jumpers and triple jumpers are particularly vulnerable to this injury (Figure 15.12).

- Symptoms and signs: Pain is felt under the heel from loading.
- Diagnosis: Diagnosis is made on the basis of tenderness from palpation under the injured part of the heel, but is clinically difficult to differentiate form plantar fasciitis. Ultrasound examination can help differentiate. Calcaneal injury should be excluded in patients with recalcitrant symptoms Reduction of the fatty tissue that covers the heel bone improves the pain, demonstrated by exam or with use of a well-fitting heel cup.
- Treatment: Recommended treatments are unloading of the injured area with shock-absorbing soles (such as Tulis), fitting special insoles with cutouts around the most painful spot, and possibly a heel cup with a shock-absorbing pad. General unloading is recommended, particularly after acute injuries. The patient often needs to walk with crutches for 2 or 3 weeks.
- Prognosis: Pain may be long term.

FOOT

Index

Note: Page numbers with italicized *f*'s and *t*'s refer to figures and tables, respectively.